Allergic Diseases

Diagnosis and Management

FIFTH EDITION

Allergic Diseases

Diagnosis and Management

EDITED BY:

ROY PATTERSON, M.D.
Ernest S. Bazley Professor of Medicine
Chief, Division of Allergy–Immunology
Department of Medicine
Northwestern University Medical School
Chief, Division of Allergy–Immunology
Northwestern Memorial Hospital
Chicago, Illinois

ASSOCIATE EDITORS:

LESLIE CARROLL GRAMMER, M.D.
Professor of Medicine
Division of Allergy–Immunology
Department of Medicine
Northwestern University Medical School
Attending Physician
Northwestern Memorial Hospital
Chicago, Illinois

PAUL A. GREENBERGER, M.D.
Professor of Medicine
Division of Allergy–Immunology
Department of Medicine
Northwestern University Medical School
Attending Physician
Northwestern Memorial Hospital
Chicago, Illinois

With 24 Additional Contributors

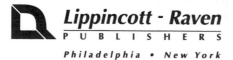

Lippincott - Raven
PUBLISHERS
Philadelphia • New York

Acquisitions Editor: *Richard Winters*
Coordinating Editorial Assistant: *Karen Frame*
Project Editor: *Ellen Campbell*
Production Manager: *Caren Erlichman*
Senior Production Coordinator: *Kevin Johnson*
Design Coordinator: *Doug Smock*
Indexer: *Alexandra Nickerson*
Printer: *Maple Press*

Fifth Edition

Library of Congress Cataloging-in-Publication Data

Allergic diseases : diagnosis and management / edited by Roy Patterson ; associate
  editors, Leslie Carroll Grammer, Paul A. Greenberger ; with 24 additional
  contributors. — 5th ed.
      p.   cm.
  Includes bibliographical references and index.
  ISBN 0–397–51609–6 (alk. paper)
  1. Allergy.   I. Grammer, Leslie Carroll.   II. Greenberger, Paul A.
  [DNLM: 1. Hypersensitivity—diagnosis.   2. Hypersensitivity—therapy.
WD 300 A43107 1997]
RC584.A34   1997
616.97—dc21
DNLM/DLC
for Library of Congress   96–49540
                                                                       CIP

Care has been taken to confirm the accuracy of the information presented and to describe generally accepted practices. However, the authors, editors, and publisher are not responsible for errors or omissions or for any consequences from application of the information in this book and make no warranty, express or implied, with respect to the contents of the publication.

The authors, editors, and publisher have exerted every effort to ensure that drug selection and dosage set forth in this text are in accordance with current recommendations and practice at the time of publication. However, in view of ongoing research, changes in government regulations, and the constant flow of information relating to drug therapy and drug reactions, the reader is urged to check the package insert for each drug for any change in indications and dosage and for added warnings and precautions. This is particularly important when the recommended agent is a new or infrequently employed drug.

Some drugs and medical devices presented in this publication have Food and Drug Administration (FDA) clearance for limited use in restricted research settings. It is the responsibility of the health care provider to ascertain the FDA status of each drug or device planned for use in their clinical practice.

9   8   7   6   5   4   3   2   1

This book is dedicated to the memory of
Ernest S. Bazley and Ernest S. Bazley, Jr.

We thank the following for support of the
Ernest S. Bazley Asthma and Allergic Diseases Center:

Gunnard Swanson

Catherine Ryan

Donna Atwater

Bank of America Illinois

Contributors

David I. Bernstein, MD
Associate Professor of Clinical Medicine
University of Cincinnati College of Medicine
Division of Immunology ML 563
231 Bethesda Avenue
Cincinnati, OH 45267-0563

Jonathan A. Bernstein, MD
Assistant Professor of Clinical Medicine
Division of Immunology
University of Cincinnati College of Medicine
Division of Immunology ML 563
231 Bethesda Avenue
Cincinnati, OH 45267-0563

Michael S. Blaiss, MD
Associate Professor of Pediatrics
Assistant Professor of Medicine
Department of Pediatrics
University of Tennessee, Memphis
777 Washington, Suite P110
Memphis, TN 38105

Bernard H. Booth, MD
Clinical Professor of Medicine
University of Mississippi
Mississippi Asthma and Allergy Clinic
9 Dell Drive
Oxford, MS 38655

Robert K. Bush, MD
Professor of Medicine (CHS)
University of Wisconsin-Madison
c/o William S. Middleton VA Hospital
2500 Overlook Terrace
Madison, WI 53705

Walter W.Y. Chang, MD
Attending Staff
St. Francis Medical Center
Queens Medical Center
Private Practice
1165 Hunakai Street
Honolulu, HI 96816-4612

Sarah Cheriyan, MD
Allergy & Asthma Clinic
Lufkin, TX 75901

Anne M. Ditto, MD
Clinical Instructor of Medicine
Division of Allergy–Immunology
Department of Medicine
Northwestern University Medical School
Chicago, IL 60611

Richard D. DeSwarte, MD
Clinical Associate Professor of Medicine
Division of Allergy–Immunology
Northwestern University Medical School
303 East Chicago Avenue
Chicago, IL 60611-3008

Jordan N. Fink, MD
Professor of Medicine
Chief, Allergy–Immunology
Medical College of Wisconsin
9000 West Wisconsin Avenue
Milwaukee, WI 53226

Leslie Carroll Grammer, MD
Professor of Medicine
Division of Allergy–Immunology
Department of Medicine
Northwestern University Medical School
MC S207
303 East Chicago Avenue, Tarry 3-713
Chicago, IL 60611

Paul A. Greenberger, MD
Professor of Medicine
Division of Allergy–Immunology
Department of Medicine
Northwestern University Medical School
MC S207
303 East Chicago Avenue, Tarry 3-705
Chicago, IL 60611

Kathleen E. Harris, BS
Senior Life Sciences Researcher
Division of Allergy–Immunology
Department of Medicine
Northwestern University Medical School
MC S207
303 East Chicago Avenue, Tarry 3-719
Chicago, IL 60611

Randy J. Horwitz, MD, PhD
Fellow, Department of Allergy/Immunology
University of Wisconsin-Madison
600 Highland Avenue, Room H6/363
Madison, WI 53792-2454

Phillip L. Lieberman, MD
Clinical Professor of Medicine and Pediatrics
Division of Allergy and Immunology
University of Tennessee College of Medicine
Memphis, TN 38163

Kris G. McGrath, MD
Associate Professor of Clinical Medicine
Northwestern University Medical School
Section Chief, Allergy and Immunology
Saint Joseph Hospital
500 North Michigan Avenue, Suite 1640
Chicago, IL 60611-3704

Roger W. Melvold, PhD
Department of Microbiology–Immunology
Northwestern University Medical School
303 East Chicago Avenue
Chicago, IL 60611–3008

W. James Metzger, MD
Professor and Section Head
Allergy, Asthma and Immunology
East Carolina University School of Medicine
Greenville, NC 27858-4354

Roy Patterson, MD
Ernest S. Bazley Professor of Medicine
Chief, Division of Allergy–Immunology
Northwestern University Medical School
MC S207
303 East Chicago Avenue, Tarry 3-711
Chicago, IL 60611-3008

Jacob J. Pruzansky, PhD
Professor Emeritus
Department of Microbiology–Immunology
Northwestern University Medical School
303 East Chicago Avenue
Chicago, IL 60611–3008

Robert E. Reisman, MD
Clinical Professor of Medicine and Pediatrics
State University of New York at Buffalo
Buffalo, NY 14214

Anthony J. Ricketti, MD
Clinical Assistant Professor
University of Medicine and Dentistry of
*   New Jersey*
Robert Wood Johnson Medical School
Director, Respiratory Care
Chief, Section of Allergy/Immunology &
*   Pulmonary Medicine*
St. Francis Medical Center
1542 Kuser Road, Suite B7
Trenton, NJ 08219

Martha A. Shaughnessy, BS
Senior Life Sciences Researcher
Division of Allergy–Immunology
Northwestern University Medical School
MC S207
303 East Chicago Avenue, Tarry 3-719
Chicago, IL 60611–3008

Raymond G. Slavin, MD
Professor of Internal Medicine and
*   Microbiology*
St. Louis University School of Medicine
Director, Division of Allergy and Immunology
St. Louis University Health Sciences Center
1402 South Grand Boulevard
St. Louis, MO 63104

Abba I. Terr, MD
Clinical Professor of Medicine
Stanford University Medical School
Director, Allergy Clinic
Division of Immunology, Room S021
Stanford University Medical Center
Stanford, CA 94305

Stephen I. Wasserman, MD
The Helen M. Ranney Professor and Chair
Department of Medicine
University of California, San Diego
402 Dickinson Street, Suite 380
San Diego, CA 92103-8811

C. Raymond Zeiss, MD
Professor of Medicine
Division of Allergy–Immunology
Northwestern University Medical School
Chief of Staff
VA Chicago Health Care System
333 East Huron
Chicago, IL 60611

Preface

The fifth edition of *Allergic Diseases: Diagnosis and Management* is published 25 years after the first edition. In this quarter of a century, we have seen growth in the worldwide population, a rising death rate from asthma, and an explosion of knowledge in the science of immunology.

Allergic diseases affect twenty percent of the population, with significant chronic illness in ten percent of the population. Many allergic diseases have complications and can result in significant health care costs and chronic morbidity with some potential fatalities. Changes in the health care delivery systems will lead to more care of allergic diseases by primary care physicians. We see a rising need for specialists in Allergy-Immunology. We hope to help all physicians provide care for allergic patients with this book.

Roy Patterson, MD
Leslie C. Grammer, MD
Paul A. Greenberger, MD

From the Preface to the First Edition

This book covers those clinical problems that are commonly seen in the daily practice of the specialty of Allergy. Because of the high incidence of hypersensitivity disease of the immediate type in the general population, reagin-mediated disease is responsible for the majority of clinical immunologic problems seen in medical practice. The theoretical and practical aspects of these IgE-mediated diseases are discussed in detail. Diseases that have clinical manifestations similar to the reagin-mediated reactions but are probably not IgE-mediated are included, because they are commonly referred to the specialist in Allergy. These diseases may include certain types of asthma, urticaria, and rhinitis. The complex problem of drug reactions, most of which are probably not IgE-mediated, is discussed in detail, because it is a common and growing problem in the clinical practice of Allergy.

The remarkable advances made in basic and clinical immunology in the past 15 years have extended the range of diseases now considered to be of immunologic origin. We have decided not to attempt to review the basic and clinical information relating to the immunology of hematology, nephrology, rheumatology, transplantation, infectious diseases, and other major areas of current interest. The consultant in the specialty of Allergy and Immunology must be familiar with these problems, but detailed information regarding them is already available in a variety of recent texts and reviews. The comprehensive practice of modern clinical allergy requires knowledge and training separate from immunology because of the importance of such aspects as pulmonary physiology in asthma, the pharmacology of therapeutic agents, and the botany and aerobiology of antigenic materials. These areas, relevant to the common allergic diseases seen in practice, are reviewed in some detail because they are less frequently encountered in recent texts dealing primarily with nonreaginic immunologic diseases.

It is the opinion of many practitioners and teachers in the field of allergy that the recent advances in basic and clinical immunology must not lead to a decline in emphasis on the common allergy problems, if only because of the high incidence of allergy and the lack of appropriate care patients may receive.

This book has been written by a group of authors who have worked together, either during their training period in Allergy, or as faculty members of the Allergy-Immunology Division of the Department of Medicine at Northwestern University Medical School. Although they were selected because of their unified approach to teaching and clinical care in allergy, they have either trained or are currently working in other medical centers; so their opinions and approaches are not restricted to those of one small group.

Contents

Chapter 5

Chapter 6

Chapter 7

Chapter 8

Chapter 9

Chapter 10

Chapter 11

Chapter 12

Chapter 13

Chapter 14

Anne M. Ditto and Leslie C. Grammer

Chapter 15

Leslie C. Grammer

Chapter 16

Roy Patterson and Sarah Cheriyan

Chapter 17

Richard D. DeSwarte and Roy Patterson

Chapter 18

Raymond G. Slavin

Chapter 19

David I. Bernstein

Chapter 20

Kris G. McGrath

Chapter 21

Chapter 22

Chapter 23

Chapter 24

Chapter 25

Chapter 26

Chapter 27

Allergic Diseases

Diagnosis and Management

Allergic Diseases, 5th Edition,
edited by Roy Patterson, Leslie Carroll Grammer, and
Paul A. Greenberger. Lippincott–Raven Publishers, Philadelphia, © 1997.

1

Review of Immunology

Roger W. Melvold

*R.W. Melvold: Department of Microbiology-Immunology
Northwestern University Medical School, Chicago, IL 60611.*

Pearls for Practitioners
Roy Patterson

- In the middle of the 20th century, knowledge of the field of immunology was sufficiently limited that a scientist could understand the whole field and participate in research in several aspects. At the end of the 20th century, no one can understand the whole field of immunology, so concentrate on areas important to your interests.
- Control of IgE-mediated allergy and other immune diseases will be increasingly carried out by biologic agents. Some of these agents will be capable of inducing allergic reactions in the person being treated.

Although immunology is a relative newcomer among the sciences, its phenomena have long been recognized and manipulated. Ancient peoples understood that survivors of particular diseases were protected from those diseases for the remainder of their lives, and the ancient Chinese and Egyptians even practiced forms of immunization. Surgeons also have long understood that tissues and organs would not survive when exchanged between different individuals (e.g., from cadaver donors) but could succeed when transplanted from one site to another within the same individual. However, only during the last century have the mechanisms of the immune systems been illuminated, at least in part. The immune system is the body's second line of defense. The first line of defense consists of several barriers such as the skin and mucous membranes, the fatty acids of the skin and the high pH of the stomach, resident microbial populations, and cells that act nonspecifically against infectious organisms.

Like the nervous and endocrine systems, the immune system is adaptive, specific, and communicative. It recognizes and responds to changes in the environment, and it displays memory by adapting or altering its responses to stimuli that have been previously encountered. It can detect the presence of millions of different substances (antigens) and has an exquisite ability to discriminate between closely related molecules. Communication and interaction, involving both direct contact and soluble mediators, must occur among a variety of lymphoid and other cells for optimal function.

The complexity of the immune system is extended by genetic differences among individuals. This is because the "repertoire" of immune responses varies among unrelated individuals in an outbred, genetically heterogeneous species such as ours. Furthermore, everyone is "immunologically incomplete" in a sense, because none can recognize and respond to all of the possible antigens that exist. Several factors contribute to this: (1) genetic or environmentally induced conditions that nonspecifically diminish immune functions; (2) variation among individuals in the genes encoding the antigen receptors of lymphocytes; (3) genetically encoded differences among individuals (often determined by the highly polymorphic genes of the human leukocyte antigen [HLA] complex), which dictate whether and how the individual responds to specific antigens; and (4) the fact that each individual's immune system must differentiate between "self" (those substances that are a normal part of the body) and "foreign" or "nonself," to avoid autoimmunity. Because self differs from one individual to the next, what is foreign also differs among individuals.

ANTIGENS

Antigens initially were defined as substances that were identified and bound by antibodies (immunoglobulins) produced by B lymphocytes. But because the specific antigen receptors of T lymphocytes are *not* immunoglobulins, the definition is broadened to include substances that can be specifically recognized by the receptors of T or B lymphocytes. It is estimated that the immune system can specifically recognize at least 10^6 to 10^7 different antigens. These include both substances that are foreign to the body (nonself) and those that are normal constituents of the body (self).

The immune system must distinguish between nonself and self antigens so that, under normal conditions, it can attack the former without damaging the latter. Thus, the immune system should be "tolerant" of self but intolerant of nonself. Autoimmune diseases arise when such distinctions are lost and the immune system attacks self antigens, a phenomenon originally described by Paul Erlich as *horror autotoxicus*. Well-known examples include rheumatoid arthritis, psoriasis, systemic lupus erythematosus, and some forms of diabetes.

Antigens can be divided into three general types, depending on the way in which they stimulate and interact with the immune system.[1-3] An immunogen can, by itself, both stimulate an immune response and subsequently be a target of that response. The terms *immunogen* and *antigen* are often, but somewhat inappropriately, used interchangeably. A hapten cannot, by itself, stimulate an immune response. But, if a hapten is attached to a larger immunogenic molecule (a "carrier"), responses can be stimulated against both the carrier and the hapten, and the hapten itself subsequently can be the target of the invoked response. A tolerogen is a substance that, after an initial exposure to the immune system, inhibits future responses against itself.

Because of the genetic diversity among individuals, a substance that is an immunogen for one person may be a tolerogen for another and may be ignored completely by the immune systems of others. Also, a substance that acts as an immunogen when administered by one route (e.g., intramuscularly) may act as a tolerogen when applied by a different route (e.g., intragastrically).

Antigens usually are proteins or carbohydrates and are found as free single molecules or as parts of larger structures (e.g., expressed on the surface of an infectious agent). Whereas some antigens are small and simple, others are large and complex, containing many different sites that can be individually identified by lymphocyte receptors or free immunoglobulins. Each individual site on an antigen that can be identified by the immune system is called an epitope or determinant (i.e., the smallest identifiable antigenic unit). Thus, a single large antigen may contain many different epitopes. In general, the more complex the molecule and the greater the number of epitopes it displays, the more potent it is as an immunogen.

Adjuvants[4] are substances that, when administered with an immunogen (or a hapten coupled to an immunogen), enhance the response against it. For example, immunogens may be suspended in mixtures (e.g., colloidal suspensions of mycobacterial proteins and oil) that induce localized inflammations and aid in arousal of the immune system.

MOLECULES OF THE IMMUNE SYSTEM

Immunoglobulin

B lymphocytes synthesize receptors (immunoglobulins) able to recognize and bind specific structures (antigens, determinants, epitopes). Each B cell, or clonally derived set of B cells, expresses only a single "species" of immunoglobulin and thus is able to recognize and bind only a single antigen.[1-3] Immunoglobulin exists either as a surface membrane-bound molecule or as a secreted molecule.

The immunoglobulin molecule is a glycoprotein composed of two identical light chains and two identical heavy chains (Fig. 1-1) linked by disulfide bonds.[5] Enzymatic cleavage of the immunoglobulin molecule creates defined fragments. Papain produces two antigen-binding fragments (Fab) and one crystallizable fragment (Fc). Pepsin, on the other hand, produces only a divalent antigen-binding fragment termed $F(ab')_2$ since the remainder of the molecule tends to be degraded and lost.

Each chain (heavy and light) contains one or more constant regions (C_H or C_L) and a variable region (V_H or V_L). Together, the variable regions of the light and heavy chains contribute to the antigen-binding sites (Fab) of the immunoglobulin molecule. The constant regions of the heavy chain (particularly in the Fc portion) determine what subsequent interactions occur between the bound immunoglobulin and other cells or molecules of the immune system. When the antigen-binding sites are filled, a signal is transmitted through the immunoglobulin molecule, which results in conformational changes in the Fc portion of the heavy chain. These conformational changes permit the Fc portion to then interact with other molecules and

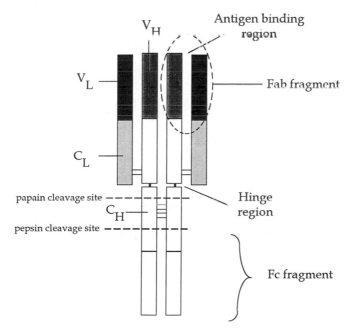

FIG. 1-1. The immunoglobulin molecule.

cells. For example, phagocytic cells bear receptors that allow them to recognize and bind the Fc portions of immunoglobulin attached to antigen, thus increasing the efficiency of phagocytosis.[6] The Fab and F(ab')$_2$ fragments are useful experimental and therapeutic tools that can bind antigens without the ensuing consequences because of the presence of the Fc region.[7]

When the Fab portion of an immunoglobulin binds to antigen, a conformational changes occur, including the Fc portion of the molecule. "Altered" Fc is recognized by receptors (Fc receptors) on macrophages and other cells, allowing them to distinguish bound from unbound immunoglobulin molecules.[8] Similarly, conformational changes in the Fc portion of bound immunoglobulin permit attachment of serum complement component C1q to initiate the classic pathway of complement activation.

The constant regions of the immunoglobulin light chains can be of two types, kappa (κ) or lambda (λ), whereas the constant regions of the heavy chains exist in five major forms (Table 1-1), each associated with a particular immunoglobulin isotype or class: C_α (IgA), C_δ (IgD), C_ε (IgE), C_γ (IgG), and C_μ (IgM). Some of these are subdividable into subclasses (e.g., IgG1, IgG2, IgG3, and IgG4). Each normal individual can generate all of the isotypes. Within a single immunoglobulin molecule, both light chains are identical and of the same type (both λ or both κ), and the two heavy chains are likewise identical and of the same isotype. IgD, IgG, and IgE exist only as basic immunoglobulin units (two heavy chains and two light chains), but serum IgM exists as a pentamer of five basic units united by a J ("joining") chain. The form of IgA found in external body fluids (e.g., tears, saliva) contains two basic units bound together by a molecule (the joining or J chain) and complexed with yet another molecule (the "secretory piece"), which allows the dimeric form of IgA to pass through epithelial cells for secretion.[9]

In addition to antigen-binding specificity, variability among immunoglobulin molecules derives from three further sources: allotypes, isotypes, and idiotypes. *Allotypes* are dictated by minor amino acid sequence differences in the constant regions of heavy or light chains that result from slight polymorphisms in the genes encoding these molecules. Allotypic differences, which typically do not affect the function of the molecule, segregate within families like typical Mendelian traits. *Isotypes*, as already discussed, are determined by more substantial differences in the heavy chain constant regions affecting the functional properties of the immunoglobulins (see Table 1-1). Finally, many antigenic determinants may be bound in more than one way, and thus there may be multiple, structurally distinct immunoglobulins with the same antigenic specificity. These differences within the antigen-binding domains of immunoglobulins that bind the same antigenic determinants are termed *idiotypes*.

Generation of Antigen-Binding Diversity Among Immunoglobulins

Each immunoglobulin chain, light and heavy, is encoded not by a single gene but by a series of genes occurring in clusters along the chromosome.[10] In humans, the series of genes encoding λ light chains, the series encoding κ light chains, and the series encoding heavy chains all are located on separate chromosomes. Within each series, the genes are found in clusters, each containing a set of similar, but not identical, genes. All of the genes are present in embryonic and germ cells, and in cells other than B lymphocytes. When a cell becomes committed to the B-lymphocyte lineage, it rearranges the DNA encoding its light and heavy chains[10–12] by clipping out and discarding some of the DNA sequences. Each differentiating B cell chooses either the λ series or the κ series (but not both). In addition, whereas both the maternally and paternally derived chromosomes carry these sets of genes, each B cell uses only one of them (*either* paternal *or* maternal) to produce a functional chain, a phenomenon termed *allelic exclusion*.

TABLE 1-1. *Immunoglobulin isotypes*

Isotype	Mol weight	Additional components	% of serum Ig	Half-life	Functions
IgA					
Monomer*	160,000		13–19	6	
Dimer[†]	385,000	J chain Secretory piece	0.3		Provides antibodies for external body fluids including mucous, saliva, and tears; effective at neutralizing infectious agents, agglutination, and (when bound to antigen) activation of the alternative complement pathway
IgD					
Monomer*,[†]	180,000		<1	3	Almost entirely found in membrane bound form; the function is unknown but may be related to maturational stages
IgE					
Monomer*,[†]	190,000		<0.001	3	IgE is bound to mast cell surfaces; subsequent binding of antigen stimulates mast cell degranulation, leading to immediate hypersensitivity responses (allergy)
IgG					
Monomer*,[†]	145,000–170,000		72–80	20	Prevalent isotype in secondary responses; in humans, subclasses are IgG1, IgG2, IgG3, IgG4
IgM					
Monomer*			—	5–10	
Pentamer[†]	970,000	J chain	6–8		Prevalent isotype in primary responses; effective at agglutination and activation of classic complement pathway

Mol, molecular; Ig, immunoglobulin.
*Membrane-bound form.
[†]Secreted form.

For the light chains, three distinct clusters of genes contribute to the synthesis of the entire polypeptide: variable genes (V_L), joining genes (J_L), and constant genes (C_L) (Fig. 1-2). In addition, each V gene is preceded by a leader sequence encoding a portion of the polypeptide that is important during the synthetic process, but is removed when the molecule becomes functional. The V_L and D_L genes are used to produce the variable domain of the light chain. This is accomplished by the random selection of a single V_L gene and a single J_L gene to be united (V_L–J_L) by splicing out and discarding the intervening DNA. Henceforth, that cell and all of its clonal descendants are committed to that particular V_L–J_L combination. Messenger RNA for the light chain is transcribed to include the V_L–J_L genes, the C_L genes, and the intervening DNA between them. Before translation, the mRNA is spliced to unite the V_L–J_L genes with a C_L gene so that a single continuous polypeptide can be produced from three genes that originally were separated on the chromosome.

For heavy chains, four distinct clusters of genes are involved (Fig. 1-3): variable genes (V_H), diversity genes (D_H), joining genes (J_H), and a series of distinct constant genes (C_μ, C_δ, C_λ, C_ε, and C_α). As with the light chain genes, each V gene is preceded by a leader sequence (L) that plays a role during synthesis but is subsequently lost. One V_H gene, one D_H gene, and one J_H gene are randomly selected, and the intervening DNA segments are excised and discarded to bring these genes together (V_H–D_H–J_H). Messenger RNA is then transcribed to include both the V_H–D_H–J_H and constant genes, but unlike light chains, the process is distinctly different in stimulated and unstimulated B lymphocytes.

Unstimulated B cells transcribe heavy chain mRNA from V_H–D_H–J_H through the C_μ and C_δ genes. This transcript does *not* contain the information from the Cγ, C_ε, or C_α genes. The mRNA is then spliced to bring V_H–D_H–J_H adjacent to either C_μ or Cδ, which permits the

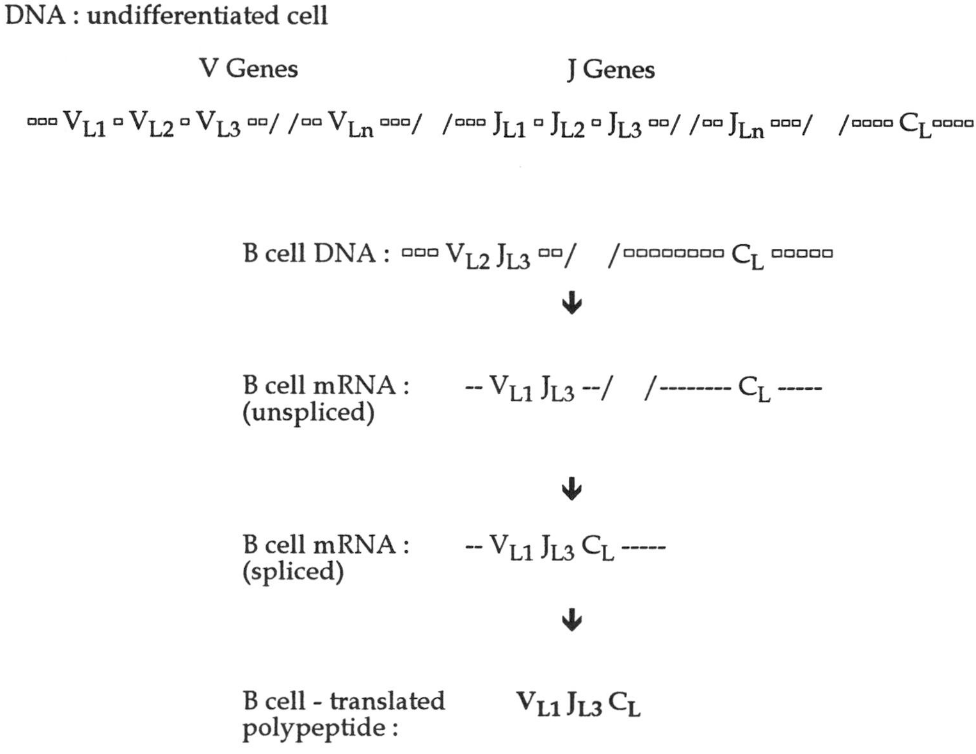

DNA : undifferentiated cell

V Genes   J Genes

□□□ V_{L1} □ V_{L2} □ V_{L3} □□/ /□□ V_{Ln} □□□/   /□□□ J_{L1} □ J_{L2} □ J_{L3} □□/ /□□ J_{Ln} □□□/   /□□□□ C_L □□□□

B cell DNA : □□□ $V_{L2} J_{L3}$ □□/   /□□□□□□□□ C_L □□□□□

⬇

B cell mRNA :   -- $V_{L1} J_{L3}$ --/   /-------- C_L -----
(unspliced)

⬇

B cell mRNA :   -- $V_{L1} J_{L3} C_L$ -----
(spliced)

⬇

B cell - translated $V_{L1} J_{L3} C_L$
polypeptide :

FIG. 1-2. Synthesis of immunoglobulin light chains.

DNA : undifferentiated cell

V Genes	D Genes	J Genes	Constant Genes

□ V_{H1} □ V_{H2} □ V_{Hn} □//□ D_{H1} □ D_{H2} □ D_{Hn} □//□ J_{H1} □ J_{H2} □ J_{Hn} □//□ C_{δ} □ C_{μ} □ C_{γ} □ C_{ϵ} □ C_{α} □

⇓

B cell DNA : □□□ V_{H2} D_{H1} J_{H2} □□/   /□□□ C_{δ} □ C_{μ} □ C_{γ} □ C_{ϵ} □ C_{α} □

⇓

naive B cell mRNA :   -- V_{H1} D_{H1} J_{H2} --/   / C_{δ} - C_{μ}
(unspliced)

⇓

naive B cell mRNA :   -- V_{H1} D_{H1} J_{H2} C_{δ} or   -- V_{H1} D_{H1} J_{H2} C_{μ}
(spliced)

⇓

naive B cell -
translated V_{H1} D_{H1} J_{H2} C_{δ} or V_{H1} D_{H1} J_{H2} C_{μ}
polypeptide :
                    (IgM)   (IgD)

FIG. 1-3. Synthesis of immunoglobulin heavy chains.

translation of a single continuous polypeptide with a variable domain (from V_H–D_H–J_H) and a constant domain (from C_{μ} or $C\delta$). Thus, the surface immunoglobulin of naive unstimulated B cells includes only the IgM and IgD isotypes.

After antigenic stimulation, B cells can undergo an isotype switch in which splicing of DNA, rather than RNA, brings the united V_H–D_H–J_H genes adjacent to a constant region gene.[13-15] This transition is controlled by cytokines secreted by T lymphocytes. Depending on the amount of DNA excised, the V_H–D_H–J_H genes may be joined to any of the different C_H genes (Fig. 1-4). As a result of the isotype switch, B cell "subclones" are generated that produce an array of immunoglobulins having identical antigen-binding specificity but with different isotypes.

Two additional sources of diversity in the variable (antigen-binding) regions of light and heavy immunoglobulin chains occur. First, "junctional diversity" results from imprecision in the cutting and splicing, which brings V, D, and J genes together; and second, somatic mutations occur and accumulate in successive "generations" of clonally derived B lymphocytes.[16-18]

T-Cell Receptor

T lymphocytes (T cells) do not use immunoglobulins as antigen receptors, but use a distinct set of genes encoding four polypeptide chains (α, β, γ, and δ), each with variable and constant domains, used to form T cell receptors (TcRs).[19-24] The TcR is a heterodimer, either an

DNA : B cell $\square\square\square$ V_{H2} D_{H1} J_{H2} $\square\square$/   /$\square\square\square$ C_δ $\square$ C_μ $\square$ C_γ $\square$ C_ε $\square$ C_α $\square\square\square$
(naive)

After antigenic stimulation, DNA between the VDJ unit and the constant genes is excised. The
excision length may vary, bringing VDJ adjacent to different constant genes.

DNA : B cell $\square\square\square$ V_{H2} D_{H1} J_{H2} C_δ $\square$ C_μ $\square$ C_γ $\square$ C_ε $\square$ C_α $\square\square\square$
(stimulated)

  mRNA   --- V_{H2} D_{H1} J_{H2} C_δ --- → translated to IgD

or

B cell DNA : $\square\square\square$ V_{H2} D_{H1} J_{H2} C_μ $\square$ C_γ $\square$ C_ε $\square$ C_α $\square\square\square$
(stimulated)

  mRNA   --- V_{H2} D_{H1} J_{H2} C_μ --- → IgM

or

B cell DNA : $\square\square\square$ V_{H2} D_{H1} J_{H2} C_γ $\square$ C_ε $\square$ C_α $\square\square\square$
(stimulated)

  mRNA   --- V_{H2} D_{H1} J_{H2} C_γ --- → IgG

or

B cell DNA : $\square\square\square$ V_{H2} D_{H1} J_{H2} C_ε $\square$ C_α $\square\square\square$
(stimulated)

  mRNA   --- V_{H2} D_{H1} J_{H2} C_ε --- → IgE

or

B cell DNA : $\square\square\square$ V_{H2} D_{H1} J_{H2} C_α $\square\square\square$
(stimulated)

  mRNA   --- V_{H2} D_{H1} J_{H2} C_α --- → IgA

FIG. 1-4. The isotype switch.

α–β or a γ–δ chain combination that recognizes and binds antigen (Fig. 1-5). This heterodimer is complexed with several other molecules (e.g., CD3, CD4, and CD8) that provide
stability and auxiliary functions for the receptor.[25–27] Unlike immunoglobulin, which can bind
to free antigen alone, TcRs bind to specific combinations of antigen plus self cell surface molecules. The self molecules are encoded by the polymorphic genes of the HLA complex[28]: class
I (encoded by the HLA-A, -B, and -C loci), and class II (encoded by the DP, DQ, and DR loci
within the D/DR region). TcRs of CD8[+] T cells recognize and bind antigen only when it is

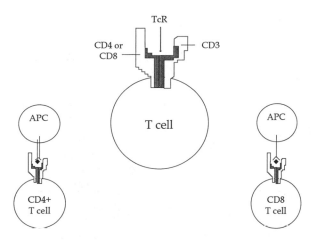

FIG. 1-5. The T cell receptor. APC, antigen-presenting cell.

associated with class I molecules, whereas those of CD4$^+$ T cells recognize and bind antigen only when it is associated with class II molecules.

Like immunoglobulin, the TcR chains contain variable and constant domains. The variable domains are encoded by a series of V, J, and sometimes D (β and δ chains only) gene clusters that undergo DNA rearrangement, and the constant regions are encoded by constant genes. TcRs do not undergo any equivalent of the isotype switch. Junctional diversity provides an additional source of variation for the variable domains of α and β chains, but not for γ and δ chains. Somatic mutation is not found in TcRs.

CD Molecules

Several cell surface molecules (cell determinant [CD] molecules) indicate the functional capacities of lymphocytes and other cells.[29] The most commonly used are those distinguishing T lymphocyte subsets.

- *CD3* is a complex of several molecules associated with the T-cell antigen receptor.[25,27] It provides support for the TcRs and is involved in transmembrane signaling. It is found on all T cells.
- *CD4* is found on T lymphocytes of the helper T (Th) and delayed hypersensitivity (Tdh) subsets.[30-33] It is found on all α–β CD4$^+$ T cells. CD4 molecules are found in association with the TcRs and recognize major histocompatibility complex (MHC) class II molecules on antigen-presenting cells (APCs). The TcRs of CD4$^+$ cells are thus restricted to recognizing combinations of antigen plus MHC class II molecules.
- *CD8* is found on T cells of the cytotoxic T lymphocytes (CTLs) and suppressor T (Ts) subsets.[30,32] It is found on all α–β CD8$^+$ T cells. CD8 molecules are found in association with the TcRs and recognize MHC class II molecules on APCs. The TcRs of CD8$^+$ cells are thus restricted to recognizing combinations of antigen plus MHC class I molecules.

HLA Molecules

The HLA is the MHC of humans.[28,34,35] It is a small region of chromosome 6 containing several (10 to 20) individual genes encoding proteins of three different types called class I, II, and III MHC molecules (Fig. 1-6).

A   Regions & Loci

Regions	D/DR	C2,C4,B$_f$	B	C	A
Loci	(see Fig. 1-6B)	C2,C4,B$_f$	HLA-B	HLA-C	HLA-A
Class	II	III	I	I	I

B   ———————————————— D/DR Region ————————————————

Subregions	DP	DQ	DR
Loci	DP1$_\alpha$ DP1$_\beta$ DP2$_\alpha$ DP2$_\beta$	DQ1$_\alpha$ DQ1$_\beta$ DQ2$_\alpha$ DQ2$_\beta$	DR$_\alpha$ DR1$_\beta$ DR2$_\beta$ DR3$_\beta$
	↘ ↙ ↘ ↙	↘ ↙ ↘ ↙	↘ ↙ ↙ ↙
Molecules Expressed	DP1 DP2 (1α-1β) (2α-2β)	DQ1 DQ2 (1α-1β) (2α-2β)	DR1 DR2 DR3 (α-1β) (α-2β) (α-3β)

Each expressed molecule (DP1, DP2, *etc.*) consists of a separately encoded α and β chain.

FIG. 1-6. The HLA complex. (**A**) Regions and loci. (**B**) The D/DR region.

- *Class I molecules* are membrane-bound glycoproteins found on all nucleated cells. They are a single large polypeptide (approximately 350 amino acids) associated with a smaller molecule (β_2-microglobulin). The HLA complex includes three distinct class I loci (HLA-A, -B, and -C), each having scores of alleles.
- *Class II molecules* consist of two membrane-bound, noncovalently linked chains (α and β) and show a much more limited cellular distribution than class I molecules. They are encoded by the DR, DP, and DQ regions of the HLA complex. They are expressed constitutively on B lymphocytes, macrophages, monocytes, and similar cells in various tissues (Kupffer cells, astrocytes, Langerhans cells of the skin). Some other cells (e.g., vascular epithelium) are able to transiently express class II molecules under particular conditions.
- *Class III molecules* are those complement molecules encoded within the HLA complex.

Cytokines

Cytokines are short-range acting soluble products that are important in the cellular communication necessary for generating immune responses.[36–41] Those produced predominantly by lymphocytes or monocytes often are referred to as lymphokines or monokines, but because so many are produced by multiple cell types, the term cytokine has gained favor. Many cytokines have been identified, although the roles of many of them are not well understood. Many of the cytokines are crucial in regulating the types of immune responses evoked by specific responses.[41–44] Those most basically involved in common immune responses are given in Table 1-2.

Complement

Complement is the composite term for several serum proteins (complement components) that can interact with one another, as well as with antibodies under some circumstances, to pro-

TABLE 1-2. *Cytokines*

Cytokine	Activities	Sources
Interleukin-1 (IL-1)	Stimulates the synthesis of IL-2 and receptors for IL-2 (IL-2R) by T lymphocytes; involved in inflammatory responses. Also known as lymphocyte activating factor (LAF).	Activated macrophages
Interleukin-2 (IL-2)	Stimulates proliferation and maturation of T lymphocytes; stimulates differentiation of B lymphocytes. Stimulates NK cells. Also known as T cell growth factor (TCGF).	CD4+ Th1 cells, some CD+ T cells
Interleukin-3 (IL-3)	Stimulates proliferation and maturation of T lymphocytes and stem cells; induces IL-1 synthesis by activated macrophages.	CD4+ T cells; some CD8+ T cells
Interleukin-4 (IL-4)	Stimulates proliferation of activated B lymphocytes and Th2 lymphocytes; stimulates differentiation of B lymphocytes producing IgE and IgG1. Down-regulates activities of CD4+ Th1 lymphocytes. Also known as B-cell growth factor (BCGF).	CD4+ Th2 T cells, mast cells
Interleukin-5 (IL-5)	Stimulates differentiation of B lymphocytes producing IgA.	CD4+ Th2 T cells
Interleukin-6 (IL-6)	Stimulates proliferation and differentiation of B lymphocytes.	CD4+ Th2 T cells, macrophages
Interleukin-10 (IL-10)	Inhibits macrophage activity, stimulates B cells and mast cells, inhibits CD4+ Th1 T cells.	CD4+ Th2 T cells
Interleukin-12 (IL-12)	Stimulates IFN-γ by NK cells.	Macrophages, B cells
Tumor necrosis factor (TNF-α)	Has toxic activity toward tumor cells. Involved in some inflammatory responses. Also known as tumor necrosis factor-alpha.	T cells, activated macrophages
Lymphotoxin (LT, TNF-β)	Has toxic activity toward tumor cells. Stimulates macrophages. Also called tumor necrosis factor-beta.	CD4+ Th1 T cells
Interferon γ (IFN-γ)	Activates macrophages, stimulates increased expression of MHC class I and II molecules, inhibits viral replication, promotes the differentiation of some B lymphocytes, and stimulates activity of NK cells. Inhibits CD4+ Th2 T cells. Also known as macrophage activating factor (MAF).	CD4+ Th1 T cells, CD8+ T cells, NK cells

NK, natural killer.

duce several different chemical signals and destructive responses.[45,46] The complement components (C1 through C9 plus B, D, and P) act on one another sequentially (the complement "cascade") (Fig. 1-7). The cascade begins with the binding of either component C1 to an antigen–antibody (Ag–Ab) complex or of component C3 to a bacterial or other membrane surface (*without* the assistance of antibody). The binding of C1 initiates what is termed the *classic pathway* (involving the subsequent binding of components C4, C2, and C3), whereas the direct binding of C3 initiates the *alternative pathway* (involving the additional binding of

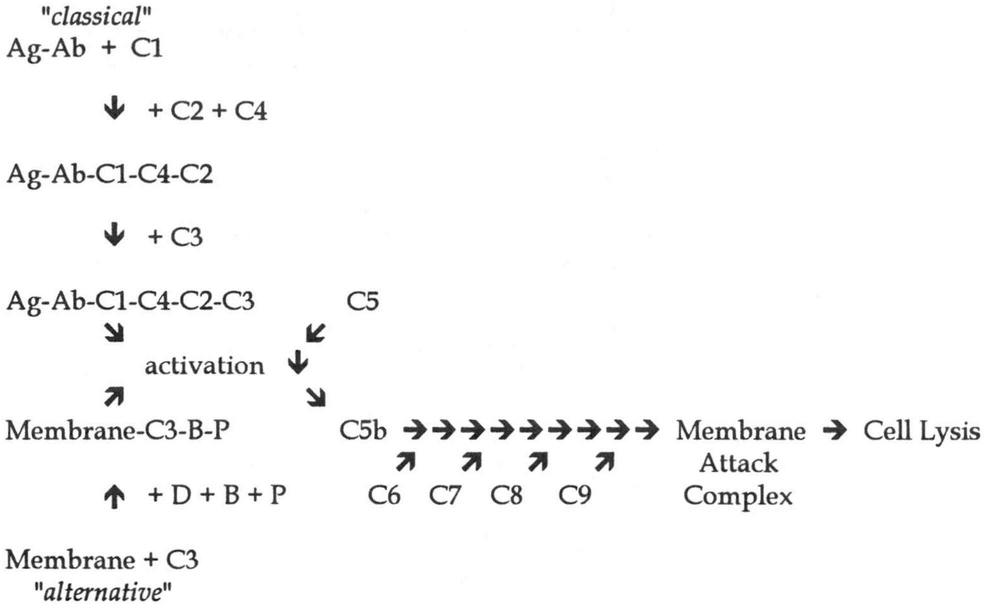

"*classical*"
Ag-Ab + C1

↓ + C2 + C4

Ag-Ab-C1-C4-C2

↓ + C3

Ag-Ab-C1-C4-C2-C3   C5
  ↘   ↙
       activation ↓
  ↗   ↘
Membrane-C3-B-P   C5b ➔➔➔➔➔➔➔➔➔ Membrane ➔ Cell Lysis
                             ↗ ↗ ↗ ↗   Attack
  ↑ + D + B + P   C6 C7 C8 C9   Complex

Membrane + C3
  "*alternative*"

FIG. 1-7. The complement cascade. Ag–Ab, antigen–antibody complex.

components D, B, and P). Both the classic and alternative pathways eventually lead to the activation and binding of component C5, followed by components C6, C7, C8, and C9. The completion of this combination of C5 through C9 is termed the *membrane attack complex* and results in the rupture of the cell surface to which it is attached.[47]

While the complement components interact with one another, each is cleaved into fragments. Some, like C5b, become enzymatically active to continue the cascade. Other fragments gain hormone-like functions and are important in stimulating various inflammatory reactions.[48] C5a (a fragment of C5) attracts neutrophils and macrophages to the site of interest. C3a (a fragment of C3) causes smooth muscle contraction and stimulates basophils, mast cells, and platelets to release histamine and other chemicals contributing to inflammation. C3b (another fragment of C3) stimulates the ingestion (opsonization) of the cells onto which the C3b is bound by monocytes and other phagocytic cells. C4a (fragment of C4) has activity similar to C5a, although it is less effective.

Antigen–Antibody Complexes

Binding of antigen with antibody is noncovalent and reversible. The strength of the interaction is termed *affinity* and determines the relative concentrations of bound versus free antigen and antibody. The formation of Ag–Ab complexes results in lattice-like aggregates of soluble antigen and antibody, and the efficiency of such binding is affected by the relative concentrations of antigen and antibody.[1–3,49] This is best illustrated by the quantitative precipitin reaction (Fig. 1-8). When there is an excess of either antibody or antigen, the Ag–Ab complexes tend to remain small and in solution. The optimal binding, and formation of large aggregates that fall out of solution, occurs when the concentrations of antibody and antigen are in "equivalence." The quantitative precipitin curve provides the basis of laboratory methods for determining the amount of antigen or antibody in, for example, a patient's serum.

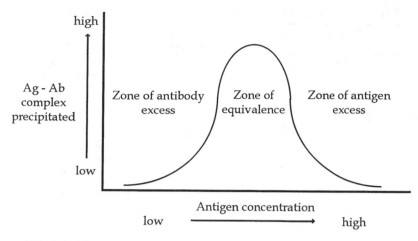

FIG. 1-8. The quantitative precipitin reaction. Ag-Ab, antigen–antibody.

CELLS OF THE IMMUNE SYSTEM

Lymphocytes (General)

The ability of the immune system to specifically recognize a diverse range of antigens resides with the lymphocytes.[1-3] The lymphocytic lineage, derived from stem cells residing within the bone marrow, includes the B lymphocytes, T lymphocytes, and "null" cells. B lymphocytes mature in the bone marrow, whereas those destined to become T lymphocytes migrate to the thymus where they mature. The bone marrow and thymus thus constitute the primary lymphoid organs of the immune system, as opposed to the secondary organs (e.g., spleen, lymph nodes, Peyer's patches) where cells later periodically congregate while they circulate throughout the body.

The ability of the immune system to identify so many different antigens is based on a division of labor: each lymphocyte (or clone of lymphocytes) is able to identify only one epitope or determinant. During its development and differentiation, each cell that is committed to becoming a B or T lymphocyte rearranges the DNA encoding its receptors (as previously described) to construct a unique antigen receptor. Thereafter, that cell and all of its clonal descendants express receptors with the same antigenic specificity. Other surface molecules and secreted products define the functional subsets of lymphocytes (Table 1-3). The specificity of an immune response lies in the fact that the entry of a foreign antigen into the body stimulates *only* those lymphocytes whose receptors recognize and bind the determinants expressed on the antigen. As a result of this specific binding and subsequent intercellular communication, a response is initiated that includes distinct phases:

1. Recognition of antigen by binding to the receptors of lymphoid cells, which is often manifested by clonal proliferation of the stimulated cells
2. *Differentiation* and *maturation* of the stimulated cells to mature functional capacity
3. *Response* against the antigen, cell, or organism by any of several methods
4. The establishment of immunologic *memory*.

Memory[50] resides in a portion of the stimulated lymphocytes that do not carry out effector functions. Instead, they remain quiescent in the system, providing an enlarged pool of "presensitized" cells. As a result, subsequent exposures to the same epitope may produce faster and

TABLE 1-3. *Cells of the human immune system: markers and functions*

Cell	Antigen receptor	Distinctive markers	Soluble products	Immunologic functions
B lymphocyte	Ig MHC class II FcR C3R	Ig IL-3	Ig	Antibody production Antigen processing Antigen presentation
T lymphocyte				
Th1	TcR	TcR CD2 CD3 CD4	IL-2 IL-3 IFN-γ LT	DTH "Helping" IgG2a B cells Inhibition of Th2 T cells Providing help of cell-mediated immunity, including inflammatory responses
Th2	TcR	TcR CD2 CD3 CD4	IL-3 IL-4 IL-5 IL-6	Providing help for B cells (other than IgG2a) Stimulation of granulocytes, mast cells, eosinophils
Tc	TcR	TcR CD2 CD3 CD8		Lysis (by direct contact) of cells altered by infection or malignancy
Ts	TcR	TcR CD2 CD3 CB8	Suppressor factors	"Negative" regulation of immune responses
NK cell	?	FcR Ly49		Lysis of transformed cells
Macrophage	None	MHC class II FcR C3R	IL-1	Phagocytosis Antigen processing and presentation Active in DTH
Mast cell & basophil	None	FcR$_e$	Histamine PAF	Immediate hypersensitivity
Neutrophil	None		Enzymes	Phagocytosis Pinocytosis (???) Inflammation
Eosinophil	None			Antiparasite activity

NK, natural killer; Ig, immunoglobulin; TcR, T-cell receptor; FcR, Fc receptor; FcR$_e$, receptor for Fc of unbound IgE; C3R, C3 receptor; PAF, platelet activating factor; IL, interleukin; IFN-γ, interferon gamma; LT, lymphotoxin; DTH, delayed type hypersensitivity; Ts, suppressor T cell; Tc, cytotoxic T cell.

higher (secondary or anamnestic) responses than were seen in the initial (primary) response. Memory can persist for long periods of time and is primarily maintained by T lymphocytes.

B Lymphocytes

Immunoglobulins recognize and bind specific antigens and determinants. Each B cell, or clonally derived set of B cells, expresses only a single species of immunoglobulin, and thus is capable of recognizing and binding to only a single epitope. Immunoglobulin can be either membrane bound or secreted, and these forms serve two different purposes:

1. As a membrane-bound component of a B-cell surface, immunoglobulin detects the presence of the antigen or epitope for which that particular B cell is specific. The binding of antigen to a B cell's surface immunoglobulin, together with "help" (proliferative and maturation factors) from T lymphocytes, induces the B cell to proliferate and mature into a terminally differentiated plasma cell, which produces and secretes large amounts of immunoglobulin.[51]

2. When secreted by plasma cells, immunoglobulin binds to the antigen of interest, "tagging" it for removal or for subsequent interaction with other cells and molecules. The binding specificities of the membrane-bound and secreted immunoglobulins from a single B cell or clonal set of B cells or plasma cells are identical.

T Lymphocytes

T lymphocytes (T cells) also bear antigen-specific surface receptors (TcRs). The TcR of most T cells is an α–β heterodimer that is complexed with several other molecules (e.g., CD3, CD4, and CD8), which provide auxiliary functions. As described earlier, the antigen receptors of T cells do not bind to antigen alone, but to specific combinations of antigen plus MHC class I or II molecules.[52-55] T cells include several different functional groups:

- *Helper T cells* (Th) initiate responses by proliferating and providing help to B cells and to other T cells (e.g., cytotoxic T lymphocytes) and participate in inflammatory responses. T cell help consists of a variety of cytokines that are required for activation, proliferation, and differentiation of cells involved in the immune response, including the Th cells themselves. Helper T cells are, in turn, composed of two broad categories, Th1 and Th2,[56-59] which secrete different sets of cytokines. These two particular subsets have been best characterized in the mouse, and comparable subsets are being identified in humans. All helper T cells, both Th1 and Th2, bear the CD4 marker and receptors, which recognize combinations of antigen plus HLA class II molecules.
  - *Th1* cells help other effector T cells (e.g., cytotoxic T lymphocytes) in carrying out cell-mediated responses. They also provide help to B cells producing immunoglobulins of the IgG2a isotype. Th1 cells are characterized by the production of interleukin (IL)-2, tumor necrosis factor-alpha, and interferon gamma (IFN-γ) (see Table 1-2). They participate in delayed typed hypersensitivity (DTH) responses, but it is unclear whether the cells doing so are a distinct subset of Th1. In addition to its help functions, IFN-γ also diminishes the activity of Th2 cells.
  - *Th2* cells provide help for B cells, with the exception of those producing IgG2a, and are characterized by the production of IL-4, IL-5, IL-6, and IL-10 (see Table 1-2). In addition to their help functions, IL-4 and IL-10 also diminish the activity of Th1 cells.

- *CTLs* can lyse other cells, which they identify as altered by infection or transformation, through direct contact[60-62] and by using a short-range acting cytolysin, which does not damage the membrane of the CTL itself. These cells, which require help from Th1 cells to proliferate and differentiate, bear CD8 molecules and TcRs recognizing the combinations of antigen plus HLA class I molecules on the surface of antigen-producing cells (where they are first stimulated), and later on the surface of cells, which they subsequently identify as "targets" for destruction. For a CTL to attack and lyse a potential target cell, it must see (on that target) the same combination of antigen plus class I molecule that provided its initial stimulation.
- *DTH T cells* (a subset of Th1) mediate an effector mechanism whereby the Tdh cells, bearing CD4 molecules and triggered by specific combinations of the antigen plus HLA class II molecules, produce cytokines that attract and activate macrophages.[58,59] The activated macrophages, which themselves do not have any specificity for antigen, then produce a localized inflammatory response arising 24 to 72 hours after an antigenic challenge.
- *Suppressor T lymphocytes* (Ts) provide negative regulation to the immune system—the counterweight to helper T cells.[63] These cells, classically defined as bearing CD8 markers and recognizing combinations of antigen plus HLA class I complex, are involved in keeping immune responses within acceptable levels of intensity, depressing them while the antigenic stimulation declines, and preventing aberrant immune responses against self antigens. The mechanisms by which suppressor T lymphocytes carry out these functions is a topic of intense debate, and some investigators question their existence altogether. Recently, some CD4+ T cells also have been implicated in suppressive activity. The mutual negative regulation of Th1 and Th2 cells is a case in point.

Although T lymphocytes with α–β TcRs also express either the CD4 or CD8 markers, those with γ–δ TcRs usually express neither. The ontogeny, distribution, and functional roles of γ–δ T lymphocytes still are unclear.[64,65]

Macrophages and Other Antigen-Presenting Cells

T cell receptors usually do not recognize antigen alone in its "natural" form, but rather bind to antigen that has been "processed" and "presented" on the surface of appropriate APCs.[66-68] These phagocytic cells[6] internalize antigen from the local environment, enzymatically degrade it into fragments (processing), and put the fragments back onto their surface in association with MHC class I and II molecules (presentation). APCs (see Table 1-3) include monocytes, macrophages, and other related tissue-specific cells that express MHC class II molecules (e.g., astrocytes in the central nervous system, Langerhans cells in the skin, Kupffer cells in the liver). In addition, B lymphocytes (which normally express class II) can efficiently process and present antigen,[69,70] as can some other cells that are capable of transient expression of class II (e.g., vascular endothelium). Also, a variety of other molecules on APCs and T cells stabilize the contact between the TcR and antigen plus MHC complex.

Null Cells

In addition to T and B cells, the lymphoid lineage includes a subset of cells that lack both of the classic lymphoid antigen receptors (immunoglobulin and TcR). This subset includes killer (K) and natural killer (NK) cells, and probably other cells such as lymphokine activated killers (LAKs) and large granular lymphocytes (LGLs), which may represent differentially activated forms of K or NK cells.[71,72] K cells bear receptors capable of recognizing the Fc portion of bound immunoglobulins. If the antigen is on the surface of a cell, the K cell uses the bound immunoglobulin to make contact with that cell and lyse it by direct contact (antibody-dependent cellular cytotoxicity. The K cell has no specificity for the antigen that is bound to the antibody, only for the Fc portion of the bound antibody. NK cells are able to distinguish between altered (by malignant transformation or by viral infection) cells and comparable normal cells, and to preferentially bind and lyse the former. The means by which they make this distinction is unknown, but their activity is heightened by IFN-γ and IL-2. NK cells may be able to recognize decreases in the levels of MHC class I molecules or other molecules on the surface of infected or malignant cells.[73] K cells may be a subset of NK cells, and the distinction between them may reflect distinct stages of differentiation, or even simply the use of different assay systems.

Mast Cells and Granulocytes

A variety of other cells are involved in some immune responses, particularly those involving inflammation (see Table 1-3). Mast cells and basophils bear receptors for the Fc portion of IgE[74], which permits them to use IgE on their own surface as an "antigen detector."[74] When antigen binds simultaneously to two or more such molecules on the surface of the same mast cell ("bridging"), a signal is transmitted into the cell that leads to degranulation and release of a variety of mediators, including histamine, which are the basis for the immediate hypersensitivity (allergic) response.[75] Neutrophils are drawn to sites of inflammation by cytokines, where their phagocytic activity, together with production of enzymes and other soluble mediators, contribute to the inflammatory response.[76] Eosinophils[77,78] are involved in immune responses against large parasites, such as roundworms, and are apparently capable of killing them by direct contact.

PRIMARY ORGANS: BONE MARROW AND THYMUS

The primordial stem cells that ultimately produce the human immune system (and other elements of the hematopoietic system) originate in the yolk sac at about 60 days after fertilization. These cells migrate to the fetal liver, and then (beginning about 80 days after fertilization) to the bone marrow, where they remain for life. These primordial hematopoietic stem cells give rise to more specialized stem cells, which lead to the erythrocytic, granulocytic, thrombocytic (platelet), myelocytic (e.g., macrophages, monocytes), and lymphocytic lineages.

Primary lymphoid organs consist of the bone marrow and thymus where B and T lymphocytes, respectively, mature. B cells undergo their development, including generation of immunoglobulin receptors while in the bone marrow. Cells of the T lymphocyte lineage, however, migrate from the bone marrow to the thymus, where they undergo development and generation of TcRs.[78,79] It is in the thymus, under the influence of thymic stroma, nurse cells, and thymic APCs, that T cells receive an initial "thymic education" with regard to what should be recognized as self.[80-82]

SECONDARY ORGANS: SPLEEN AND LYMPH NODES

The secondary organs (e.g., spleen, lymph nodes, Peyer's patches) provide sites where recirculating lymphocytes and APCs enter after passage through diverse parts of the body, "mingle" in close proximity for a period of time, and then leave again to recirculate. This intimate contact between recirculating cells facilitates the close interactions needed to initiate immune responses and generate appropriately sensitized cells whose activities are then expressed throughout the body.[1-3] Thus, most immune responses are initiated in the secondary organs.

INTERACTIONS IN IMMUNE RESPONSES

Antibody Responses

Antibody responses against 99% or more of antigens (T-dependent antigens) require the involvement of T lymphocytes. Thus, T-dependent antigens are distinguished from the relatively few T-independent (TI) antigens, which can provoke antibody production in their absence. The TI antigens fall into two general categories: TI-1 antigens (e.g., a variety of lectins), which are mitogenic, inducing proliferation and differentiation through binding to B-cell surface molecules other than immunoglobulins; and TI-2 antigens, which have regular repeating structures (e.g., repetitive carbohydrate moieties as found in dextran) capable of cross-linking multiple immunoglobulin molecules *on the surface of the same B cell.*

Antibody responses to the most antigens are T dependent and require interactions between APCs (e.g., macrophages), T lymphocytes, and B lymphocytes,[51,83-87] as illustrated in Figure 1-9. B lymphocytes responding to T-dependent antigens require two signals for proliferation and differentiation: (1) the binding of their surface immunoglobulin by appropriate specific antigen, and (2) binding of cytokines (e.g., IL-4 and other "helper factors") produced by activated helper T cells.[88-90] The help provided by T cells acts only over a short range, and thus the T and B cells must be in fairly intimate contact for these interactions to successfully occur. The involvement of APCs, such as macrophages or even B cells themselves, is essential for the activation of helper T cells, and also provides a means of bringing T and B cells into proximity.

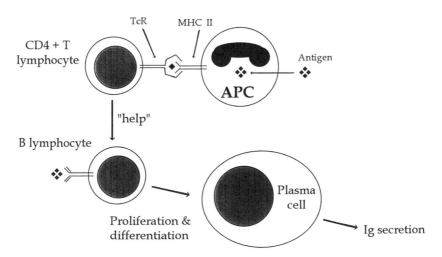

FIG. 1-9. Interactions in antibody production. APC, antigen-presenting cell; TcR, T-cell receptor; MHC, major histocompatibility complex; Ig, immunoglobulin.

Cellular Responses

The mixed lymphocyte response (MLR) is an in vitro measure of T-cell proliferation, primarily involving CD4[+] helper T cells, which is often used as a measure of the initial phase (recognition–proliferation) of the cellular response. Splenic or lymph node T cells from the individual in question (responder) are mixed with lymphocytes from another individual (sensitizer) against whom the response is to be evaluated. The sensitizing cells usually are treated (e.g., with mitomycin or irradiation) to prevent them from proliferating. The two cell populations are incubated together for 4 to 5 days, after which tritiated thymidine is added to the culture for a few hours. If the responder cells are actively proliferating as a result of the recognition of foreign antigens on the sensitizing cells, significant increases of thymidine incorporation (over control levels) can be measured. The strongest MLR responses typically occur when the responding and sensitizing cells bear MHC class II molecules not present on the responding cells, although primary significant MLR responses also are often observed for MHC class I differences only, and even for some non-MHC differences, such as Mls in the mouse.[91] If the responder was appropriately sensitized in vivo before the MLR, significant responses to other non-MHC alloantigens often is seen as well. The MLR is a special subset of T-proliferative assays, one which is directed at genetically encoded alloantigens between two populations of lymphocytes. The same principle can, however, be used to assess the proliferation of T cells against antigen in other forms (e.g., soluble antigen on the surface of APCs).

Cell-mediated lysis is the response function of cytotoxic T lymphocytes. After appropriate stimulation (by antigen in conjunction with class I MHC molecules on the surface of APC, together with help from Th1 cells), CTLs proliferate and differentiate to become capable of binding and destroying target cells through direct cell-to-cell contact (Fig. 1-10). Clonally derived

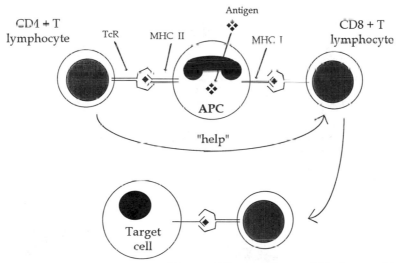

Mature CTL recognizes and binds same [Ag + MHC class I] as originally seen on APC. Lysis of target cell ensues.

FIG. 1-10. Cytotoxic T lymphocytes. TcR, T-cell receptor; MHC, major histocompatibility complex; CTL, cytotoxic T lymphocyte; APC, antigen-presenting cell; Ag, antigen.

CTLs can lyse only those cells that bear the same combination of antigen plus class I molecules originally recognized on the APC by the original CTL from which the clone was derived.

DTH is an in vivo activity of inflammatory Th1 (or Tdh) cells (Fig. 1-11). Individuals who have been presensitized against a particular antigen, then later challenged intradermally with a small amount of the same antigen, display local inflammatory responses 24 to 72 hours later at the site of challenge, as in the tuberculin skin test (Mantoux test). The response is mediated by CD4$^+$ Th1 cells, previously sensitized to a combination of antigen plus class II. On subsequent exposure to the same antigen plus class II molecule, the Th1 responds by secreting a series of cytokines (see Table 1-2), which attract macrophages to the site of interest and activate them. The activated macrophages then destroy and phagocytize the antigenic stimulus, but because macrophages are not antigen specific, they often destroy normal cells and tissues in the local area ("innocent bystander" destruction).

THE IMMUNE SYSTEM: A DOUBLE-EDGED SWORD

The immune system evolved to protect the body from a variety of external (infectious agents or harmful molecules) and internal (malignant cells) threats. In this regard, the immune system provides the body with a means of minimizing or preventing disease. This is most clearly manifested by the problems encountered by individuals who have defects in immune function (immunodeficiency disease) resulting from genetic, developmental, infective, or therapeutic causes. Because of its destructive potential, however, the immune system is capable of causing, rather than preventing, disease when confronted with inappropriate antigenic stimulation or loss of regulatory control.

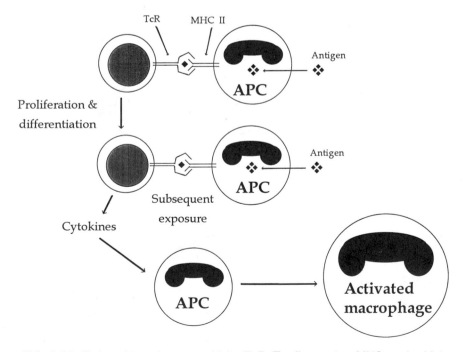

FIG. 1-11. Delayed type hypersensitivity. TcR, T-cell receptor; MHC, major histocompatibility complex; APC, antigen-presenting cell.

Transplantation

Transplantation requires the ability to replace damaged or diseased body parts by transplanting organs from one individual to another. Unfortunately, the immune system is adept at recognizing nonself and rejecting transplanted organs from donors differing genetically from the recipient.[92,93] The cell surface molecules that trigger the rejection response are termed *histocompatibility antigens* and are divided into two primary categories: major (encoded by MHC class I and II genes), and minor (scores, possibly hundreds, of antigens encoded by widely diverse genes scattered across the chromosomes). Because a genetically perfect match between host and donor is only rarely found (i.e., identical twins), transplant surgeons usually attempt to minimize or prevent the immune response of the recipient against the transplanted organ. Some of these problems are minimized by attempting to find the closest genetic match between donor and recipient using tissue typing, but in humans this is possible only for the HLA system. It would be best if only the ability of the immune system to react to the antigens on the transplanted organ could be diminished (i.e., induction of antigen-specific immunologic tolerance), leaving the rest of the immune system intact. Currently, practitioners must rely on drugs that depress the immune system in a relatively nonspecific fashion, thus leading to complications such as overwhelming opportunistic infections. Recently, some agents (i.e., cyclosporin and FK506) have been found to diminish immune responses in a more specific fashion, but their long-term use may have secondary complications, especially after long-term use.

Autoimmunity

Autoimmune diseases involve the development of antibody or cell-mediated immune responses directed against self antigens.[94] There are several possible scenarios under which such undesirable responses might be initiated.

Autoimmune responses arise when antigens that are normally sequestered from the immune system (e.g., in immunologically privileged sites) are exposed, for example, as a result of trauma. Having never been "seen" previously by the immune system as it developed its sense of "self versus nonself," such antigens are seen as foreign. Secondly, the interaction of self molecules with small reactive chemicals (e.g., haptens) or with infectious agents may produce alterations in a self molecule (altered antigen or neoantigen), which results in it now being seen as nonself. Thirdly, immune responses against determinants on infectious agents may generate clones of lymphocytes with receptors capable of cross-reacting with self antigens (cross-reactive antigens). A classic example is rheumatic fever, which results from immune responses against *Streptococcal* antigens, which are cross-reactive with molecules found on heart tissue. Finally, some autoimmune responses, especially those that tend to develop in later life, may result from senescence of inhibitory mechanisms, such as suppressor T lymphocytes. For example, the onset of systemic lupus erythematosus often is associated with a decline in suppressor T cell function. In some such diseases, an individual's risk is affected by that individual's HLA genes.[1-3,95]

Immune Complex Diseases

The humoral immune response generally is efficient at eliminating foreign antigens by the formation of Ag–Ab complexes, which are then cleared by the reticuloendothelial system. There are, however, cases where Ag–Ab complexes (involving IgG and IgM antibodies) reach such high concentrations that they precipitate out of solution and accumulate in tissues (often unrelated to the source of the antigen), leading to systemic or localized inflammation while the complexes bind and activate serum complement components, attract phagocytic cells such as macrophages and neutrophils, and induce the release of proteolytic enzymes and other mediators of inflammation. Attempts to clear depositions of Ag–Ab complexes often damage the tissues or organs involved. Such situations most often arise as a secondary effect of situations where there is a persistence of antigen (e.g., chronic infection, cancer, autoimmunity, or frequent repeated administration of an external reagent) leading to continual stimulation of the immune system and production of high titers of antibodies against the persisting antigen. Among the most commonly damaged sites are the kidneys (glomerulonephritis), where the filtration apparatus tends to accumulate deposited complexes; synovial membranes of the joints (rheumatoid arthritis); the skin (rashes); and the endothelial walls of blood vessels (arteritis).

Contact Dermatitis

Contact dermatitis is an example of a normally protective T-cell–mediated immune response that can be harmful under certain circumstances. Contact dermatitis is a DTH response, usually caused by the presence of small chemically reactive antigens (e.g., heavy metals or, as in the case of poison ivy, plant lipids such as catechol) that bind to self proteins (e.g., MHC class II molecules) on the skin and produce neoantigens.

Allergies and Anaphylaxis (Immediate Hypersensitivity)

Allergies and anaphylaxis antigen-specific immunologic reactions involving IgE antibodies bound (by their Fc domain) to the membranes of mast cells and basophils.[74] When antigen is bound, resulting in cross-linking of the IgE molecules, the mast cells are stimulated to degranulate and release histamine, serotonin, platelet-activating factors, and other mediators of immediate hypersensitivity.[95] Immediate hypersensitivity develops against a wide array of environmental substances and is localized (e.g., itching, tearing) or systemic (e.g., involving the circulatory system). The latter may be life-threatening if severe. Treatment involves the prompt application of pharmaceutical antagonists (e.g., epinephrine, antihistamines) of histamine and serotonin.

TOLERANCE

In many cases, it is desirable to deliberately diminish or eliminate immune responses. For example, the host response against transplanted tissues or organs, autoimmune responses, and asthmatic or allergic responses all represent situations where undesirable immune responses have been initiated. There are basically two methods for achieving this aim: nonspecific and specific.

Immunosuppression is the elimination of all immune responses, regardless of the specificity of those responses. This may occur naturally, as in the case of individuals who are deficient in immune function for genetic reasons (e.g., severe combined immunodeficiency disease) or as the result of infection (e.g., AIDS). Alternatively, it may be intentionally imposed by the application of radiation, drugs, or other reagents (e.g., antilymphocyte sera). Such procedures, however, impose a new set of risks because their "nonspecificity" leave the patient or experimental animal open to infections by opportunistic pathogens. Attempts to diminish these consequences involve the development of reagents with narrower effects, including drugs such as cyclosporin and FK506, or the application of antibodies specific for only particular subsets of lymphocytes.[96] *Immunologic tolerance* is the specific acquired inability of individuals to respond to an immunogenic determinant toward which they would normally respond. Tolerance is more desirable than immunosuppression because it eliminates or inactivates only those lymphocytes that are specific for a particular determinant, leaving the remainder of the immune system intact to deal with opportunistic infections.

The natural induction of tolerance during the development of the immune system prevents immune responses against self antigens ("self tolerance"), thus preventing autoimmunity.[97] Experimentally, tolerance can be induced in immunocompetent adult animals by manipulation of a variety of factors including age, the physical nature and dose of antigen, and the route by which the antigen is administered.[98,99] Tolerance may be induced in both T lymphocytes and B lymphocytes, although tolerance of T cells generally requires lower doses of antigen and is effective for a longer period of time. In addition, because of the requirement of B lymphocytes for T-cell help, the induction of tolerance in T cells often also diminishes corresponding humoral responses.

The means by which specific tolerance is induced and maintained involve three general mechanisms, all of which occur in various situations. Clonal deletion or abortion is the actual elimination of those clones of lymphocytes that encounter the specific antigen under particular conditions. Clonal anergy is the functional inactivation of those clones of lymphocytes that encounter the specific antigen in a tolerogenic form. This may be reversible. Antigen-specific suppressor T cells (classically, CD8+ cells, although CD4+ T cells also have been implicated) inhibit the antigen-specific induction or expression of immune responses by other T or B lymphocytes. The association of autoimmune disorders with advancing age often is attributed to age-related declines in suppressor T cells.

The immune system is an amazing biologic system. Precise interactions must occur between an almost bewildering array of cells and molecules, in appropriate sequences and quantities. Moreover, these highly specific cells and molecules must find one another, after patrolling throughout the entire body, to coordinate their activities. It seems incredible that it all works so well so much of the time. It can malfunction, however, with potentially harmful consequences, and the process of learning how to correct and alleviate these occasions is ongoing.

REFERENCES

1. Klein J. Immunology. Boston: Blackwell Scientific Publications, 1990.
2. Roitt I. Essential immunology. 7th ed. Boston: Blackwell Scientific Publications, 1991.
3. Travers P, Janeway CA Jr. Immunobiology: the immune system in health and disease. New York: Garland Publishing, 1994.
4. Audibert FM, Lise LD. Adjuvants: current status, clinical perspectives and future prospects. Immunol Today 1993;14:281.
5. Alzari PM, Lascombe PW, Poljak RJ. Three-dimensional structure of antibodies. Annu Rev Immunol 1988;6:555.
6. Van Oss CJ. Phagocytosis: an overview. Methods Enzymol 1986;132:3.
7. Adair JR. Engineering antibodies for therapy. Immunol Rev 1992;130:5.
8. Morgan EL, Weigle WO. Biological activities residing in the Fc portion of immunoglobulin. Adv Immunol 1987;40:61.
9. Underdown BJ, Schiff JM. Immunoglobulin A: strategic defense initiative at the mucosal surface. Annu Rev Immunol 1986;4:389.
10. Tonegawa S. Somatic generation of antibody diversity. Nature 1983;302:575.
11. Yancopoulos GD, Alt FW. Regulation of the assembly and expression of variable-region genes. Annu Rev Immunol 1986;4:339.
12. Alt FW, Oltz EM, Yound F, et al. VDJ recombination. Immunol Today 1992;13:306.

13. Esser C, Radbruch A. Immunoglobulin class switching: molecular and cellular analysis. Annu Rev Immunol 1990;8:717.
14. Harriman W, Völk H, Defranoux N, et al. Immunoglobulin class switch recombinations. Annu Rev Immunol 1993;11:361.
15. Radbruch A, Burger C, Klein S, et al. Control of immunoglobulin class switch recombination. Immunol Rev 1986;89:69.
16. Rudikoff S, Pawlita M, Pumphrey J, et al. Somatic diversifications of immunoglobulins. Proc Natl Acad Sci USA 1984;81:2162.
17. Sablitzky F, Wildner G, Rajewsky K. Somatic mutation and clonal expansion of B cells in an antigen-driven immune response. EMBO J 1985;4:345.
18. Berek C, Milstein C. Mutation drift and repertoire shift in the maturation of the immune response. Immunol Rev 1987;96:23.
19. Allison JP, Lanier LL. The structure, function and serology of the T-cell antigen receptor complex. Annu Rev Immunol 1987;5:503.
20. Ashwell JD, Klausner RD. Genetic and mutational analysis of the T cell antigen receptor. Annu Rev Immunol 1990;8:139.
21. Kronenberg M, Siu G, Hood LE, et al. The molecular genetics of the T-cell antigen receptor and T-cell antigen recognition system. Annu Rev Immunol 1986;4:529.
22. Matis L. The molecular basis of T-cell specificity. Annu Rev Immunol 1990;8:65.
23. Raulet DH. The structure, function, and molecular genetics of the γ/δ T cell receptor. Annu Rev Immunol 1989;7:175.
24. Wilson RK, Lai E, Concannan P, et al. Structure, organization and polymorphism of murine and human T-cell receptor α and β chain gene families. Immunol Res 1988;101:149.
25. Clevers H, Alarcon B, Wileman T, et al. The T cell receptor/CD3 complex: a dynamic protein ensemble. Annu Rev Immunol 1988;6:629.
26. Goodman JL, Sercarz EE. The complexity of structures involved in T-cell activation. Annu Rev Immunol 1983;1:465.
27. Weiss A, Imboden J, Hardy K, et al. The role of the T3/antigen receptor complex in T-cell activation. Annu Rev Immunol 1986;4:593.
28. Klein J. Natural history of the major histocompatibility complex. New York: John Wiley & Sons, 1986.
29. Schlossman SF, Boumsell L, Gilks W, et al. CD antigens 1993. Immunol Today 1994;15:98.
30. Bierer BE, Sleckman BP, Ratnofsky SE, et al. The biological roles of CD2, CD4, and CD8 in T-cell activation. Annu Rev Immunol 1989;7:579.
31. Biddison WE, Shae S. CD4 expression and function in HLA class II–specific T cells. Immunol Rev 1989;109:5.
32. de Vries JE, Yssel H, Spits H. Interplay between the TCR/CD3 complex and CD4 or CD8 in the activation of cytotoxic T lymphocytes. Immunol Rev 1989;109:119.
33. Janeway CA Jr, Carding S, Jones B, et al. CD4+ T cells: specificity and function. Immunol Rev 1988;101:39.
34. Bjorkman PJ, Saper MA, Samraoui B, et al. Structure of the human class I histocompatibility antigens. Nature 1987;329:506.
35. Klein J, Takahata N. The major histocompatibility complex and the quest for origins. Immunol Rev 1990;113:5.
36. Dinarello CA. Interleukin-1 and its biologically related cytokines. Adv Immunol 1989;44:153.
37. Balkwill FR, Burke F. The cytokine network. Immunol Today 1989;10:299.
38. Gardner P. IL-6: an overview. Annu Rev Immunol 1990;8:253.
39. Moore KW, O'Garra A, de Waal R, et al. IL-10. Annu Rev Immunol 1993;11:165.
40. Trinchieri G. Interleukin-12: a proinflammatory cytokine with immunoregulatory functions that bridge innate resistance and antigen-specific adaptive immunity. Annu Rev Immunol 1995;13:251.
41. Mosmann TR, Moore KW. The role of IL-10 in cross-regulation of T_H1 and T_H2 responses. Immunol Today 1991;12:A49.
42. Dallman MJ, Wood KJ, Hamano K, et al. Cytokines and peripheral tolerance to alloantigens. Immunol Rev 1993;133:5.
43. Sher A, Gazzinelli RT, Oswald IP, et al. Role of T-cell derived cytokines on the downregulation of immune responses in parasitic and retroviral infection. Immunol Rev 1992;127:183.
44. Hayday AC, Bottomly K. Cytokines in T-cell development. Immunol Today 1991;12:239.
45. Fearon DT. Activation of the alternative complement pathway. Crit Rev Immunol 1979;1:1.
46. Porter RR, Reid KBM. Activation of the complement system by antigen-antibody complexes: the classical pathway. Adv Protein Chem 1979;33:1.
47. Muller-Eberhard HJ. The membrane attack complex of complement. Annu Rev Immunol 1986;4:503.
48. Damaran B. Biological activities of complement-derived peptides. Rev Physiol Biochem Pharmacol 1987;108:151.
49. Colman PM. Structure of antibody-antigen complexes: implications for immune recognition. Adv Immunol 1988;43:99.
50. Gray D. Immunological memory. Annu Rev Immunol 1993;11:49.
51. Vitetta ES, Fernandez-Botran R, Myers CD, et al. Cellular interactions in the humoral immune response. Adv Immunol 1989;45:1.

52. Schwartz RH. T-lymphocyte recognition of antigen in association with gene products of the major histocompatibility complex. Annu Rev Immunol 1985;3:213.
53. Blackman MA, Kappler JW, Marrack P. T cell specificity and repertoire. Immunol Rev 1988;101:5.
54. Hedrick SM. Specificity of the T cell receptor for antigen. Adv Immunol 1988;43:193.
55. Kourilsky P, Claverie J-M. MHC–antigen interaction: what does the T cell receptor see? Adv Immunol 1989;45:107.
56. Bottomly K. A functional dichotomy in CD4+ T lymphocytes. Immunol Today 1988;9:268.
57. Mosmann TR, Coffman RL. Th1 and Th2 cells: different patterns of lymphokine secretion lead to different functional properties. Annu Rev Immunol 1989;7:145.
58. Street NE, Mosmann TR. Functional diversity of T lymphocytes due to secretion of different cytokine patterns. FASEB J 1991;5:171.
59. Fitch FW, McKisic MD, Lancki DW, et al. Differential regulation of murine T lymphocyte subsets. Annu Rev Immunol 1993;11:48.
60. Henkart PA. Mechanism of lymphocyte-mediated cytotoxicity. Annu Rev Immunol 1985;3:31.
61. Peters PJ, Geuze HJ, van der Donk HA, et al. A new model for lethal hit delivery by cytotoxic T lymphocytes. Immunol Today 1990;11:28.
62. Townsend ARM, Bodmer H. Antigen recognition by class I–restricted T lymphocytes. Annu Rev Immunol 1989;7:601.
63. Asherson GL, Colizzi V, Zembala M. An overview of T-suppressor cell circuits. Annu Rev Immunol 1986;4:37.
64. Haas W, Periera P, Tonegawa S. Gamma/delta cells. Annu Rev Immunol 1993;11:637.
65. Porcelli S, Brenner MB, Band H. Biology of the human γδ T-cell receptor. Immunol Rev 1991;120:137.
66. Germain RN, Margulies DH. The biochemistry and cell biology of antigen processing and presentation. Annu Rev Immunol 1993;11:403.
67. Harding CV, Leyva-Cobian F, Unanue ER. Mechanisms of antigen processing. Immunol Rev 1988;106:77.
68. Chain BM, Kaye PM, Shaw M-A. The biochemistry and cell biology of antigen processing. Immunol Rev 1988;106:33.
69. Lanzavecchia A. Receptor-mediated antigen uptake and its effect on antigen presentation to class II–restricted T lymphocytes. Annu Rev Immunol 1990;8:773.
70. Pierce SK, Morris JF, Grusby MJ, et al. Antigen-presenting function of B lymphocytes. Immunol Rev 1988;106:149.
71. Kaplan J. NK cell lineage and target specificity: a unifying concept. Immunol Today 1987;7:10.
72. Trinchieri G. Biology of natural killer cells. Adv Immunol 1989;47:187.
73. Moretta L, Ciccione E, Moretta A, et al. Allorecognition by NK cells: nonself or no self? Immunol Today 1992;13:300.
74. Metzger H. The receptor with high affinity for IgE. Immunol Rev 1992;125:37.
75. Stevens RL, Austin KF. Recent advances in the cellular and molecular biology of mast cells. Immunol Today 1989;10:381.
76. Bach MK. Mediators of anaphylaxis and inflammation. Annu Rev Microbiol 1982;36:371.
77. Gleich GJ. Current understandings of eosinophil function. Hosp Practice 1988;23:137.
78. Haynes BF, Denning SM, Singer KH, et al. Ontogeny of T-cell precursors: a model for the initial stages of human T-cell development. Immunol Today 1989;10:87.
79. Nikolic-Zugic J. Phenotypic and functional stages in the intrathymic development of αβ T cells. Immunol Today 1991;12:65.
80. Meuller DL, Jenkins MK, Schwartz RH. Clonal expansion vs functional clonal inactivation. Annu Rev Immunol 1989;7:445.
81. Sprent J, Lo D, Gao E-K, et al. T cell selection in the thymus. Immunol Rev 1988;101:173.
82. Von Boehmer H, Teh HS, Kisielow P. The thymus selects the useful, neglects the useless and destroys the harmful. Immunol Today 1989;10:57.
83. Coffman RL, Seymour BWP, Lebman DA, et al. The role of helper T cell products in mouse B cell differentiation and isotype regulation. Immunol Rev 1988;102:5.
84. Randolph RJ, Snow EC. Cognate interactions between helper T cells and B cells. Immunol Today 1990;11:361.
85. Singer A, Hodes RJ. Mechanism of T-cell B-cell interaction. Annu Rev Immunol 1983;1:211.
86. Vitetta ES, Bossie A, Botran RF, et al. Interaction and activation of antigen-specific T and B cells. Immunol Rev 1987;99:193.
87. Berek C, Milstein C. The dynamic nature of the antibody repertoire. Immunol Rev 1988;105:5.
88. Finkelman FD, Katona IM, Urba JF Jr, et al. Lymphokine control of in vivo immunoglobulin isotype selection. Annu Rev Immunol 1990;8:303.
89. Melchers F, Anderson J. Factors controlling the B-cell cycle. Annu Rev Immunol 1986;4:13.
90. Hamaoka T, Ono S. Regulation of B-cell differentiation: interactions of factors and corresponding receptors. Annu Rev Immunol 1986;4:167.
91. Abe R, Hodes RJ. Properties of the Mls system: a revised formulation of Mls genetics and an analysis of T-cell recognition of Mls determinants. Immunol Rev 1989;107:5.
92. Mason DW, Morris PJ. Effector mechanisms in allograft rejection. Annu Rev Immunol 1986;4:119.
93. Clift RA, Storb R. Histoincompatible bone marrow transplants in humans. Annu Rev Immunol 1987;5:43.
94. Shoenfeld Y, Isenberg DA. The mosaic of autoimmunity. Immunol Today 1989;10:123.

95. Charron D. The molecular basis of human leukocyte antigen class II disease associations. Adv Immunol 1989;47:187.
96. Sutton BJ, Gould HJ. The human IgE network. Nature 1993;366:421.
97. Waldmann H. Manipulation of T-cell responses with monoclonal antibodies. Annu Rev Immunol 1989;7:407.
98. Marrack P, Hugo P, McCormack J, et al. Self-ignorance in the peripheral T-cell pool. Immunol Rev 1993;13:119.
99. Weiner HL, Friedman A, Miller A, et al. Oral tolerance: immunologic mechanisms and treatment of animal and human organ-specific autoimmune diseases by oral administration of autoantigens. Annu Rev Immunol 1994;12:809.

Allergic Diseases, 5th Edition,
edited by Roy Patterson, Leslie Carroll Grammer, and
Paul A. Greenberger. Lippincott–Raven Publishers, Philadelphia, © 1997.

2

Immunology of IgE-Mediated and Other Hypersensitivity States

C. Raymond Zeiss and Jacob J. Pruzansky

C.R. Zeiss: Division of Allergy-Immunology,
Northwestern University Medical School, Chicago, IL 60611.
J.J. Pruzansky: Department of Microbiology-Immunology,
Northwestern University Medical School, Chicago, IL 60611.

Pearls for Practitioners
Roy Patterson

- Demonstrating IgE antibody by skin tests or in vitro tests does not make a diagnosis of IgE-mediated disease. These tests show only the *presence* of IgE antibody. This is one of the most misunderstood and misused aspects of immediate-type allergy. The diagnosis is made by correlating the presence of IgE antibody and the exposure and response of the patient to the allergen.
- Immediate-type skin tests are a more sensitive test for IgE antibody than in vitro tests because the in vitro skin test is magnified by the release of highly potent bioactive mediators from mast cells activated by allergen reacting with IgE antibody on the mast cell surface. Both prick and intradermal tests (if prick test results are negative) are required to exclude IgE antibody by skin tests.
- It is unlikely that IgE antibody production will be inhibited by new techniques in the next decade. Current therapies must be understood and used.

HISTORICAL REVIEW OF IgE-MEDIATED HYPERSENSITIVITY

In 1902, Richet and Portier described the development of anaphylaxis in dogs given sea anemone toxin; subsequently, anaphylaxis was described in humans after the injection of horse serum to achieve passive immunization against tetanus and diphtheria. In 1906, Clemons von Pirquet correctly predicted that immunity and hypersensitivity reactions would depend on the interaction between a foreign substance and the immune system, and that immunity and hypersensitivity would have similar underlying immunologic mechanisms.[1]

The search for the factor responsible for immediate hypersensitivity reactions became a subject of intense investigation over several years. In 1921, Prausnitz and Küstner[2] described the transfer of immediate hypersensitivity (to fish protein) by serum to the skin of a normal individual. This test for the serum factor responsible for immediate hypersensitivity reactions was termed the Prausnitz-Küstner test. Variations of this test remained the standard for measuring skin sensitizing antibody over the next 50 years.

In 1925, Coca and Grove[3] extensively studied the skin sensitizing factor from sera of patients with ragweed hay fever. They called skin sensitizing antibody *atopic reagin* because of its association with hereditary conditions and because of their uncertainty as to the nature of the antibody involved. Thereafter, this factor was called atopic reagin, reaginic antibody, or skin sensitizing antibody. This antibody clearly had unusual properties and could not be measured readily by standard immunologic methods. Major research efforts from the 1920s through the 1960s defined its physical–chemical properties and measured its presence in allergic individuals. Stanworth[4] and Sehon and Gyenes[5] detailed the history of this effort. Estimates indicated that reaginic antibody was present in serum in less than microgram-per-milliliter quantities, had an electrophoretic mobility in the fast gamma region, and had a sedimentation constant higher than that of IgG. Additionally, many immunologists believed that reaginic antibody belonged to a class of immunoglobulins called IgA.

In 1967, the Ishizakas[6] discovered that skin sensitizing antibody belonged to a unique class of immunoglobulin, which they called IgE. The Ishizakas[6] had been studying IgA antibody against blood group substances and found that IgA antibody against blood group substance A had no capacity to sensitize human skin. This was strong evidence against IgA being the carrier of reaginic activity. In subsequent elegant studies using immunologic techniques, they clearly demonstrated that reagin-rich serum fractions from a patient with ragweed hay fever belonged to a unique class of immunoglobulin.[6] Shortly thereafter, the Swedish researchers Johansson and Bennich discovered a new myeloma protein, termed IgND, which had no antigenic relation to the other immunoglobulin classes. In 1969, cooperative studies between these workers and Ishizakas confirmed that the proteins were identical and that a new class of immunoglobulin, IgE, had been discovered.[7]

PHYSIOLOGY OF IgE

IgE Structure and IgE Receptors

The immunochemical properties of IgE are shown in Table 2-1 in contrast to those of the other immunoglobulin classes. IgE is a glycoprotein that has a molecular weight of 190,000 with a sedimentation coefficient of 8S. Like all immunoglobulins, they have a four-chain structure with two light chains and two heavy chains. The heavy chains contain five domains (one variable and four constant regions) that carry unique, antigenic specificities termed the epsilon (ε) determinants (Fig. 2-1*A*). These unique antigenic structures determine the class specificity of this protein. Digestion with papain yields the Fc fragment, which contains the epsilon antigenic determinants, and two Fab fragments. The Fab fragments contain the antigen combining sites. The tertiary structure of the Fc fragment is responsible for the protein's ability to fix to the FcεR1 receptors on mast cells and basophils.[8]

The FcεR1 receptor is the high-affinity receptor for IgE found on mast cells, basophils, and on human skin Langerhans cells.[9] Cross-linking of high-affinity receptor bound IgE by allergen results in the release of mediators from mast cells and basophils. Molecular biologic techniques have been used to clone the gene encoding the ε chain of human IgE (ND).[10] Several recombinant fragments of the ε chain have been used as a probe to localize the ε chain site that binds to the FcεR1 receptor.[11] This site has been localized mainly to the Cε2 and part of the Cε3 heavy chain domains.[12] The high-affinity receptor for IgE is composed of an alpha chain, beta chain, and two gamma chains, and it is the alpha chain that binds IgE[13] (see Fig.2-1*B*). The beta and gamma chains are involved in signal transduction when the receptors are aggregated by the cross-linking of IgE, resulting in mediator release.

TABLE 2-1. *Immunoglobulin isotypes*

Isotype	No. of C$_H$ domains	Additional components	Percentage of serum Ig	Approximate half-life (d)	Functions
IgA					
Monomer*	3	J chain	13–19	6	Provides antibodies for external body fluids, including mucus, saliva, and tears; effective at neutralizing infectious agents, agglutination, and (when bound to antigen) activation of the alternative complement pathway
Dimer†	3	Secretory piece	0.3		
IgD					
Monomer*†	3		<1	3	Almost entirely found in membrane-bound form; the function is unknown, but may be related to maturational stages
IgE					
Monomer*†	4		<0.001	3	IgE is bound to mast cell surfaces; subsequent binding of antigen stimulates mast cell degranulation, leading to immediat hyper-sensitivity responses (allergy)
IgG					
Monomer*†	3		72–80	20	Found in four subclasses IgG1, IgG2, IgG3, and IgG4. Prevalent isotype in secondary responses
IgM					
Monomer*	4		—	5–10	Prevalent isotype in primary responses; effective at agglutination and activation of classical complement pathway
Pentamer†	4	J chain	6–8		

*Membrane-bound form.
†Secreted form.

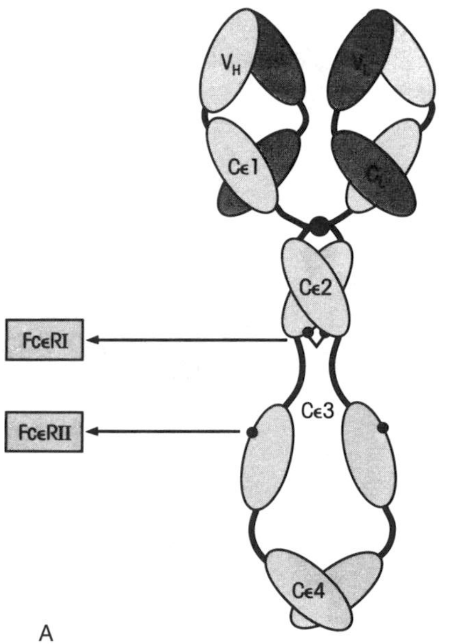

V_H
V_L
Cϵ1
C_L
Cϵ2
Cϵ3
Cϵ4
FcϵRI
FcϵRII

A

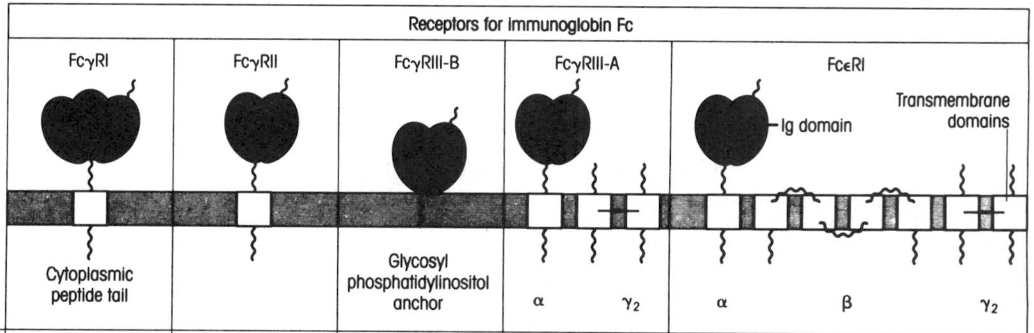

Receptors for immunoglobin Fc
FcγRI
FcγRII
FcγRIII-B
FcγRIII-A
FcϵRI
Ig domain
Transmembrane domains
Cytoplasmic peptide tail
Glycosyl phosphatidylinositol anchor
α
γ2
α
β
γ2

	FcγRI	FcγRII	FcγRIII-B	FcγRIII-A	FcϵRI
Affinity (M^{-1})	hi 10^9	lo<10^7	lo<10^7	lo<10^7	v.hi 10^{10}
Bind monomeric IgG	++	–	–	–	–
Bind aggregated IgG	+++	++	++	++	–
Bind monomeric IgE	–	–	–	–	+++
Present on:					
Monocycles	+	+	–	+*i*	–
Macrophages	+	+	–	+	–
Neutrophils	+*i*	+	+	–	–
NK cells	–	–	–	+	–
B cells	–	+	–	–	–
Mast cells	–	?	?	?	+

B

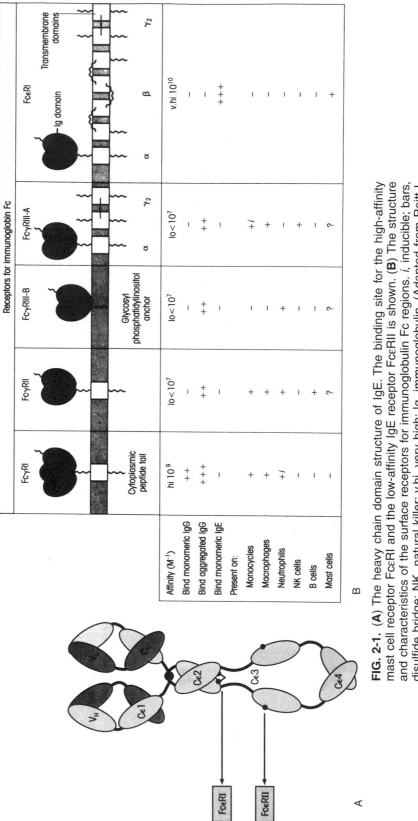

FIG. 2-1. (**A**) The heavy chain domain structure of IgE. The binding site for the high-affinity mast cell receptor FcεRI and the low-affinity IgE receptor FcεRII is shown. (**B**) The structure and characteristics of the surface receptors for immunoglobulin Fc regions. *i*, inducible; bars, disulfide bridge; NK, natural killer; v.hi, very high; Ig, immunoglobulin. (Adapted from Roitt I. Essential immunology. 8th ed. Oxford: Blackwell Scientific Publications, 1994:57, 61.)

A low-affinity FcεR2 receptor (CD23) has been localized to B lymphocytes, monocytes and macrophages, and platelets and eosinophils. The receptor has an A form found only on B lymphocytes and a B form found on all cells expressing CD23. The expression of this receptor is markedly up-regulated on all cell types by interleukin (IL)-4. Binding of IgE to this receptor places IgE at the center of activation of many important effector cells.[14] The FcεR2 receptor is cleaved into soluble products that retain the ability to bind IgE and have a role in the regulation of IgE synthesis. The natural ligand for CD23 has been found to be CD21, a receptor for Epstein-Barr virus and a complement receptor found on T cells, dendritic cells, and B cells, which may be responsible for cell–cell interactions.[15]

Sites of IgE Production, Turnover, and Tissue Localization

With the advent of a highly specific reagent for detecting IgE, antibody against the Fc portion of IgE (anti-IgE), the sites of production of this immunoglobulin could be examined by fluorescent-labeled anti-IgE. It was found that lymphoid tissue of the tonsils, adenoids, and the bronchial and peritoneal areas contained IgE-forming plasma cells. In contrast, IgE-forming plasma cells were sparse in the spleen and subcutaneous lymph nodes. IgE-forming plasma cells also were found in the respiratory and intestinal mucosa.[16] This distribution is similar to that of IgA. However, unlike IgA, IgE is not associated with a secretory piece, although IgE is found in respiratory and intestinal secretions. The traffic of IgE molecules from areas of production to the tissues and the circulation has not been established. Areas of production in the respiratory and intestinal mucosa are associated with the presence of tissue mast cells.[17]

With the development of techniques to measure total IgE in the blood and the availability of purified IgE protein, investigators were able to study the metabolic properties of this immunoglobulin in normal persons.[18] The mean total circulating IgE pool was found to be 3.3 μg per kg of body weight, in contrasted to the total circulating IgG pool of approximately 500,000 μg per kg of body weight. IgE has an intravascular half-life of only 2.3 days. The rate of IgE production was found to be 2.3 μg/kg/day.

It had been known for several years that the half-life of reaginic antibody in human skin as determined by passive transfer studies was approximately 14 days. This was reconfirmed with studies that investigated the disappearance of radiolabeled IgE in human skin. The half-life in the skin was found to be between 8 and 14 days.[6] The basophil and mast cell–bound IgE pool needs to be investigated thoroughly, but it has been estimated that only 1% of the total IgE is cell bound. Direct quantification of specific IgE in the blood, in contrast to specific IgE on the basophil surface, indicates that for every IgE molecule on the basophil, there are 100 to 4000 molecules in circulation.[19]

Regulation of IgE Production

Major advances in the understanding of IgE synthesis have risen from human and animal studies.[20–25] Tada[20] studied the production of IgE antibody in rats and found that IgE antibody production is regulated by cooperation between T lymphocytes (T cells) and B lymphocytes (B cells). The T cells provide the helper function, and the B cells are the producers of IgE antibody. Tada[20] also demonstrated that interventions that decrease T-cell activity may result in prolongation and enhancement of IgE formation.

In human systems, it became clear that IgE production from B cells required T-cell signals that were unique to the IgE system.[21] In 1986, Coffman and Carty[22] defined the essential role of IL-4 in the production of IgE. The pathway to IgE production is complex, requiring not only IL-4 but T- and B-cell contact, MHC complex restriction, adhesion molecules, expression of FcεR2 receptors, and the terminal action of IL-5 and IL-6.[23]

IL-4 acts on precursor B lymphocytes and is involved in the class switch to gamma (ε) heavy chain production.[24] IL-4 is not sufficient by itself to complete the switch to epsilon messenger RNA, and several second signals have been described that result in productive messenger RNA transcripts.[25,26] A key physiologic second signal is provided by CD4+ T-helper cell contact. This contact signal is provided by CD40 ligand on activated T cells, which interacts with the CD40 receptor on IL-4 primed B cells and completes isotype switching to IgE.[24]

Another cytokine, interferon gamma (IFN-γ) suppresses IgE production acting at the same point as IL-4. IFN-γ–secreting T cells (Th1 cells) are responsible for IgE suppression, and IL-4–secreting T cells (Th2 cells) are responsible for inducing IgE synthesis.[24]

In addition, several cytokines (IFN-α, transforming growth factor B, IL-8, IL-12) have been reported to suppress IgE synthesis.[23] This complex set of interactions is shown in Figure 2-2. During terminal differentiation of IgE B cells to plasma cells producing IgE, IgE binding factors have been described that either enhance or suppress IgE synthesis.[27] In addition, soluble fragments of the FcεR2 receptor (CD23) may enhance IgE production.[15]

During the secondary IgE response to allergen, allergen-specific B-lymphocytes capture allergen by surface IgE, internalize and degrade it, and present it to T cells as peptides complexed to MHC class II molecules. This leads to T cell–B cell interaction, mutual exchange of cytokine and cell contact signals, and enhanced allergen-specific IgE production.

THE ROLE OF IgE IN HEALTH AND DISEASE

The fetus is capable of producing IgE by 11 weeks' gestation. Johansson and Foucard[28] measured total IgE in sera from children and adults. They found that cord serum contained 13 to 202 ng/mL, and that the concentration of IgE in the cord serum did not correlate with the serum IgE concentration of the mother, which confirmed that IgE does not cross the placenta. In children, IgE levels increase steadily and peak between 10 and 15 years of age. Johansson

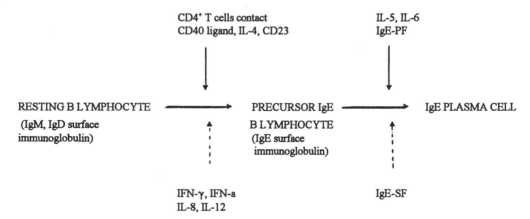

FIG. 2-2. Factors influencing B-lymphocyte differentiation to IgE-forming plasma cells. CD23, soluble FcεR2 receptor; PF, potentiating factor; SF, suppressor factor; IL, interleukin; dashed lines, inhibition. (Adapted from Leung YM. Mechanisms of the human allergic response: clinical implications. Pediatr Clin North Am 1994;41:727; and Ishizaka K. Regulation of the IgE antibody response. Int Arch Allergy Appl Immunol 1989;88:8.)

and Foucard illustrate well the selection of population groups for determining the normal level of serum IgE. Studies of healthy Swedish and Ethiopian children showed a marked difference in mean IgE levels: Swedish children had a mean of 160 ng/mL, and Ethiopian children had a mean of 860 ng/mL.[29] Barbee and coworkers[30] studied the IgE levels in atopic and nonatopic persons aged from 6 to 75 years in Tucson. IgE levels peaked in persons aged 6 to 14 years and gradually declined with advancing age; male subjects had higher levels of IgE than female subjects (Fig. 2-3).

Several roles for the possible beneficial effect of IgE antibody have been postulated. The presence of IgE antibody on mast cells in the tissues that contain heparin and histamine points to a role for IgE in controlling the microcirculation, and a role for the mast cell as a "sentinel" or first line of defense against microorganisms has been advanced. The hypothesis is that IgE antibody specific for bacterial or viral antigens could have a part in localizing high concentrations of protective antibody at the site of tissue invasion.[31,32]

The role of IgE antibody has been studied extensively in an experimental infection of rats with the parasite *Nippostrongylus brasiliensis*. IgE antibody on the surface of mast cells in the gut may be responsible for triggering histamine release and helping the animal to reduce the worm burden.[33] In experimental *Schistosoma mansoni* infection in the rat, IgE is produced at high levels to schistosome antigens. IgE complexed to these antigens has a role in antibody-dependent cell-mediated cytotoxicity, whereas eosinophils, macrophages, and platelets are effector cells that damage the parasite.[34] IgE and IgE immune complexes are bound to these effector cells by the IgE FcεR2 receptor, which has a high affinity for IgE immune complexes. Effector cells triggered by FcεR2 receptor aggregation result in release of oxygen metabolites, lysosomal enzymes, leukotrienes, and platelet-activating factor. These observations in animals have relevance to human populations, where the IgE inflammatory cascade may protect against helminth infections.[34]

IgE in Disease

Several early studies evaluated the role of IgE in patients with a variety of allergic diseases.[28] Adults and children with allergic rhinitis and extrinsic asthma tend to have higher total serum IgE levels. Approximately 50% of such patients have total IgE levels that are two standard deviations above the mean of a normal control group. Significant overlap of total serum IgE levels in normal persons and in patients with extrinsic asthma and hay fever has been demonstrated. Therefore, the total serum IgE level is not a specific or sensitive diagnostic test for the presence of these disorders.

Total serum IgE has been found to be markedly elevated in atopic dermatitis, with the serum IgE level correlating with the severity of the eczema and with the presence of allergic rhinitis, asthma, or both. Patients with atopic dermatitis without severe skin disease or accompanying asthma or hay fever may have normal IgE levels (Fig. 2-4). Total IgE levels have been found to be markedly elevated in allergic bronchopulmonary aspergillosis.

The expression of the atopic state is dependent on genes that control both total IgE production and specific IgE responsiveness to environmental allergens. High serum IgE levels have been shown to be under the control of a recessive gene, and specific allergen responses are associated with HLA antigens.[35,36] The chromosomal location and identification of these genes are under intense investigation but currently are uncertain.[36]

Extensive evidence has accumulated that may define the underlying immunologic basis for the atopic phenotype, that is, individuals with extrinsic asthma, allergic rhinitis, and atopic eczema.[24] The reciprocal action of IL-4 and IFN-γ on IgE production led to several studies on

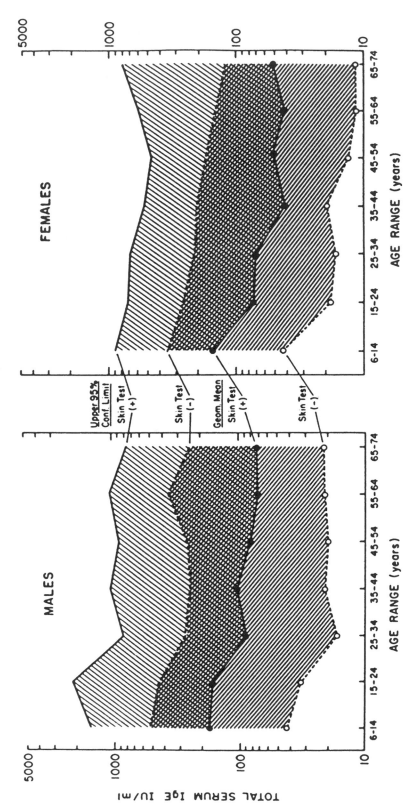

FIG. 2-3. Serum IgE as function of age and sex among whites in the United States. Geometric means and upper 95% confidence intervals are plotted against age for males and females with positive and negative results from skin tests. Double cross-hatched area represents overlap of total IgE levels between the two groups of subjects. Age-related declines in serum IgE are significant in all groups. (Knauer KA, Adkinson NF. Clinical significance of IgE. In: Middleton E, Reed CE, Ellis EJ, eds. Allergy principles and practice. St Louis: CV Mosby, 1983.)

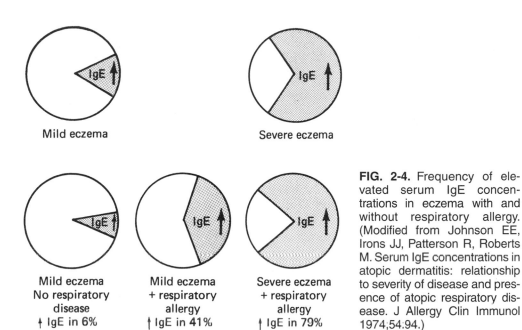

FIG. 2-4. Frequency of elevated serum IgE concentrations in eczema with and without respiratory allergy. (Modified from Johnson EE, Irons JJ, Patterson R, Roberts M. Serum IgE concentrations in atopic dermatitis: relationship to severity of disease and presence of atopic respiratory disease. J Allergy Clin Immunol 1974;54:94.)

the T-cell origin of these cytokines. Mosmann and Coffman[37] described two distinct types of T helper cells in murine systems and defined them as Th1 or Th2 cells by the pattern of cytokine secretion. Th1 cells produced IL-2, IFN-γ, and lymphotoxin. Th2 cells produced IL-4, IL-5, IL-6, and IL-10. A significant body of evidence has defined the role of Th2 cells in the human atopic state related to IL-4 production, IgE synthesis, and the maturation and recruitment of eosinophils by IL-5 and the maturation of IgE B cells by IL-5 and IL-6.[37] T cells having the Th2 cytokine profile have been cloned from individuals with a variety of atopic diseases,[24] have been identified in the airway of atopic asthmatics, and have been implicated as fundamental to persistent airway inflammation in asthma.[38–40]

Once a Th2 response is established, there is down-regulation of Th1 cells by the cytokines IL-4 and IL-10. Th1 cells are capable of down-regulating Th2 cytokine secretion through the reciprocal action of IFN-γ on Th2 cells, a physiologic control that is abrogated by the predominant Th2 cell response in the atopic state.

The recent observation that mast cells and basophils produce IL-4, leading to IgE synthesis,[23] adds an additional amplification loop that maintains the atopic state with continued exposure to allergen, leading to mast cell and basophil activation and mediator and cytokine release with enhanced and sustained IgE production.

Studies of the interaction of histamine releasing factor (HRF) and human basophil histamine release discovered that there may be two kinds of IgE: IgE that reacts with HRF (IgE+) and IgE that does not (IgE–).[41] The amino acid sequence of this HRF has been determined.[42] These observations may add to the role of IgE in several diseases where no definable allergen is present.

Measurement of Specific IgE

Since the discovery of IgE in 1967, it is not only possible to measure total IgE in the serum but also to measure IgE antibody against complex as well as purified allergens. One of the first methods described by Wide and coworkers[43] was the radioallergosorbent test (RAST). Allergen is covalently linked to solid-phase particles, and these solid-phase particles are incubated with the patient's serum, which may contain IgE antibody specific for that allergen. After a period of incubation, the specific IgE present binds firmly to the solid phase. The solid phase then is washed extensively, and the last reagent added is radiolabeled anti-IgE antibody. The bound anti-IgE reflect amounts of specific IgE bound to the allergen. The results usually are given in RAST units or in units where a standard serum containing significant amounts of IgE specific for a particular allergen is used as a reference.

Specific IgE antibody detected by RAST in the serum of patients whose skin test results are positive to an allergen have been shown to cover a wide range. From 100-fold to 1000-fold differences in RAST levels against a specific allergen are found in skin-reactive individuals. In studies of large groups of patients, there is a significant correlation between the RAST result, specific IgE level, and skin test reactivity. However, individuals with the same level of specific IgE antibody to ragweed allergen may vary 100-fold in their skin reactivity to that allergen.[44]

The IgE antibody, as measured by RAST, has been shown to correlate with bronchial challenge, endpoint skin test titrations, and symptom scores for a variety of allergens. For most of the allergens studied, a reasonably good overall correlation between RAST levels and these other measures of reactivity has been found. However, in a given person, the RAST level does not predict a patient's sensitivity because these measures of sensitivity vary widely for any given RAST level.

The RAST concept has been extended to the use of fluorescent- and enzyme-labeled anti-IgE, which obviates the need for radiolabeled materials.

It is possible to estimate the absolute quantity of specific IgE antibody per milliliter of serum against complex and purified allergens.[45,46] Using one of these methods to measure IgE antibody against ragweed allergens, Gleich and coworkers[45] defined the natural rise and fall of ragweed-specific IgE over a 1-year period. In this population of ragweed-sensitive individuals, the IgE antibody specific for ragweed allergens varied from 10 to 1000 ng/mL. A marked rise of specific IgE level occurred after the pollen season, with a peak in October followed by a gradual decrease. Specific IgE level reached a low point just before the next ragweed season in August (Fig. 2-5).

It is possible to measure basophil-bound, total, and specific IgE against ragweed antigen E. There are between 100,000 and 500,000 molecules of total IgE per basophil,[47] and between 2500 and 50,000 molecules of specific IgE per basophil.[19]

Although RAST and other specific IgE measurement technologies have clarified the relationships between specific IgE in the serum and patients' clinical sensitivity, these tests do not replace skin testing with the allergens in clinical practice.

OTHER HYPERSENSITIVITY STATES

All immunologically mediated hypersensitivity states had been classified into four types by Gell and Coombs in 1964. This classification has been a foundation for an understanding of the immunopathogenesis of clinical hypersensitivity syndromes.[48] This schema depends on the location and class of antibody that interacts with antigen resulting in effector cell activation and tissue injury.

In type I, or immediate hypersensitivity, allergen interacts with IgE antibody on the surface of mast cells and basophils, resulting in the cross-linking of IgE, FcεR1 receptor apposition, and mediator release from these cells. Only a few allergen molecules, interacting with

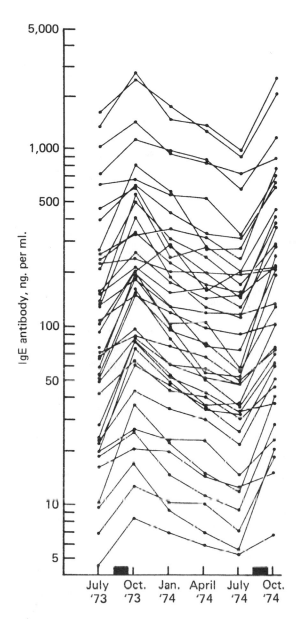

FIG. 2-5. Levels and changes of IgE antibodies to ragweed allergens in 40 untreated allergy patients. The ragweed pollination season is indicated by the black bar on the abscissa. (Gleich GJ, Jacob GL, Unginger JW, Henderson LL. Measurement of the absolute levels of IgE antibodies in patients with ragweed hay fever. J Allergy Clin Immunol 1977; 60:188.)

cell-bound IgE, lead to the release of many mediator molecules, resulting in a major biologic amplification of the allergen–IgE antibody reaction. Clinical examples include anaphylaxis, allergic rhinitis, and extrinsic asthma.

In type II, or cytotoxic injury, IgG or IgM antibody is directed against antigens on the individual's own tissue. Binding of antibody to the cell surface results in complement activation, which signals white blood cell influx and tissue injury.

In addition, cytotoxic killer lymphocytes, with Fc receptors for IgG, can bind to the tissue-bound IgG, resulting in antibody-dependent cellular cytotoxicity. Clinical examples include lung and kidney damage in Goodpasture's syndrome, acute graft rejection, hemolytic disease of the newborn, and certain bullous skin diseases.

In type III, or immune complex disease, IgG and IgM antigen–antibody complexes of a critical size are not cleared from the circulation and fix in small capillaries throughout the body. These complexes activate the complement system, which leads to the influx of inflammatory white blood cells, resulting in tissue damage. Clinical examples include serum sickness (after foreign proteins or drugs), lupus erythematosus, and glomerulonephritis after common infections.

In type IV, or delayed type hypersensitivity, the T-cell antigen receptor on Th1 lymphocytes binds to tissue antigens, resulting in clonal expansion of the lymphocyte population and T-cell activation with the release of inflammatory lymphokines. Clinical examples include contact dermatitis (e.g., poison ivy) and tuberculin hypersensitivity in tuberculosis and leprosy.

REFERENCES

1. Von Pirquet C. Allergie. Münch Med Wochenschr 1906;53:1457.
2. Prausnitz C, Küstner H. Studien über ueberempfindlichkeit. Centralbl. Bakteriol 1921;86:160.
3. Coca AF, Grove EF. Studies in hypersensitiveness. XIII. A study of atopic reagins. J Immunol 1925;10:444.
4. Stanworth DR. Reaginic antibodies. Adv Immunol 1963;3:181.
5. Sehon AH, Gyenes L. Antibodies in atopic patients and antibodies developed during treatment. In: Samter M, ed. Immunological diseases. 2nd ed. Boston: Little, Brown, 1971:785.
6. Ishizaka K, Ishizaka T. Immunology of IgE mediated hypersensitivity. In: Middleton E, Reed CE, Ellis EJ, eds. Allergy principles and practice. 2nd ed. St Louis: CV Mosby, 1983:52.
7. Bennich H, Ishizaka K, Ishizaka T, et al. Comparative antigenic study of E globulin and myeloma IgND. J Immunol 1969;102:826.
8. Bennich H, Johansson SGO. Structure and function of human immunoglobulin E. Adv Immunol 1971;13:1.
9. Wang B, Reiger A, Kigus O, et al. Epidermal Langerhans cells from normal human skin bind monomeric IgE via FceR1. J Exp Med 1992;175:1353.
10. Kenten JH, Molgaard HV, Hougton M, et al. Cloning and sequence determination of the gene for the human e chain expressed in a myeloma cell line. Proc Natl Acad Sci USA 1982;79:6661.
11. Geha RS, Helm B, Gould H. Inhibition of the Prausnitz- Küstner reaction by an immunoglobulin e-chain fragment synthesized in *E. coli*. Nature 1985;315:577.
12. Helm B, Marsh P, Vercelli D, et al. The mast cell binding site on human immunoglobulin E. Nature 1988;331:180.
13. Metzger H. The receptor with high affinity for IgE. Immunol Rev 1992;125:37.
14. Delespesse G, Sarfati M, Wu CY, Fournier S, Letellier M: The low-affinity receptor for IgE. Immunol Rev 1992;125:77.
15. Bonnefoy J-Y, Pochon S, Aubry J-P, et al. A new pair of surface molecules involved in human IgE regulation. Immunol Today 1992;14:1.
16. Tada T, Ishizaka K: Distribution of gamma E-forming cells in lymphoid tissues of the human and monkey. J Immunol 1970;104:377.
17. Callerame ML, Londemi JJ, Ishizaka K, et al. Immunoglobulins in bronchial tissues from patients with asthma, with special reference to immunoglobulin E. J Allergy 1981;47:187.
18. Waldmann TM, Iio A, Ogawa M, et al. The metabolism of IgE: studies in normal individuals and in a patient with IgE myeloma. J Immunol 1976;117:1139.
19. Zeiss CR, Pruzansky JJ, Levitz D, et al. The quantitation of IgE antibody specific for ragweed antigen E on the basophil surface in patients with ragweed pollenosis. Immunology 1978;35:237.
20. Tada T. Regulation of reaginic antibody formation in animals. Prog Allergy 1975;19:122.
21. Lebman DA, Coffman RL. Interleukin-4 causes isotype switching to IgE in T cell–stimulated clonal B cell cultures. J Exp Med 1988;168:853.
22. Coffman RL, Carty J. A T-cell activity that enhances polyclonal IgE production and its inhibition by interferon-γ. J Immunol 1986;136:949.
23. Leung YM. Mechanisms of the human allergic response: clinical implications. Pediatr Clin North Am 1994;41:727.
24. Maggi E, Romagnani S. Role of T-cells and T-cell derived cytokines in the pathogenesis of allergic diseases. Ann N Y Acad Sci 1994;725:2.
25. Gauchat J-F, Lebman DA, Coffman RL, et al. Structure and expression of germline e transcripts in human B cells induced by interleukin-4 to switch to IgE production. J Exp Med 1990;172:463.
26. Vercelli D, Geha RS. Regulation of IgE synthesis: from the membrane to the genes. Springer Semin Immunopathol 1993;15:5.
27. Ishizaka K. Regulation of the IgE antibody response. Int Arch Allergy Appl Immunol 1989;88:8.
28. Johansson SGO, Foucard T. IgE in immunity and disease. In: Middleton E, Reed CE, Ellis EJ, eds. Allergy principles and practice. 1st ed. St Louis: CV Mosby, 1978:551.

29. Johansson SGO, Mellbin T, Vahlquist G. Immunoglobulin levels in Ethiopian preschool children with special reference to high concentrations of immunoglobulin E (IgND). Lancet 1968;1:1118.
30. Barbee RA, Halonen M, Lebowitz M, Burrows B: Distribution of IgE in a community population sample: correlation with age, sex, allergen skin test reactivity. J Allergy Clin Immunol 1981;68:106.
31. Lewis RA, Austen KF. Mediation of local homeostasis and inflammation by leukotrienes and other mast-cell dependent compounds. Nature 1981;293:103.
32. Steinberg P, Ishizaka K, Norman PS. Possible role of IgE-mediated reaction in immunity. J Allergy Clin Immunol 1974;54:359.
33. Dineen JK, Ogilvie BM, Kelly JD. Expulsion of *Nippostrongylus brasiliensis* from the intestine of rats: collaboration between humoral and cellular components of the immune response. Immunology 1973;24:467.
34. Dessaint JP, Capron A. IgE inflammatory cells: the cellular network in allergy. Int Arch Allergy Appl Immunol 1989;90:28.
35. Marsh DG, Huang S-K. Molecular genetics of human immune responsiveness to pollen allergens. Clin Exper Allergy 1991;21:168.
36. Blumenthal M. Searching for the asthma and allergy gene: the current status of our knowledge. ACI News 1995;7:15.
37. Mosmann TR, Coffman RL. Th1 and Th2 cells: different patterns of lymphokine secretion lead to different functional properties. Annu Rev Immunol 1989;7:145.
38. Wierenga EA, Snoek M, deGroot C, et al. Evidence for the compartmentalization of functional subsets of CD4$^+$ T lymphocytes in atopic patients. J Immunol 1990;144:4651.
39. Robinson DS, Hamid Q, Ying S, et al. Predominant Th2-like bronchoalveolar T-lymphocyte population in atopic asthma. N Engl J Med 1992;326:298.
40. Busse WW, Coffman RL, Gelfand EW, Kay AB, Rosenwasser LJ. Mechanisms of persistent airway inflammation in asthma: a role for T cells and T-cell products. Am J Respir Crit Care Med 1995;152:388.
41. MacDonald SM, Lichtenstein LM, Proud O, et al. Studies of IgE dependent histamine releasing factors: heterogenicity of IgE. J Immunol 1987;139:506.
42. MacDonald SM, Rafnar T, Langdon J, Lichtenstein LM. Molecular identification of an IgE-dependent histamine releasing factor. Science 1995;269:688.
43. Wide L, Bennich H, Johansson SGO. Diagnosis of allergy by an *in vitro* test for allergenic antibodies. Lancet 1967; 2:1105.
44. Norman P. Correlations of RAST and in vivo and in vitro assays. In: Evans R III, ed. Advances in diagnosis of allergy: RAST. Miami: Symposia Specialists, 1975:45.
45. Gleich GJ, Jacobs GL, Yunginger JW, et al. Measurement of the absolute levels of IgE antibodies in patients with ragweed hay fever: effect of immunotherapy on seasonal changes and relationship to IgG antibodies. J Allergy Clin Immunol 1978;60:188.
46. Zeiss CR, Pruzansky JJ, Patterson R, et al. A solid phase radioimmunoassay for the quantitation of human reaginic antibody against ragweed antigens. J Immunol 1973;110:414.
47. Conroy MC, Adkinson NF, Lichtenstein LM. Measurement of IgE on human basophils: relation to serum IgE and anti-IgE induced histamine release. J Immunol 1977;118:1317.
48. Roitt I. Hypersensitivity. In: Essential immunology. 8th ed. London: Blackwell Scientific Publications, 1994:313.

Allergic Diseases, 5th Edition,
edited by Roy Patterson, Leslie Carroll Grammer, and
Paul A. Greenberger. Lippincott–Raven Publishers, Philadelphia, © 1997.

3

Models of Asthma

Roy Patterson and Kathleen E. Harris

R. Patterson and K.E. Harris: Division of Allergy-Immunology, Northwestern University Medical School, Chicago, IL 60611-3008.

Pearls for Practitioners
Roy Patterson

- Naturally occurring allergy in several species of monkey simulates IgE-mediated allergy in humans.
- Allergy in individual monkeys (as in humans) varies in severity and duration of allergy, but persists for years in most primates.
- In my opinion, a cure for IgE-mediated allergy in monkeys will result in a cure for allergy in humans.
- Monkeys with asthma have hyperactive airways, like humans with asthma.
- Canine IgE sensitizes primate mast cells, but the reverse does not occur. Thus, the Fc portion of primate IgE fits the Fc receptor of canine mast cells, but the reverse does not fit.
- IgE-mediated allergy in dogs is manifested primarily by a highly pruritic dermatitis.
- Flea allergy in dogs is important. Sometimes the canine fleas affect humans, causing papular urticaria.

The theories and proposed mechanisms of common allergic diseases and asthma have evolved over the last century. Although various clinical manifestations of these diseases can be well controlled by immunologic management (i.e., allergen avoidance), pharmacotherapy, or both, the basic abnormalities of many clinical diseases classified as allergic diseases are not understood. Among the latter are asthma, non-IgE–mediated chronic rhinitis, idiopathic urticaria, idiopathic angioedema, and idiopathic anaphylaxis. This chapter broadly covers the history and evolution of major theories and in vitro and in vivo models thought to duplicate features of human allergic diseases. These models can be used to explain mechanisms of allergic diseases, to confirm theories, or to demonstrate laboratory systems for evaluating pharmacologic therapies before use in humans.

Although IgE was not identified as the immunoglobulin responsible for immediate-type allergic reactions in humans until 1967 by the Ishizakas,[1] a significant understanding of the basis of allergic reactions had already developed. It was recognized that allergic antibody was different from the major protective antibody (subsequently identified as IgG), that it resulted in histamine release, and that it had various distinct and well-defined physical and chemical properties such as heat lability at 56°C. Allergen injection therapy had been known to reduce the severity of allergic rhinitis since the early decades of this century, and this appeared to result from the production of a different form of antibody, a protective antibody, which was termed *blocking antibody*.[2] This background information thus was already available when IgE was discovered,[1] and a more complete understanding of allergic rhinitis, allergic conjunctivitis, and human anaphylaxis rapidly began to unfold.

The disease known as asthma has been more difficult to analyze and may even constitute more than one disease. Characterized clinically as intermittent wheezing, physiologically as reversible obstructive airway disease, and pharmacologically as being responsive to beta agonists, the basic abnormality in asthma remains unknown. Thus, although asthma has been known as a disease for thousands of years (referred to in the Papyrus of Ebers and the Talmud[3]) and is well managed by modern pharmacotherapy, no single, unifying pathophysiologic mechanism has been identified.

Recently, the concept of asthma being an inflammatory disease of the airways for many patients has received major attention. The efficacy of corticosteroids in controlling asthma was established over three decades ago. Topical inhaled corticosteroids are front-line therapy for most cases of chronic asthma, and the logical explanation for this therapeutic success is controlling airway inflammation.

Because of the lack of complete understanding of asthma and the absence of asthma as a defined, naturally occurring state in animals, the animal models used may only mimic certain features of asthma with varying degrees of relevance to human disease. The types of models available for study are reviewed here with emphasis on which component of human asthma the model appears to simulate best.

ANIMAL MODELS OF ACUTE ASTHMA

Acute allergic asthma in humans is the abrupt onset of wheezing dyspnea subsequent to the environmental exposure to inhaled proteins such as animal dander. Pulmonary function studies demonstrate acute obstruction to airflow, particularly during expiration. This bronchospastic type of response can be simulated in a variety of laboratory animals sensitized by immunization, either systemically or by aerosol with heterologous proteins. Systemic challenge with the foreign protein after sensitization results in anaphylaxis, or, if the protein is aerosolized, bronchospasm. In the latter case, certain features of asthma are mimicked. The inhaled protein, acting as an antigen, reacts with IgE or analogous antibody bound to receptors on mast cells and releases a variety of bronchoactive substances synthesized or stored in these cells. The result is allergen-induced bronchospasm or airway anaphylaxis that can be induced in such species as guinea pigs,[4,5] rats,[6] and dogs.[7] Such airway responses may be simulated by mast cell–derived products such as aerosolized histamine,[8] leukotriene (LT) D_4,[9] prostaglandin (PG) $F_{2\alpha}$,[10] PGD_2, acetylcholine,[8] and bradykinin.[11] Smooth muscle from such animals studied in vitro contracts when stimulated by antigen or the agonists just listed. Such in vivo or in vitro models may be used to study compounds capable of inhibiting antigen-induced mast cell degranulation or compounds (termed *receptor antagonists*) that block the action of released mediators at the level of the bronchial smooth muscle. These models have significant potential for studying selected agonists, but there may be marked limitations when extrapolated to human asthma. This is most clearly exemplified by H_1-receptor histamine antagonists. Compounds of this class block the effect of histamine—released from mast cells by antigen—on isolated guinea pig airways and also block antigen-induced airway responses in guinea pigs. However, H_1-receptor histamine antagonists have, with rare exception, no therapeutic effect in human asthma. In summary, acute antigen-induced bronchospasm in purposefully sensitized laboratory animals may be valuable in pharmacologic study but offers limited applicability to human asthma.

ATOPY IN ANIMALS

The atopic state in humans has been variously defined by different investigators. The most restrictive definition is the presence of an atopic disease (allergic rhinitis, allergic asthma, atopic dermatitis), significant eosinophilia, and IgE antibody against various inhalant and food allergens. The least restrictive definition is the presence of IgE antibody against one allergen demonstrated by immediate-type skin test. Using the range of these two definitions, the incidence rate of atopy in a human population varies from about 10% to 40% of the population (using the most to the least restrictive definition, respectively). Thus, evaluating the research related to the state of "atopy" in humans must include evaluating the definition of atopy used by each investigator.

When evaluating the occurrence of atopy in animals, the most restrictive definition should be used, that is, that of IgE antibody to the antigen and clinical disease related to environmental exposure. Using that restricted definition, the only species other than humans in which the atopic state exists is the dog. The major clinical manifestation in dogs, as a result of environmental exposure, is a highly pruritic, seasonal eczema occasionally associated with allergic rhinitis and conjunctivitis.[12] The immunoreactant is the canine analogue of IgE, and immediate-type local cutaneous reactions are seen with appropriate intradermal allergen skin tests. Serum from such dogs passively sensitizes normal dog skin or bronchi.[13] These allergic dogs respond with bronchospasm to an aerosolized allergen challenge with the appropriate antigen and have been used as a model of allergic asthma.[14] This model is limited because few allergic dogs are available. Although this allergic disease in dogs is not rare, these animals are valued pets and, thus, rarely are available for laboratory study. An inbred strain of dogs with IgE-mediated allergy has not been developed despite at least two attempts. A more readily available IgE-mediated response in dogs is the one in which a roundworm intestinal parasite *Ascaris suum*[15] is used as the antigen. Since most dogs have been infected with parasites during early life, including *Ascaris* sp, they have either high serum levels of IgE antibody or, if serum levels to this antibody are low, they often can be boosted by reexposure, such as by aerosol challenge with *Ascaris* antigen. Thus, a large animal model of an IgE-mediated bronchospastic response is readily available. The model has several limitations, including the high degree of variability in airway responses, even in the same animal after successive airway challenges. The predictability of pharmacologic agents capable of blocking airway responses in this model has limited application to humans.

Sheep also demonstrate IgE-mediated responses to *Ascaris* antigen and have been relied on heavily as a model for various IgE-triggered respiratory studies.[16] This model is about equally valuable as the dog model in laboratory research.

THEORIES OF ASTHMA AND ANIMAL MODELS

Asthma as a Psychosomatic Illness

The theory of the early 1900s that asthma had a psychological origin has been discarded for lack of documentation. Stress exacerbates the problems associated with any chronic disease, including asthma. Investigators studying asthma do not accept that psychological features are the basic cause of this disease. Evaluating this theory in an animal model has never been possible.

Asthma as a Neurogenic Disease

A theory popularized in the middle 1900s proposed that the abnormalities associated with asthma, such as increased mucous production and bronchospasm, were the result of abnormalities of the parasympathetic nervous system. Major investigational efforts studied the hypothesis that asthma was mediated by hyperactivity of cholinergic innervation of the airways.[17] Certain vagal stimulation of animals could simulate abnormalities suggestive of asthma. Analogues of acetylcholine simulate features of asthma in animals and humans, and antagonists of acetylcholine were evaluated for effectiveness in controlling asthma. Clinical application of such therapy has little benefit for controlling asthma for most patients; thus, animal research in this area recently has decreased, and the vagal mediation theory of asthma has been deemphasized.

Similarly, the beta adrenergic receptor blockade theory of asthma of Szentivanyi[18] postulated that asthma and other atopic diseases result from a defect in the beta adrenergic receptors that mediate epinephrine or norepinephrine-induced relaxation of airway smooth muscle. This was not substantiated by laboratory animal research, and the widespread use of pharmacologic beta adrenergic receptor blockers without a significant concomitant problem with induction or potentiation of asthma prevents this theory from being a major consideration.

"Infectious" Asthma

The infectious asthma approach does not postulate that asthma is the result of specific transmissible bacteria, but rather that a form of allergy occurs in patients with nonallergic asthma. The theory was based on the concept that all asthma is the result of immunologic hypersensitivity reactions. In the absence of other inhalant allergens and because of frequent exacerbations of asthma after respiratory infections, patients were presumed to have an allergic reaction to bacteria growing in their airway secretions. This resulted in prolonged clinical attempts to "desensitize" patients by injection of sterile-killed preparations of common bacterial organisms cultured from the respiratory tract during asthma exacerbations. Although the exacerbation of asthma clearly is associated with respiratory infections (usually viral), the absence of evidence for this mechanism in humans or animals led to a decline in interest in the theory and in "bacterial vaccine" injection therapy. The importance of virally induced exacerbation in humans clearly is evident, but animal models are only beginning to be developed in this area.

Mast Cells and Bioactive Mediators

The scientifically accepted mechanism of allergic rhinitis is that IgE-sensitized mast cells are triggered by allergens absorbed through the nasal mucosa. This results in mast cell activation and degranulation releasing a variety of potent bioactive mediators. Extension of this concept explains food anaphylaxis (e.g., caused by peanuts) and IgE-mediated drug anaphylaxis (e.g., caused by penicillin injection).[19] In these anaphylaxis examples, the food or drug allergen is absorbed through the gastrointestinal mucosa and combines with serum proteins, giving rise to IgE antibody production, which results in activation of widely disbursed mast cells and anaphylaxis.

The release of mast cell–bioactive mediators by allergen has been the major theory for explaining the basic abnormality of asthma. Supporting this theory are the clearly defined cases of inhalant, IgE-mediated allergic asthma (animal dander, mold spores, trimellitic anhydride); the control of such patients by avoiding the allergen; and the pharmacologic control by mast cell "stabilizers" such as sodium cromolyn. The fact that IgE-triggered asthma differs pharmacologically from allergic rhinitis is clear from the absence of the significant effect of H_1-receptor histamine antagonists in asthma, in contrast to their apparent efficacy in allergic rhinitis. In the early 1950s, recognition that histamine played a less significant role in asthma than in rhinitis led to a search for other bioactive mediators. Leading contestants included a chemically undefined material termed *slow reacting substance of anaphylaxis*,[20] which was subsequently renamed *leukotrienes* when the structure was determined. LTD_4 and LTE_4 are considered to be the major agonists in human asthma. Studying the origin and biosynthetic pathways of these mediators has defined the products of arachidonic acid metabolism through the lipoxygenase and cyclooxygenase pathways.[21] Several of the products of the lipoxygenase pathway (LTB_4, LTC_4, and LTD_4) and the cyclooxygenase pathway (thromboxane, PGD_2) may be major bioactive mediators responsible for asthma. Other bioactive substances that have generated interest include platelet-activating factor (PAF)[22] and bradykinin.[23] Receptor antagonists have been generated, and enzyme inhibition is in various stages of development for several of these mediators. Whether any of these will alter the management of asthma depends not only on the appropriate prelicensing clinical trials, but also on extensive use in the clinical setting. Guidelines of optimal therapeutic goals for new pharmacologic approaches to asthma are listed in Table 3-1.

The Sensory Nerve Fiber Theory of Asthma

One of the newer theories for this old disease is that the airway smooth muscle may be altered by the overactivity of the so-called nonadrenergic noncholinergic excitatory (NANCe) nervous system.[24] The airways of most mammalian species, including humans, are innervated by four distinct nervous systems, each of which releases a distinct neurotransmitter. These systems, along with their neurotransmitters, are as follows: (1) parasympathetic (acetylcholine);

TABLE 3-1. *Spectrum of pharmacologic actions desirable for controlling asthma*

Correction of the Presumed Basic Abnormalities of Asthma

Reduce the hyperactive airway to normal reactivity

Control the inflammation of the airway

Prevent bronchospasm

Prevent allergen-induced asthma

Prevent nocturnal asthma

Clinical Therapeutic Goals

Prevent (or reverse) asthma from exercise, cold air, allergens, and infections

Be as effective as corticosteroids with no corticosteroid side effects

Pharmacotherapeutic Goals

Preventive therapy is better than symptomatic treatment

Optimal compliance is essential; this is best achieved by the following:

Limited no. of medications, especially in pediatric, adolescent, and geriatric patients

Limited no. of doses of medication

Absence of side effects

Once daily dosing

(2) sympathetic (norepinephrine); (3) nonadrenergic noncholinergic inhibitory (vasoactive intestinal polypeptide *or* peptide histidine methionine *or* peptide histidine isoleucine); and (4) nonadrenergic noncholinergic excitatory (neurokinin A, substance P, calcitonin gene related peptide). The last two "peptidergic systems" were discovered relatively recently, and an understanding of their roles in asthma remains to be determined. Regarding the NANCe system, one hypothesis postulates that these nerves contribute to airway hyperresponsiveness— a phenomenon that is widely believed to underpin asthma (both allergic and nonallergic).

These hypotheses are complex and difficult to apply to humans with asthma. Applying them to the study of animal models of asthma has been just as difficult because of the limitations of these animal models. Currently, interest is declining in the potential applicability of these hypotheses of neurogenic asthma to either animal models or human asthma.

THE PRIMATE MODEL OF ASTHMA

The endpoint analysis of both theory and pharmacologic control of asthma depends on the clinical use and clear demonstration of the successful control of patients' illness in the varying spectrum of severity of human asthma.

In drug development, the centimillions of dollars required for basic research and the clinical trials before final marketability would best be studied in an animal model for possible prediction of therapeutic effectiveness. Perhaps the best animal model for studying certain features of asthma—both in theory and for evaluating potential pharmacologic agents—is the rhesus monkey model of asthma. This model is briefly summarized here.

About 20% of adult *Macaca mulatta* rhesus monkeys have naturally occurring IgE antibody against *Ascaris* antigen (using *Ascaris suum* as a source), presumably as a residual of infection with *Ascaris* in the wild. About 5% of monkeys with IgE antibody have acute asthma–type airway responses to airway challenge with *Ascaris* antigen and, thus, approximately 1% of the monkey population have IgE antibody and asthma-type responses, an incidence rate similar to the human population.[25] These allergic monkeys are a primary model of allergic human asthma.

As in humans, the IgE antibody and the airway responsiveness have a long duration (years) but may disappear spontaneously. The animals with antigen airway reactivity also demonstrate airway hyperresponsiveness to histamine[26] and analogues of acetylcholine and $PGF_{2\alpha}$.[27] This airway hyperresponsiveness is not present in animals with IgE antibody but no antigen airway reactivity, but may be seen in some monkeys with no IgE antibody (as in human asthma unrelated to IgE-mediated allergy). These animals have bronchial lumen mast cells that respond with histamine release to antigen challenge.[28] Their airway responses to $PGF_{2\alpha}$,[29] PGE_1,[30] PGD_2,[31] LTD_4,[32] and PAF[33] and their use in analysis of receptor antagonists of LTD_4 and PAF[34–36] have been studied. Although no naturally occurring clinical asthma has been reported in these animals in the wild or in zoos, we believe that it likely occurs, just as dogs with IgE antibody against environmental allergens have clinical dermatitis.

The potential use of this primate model extends from development of analytical models of the late phase asthmatic response, allergic and inflammatory reactions in the airway evaluated by bronchial alveolar lavage, the potential role of neurokinins in the asthmatic response, and induction of the hyperactive airway state in primates. A major positive and negative feature of this model is that individual monkeys (like humans) vary in the severity of the asthmatic response. Thus, longitudinal studies of individual animals offer great value, but grouping animals with marked variability in asthma offers a significant problem in interpreting results.

RECENT OBSERVATIONS

The following are the most recent observations on the colony of rhesus monkeys in the Allergy-Immunology Division at Northwestern University (Chicago). Cutaneous testing and airway challenge have reconfirmed the long duration of the presence of IgE antibody against *Ascaris* antigen.[37] This is present for years, but individual animals vary in degree of reactivity. Certain animals lose airway reactivity to antigen as they mature, which is similar to humans who "outgrow" asthma. Some animals have cutaneous reactivity without asthma, like many humans. Thus, the state of naturally occurring IgE antibody in rhesus monkeys is markedly similar to the human analogue.

A recent observation of major interest is that aerosolized substance P, followed by aerosolized *Ascaris* antigen, can induce asthma to antigen alone in animals that have lost the asthmatic response or in animals that had cutaneous reactivity but no airway response to antigen.[38]

The presence of allergy to house dust mites in the colony of monkeys has been documented and offers a major variation of this research model with this naturally occurring important environmental aeroallergen.[39]

Finally, an unexpected research result is that aerosolized substance P followed by aerosolized *Ascaris* allergen significantly reduced IgE antibody reactivity to *Ascaris* antigen.[40] Although it had already been recognized that neuromodulation of the immune system is a major new research area, the implications of extending this observation from allergic subhuman primates to the human allergic state illustrates the great potential for future research in atopic diseases.

REFERENCES

1. Ishizaka K, Ishizaka T, Terry WD. Antigenic structure of gamma E globulin and reaginic antibody. J Immunol 1967;99:849.
2. Cooke RA, Barnard JH, Hebald S, et al. Serologic evidence of immunity with coexisting sensitization in a type of human allergy (hayfever). Exp Med 1935;62:733.
3. Brothwell D, Sandison AT. Diseases in antiquity. Springfield, IL: Charles C Thomas, 1967;214, 492.
4. Feinberg SM, Malkiel S. Protective effect of cortisone on induced asthma in the guinea pig. Proc Soc Exp Biol Med 1952;81:104.
5. Wiestar MJ, Tepper JS, Weber MF, Menache MG. Histamine and methacholine aerosol bronchial challenge in awake guinea pigs. J Pharmacol Exp Ther 1990;253:27.
6. Carswell F, Oliver J. The respiratory response in sensitized rats to aerosol challenge. Immunology 1978;34:465.
7. Patterson R. Laboratory models of reaginic allergy. Prog Allergy 1969;13:332.
8. Krell RD, Chakrin LW, Christian P, Giannone E, McCoy J, Osborn R. Canine airway responses to acetylcholine, prostaglandin F$_{2\alpha}$, histamine, and serotonin after chronic antigen exposure. J Allergy Clin Immunol 1976;58:664.
9. Russi EW, Abraham WM, Chapman GA, Stevenson JS, Codias E, Wanner A. Effects of leukotriene D$_4$ on mucociliary and respiratory function in allergic and nonallergic sheep. J Appl Physiol 1985;59:1416.
10. Strandberg K, Hedquist P. Airway effects of slow reacting substance, prostaglandin F$_2$ alpha and histamine in the guinea pig. Acta Physiol Scand 1975;94:105.
11. Hogan MB, Harris KE, Patterson R. A bradykinin antagonist inhibits the early phase IgE mediated allergen induced airway response in primates (submitted for publication).
12. Patterson R. Investigations of spontaneous hypersensitivity in the dog. J Allergy 1960;31:351.
13. Patterson R, Sparks DB. The passive transfer to normal dogs of skin reactivity, asthma and anaphylaxis from a dog with spontaneous ragweed pollen hypersensitivity. J Immunol 1962;88:262.
14. Patterson R, Mellies CJ, Kelly JF, Harris KE. Airway responses of dogs with ragweed and ascaris hypersensitivity. Chest 1974;65:488.
15. Booth B, Patterson R, Talbot C. Immediate-type hypersensitivity in dogs: cutaneous, anaphylactic, and respiratory responses to *Ascaris*. J Lab Clin Med 1970;76:181.
16. Wanner A, Mezey RJ, Reinhart M, Eyre P. Antigen-induced bronchospasm in conscious sheep. J Appl Physiol 1979;47:917.
17. Gold WM. Vagally-mediated reflex bronchoconstriction in allergic asthma. Chest 1973;63(Suppl):11S.
18. Szentivanyi A. The beta-adrenergic theory of the atopic abnormality in bronchial asthma. J Allergy 1968;42:203.
19. Levine BB. Immunochemical mechanisms of drug allergy. Annu Rev Med 1966;17:23.

20. Orange RP, Austen WG, Austen KF. Immunological release of histamine and slow reacting substance of anaphylaxis from human lung. I. Modulation by agents influencing cellular levels of cyclic 3′,5′AMP. J Exp Med 1971;134:1368.
21. Samuelsson B. Leukotrienes: mediators of immediate hypersensitivity reactions and inflammation. Science 1983;220:568.
22. Barnes PJ, Chung KF, Page CP. Platelet activating factor as a mediator of allergic disease. J Allergy Clin Immunol 1988;81:919.
23. Proud D, Togias A, Naclerio RM, Crush SA, Norman PS, Lichtenstein LM. Kinins are generated *in vivo* following nasal airway challenge of allergic individuals with allergen. J Clin Invest 1983;72:1678.
24. Barnes PJ. Neural control of human airways in health and disease. Am Rev Respir Dis 1986;134:1289.
25. Patterson R, Kelly JF. Animal models of the asthmatic state. Annu Rev Med 1974;25:53.
26. Krell RD. Airway hyperreactivity to pharmacologic agents in rhesus monkeys cutaneously hypersensitive to *Ascaris* antigen. Life Sci 1976;19:1777.
27. Patterson R, Harris KE, Suszko IM, Roberts M. Reagin-mediated asthma in rhesus monkeys and relation to bronchial cell histamine release and airway reactivity to carbocholine. J Clin Invest 1976;57:586.
28. Patterson R, Ts'ao C, Suszko IM. Antigen-reactive, histamine-releasing cells in the bronchial lumens of three species. In: Bouhuys A, ed. Lung cells in disease. New York: Elsevier/North–Holland Biomedical Press, 1976:239.
29. Patterson R, Harris KE. The qualitative evaluation of airway responses to immunologic and pharmacologic stimuli in rhesus monkeys. J Allergy Clin Immunol 1978;61:261.
30. Patterson R, Harris KE. Effect of PGE_1 on immediate-type immunologic and pharmacologic respiratory responses of the rhesus monkey. J Lab Clin Med 1977;90:18.
31. Patterson R, Harris KE, Greenberger PG. Effect of prostaglandin D_2 and I_2 on the airways of rhesus monkeys. J Allergy Clin Immunol 1980;65:269.
32. Patterson R, Harris KE, Smith LJ, et al. Airway responses to leukotriene D_4 in rhesus monkeys. Int Arch Allergy Appl Immunol 1983;71:156.
33. Patterson R, Harris KE. Activity of aerosolized and intracutaneous synthetic platelet activating factor (AGEPC) in rhesus monkeys with IgE-mediated airway responses and normal monkeys. J Lab Clin Med 1983;102:933.
34. Patterson R, Harris KE, Krell RD. Effect of a leukotriene D_4 (LTD_4) antagonist on LTD_4 and *Ascaris* antigen-induced airway responses in rhesus monkeys. Int Arch Allergy Appl Immunol 1988;86:440.
35. Patterson R, Harris KE, Handley DA, Saunders RN. Evaluation of the effect of a platelet activating factor antagonist on platelet activating factor and ascaris antigen-induced airway responses in rhesus monkeys. J Lab Clin Med 1987;110:606.
36. Patterson R, Harris KE, Bernstein PR, Krell RD, Handley DA. Effects of combined receptor antagonists of leukotriene D_4 (LTD_4) and platelet-activating factor (PAF) on rhesus airway responses to LTD_4, PAF and antigen. Int Arch Allergy Appl Immunol 1989;88:462.
37. Patterson R, Harris KE. IgE mediated rhesus monkey asthma: natural history and individual animal variation. Int Arch Allergy Applied Immunol 1992;97:154.
38. Patterson R, Harris KE. Substance P and IgE mediated allergy. I. Transient increase in airway responsiveness to allergen in primates. Allergy Proc 1993;14:49.
39. Hogan MB, Harris KE, Patterson R. A naturally occurring model of immunoglobulin E antibody–mediated hypersensitivy in laboratory animals. J Lab Clin Med 1994;123:899.
40. Patterson R, Harris KE. Substance P and IgE mediated allergy. II. Reduction of rhesus IgE antibody following aerosol exposure to substance P and allergen. Allergy Proc 1993;14:53.

Allergic Diseases, 5th Edition,
edited by Roy Patterson, Leslie Carroll Grammer, and
Paul A. Greenberger. Lippincott–Raven Publishers, Philadelphia, © 1997.

4

Biochemical Mediators of Allergic Reactions

Stephen I. Wasserman

*S.I. Wasserman: Department of Medicine,
University of California San Diego Medical Center, San Diego, CA 92103*

Pearls for Practitioners
Roy Patterson

- The amount of IgE in a human approximates 1/10,000 of the IgG. The reason that IgE antibody in such small amounts causes severe local or potentially fatal anaphylactic reactions is the explosive magnification of the reaction by the biochemical mediators released in an IgE-mediated reaction.
- Idiopathic anaphylaxis, urticaria, and angioedema presumably are caused by the same biochemical mediators released in an IgE-mediated reaction. The difference is that internal factors such as histamine releasing factors or IgG anti IgE initiate the reaction rather than external allergens.

Recent research has expanded the understanding of the cells and mediators relevant to diseases of immediate-type hypersensitivity. The biologically active molecules responsible have been identified, and a thorough biochemical and structural elucidation of diverse lipid mediators has been accomplished. The activity of mediator-generating cells and their diverse products has been assigned a central role in both IgE-mediated acute and prolonged inflammatory events. This chapter places in perspective the mediator-generating cells, the mediators themselves, and these newer concepts of their roles in pathobiologic and homeostatic events.

MEDIATOR-GENERATING CELLS

Mast cells and basophilic polymorphonuclear leukocytes (basophils) constitute the two IgE-activated mediator-generating cells.[1] Mast cells are heterogeneous, and both connective tissue and mucosal types have been recognized[2] (Table 4-1). The latter predominate in the lamina propria of the gastrointestinal tract and in the peripheral airways and alveolar septa. Both occur in the upper airway and nose, and the connective tissue subtype dominates in the skin.[3]

Mast cells are richly distributed in the deeper region of the central nervous system, the upper and lower respiratory epithelium, the bronchial lumen, the gastrointestinal mucosa and submucosa, bone marrow, and skin.[4,5] They are especially prominent in bone, dense connective tissue adjacent to blood vessels (particularly small arterioles and venules), and peripheral

TABLE 4-1. *Human mast cell heterogeneity*

Characteristic	MC^T	MC^{TC}
Location	Lungs and gastrointestinal mucosa	Skin and gastrointestinal submucosa
Protease	Tryptase	Tryptase–chymase
Granule structure	Scrolls	Grating–lattices
Growth factor dependent	Yes	No
Formalin sensitivity	Yes	No
Proteoglycan	Heparin*	Heparin*
Secretogogue response (morphine, substance P, C5a, compound 48/80, f-met-peptide)	No	Yes
Temperature for degranulation	37°C	23–30°C
Migratory	Yes	No

MC^T, mast cell (mucosal type); MC^{TC}, mast cell (connective tissue type).
*Structurally different.
Adapted from Bernstein JA, Lawrence ID. The mast cell: a comprehensive, updated review. Allergy Proc 1990;11:209.

nerves. In the skin, the lungs, and gastrointestinal tract, mast cell concentrations approximate 10,000 to 20,000 cells/mm.[6] They develop from CD34+ bone marrow precursors through the action of stem cell factor (kit-ligand SCF), which binds to a specific receptor (c-kit). Precursor cells exit the marrow and terminally differentiate in tissues under a variety of local influences,[7,8] stimulated by interleukin (IL)-3, IL-4, IL-9, IL-10, and factors from fibroblasts, but inhibited by transforming growth factor B.[9–11] Mast cells are large (10 to 15 mm in diameter) and possess a ruffled membrane, numerous membrane-bound granules (0.5 to 0.7 mm in diameter), mitochondria, a mononuclear nucleus, and scant rough endoplasmic reticulum. Ultrastructurally, human mast cell granules display whorl and scroll patterns.[12]

Basophils, most closely related to eosinophils, are circulating leukocytes whose presence in tissue is unusual except in disease states.[1] They originate in bone marrow and constitute 0.1% to 2.0% of the peripheral blood leukocytes. Basophils possess a polylobed nucleus and differ from mast cells in their tinctorial properties, their relatively smooth cell surface, and their granule morphologic makeup, which is larger and less structured than that of the mast cell. They do not respond to SCF but respond to IL-3 and granulocyte-macrophage colony-stimulating factor (GM-CSF).

ACTIVATION OF MAST CELLS AND BASOPHILS

Mast cells and basophils possess numerous high-affinity intramembranous receptors (FcεRI) for the Fc portion of IgE. The bridging of two or more such Fc receptors by antigen cross-linking of adjacent surface IgE molecules leads to cell activation and rapid release of preformed granular constituents and the generation of unstored mediators. Mast cell responsiveness may be heightened by exposure to SCF or other cytokines[13,14] whereas basophils are primed to respond by GM-CSF, IL-1, and IL-3.[15] Other important secretagogues include a family of histamine releasing factors[16] and complement fragments C3a and C5a.

The secretagogue-induced activation of mediator release is noncytolytic, a process termed *stimulus-secretion coupling*. In vitro, extremely complex intertwined and potentially interacting systems have been identified, some of which may play roles in cell activation.

An additional complexity is added as stored granule-associated mediators are regulated independently from unstored newly generated mediators. In IgE-mediated activation receptor bridging is accompanied by protein tyrosine phosphorylation, an increase in intracellular calcium, protein kinase C translocation, G protein activation, and cyclic adenosine monophosphate generation. At the same time, membrane phospholipids are metabolized to generate monoacylglycerols, diacylglycerols, and phosphorylated inositol species, which facilitate protein kinase C function and liberate Ca^{2+} from intracellular sites. While these biochemical events are underway, adenosine triphosphate (ATP) is broken down and adenosine is liberated, which, in turn, activates a mast cell adenosine receptor to enhance granule release. Finally, the cell gains control over mediator release, the process stops, and the cell regranulates.[17]

MEDIATORS

Whatever their final metabolic interrelationships, the early biochemical processes lead to the generation of a heterogenous group of molecules termed *mediators*.[18] Some mediators are preformed and are stored in the granules of the cell; others are generated only after cell activation and originate in the cytosol or membrane. Mediators are classified in this chapter by their proposed actions (Tables 4-2 and 4-3), although some mediators subserve several functions.

Spasmogenic Mediators

Histamine, generated by decarboxylation of histidine, was the first mast cell mediator to be identified, and it is the sole preformed mediator in this functional class. It is bound to the proteoglycans of mast cell and basophil granules (5 and 1 mg/10^6 cells, respectively).[19,20] Histamine

TABLE 4-2. *Mast cell vasoactive and spasmogenic mediators*

Mediator	Other actions
Histamine	Alters cell migration Generates prostaglandins Increases mucus production Activates suppressor T lymphocytes
PAF	Activates platelets Attracts and activates eosinophils
PGD$_2$	Prevents platelet aggregation Alters cell migration
Sulfidopeptide leukotrienes (C$_4$, D$_4$, E$_4$)	Increase mucus production Generate prostaglandins
Adenosine	Prevents platelet aggregation Enhances mediator release Inhibits neutrophil superoxide production

PAF, platelet-activating factor; PGD$_2$, prostaglandin D$_2$.

circulates at concentrations of approximately 300 pg/mL with a circadian maximum in the early morning hours.[21] Histamine excretion exceeds 10 mg/24 hours; a small fraction excreted is the native molecule, and the remainder is imidazole acetic acid or methyl histamine. Histamine interacts with specific H_1, H_2, and H_3 receptors.[22–24] H_1 receptors predominate in the skin and smooth muscle; H_2 receptors in the skin, lungs, stomach, and a variety of leukocytes; and H_3 receptors predominate in the brain. The biologic response to histamine reflects the ratio of these receptors in a given tissue. H_1 histamine effects include contraction of bronchial and gut musculature, vascular permeability, pulmonary vasoconstriction, and nasal mucus production. By its H_2 pathway, histamine dilates respiratory musculature, enhances airway mucus production, inhibits basophil and skin (but not lung) mast cell degranulation, and activates suppressor T lymphocytes. Both H_1 and H_2 actions are required for the full expression of pruritus, cutaneous vasodilation, and cardiac irritability. The H_3 actions of histamine suppress central nervous system histamine synthesis. Increased levels of histamine are seen in physical urticaria, anaphylaxis, systemic mastocytosis, and antigen-induced rhinitis and asthma.

Platelet-Activating Factor

Platelet-activating factor (PAF) is a lipid identified structurally as 1-alkyl-2-acetyl-sn-glyceryl-3-phosphorylcholine.[25] This mediator is generated by mast cells, eosinophils, and monocytes. Degradation of PAF occurs by the action of acetyl hydrolase to remove acetate from the sn-2 position.

PAF causes aggregation of human platelets, wheal-and-flare permeability responses, and eosinophil chemotaxis[26]; contracts pulmonary and gut musculature; induces vasoconstriction; and is a potent hypotensive agent. Effects mediated by PAF also include pulmonary artery hypertension, pulmonary edema, an increase in total pulmonary resistance, and a decrease in dynamic compliance. PAF also is capable of inducing prolonged increase in nonspecific bronchial hyperreactivity in vivo.[27]

Oxidative Products of Arachidonic Acid

Arachidonic acid is a C20:4 fatty acid component of mast cell membrane phospholipids, from which it may be liberated by the action of phospholipase A_2 or by the concerted action of phospholipase C and diacylglycerol lipase. At least 20 potential end products may be generated from arachidonic acid by the two major enzymes, 5-lipoxygenase and cyclooxygenase, which regulate its fate.

Cyclooxygenase Products

In human mast cells, prostaglandin (PG) D_2 is the predominant cyclooxygenase product generated. The production of PGD_2 from PGH_2 is glutathione dependent and is blocked by nonsteroidal antiinflammatory drugs and dapsone. It is a potent vasoactive and smooth muscle reactive compound that causes vasodilation on injection into human skin, induces gut and pulmonary muscle contraction, and inhibits platelet aggregation in vitro.[28] PGD_2 is thought to be responsible for flushing and hypotension in some patients with mastocytosis.[29]

Immediate IgE antigen–activated PGD_2 production is dependent on the constitutive expression of cyclooxygenase 1, whereas later and more prolonged PGD_2 synthesis occurs after antigen challenge of sensitized cells that are stimulated with SCF and IL-10.[30]

TABLE 4-3. *Mast cell mediators affecting cell migration*

Mediator	Cell target
High molecular weight NCF	Neutrophils
ECF-A	Eosinophils
ECF oligopeptides	Eosinophils (secondary mononuclear)
T-lymphocyte chemotactic factors	T cells
Histamine	Nonselective
PGD$_2$	Eosinophils and neutrophils
Leukotriene B$_4$	Neutrophils
Leukotriene E$_4$	Eosinophils
PAF	Eosinophils and neutrophils
Lymphocyte chemokinetic factor	T and B cells

NCF, neutrophil chemotactic factor; ECF-A, eosinophil chemotactic factor of anaphylaxis; PGD$_2$, prostaglandin D$_2$; PAF, platelet-activating factor.

Lipoxygenase Products

Human mast cells generate 5-lipoxygenase products of arachidonic acid, starting with an unstable intermediate, 5-HPETE (which may be reduced to the monohydroxy fatty acid), 5-HETE, or (through leukotriene synthetase) to LTC4 by addition of glutathione. The initial product of this pathway is LTC$_4$, from which LTD$_4$ may be generated by the removal of the terminal glutamine, and LTE$_4$ by the further removal of glycine. The biologic activity of the sulfidopeptide leukotrienes occurs by specific receptor recognition. Degradation is rapid and is accomplished by various oxygen metabolites. Clinically useful inhibitors of 5-lipoxygenase or LTD$_4$ receptors are available and demonstrate efficacy in clinical asthma.[31]

Leukotrienes are potent and possess a broad spectrum of biologic activity.[32] They induce wheal-and-flare responses that are long lived, and are accompanied histologically by endothelial activation and dermal edema. In the airway, they enhance mucus production and cause bronchoconstriction, especially by affecting peripheral units. In humans, LTD$_4$ is most active, LTC$_4$ is intermediate, and LTE$_4$ is the least potent. LTE$_4$ has been implicated as an inducer of nonspecific bronchial hyperreactivity.[33] All depress cardiac muscle and diminish coronary flow rates. LTC$_4$ and LTD$_4$ have been recovered from nasal washings and bronchial lavage fluids of patients with allergic rhinitis or asthma.

Adenosine

The nucleoside adenosine generated from the breakdown of ATP is released from mast cells on IgE-mediated activation.[34] In humans, circulating blood levels of adenosine are 0.3 μm and are increased after hypoxia or antigen-induced bronchospasm. Adenosine is a potent vasodilator, inhibits platelet aggregation, and causes bronchospasm on inhalation by asthmatics. Adenosine, acting through a cell surface receptor, enhances mast cell mediator release in vitro and potentiates antigen-induced local wheal-and-flare responses in vivo. Adenosine binding to its receptor is inhibited by methylxanthines.

Chemotactic Mediators

Several chemotactic molecules have been characterized by activities generated during IgE-dependent allergic responses. Most remain incompletely characterized.

Neutrophil Chemotactic Factors

High molecular weight (HMW) factors are the most prominent neutrophil-directed activities noted. HMW-NCF (neutrophil chemotactic factor) is released into the circulation soon after mast cell activation.[35] Its release in asthmatics is antigen dose dependent, inhibited by cromolyn, and accompanied by transient leukocytosis.

LTB$_4$ and PAF are potent chemotactic agents capable of inducing neutrophil exudation into human skin, and induce production of oxygen radicals and lipid mediators. Histamine also alters neutrophil chemotactic responses.

Eosinophil Chemotactic Factors

The most potent and selective eosinophil-directed agent is PAF,[26] which induces skin or bronchial eosinophilia. Other less active eosinophil-directed mast cell products include the tetrapeptides Val or ala-gly-ser-glu (eosinophil chemotactic factor of anaphylaxis [ECF-A])[36] and others having a molecular weight of 1000 to 3000. The latter ones have been found in the blood of humans after induction of physical urticaria or allergic asthma. ECF-A is capable of inducing PAF production by eosinophils.[37]

Mediators With Enzymatic Properties

Two important proteases are found in human mast cells and not basophils. Tryptase,[38] a tryptic protease of 140,000 daltons is present in all human mast cells. It constitutes nearly 25% of mast cell granular protein and is released during IgE-dependent reactions. It is capable of cleaving kininogen to yield bradykinin, diminish clotting activity, and to generate and degrade complement components such as C3a and a variety of other peptides. Tryptase is not inhibited by plasma antiproteases, and thus its activity may be persistent. It is present in plasma in patients experiencing anaphylaxis (in which case it may prove a valuable clinical diagnostic marker[39]) and in those with systemic mastocytosis. Its effects are not clear, but it enhances smooth muscle reactivity and is a mitogen for fibroblasts.[18,40]

A chymotryptic protease termed *chymase* is present in a subclass of human mast cells, particularly those in the skin and on serosal surfaces, and has thus been used as a marker to identify connective tissue mast cells. It cleaves angiotensinogen to yield angiotensin and activates IL-1.[41] Other enzymes found in mast cells include carboxypeptidase and acid hydrolases.[42]

Structural Proteoglycans

The structural proteoglycans include heparin and various chondroitin sulfates.

Heparin

Heparin is a highly sulfated proteoglycan that is contained in amounts of 5 pg/10^6 cells in human mast cell granules[43] and is released on immunologic activation. Human heparin is an anticoagulant proteoglycan and a complement inhibitor, and it modulates tryptase activity. Human heparin also may be important in angiogenesis by binding angiogenic growth factors and preventing their degradation.

Chondroitin Sulfates

Human basophils contain approximately 3 to 4 pg of chondroitin 4 and 6 sulfates, which lack anticoagulant activity and bind less histamine than heparin. Human lung mast cells contain oversulfated proteoglycans chondroitin sulfates D and E, which accounts for the different staining characteristics of these mast cells.

Cytokines

Although cytokines traditionally have been viewed as products of monocyte-macrophages or lymphocytes, it has become clear that mast cells themselves generate several products, including tumor necrosis factor-alpha (TNF-α),[44] IL-3, IL-4, IL-5, IL-6, and GM-CSF.[45,46] These molecules may be central to local regulation of mast cell growth and differentiation and also may provide new functions for mast cells in health and disease.

MEDIATOR INTERACTIONS

The mediators generated and released after mast cell activation have been isolated, identified, and characterized as individual factors, whereas physiologic and pathologic events reflect their combined interactions. Given the number of mediators, the knowledge that many have yet to be purified (or even identified), and the lack of understanding of appropriate ratios of mediators generated or released in vivo, it is not surprising that there are no reliable data regarding these interactions in health or disease. The number and type of mast cell mediator interactions are potentially enormous, and their pathobiologic consequences are relevant to a variety of homeostatic and disease processes. The best clues to the interaction of mediators are the known physiologic and pathologic manifestations of allergic diseases. Hopefully, the valuable tool of gene knockouts in mice will elucidate critical individual and interactive roles of these molecules.

THE ROLE OF THE MAST CELL AND ITS MEDIATORS IN TISSUE

The most compelling evidence for the role of mast cells and mediators in tissue is derived from experiments in which IgE-dependent mast cell activation in skin or lung tissue is caused by specific antigen (or antibody to IgE). The participation of other immunoglobulin classes, and thus of other inflammatory pathways, is excluded in such studies by using purified IgE to sensitize nonimmune individuals. Activation of cutaneous mast cells by antigen results initially in a pruritic wheal-and-flare reaction that begins in minutes and persists for 1 hour to 2 hours, followed in 6 to 12 hours by a large, poorly demarcated, erythematous, tender, and indurated lesion.[47] Histologic analysis of the initial response shows mast cell degranulation, dermal edema, and endothelial cell activation.

The late reaction is characterized by edema; by infiltration of the dermis by neutrophils, eosinophils, basophils, lymphocytes, and mononuclear leukocytes; and in some instances by hemorrhage, blood vessel wall damage, and fibrin deposition of sufficient severity to warrant the diagnosis of vasculitis. A similar dual-phase reaction is experienced by allergic persons who inhale antigen. Such challenges result in an immediate bronchospastic response followed by recovery, and, 6 hours to 24 hours later, by a recrudescence of asthmatic signs and symptoms.[48] The mediators responsible for these pathophysiologic manifestations have not been delineated fully, but clues to their identity can be derived from knowledge of the effects of pharmacologic manipulation, by the identification of mediators in blood or tissue fluid obtained when the inflammatory response occurs, and by the known effects of isolated mediators.

Pharmacologic intervention suggests that the initial phase is mast cell dependent in both skin and lung tissues. The initial response in skin may be inhibited by antihistamines, and in the lungs by cromolyn. In both tissues, corticosteroid effectively inhibits only the late response, reflecting its inflammatory nature. Histamine, TNF-α, tryptase, LTD_4, PGD_2, IL-5, and eosinophil chemotactic activity are found soon after challenge. The late response is associated with leukocyte infiltration but not with a unique profile of released mediators. The exact genesis of the early and late reactions is speculative. The concerted action of the spasmogenic mediators histamine, adenosine, PGD_2, leukotrienes, and PAF seems sufficient to account for all of the immediate pathophysiologic (anaphylactic) responses to antigen. This concept is supported by the knowledge that the early response occurs before a significant influx of circulating leukocytes.

However, mast cell mediators or mediators from antigen-reactive T lymphocytes, epithelial cells, or macrophages may induce such changes, either directly or indirectly. In response to mediators, vascular endothelium, fibroblasts, and a variety of connective tissue and epithelial cells then could generate other inflammatory and vasoactive mediators. The late phases in lung and skin tissue are likely to represent the residue of the early response as well as the contribution of active enzymes, newly arrived plasma inflammatory cascades, various cytokines (particularly those inducing endothelial expression of adhesion molecules), and the influx of activated circulating leukocytes. Of direct relevance to leukocyte recruitment are GM-CSF, IL-3, and especially IL-5, which promote eosinophil growth, differentiation, migration, adherence, and activation.[49,50] The late inflammatory response is relevant to the progression of asthma in that patients experiencing the late responses have exacerbation of their nonspecific bronchial hyperreactivity, whereas this phenomenon does not occur after isolated early responses.

HOMEOSTATIC ROLE OF MAST CELLS

Mast cell mediators likely are important in maintaining normal tissue function. Because mast cells are positioned near small blood vessels and at the host–environment interface, and are thus at crucial sites for regulating local nutrient delivery and for the entry of noxious materials, the potential regulatory role of mediators is obvious. They are likely to be especially important in the regulation of flow through small blood vessels, impulse generation in unmyelinated nerves, and smooth muscle and bone structural integrity and function. The ability to recruit and activate plasma proteins and cells also may provide preimmune defense against host invasion by infectious agents. Such a role is most apparent in parasitic infestation but also is likely in the case of other insults. Moreover, the recognition of mast cell heterogeneity implies that differences in mast cells relate to locally important biologic requirements.

Although the precise homeostatic and pathophysiologic role of mast cell mediators is understood imprecisely, the broadening understanding of their chemical nature and function provides a useful framework for addressing their role in health and disease.

REFERENCES

1. Galli SJ, Austen KF. Mast cell and basophil differentiation in health and disease. New York: Raven Press, 1989.
2. Bernstein JA, Lawrence ID. The mast cell: a comprehensive, updated review. Allergy Proc 1990;11:209.
3. Irani AA, Schechter NM, Craig SS, Schwartz LB. Two types of human mast cells that have distinct neutral protease compositions. Proc Acad Sci USA 1986;83:4464.
4. Benyon RC, Church MK, Clegg LS, Holgate ST. Dispersion and characterization of mast cells from human skin. Int Arch Allergy Appl Immunol 1986;79:332.
5. Fox CC, Dvorak AM, Peters SP, Kagey-Sobotka A, Lichtenstein LM. Isolation and characterization of human intestinal mucosal mast cells. J Immunol 1985;135:483.
6. Mikhail GR, Miller-Milinska A. Mast cell population in human skin. J Invest Dermatol 1964;43:249.
7. Valent P, Spanblochl E, Sperr WR, et al. Induction of differentiation of human mast cells from bone marrow and peripheral blood mononuclear cells by recombinant human stem cell factor/kit-ligand in long-term culture. Blood 1990;80:2237.
8. Galli SJ, Tsai M, Wershil BK. The c-kit receptor, stem cell factor, and mast cells: what each is teaching about the others. Am J Pathol 1993;142:965.
9. Thompson-Snipes L, Dhar V, Bond MW, Mosman TR, Moore KW, Rennich DM. Interleukin 10: a novel stimulatory factor for mast cells and their progenitors. J Exp Med 1991;173:507.
10. Smith CA, Rennick DM. Characterization of a murine lymphokine distinct from interleukin-2 and interleukin-3 possessing a T-cell growth factor activity and a mast cell growth factor activity that synergizes with IL-3. Proc Natl Acad Sci USA 1986;83:1857.
11. Broide DH, Wasserman SI, Alvaro-Garcia J, Zvaifler NJ, Firestein GS. TGF-B selectively inhibits IL-3 dependent mast cell proliferation without affecting mast cell function or differentiation. J Immunol 1989;143:1591.
12. Dvorak AM. The fine structure of human basophils and mast cells. In: Holgate ST, ed. Mast cells, mediators and disease. London: Kluwer Academic Publishers, 1988:29.
13. Coleman JW, Holliday MR, Klimber I, Zsebokm, Galli SJ. Regulation of mouse peritoneal mast cell secretory function by stem cell factor, IL-3, IL-4. J Immunol 1993;150:556.
14. Alam R, Welter JB, Forsythe PA, Grant A. Comparative effect of recombinant IL-1, 2, 3, 4, and 6, IFN gamma, granulocyte-macrophage colony stimulating factor, tumor necrosis factor-alpha, and histamine from basophils. J Immunol 1989;142:3431.
15. MacDonald SM, Lichtenstein LM, Proud D, Lichtenstein LM. Studies of IgE dependent histamine releasing factors: heterogeneity of IgE. J Immunol 1987;139:506.
16. Siriganian RP. Mechanism of IgE-mediated hypersensitivity. In: Middleton E, Reed CE, Ellis EF, Adkinson NJ, Yuninger JW, Busse WW, eds. Allergy: principles and practice. 4th ed. St Louis: CV Mosby, 1993.
17. Schwartz LB. Mast cells: function and contents. Curr Opin Immunol 1994;6:91.
18. Paterson NAM, Wasserman SI, Said JW, Austen KF. Release of chemical mediators from partially purified human lung cells. J Immunol 1976;117:1356.
19. MacGlashan DW, Lichtenstein LM. The purification of human basophils. J Immunol 1980;124:219.
20. Barnes P, Fitzgerald G, Brown M, Dollery C. Nocturnal asthma and changes in circulating epinephrine, histamine, and cortisol. N Engl J Med 1980;303:263.
21. Black JW, Duncan WA, Durant CJ, et al. Definition and antagonism of histamine H2-receptors. Nature 1972;236:385.
22. Marquardt DL. Histamine. Clin Rev Allergy 1983;1:343.
23. West RE, Zweig A, Shih N-Y, et al. Identification of two H_3-histamine receptor subtypes. Mol Pharmacol 1990;38:610.
24. O'Flaherty JT, Wykle RL. Biology and biochemistry of platelet-activating factor. Clin Rev Allergy 1983;1:353.
25. Wardlaw A, Moqbel R, Cromwell O, et al. Platelet activating factor: a potent chemotatic and chemokinetic factor for eosinophils. J Clin Invest 1986;78:1701.
26. Cuss FM, Dixon CM, Barnes PJ. Effects of platelet activating factor on pulmonary function and bronchial responsiveness in man. Lancet 1986;ii:189.
27. Hardy CC, Robinson C, Tattersfield AE, Holgate ST. The bronchoconstrictor effects of inhaled prostaglandin D_2 in normal and asthmatic men. N Engl J Med 1984;311:209.
28. Roberts LJ, Sweetman BJ, Lewis RA, et al. Increased production of prostaglandin D_2 in patients with systemic mastocytosis. N Engl J Med 1980;303:1400.

29. Murakami M, Bingham CO, Mastumoto R, Austen KF, Arm JP. IgE- dependent activation of cytokine primed mouse cultured mast cells induces a delayed phase of prostaglandin D_2 generation via prostaglandin endoperoxidase synthase 2. J Immunol 1995;155:4445.

30. Israel E, Rubin P, Kemp JP, et al. The effect of inhibition of 5-lipoxygenase by Zileuton in mild to moderate asthma. Ann Intern Med 1993;119:1059.

31. Lewis RA, Austen KF, Sherman RJ. Leukotrienes and the products of the 5-lipoxygenase pathway: biochemistry and relation to pathobiology in human diseases. N Engl J Med 1990;323:645.

32. Henderson WR Jr. The role of leukotrienes in inflammation. Ann Intern Med 1994;121:686.

33. Marquardt DL, Gruber HE, Wasserman SI. Adenosine release from stimulated mast cells. J Allergy Clin Immunol 1984;73:115.

34. Atkins PC, Norman M, Werner H, Zweiman B. Release of neutrophil chemotactic activity during immediate hypersensitivity reactions in humans. Ann Intern Med 1976;86:415.

35. Goetzl EJ, Austen KF. Purification and synthesis of eosinophilotactic tetrapeptides of human lung tissue: identification as eosinophil chemotactic factor of anaphylaxis (ECF-A). Proc Natl Acad Sci USA 1975;72:4123.

36. Lee TC, Lenihan DJ, Malone B, Roddy LL, Wasserman SI. Increased iosynthesis of platelet activating factor in activated human eosinophils. J Biol Chem 1994;259:5526.

37. Johnson DA, Barton GJ. Mast cell tryptases: examination of unusual characteristics by multiple sequence alignment and molecular modeling. Protein Sci 1992;1:370.

38. VanderLinden PG, Hack CE, Poortman J, Vivie-Kipp YC, Struyvenberg A, Vanderzwan JK. Insect sting challenge in 138 patients: relation between clinical severity of anaphylaxis and mast cell activation. J Allergy Clin Immunol 1992;90:110.

39. Ruoss SJ, Hartmann T, Caughey GH. Mast cell tryptase is a mitogen for cultured fibroblasts. J Clin Invest 1991;88:493.

40. Mizutani H, Schechter N, Lazarus G, Black RA, Kripper TS. Rapid and specific conversion of precursor interleukin 1B to an active IL-1 species by human mast cell chymase. J Exp Med 1991;174:821.

41. Goldstein SM, Kaempfer CE, Kealey JT, Wintroub BU. Human mast cell carboxypeptidase: purification and characterization. J Clin Invest 1989;83:1630.

42. Metcalfe DD, Lewis RA, Silbert JE, Rosenberg RD, Wasserman SI, Austen KF. Isolation and characterization of heparin from human lung. J Clin Invest 1979;64:1537.

43. Walsh LJ, Trinchieri G, Waldorf HA, Whitaker D, Murphy GF. Human dermal mast cells contain and release tumor necrosis factor alpha which induces endothelial leukocyte adhesion molecule I. Proc Natl Acad Sci USA 1991;88:4220.

44. Bradding P, Feather IH, Howarth PH, et al. Interleukin 4 is localized to and released by human mast cells. J Exp Med 1992;176:1386.

45. Bradding P, Feather IH, Wilson S. Immunolocalization of cytokines in the nasal mucosa of normal and perennial rhinitic subjects: the mast cell as a source of IL-4, IL-5 and Il-6 in human allergic mucosal inflammation. J Immunol 1993;151:3853.

46. Dolovitch J, Hargreaves FE, Chalmers R, et al. Late cutaneous allergic responses in isolated IgE-dependent reactions. J Allergy Clin Immunol 1973;52:38.

47. MacDonald SM, Naclerio RM, Plaut M, Warner J, Kagey-Sabotka A, Lichtenstein LM. Human late-phase reactions. In: Kay AB, ed. Allergy and inflammation. London: Academic Press, 1987.

48. Fabian I, Kletter Y, Mor S, Geller-Bernstein C, et al. Activation of human eosinophil and neutrophil functions by hemopoietic growth factors: comparisons of IL-1, IL-3, IL-5 and GM-CSF. Br J Haemotol 1992;80:137.

49. Resnick MB, Weller PF. Mechanisms of eosinophil recruitment. Am J Respir Cell Mol Biol 1993;8:349.

50. Neeley SP, Hamann KJ, White SR, Boranowski SL, Burch RA, Leff RA. Selective regulation of expression of surface adhesion molecules Mac-1, L-selectin and VLA-4 on human eosinophils and neutrophils. Am J Respir Cell Mol Biol 1993;8:633.

Allergic Diseases, 5th Edition,
edited by Roy Patterson, Leslie Carroll Grammer,
and Paul A. Greenberger. Lippincott–Raven Publishers, Philadelphia, © 1997.

5

Antihistamines

Jonathan A. Bernstein

*J.A. Bernstein: Department of Internal Medicine, Division of Immunology,
University of Cincinnati College of Medicine, Cincinnati, OH 45267-0563.*

Pearls for Practitioners
Roy Patterson

- For half a century, there have been dozens of antihistamines or antihistamine-decongestant preparations on the market. It is best to know three or four well in terms of effectiveness, dosage, and side effects. If these don't work, other approaches to treatment of allergic disease must be used.

- Side effects of antihistamines, such as drowsiness, often disappear with regular use.

- Tolerance to the effect of antihistamines occurs, and substitution with a different class of agent will resolve this.

- Antihistamines do not control all cases of allergy. Years ago it was thought that insufficient concentrations of H_1 blockers at the local site were the explanation. Now it is thought that other bioactive mediators of allergic inflammation are the best explanation.

- About four decades ago, antihistamines went through a period of topical application to the skin. The clinical benefit was minimal, but there was a high incidence of contact dermatitis to the topical antihistamine.

Histamine receptor antagonists (antihistamines) are categorized in terms of their structure, pharmacokinetics, pharmacodynamics, and clinical use. Second-generation, nonsedating H_1-antagonists, many of which have been derived from first-generation agents, have added a new dimension to the treatment of allergic disorders. Recently, a new field of pharmacoepidemiology also has emerged as a result of postmarketing surveillance of these newer H_1-antagonists. Investigations into the adverse drug reactions associated with the second-generation agent, terfenadine, have served as a prototype for the design of future long-term surveillance studies monitoring the safety of drugs in a variety of clinical situations.

HISTORICAL PERSPECTIVE

Histamine, or β-imidazolylethylamine, was first synthesized by Windaus and Vogt in 1907.[1] The term *histamine* was adopted because of its prevalence in animal and human tissues (*hist*: relating to tissue) and its amine structure[2,3] (Fig. 5-1*A*). Dale and Laidlaw,[4] in 1910, were the first to recognize histamine's role in anaphylaxis when they observed a dramatic bron-

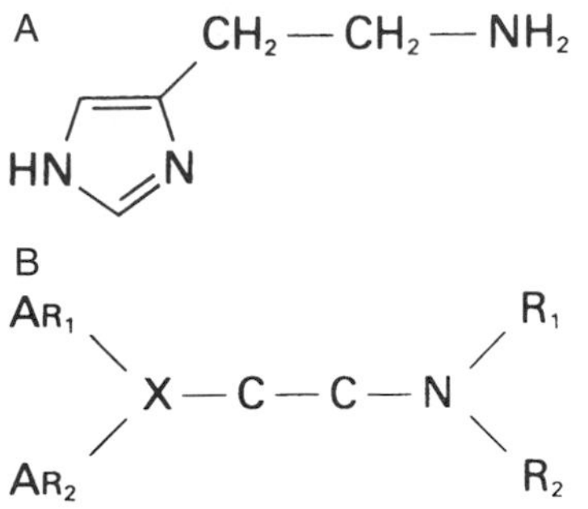

A $CH_2 - CH_2 - NH_2$

HN   N

B
AR_1 R_1

            $X - C - C - N$

AR_2 R_2

FIG. 5-1. Structure of histamine (**A**) and basic structure of H_1 antagonists (**B**).

chospastic and vasodilatory effect in animals injected intravenously with this compound. Subsequently, histamine was found to be stored as a preformed mediator in the cytoplasmic granules of tissue mast cells and circulating basophils.[5,6]

Originally, histamine's classic physiologic actions of bronchoconstriction and vasodilation were believed to be responsible for the symptoms of allergic diseases through its action at one histamine receptor. In 1966, Ash and Schild[7] were the first to recognize that histamine-mediated reactions occurred through more than one receptor, based on observations that histamine had an array of actions such as contraction of guinea pig ileal smooth muscle, inhibition of rat uterine contractions, and suppression of gastric acid secretion. This speculation was confirmed by Black and coworkers[8] in 1972, who used the experimental histamine antagonists, mepyramine and burinamide, to block histamine-induced reactions in animals. They observed that each of these antagonists inhibited different physiologic responses, suggesting that there were at least two histamine receptors, now referred to as H_1 and H_2.[8] Recently, Arrang and associates[9] discovered a third histamine receptor (H_3) with unique physiologic properties, raising the possibility that additional, yet unrecognized, histamine receptors exist. Table 5-1 summarizes the pharmacodynamic effects after activation of the known histamine receptors and their common agonists and antagonists.[9–15]

The first histamine antagonist was accidentally discovered in 1937 by Bovet and Staub, who found that a drug originally being studied for its adrenergic antagonistic properties in guinea pigs also had potent antihistaminic activity.[3] By 1942, safe and effective antihistamines developed for human use became available. Many of these agents, such as pyrilamine maleate, tripelennamine, and diphenhydramine, currently are widely prescribed.[3]

H_2-histamine antagonists were first synthesized in 1969 for developing a drug capable of inhibiting gastric acid secretion.[13] These agents have a closer structural resemblance to histamine because most are simple modifications of the histamine molecule itself.[3] However, histamine's affinity for H_1-receptors is tenfold greater than for H_2-receptors.[3]

H_1-RECEPTOR HISTAMINE ANTAGONISTS

First-Generation Agents

Structure

The chemical structure of H_1-antagonists differs substantially from histamine (see Fig. 5-1*B*). Histamine is composed of a single imidazole heterocyclic ring linked to an ethylamine group, whereas H_1-antagonists consist of one or two heterocyclic or aromatic rings

TABLE 5-1. *Histamine receptor*

	H$_1$	H$_2$	H$_3$
Location	Bronchial & gastrointestinal smooth muscle, brain	Gastric mucosa, uterus, brain	Brain, bronchial smooth muscle
Function	↑ Vascular permeability	↑ Gastric acid secretion	Vasodilation of cerebral vessels; prevents excessive broncho-constriction
	↑ Pruritus Constrict smooth muscle	Bronchial smooth muscle relaxation	
	↑ Cyclic GMP	↑ Cyclic AMP	
	↑ Prostaglandin generation	↑ Mucous secretion	
	↓ Atrioventricular node conduction time	Esophageal relaxation	
	Activation of airway vagal afferent nerves	Stimulation of T-suppressor cells	
	↑ Hypotension	↓ Basophil histamine release	
	↑ Flushing	↓ Neutrophil and basophil chemotaxis and enzyme release	
	↑ Headache	↑ Hypotension	
	↑ Tachycardia	↑ Flushing	
	↑ Release of mediators of inflammation*	↑ Headache	
	↑ Recruitment of inflammatory cells*	↑ Tachycardia	
Agonists	2-Methylhistamine	4 (5)-Methylhistamine	α-Methylhistamine
	Betahistine	Betazole	
	2-Pyridylethylamino	Dimaprit	
	2-Thiazolylethylamine	Impromidine	
Antagonists	Chlorpheniramine	Cimetidine	Thioperamide
	Diphenhydramine	Ranitidine	Impromidine
	Hydroxyzine	Famotidine	
	Terfenadine	Nizatidine	
	Astemizole	Etintidine	
	Loratadine		
	Cetirizine		

GMP, guanosine monophosphate; AMP, adenosine monophosphate.
*Not antagonized by all H$_1$-receptor antagonists.

joined to a "linkage atom" (nitrogen, oxygen, or carbon)[3] (Table 5-2). The linkage atom is important in structurally differentiating these groups of agents, whereas the number of alkyl substitutions and heterocyclic or aromatic rings determines their lipophilic nature. The ethylenediamines, phenothiazines, piperazines, and piperidines all contain nitrogen as their linkage atom, whereas the ethanolamines contain oxygen and the alkylamines contain carbon as their linkage atoms.[3,16]

TABLE 5-2. *Classification of common H₁ (first-generation) antagonists*

Structural class/Linkage atom	Generic name	Trade name
Ethanolamines/O (oxygen)	Diphenhydramine hydrochloride	Benadryl
	Dimenhydrinate	Dramamine
	Clemastine fumorate	Tavist
Alkylamines/C (carbon)	Chlorpheniramine maleate	Chlortrimeton, Teldrin
	Brompheniramine maleate	Dimetane
	Dexchlorpheniramine maleate	Polaramine
	Dexbrompheniramine maleate	Drixoral*
	Triprolidine HCl	Actifed*
	Chlorpheniramine tannate/pyrilamine tannate	Rynatan†
	Pheniramine maleate/pyrilamine maleate	Triaminic TR†
Ethylenediamines/N (nitrogen)	Tripelennamine HCl	Pyribenzamine HCl
	Tripelennamine citrate	PBZ
	Pyrilamine maleate	Allertoc
	Antazoline phosphate	Vasocon-A
Piperazines/N (nitrogen)	Hydroxyzine HCl	Atarax/Vistaril
	Meclizine HCl	Antivert/Bonine
Phenothiazines/N (nitrogen)	Promethazine HCl	Phenergan
	Trimiprazine tartrate	Temaril
Piperidines/N (nitrogen)	Cyproheptadine HCl	Periactin
	Azatadine maleate	Optamine/Trinalin*

*With decongestant.
†Combination ethylenediamine/alkylamine compound.
From Simons FER. H₁ receptor antagonists: chemical pharmacology and therapeutics. J Allergy Clin Immunol 1989;84:845.

Pharmacokinetics

Accurate pharmacokinetic data on first-generation antihistamines are available in children and adults because of sensitive detection techniques such as gas-liquid chromatography, mass spectrometry, and high-performance liquid chromatography.[3,10,16] Generally, these compounds are rapidly absorbed orally or intravenously, resulting in peak serum concentrations within 2 to 3 hours and symptomatic relief within 30 minutes. They have large volumes of distribution, slow clearance rates, and are metabolized primarily by hydroxylation in the hepatic cytochrome p450 system. Most of the parent drug is excreted as inactive metabolites in the urine within 24 hours of dosing. As a rule, serum half-lives are longer in adults than they are for children. Their lipophilic nature allows them to cross the placenta and the blood–brain barrier. This access into the central nervous system is responsible for most of the patients' side effects. These agents also are excreted in breast milk.[3,10,16] Table 5-3 summarizes pharmacokinetic data for the most commonly used first-generation agents.[17–21]

Pharmacodynamics

The first-generation H₁-antagonists compete with histamine for binding to histamine receptors. This competitive inhibition is reversible and, therefore, highly dependent on free drug plasma concentrations. While these agents are metabolized and excreted into the urine as inactive metabolites, the histamine receptors become desaturated, allowing surrounding histamine to bind. This mechanism emphasizes the need to instruct patients on using these agents

TABLE 5-3. *Pharmacokinetics of representative H₁-receptor antagonists*

H₁-Receptor antagonist	Time to peak level (h)†	Half-life‡	Clearance rate (mL/min/kg)
First generation			
Chlorpheniramine	2.8±0.8	27.9±8.7 h	1.8±0.1
Hydroxyzine	2.1±0.4	20.0±4.1 h	9.8±3.2
Diphenhydramine	1.7±1.0	9.2±2.5 h	23.3±9.4
Second generation			
Terfenadine	0.78–1.1	16–23 h	NA
Terfenadine carboxylate§	3	17 h	598–697 mL/min
Fexofenadine§	1–3	13–16 h	NA
Astemizole	0.5±0.2 to 0.7±0.3	1.1 d	1500 mL/min
N-Desmethylastemizole§	NA	9.5 d	NA
Loratadine	1.0±0.3	11.0±9.4 h	202
Descarboethozyloratadine§	1.5±0.7	17.3±6.9 h	NA
Cetirizine¶	1.0±0.5	7.4±1.6 h	1.0±0.2
Acrivastine	0.85–1.4	1.4–2.1 h	4.56
Ketotifen¶	3.6±1.6	18.3+6.7 h	NA
Azelastine	5.3±1.6	22±4 h	8.5±3.2
Demethylazelastine¶	20.5	54±15 h	NA

*Values are for healthy young adults; plus-minus values are means ± SD. See references 1 and 23 through 32 for further information.

†Time from oral intake to peak plasma concentration.

‡Plasma elimination half-life.

§Metabolite of the parent compound.

¶Currently not approved for use in the United States.

From Simons FER, Simons KJ. The pharmacology and use of H₁-receptor-antagonist drugs. N Engl J Med 1994;330:1663.

on a regular basis to achieve a maximal therapeutic benefit.[3,22] Interestingly, smaller doses of H₁-antagonists have been found to inhibit mast cell activation in vitro, whereas larger doses cause mast cell activation and histamine release.[23]

Pharmacy

Table 5-4 summarizes the children and adult dosing schedules of the three most commonly prescribed first-generation antihistamines.[10,17,24] Before the availability of pharmacokinetic data, these agents were believed to have short half-lives, requiring frequent dosing intervals to be effective.[22] Since chlorpheniramine, brompheniramine, and hydroxyzine have half-lives greater than 20 hours in adults, it may be feasible to administer these agents only once or twice a day to achieve similar efficacy.[18,19,21] The availability of sustained-release preparations of agents with shorter half-lives also has allowed less frequent dosing, thereby improving patient compliance and minimizing side effects. Whether treatment with sustained-released formulations of conventional agents with shorter half-lives offers any advantages over conventional agents with longer half-lives when similarly dosed remains unclear.[25–27]

TABLE 5-4. *Formulations and dosages of representative H₁-receptor antagonists*

H₁-Receptor antagonist	Formulation	Recommended dosage*
First generation		
Chlorpheniramine maleate (Chlor-Trimeton)	Tablets: 4 mg, 8 mg,[†] 12 mg[†] Syrup: 2.5 mg/5 mL Parenteral solution: 10 mg/mL	Adult: 8–12 mg 2×/d[‡] Child: 0.35 mg/kg/24 h
Hydroxyzine hydrochloride (Atarax)	Capsules: 10 mg, 25 mg, 50 mg Syrup: 10 mg/5 mL	Adult: 25–50 mg 2×/d (or once a day at bedtime) Child: 2 mg/kg/24 h
Diphenhydramine hydrochloride (Benadryl)	Capsules; 25 mg, 50 mg Elixir: 12.5 mg/5 mL Syrup: 6.25 mg/5 mL Parenteral solution: 50 mg/mL	Adult: 25–50 mg 3×/d Child: 5 mg/kg/24 h
Second generation		
Terfenadine (Seldane)	Tablets: 60 mg, 120 mg[§] Suspension: 30 mg/5 mL[§]	Adult: 60 mg 2×/d or 120 mg/d Child: 3–6 y, 15 mg 2×/d 7–12 y, 30 mg 2×/d
Fexofenadine (Allegra)	Tablets: 60 mg	Adult and child > 12 y: 60 mg 2x/d
Astemizole (Hismanal)	Tablets: 10 mg Suspension: 10 mg/5 mL[§]	Adult: 10 mg/d Child: 0.2 mg/kg/d
Loratadine (Claritin)	Tablets: 10 mg Syrup: 1 mg/mL	Adult: 10 mg/d Child: 2–12 y, 5 mg/d; >12 y and >30 kg, 10 mg/d
Cetirizine hydrochloride (Zyrtec)	Tablets: 5 mg, 10 mg	Adult: 5–10 mg/d
Acrivastine (Semprex)	Tablets: 8 mg	Adult: 8 mg 3×/d
Ketotifen fumarate (Zaditen)[§]	Tablets: 1 mg, 2 mg[†]	Adult with urticaria: 4 mg/d Child >3 y: 1 mg 2×/d or 2 mg/d[‡]
Azelastine hydrochloride (Astelin)[§]	0.1% Nasal solution: 0.137 mg/spray	Topical: 2 sprays/nostril/d or 2×/d
Levocabastine hydrochloride (Livostin)	Microsuspension: 0.5 mg/mL	Topical: 2 sprays, (50 µg each)/nostril 2–4×/d or 1 drop (0.15 µg) in each eye 2–4×/d

*The dose for a child should be given if the patient weighs 40 kg (90 lb) or less.
[†]A tablet of this size is a timed-release formulation.
[‡]The timed-release formulation should be given.
[§]Currently not approved for use in the United States.
From Simons FER, Simons KJ. The pharmacology and use of H₁-receptor-antagonist drugs. N Engl J Med 1994;330:1663.

Second-Generation Agents

Structure

Since the new nonsedating class of antihistamines do not fit into one of the existing structural classification categories of first-generation antagonists, they have been placed into a separate category referred to as second-generation antagonists. Their structural and pharmacokinetic profiles are responsible for their milder side effects and better tolerance among patients.[3,28,29] Table 5-5 lists the chemical derivations of these agents in addition to other similar compounds

TABLE 5-5. *Chemical derivations for second-generation*
H_1 antagonists and dual-action antihistamines

Antihistamines	Chemical family derivation
Terfenadine[*,†] (Seldane, Merrel Dow, Cincinnati)	Butyrophenone related to haloperidol
Fexofenadine (Allegra)	Acid metabolite of terfenadine
Astemizole[*] (Hismanal)	Aminopiperidinyl-benzimidazole
Loratadine (Claritin)	Piperidine derivative of azatadine
Cetirizine	Cyclizine derivative of hydroxyzine
Acrivastine	Acrylic acid derivative of tripolidine
Mequitazine	Derivative of phenothiazine
Temelastine (SKF 93944)	Derivative of pyrilamine
Levocabastine (R 50547)	Stereoisomer of a cyclohexylpiperdine
Azelastine[‡]	Phthalazinone derivative
Ketotifen[‡]	Benzocycloheptathiophene
Oxatamide[‡]	Related to cinnarizine

[*]Available in the United States.
[†]With decongestant.
[‡]Dual-action antihistamines.

undergoing investigation, and Figure 5-2 illustrates their structures in comparison with first-generation agents.[10,30,31] The five currently available agents in the United States are terfenadine, fexofenadine, astemizole, loratadine, and cetirizine. The latter agent is classified as a low-sedating agent whereas the former agents are nonsedating.

Pharmacokinetics

The pharmacokinetic data available for second-generation agents are summarized in comparison with first-generation agents in Table 5-3.[17,29,32–38] Terfenadine, astemizole, and loratadine are well absorbed from the gastrointestinal tract, with peak serum concentrations occurring within 1 to 2 hours after oral administration.[17,32,33] Data in humans on volumes of distribution for these agents are not available.[3,17] However, after ingestion, these agents undergo extensive metabolism in the liver. Astemizole undergoes oxidative dealkylation, aromatic hydroxylation, and glucoronidation through the p450-CYP3A4 pathway to form several metabolites.[39] The major active metabolite of astemizole is N-desmethylastemizole, which has a half life of 9.5 days. Terfenadine is exclusively metabolized by oxidation and oxidative N-dealkylation through the p450-CYP3A4 pathway to form an active acid metabolite (MDL 16,455; fexofenadine) and an inactive metabolite (MDL 4829), respectively.[38] The acid metabolite has one third of the original antihistaminic activity of the parent compound.[32,40] Most ($\geq 60\%$) of astemizole and terfenadine's metabolites are eliminated in the feces and bile.[32,39] Most of fexofenadine is excreted in the feces and urine unmetabolized. Astemizole is unique because it has a slower elimination half-life of 18 to 20 days compared with terfenadine, which has a half-life of 4.5 hours, although terfenadine's antihistaminic effect lasts longer than its measured half-life.[39,40] Although the half-life of terfenadine for children is only 2 hours, it is equally effective pharmacodynamically in comparison with adults.[41] Loratadine also undergoes extensive hepatic metabolism through the p450-CYP3A4 pathway to form its active metabolite, descarboethoxyloratadine.[37,38] This drug differs from terfenadine and astemizole in that it is also metabolized by an alternate isoenzyme,

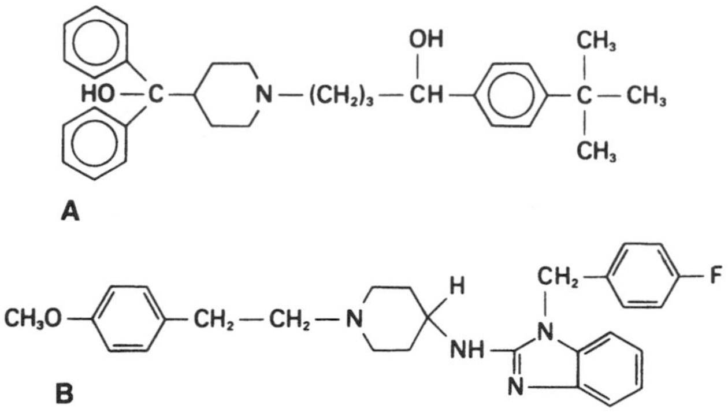

FIG. 5-2. Chemical structures of two currently available second-generation H₁ antagonists.

CYP2D6, if p450-CYP3A4 is inhibited.[38] This alternative metabolic pathway prevents drug accumulation in individuals with hepatic disease or taking concomitant drugs with microsomal oxygenase inhibitory activity.[38] Cetirizine is primarily excreted in the urine, 50% as unchanged drug. It is not significantly metabolized in the liver. Dosing adjustments are recommended for renally impaired individuals.

The understanding of drug metabolism was greatly enhanced in 1990 when the Food and Drug Administration (FDA) became aware of numerous reports associating terfenadine with malignant cardiac arrhythmias such as torsade de pointe.[38] By July 1992, 44 reports of adverse cardiovascular events had been reported, 9 resulting in death, 3 of which occurred after an overdose of terfenadine.[38] Studies delving into this problem found that terfenedine blocked the delayed rectifier current (Ik), which prolonged normal cardiac repolarization and was manifested as an increased QT_c interval on electrocardiograms.[38] It was later found that both astemizole and its active metabolite, desmethylastemizole, also inhibited the Ik, leading to QT_c prolongation. Retrospective analysis of case reports citing terfenadine-induced cardiovascular events has been helpful in defining risk factors in patients prone to these cardiac side effects.[38] These risk factors include drug overdose (i.e., most events and fatalities occurred at dosages 6 to 60 times the recommended dose), concomitant use of drugs that inhibit CYP3A4 (e.g,. macrolide antibiotics excluding azithromycin and oral antifungal agents), hepatic dysfunction, alcohol abuse, electrolyte abnormalities (e.g., hypomagnesemia and hypokalemia), and several preexisting cardiovascular diseases.[38] Loratadine has not been demonstrated to induce these cardiovascular side effects, most likely because it is metabolized by two isoenzymes (CYP2D6 and CYP3A4).[38] Loratidine and cetirizine can be safely taken with macrolide antibiotics (i.e., erythromycin) and oral antifungal agents (i.e., ketoconazole).[38] Terfenadine and astemizole are safe and effective drugs that can be used in most clinical circumstances. The acid metabolite of terfenadine, fexofenadine, which also does not effect the Ik or cause QT_c prolongation, has recently been released in the United States for clinical use.

Pharmacodynamics

In contrast to first-generation agents, second-generation agents do not operate by simple competitive inhibition. Instead, these agents bind to and dissociate from H₁-receptors slowly, in a noncompetitive fashion. They are not displaced from H₁-receptors in the presence of high histamine concentrations.[29,42] The second-generation antagonists are potent suppressors of the wheal-and-flare response.[38,43,44] Their lipophobic properties prevents them from crossing the blood–brain barrier, and thus their activity on H₁-receptors is restricted to the peripheral nervous system.[30,45] They have little affinity for non–H₁-receptors.[3,42,43]

Pharmacy

Second-generation antihistamines are available only as oral formulations. They all have convenient dosing once or twice daily (see Table 5-4).[10,17] Studies have shown that a single dose of terfenadine (120 mg) is equally effective as 60 mg twice a day at improving allergic rhinitis symptom scores and suppressing histamine-induced wheal-and-flare responses.[46,47] Astemizole and loratadine should be given on an empty stomach to avoid problems with absorption. Terfenadine, fexofenadine, and cetirizine are not significantly affected by food. All five agents have an antihistaminic potency comparable with each another and with first-generation antihistamines.

DUAL-ACTION ANTIHISTAMINES

Several agents currently unavailable for clinical use in the United States have been found to have numerous clinical effects in addition to their antihistaminic properties. The derivations of these compounds are summarized in Table 5-5.[3,30,31] Although many of their mechanisms of action are unknown, they have been hypothesized to act on mast cells and basophils by preventing calcium influx or intracellular calcium release, which interferes with activation and release of potent bioactive mediators.[48–51] Busse and coworkers[52] have shown that azelastine inhibits superoxide generation by eosinophils and neutrophils, which may represent one of its important antiinflammatory mechanisms. These drugs can bind to H_1-receptors in a competitive and noncompetitive fashion.[3,53,54] In addition to their calcium antagonistic activity, they have variable amounts of antiserotonin, anticholinergic, and antileukotriene activities.[55–61] Pharmacokinetic information for these agents is summarized in Table 5-3.[17]

OTHER AGENTS WITH ANTIHISTAMINE PROPERTIES

Tricyclic antidepressants, originally synthesized for their antihistaminic properties in the 1950s, were never fully developed as antihistamines once they were recognized as having impressive antidepressant effects.[63] Because doxepin has a high H_1-receptor affinity, it has become an acceptable alternative agent for treating chronic idiopathic urticaria.[64] Interestingly, the observation that the butyrophenone antipsychotic haloperidol also had antihistaminic properties eventually led to the development of the derivative, terfenadine.[31,40]

Two H_1-antagonists, acrivastine and cetirizine, have been extensively studied. Acrivastine, a metabolite of triprolidine, recently has been released for use in the United States in combination with a decongestant (Semprex). Although it does not qualify as a true nonsedating antihistamine when compared with second-generation agents, it generally causes less sedation compared with many first-generation agents[17] (see Tables 5-3 through 5-5). Cetirizine, a metabolite of hydroxyzine, has recently been approved by the FDA as a low-sedating second-generation agent[17] (see Tables 5-3 through 5-5).

CLINICAL USE OF ANTIHISTAMINES

The ideal H_1-receptor antagonist should provide complete and rapid relief of allergic symptoms, have a moderate duration of action, and be devoid of adverse effects. Unfortunately, this type of agent does not exist.[65] In general, first- and second-generation agents have fairly comparable antihistaminic effects in relieving common allergic symptoms, and they all have poor decongestant capabilities.[22,66–70] H_1-antagonists have proven useful in treating allergic rhinitis, allergic conjunctivitis, atopic dermatitis, urticaria, asthma, and anaphylaxis.[10,17] The treatment of these disorders is discussed in different sections of this book.

Numerous studies have compared the antihistaminic efficacy of second-generation antagonists with that of first-generation antagonists in the treatment of allergic rhinitis. Results have uniformly shown these agents to be more effective than placebos but just as effective to first-generation agents, such as chlorpheniramine, using comparable dosing schedules.[66,71–76] Studies comparing second-generation agents with one another found no dramatic differences in their clinical effects, but only astemizole and cetirizine have labeling indications for this use.[77–83]

Preliminary studies suggest that a topical eye preparation of the potent H_1-antagonist, levocabastine, available in the United States as Livostin, is more effective than conventional agents for treating allergic conjunctivitis.[84] Hydroxyzine and diphenhydramine still are considered by most clinicians to be the most effective agents in the treatment of allergic skin disorders because of their greater antipruritic and sedative effects.[21,44,85] One exception is cold-induced urticaria for which cyproheptadine is the treatment of choice.[86] All of the second-generation agents have been useful for treating patients with chronic idiopathic urticaria, but only astemizole and cetirizine have labeling indications for this use.[87,88]

The most recent position paper from the American Academy of Allergy and Immunology addressing the use of antihistamines in asthmatics has cleared the controversy surrounding their use in patients with this disease.[89] Previously, the anticholinergic properties (i.e., dryness of the airways) of these antagonists were believed to exacerbate patients' asthma.[90] It is now known that antihistamines, including some of the dual-action compounds, may actually be beneficial in treatment asthma because of their bronchodilator effect.[90–94] Although these agents are not considered to be first-line therapy for asthma, they certainly are not contraindicated in asthma patients who require them for concomitant allergic problems.[89] The *Physicians' Desk Reference* subsequently has modified warnings stating they should be used cautiously in patients with concomitant asthma.[24]

Antihistamines are important adjuncts in the management of anaphylaxis but should never replace the first-line therapy, which by general consensus is epinephrine.[10]

Antihistamines should be used cautiously during pregnancy because of the risk of teratogenicity.[10] Long-term clinical experience using antihistamines during pregnancy shows that tripelennamine, chlorpheniramine, and diphenhydramine cause no greater risk for birth defects than is experienced by the normal population.

Antihistamines are useful in treating nonallergic disorders such as nausea, motion sickness, vertigo, extrapyramidal symptoms, anxiety, and insomnia.[3] Studies evaluating these agents in the treatment of children with otitis media and upper respiratory infections found that they are not significantly beneficial when used as solo agents.[95–97] However, children with recurrent otitis media and a strong family history for allergies should be evaluated by an allergist to identify potential environmental triggers and to implement treatment with a combination of antihistamines, decongestants, and topical intranasal corticosteroids or cromolyn sodium to reduce inflammation and secretions, which could contribute to these recurrent infections.

The use of second-generation over first-generation antagonists as first-line agents is still considered premature by many experts. If a first-generation agent is taken on a regular basis at bedtime, its sedative side effects often are well tolerated by many patients. Of equal importance are their substantially lower cost. However, many patients do not tolerate these agents and require treatment with second-generation nonsedating agents. These agents have been well documented to cause less impairment of cognitive and psychomotor skills such as learning, reaction times, driving, memory, tracking, perception, recognition, and processing.[38] Impairment of these functions increases indirect costs associated with the treatment of allergic rhinitis. Indirect costs include missed days from work or school and decreased concentration and performance while at work, resulting in overall decreased productivity.[38]

ADVERSE EFFECTS OF H₁-ANTAGONISTS

The numerous side effects of first-generation antihistamines have been attributed to their ability to cross the blood–brain barrier. These side effects vary in severity among the structural subclasses. For instance, the ethylenediamines (e.g., Pyribenzamine HCl) have more pronounced gastrointestinal side effects, whereas the ethanolamines (e.g., Benadryl) have increased antimuscarinic activity and cause a greater degree of sedation in patients. The alkylamines (e.g., Chlor-Trimeton) have milder CNS side effects and generally are the best tolerated among the first-generation agents.[98]

Specific side effects of first-generation agents include impaired cognition, slowed reaction times, decreased alertness, confusion, dizziness, tinnitus, anorexia, nausea, vomiting, epigastric distress, diarrhea, and constipation. Associated anticholinergic side effects include dry mouth, blurred vision, and urinary retention.[98] First-generation agents also potentiate the effects of benzodiazepines and alcohol.[10,98] Cyproheptadine, a piperidine, has the unique effect of causing weight gain in some patients.[16]

Intentional and accidental overdose, although uncommon, has been reported with these drugs.[10,14,99] Adults usually manifest symptoms of CNS depression, whereas children may exhibit an excitatory response manifested as hyperactivity, irritability, insomnia, visual hallucinations, and seizures. Even with normal doses, it is not unusual for children to experience a paradoxic excitatory reaction. Malignant cardiac arrhythmias have been known to occur with overdoses, emphasizing the need to act expeditiously to counteract the toxic effect of these agents.[10,14,98,99] Caution should be exercised using antihistamines in elderly patients or in those with liver dysfunction because of their slower clearance rates and increased susceptibility to overdose.[10,14,100] Because these agents are secreted in breast milk, caution should be exercised when using these agents in lactating women to avoid adverse effects in the newborn.[98]

The second-generation agents have substantially fewer associated side effects. Sedation and the side effects associated with first-generation agents has been noted to occur, but to no greater extent than with placebos.[10,14,101] Astemizole, like cyproheptadine, has been associated with increased appetite and weight gain.[10] As discussed earlier, terfenadine and astemizole have been reported to cause rare episodes of torsade de pointes leading to cardiac arrest.[10,17,38,102] Loratadine has a similar side effect profile to the other two second-generation agents, but it has not been found to cause cardiotoxicity.[38] Cetirizine may cause mild sedation in some individuals but has not been associated with cardiotoxicity.

TOLERANCE

Tolerance to antihistamines is a common concern of patients taking these agents chronically. This phenomenon has been speculated to occur because of autoinduction of hepatic metabolism resulting in an accelerated clearance rate of the antihistamine.[103] However, studies have failed to confirm this hypothesis, and most reports of tolerance to antihistamines are believed to be secondary to patient noncompliance because of the drugs' intolerable side effects or breakthrough symptoms caused by severity of disease.[104–107] Short-term studies evaluating tolerance to second-generation agents found no change in their therapeutic efficacy after 6 to 8 weeks of regular use.[108,109] Studies lasting up to 12 weeks found no evidence that second-generation agents cause autoinduction of hepatic metabolism leading to rapid excretion rates and drug tolerance.[38] The clinical efficacy of these agents in the skin and treatment of allergic rhinitis does not decrease with chronic use.

SYMPATHOMIMETICS

Many of the first-generation antihistamines, and now the second generations (Seldane D, Claritin D, Claritin D 24-hour) have been formulated in combination with a decongestant. The decongestants currently used in most preparations predominantly include phenylpropanolamine HCl, phenylephrine HCl, and pseudoephedrine HCl. These agents have saturated benzene rings without 3- or 4-hydroxyl groups, which is the reason for their weak β-adrenergic effect, improved oral absorption, and duration of action. Compared with other decongestants, these agents have less of an effect on blood pressure and are less likely to cause CNS excitation manifested as insomnia or agitation.[110]

H_2-ANTAGONISTS

H_2-antagonists are weak bases with water-soluble hydrochloride salts and tend to be less lipophilic than H_1-antagonists.[3,13–15] The early agents, which were developed for their gastric acid inhibitory properties, either were not strong enough for clinical use or hazardous because of serious associated side effects (e.g., neutropenia, bone marrow suppression).[111,112] Cimetidine (Tagamet, SmithKline, Philadelphia) was introduced to the United States in 1982 and has proven safe and effective in treating peptic ulcer disease.[13–15] Cimetidine and oxmetidine resemble the earliest agents structurally, since they have an imidazole ring similar to histamine's structure. The newer agents vary structurally by having different internal ring components. For example, ranitidine (Zantac) has a furan ring, whereas famotidine (Pepcid) and nizatidine (Axid) are composed of thiozole rings.[13–15] H_2-antagonists act primarily by competitive inhibition of the H_2 receptors, with the exception of famotidine, which works noncompetitively.[15] The four available H_2-antagonists all have potent H_2-antagonistic properties, varying mainly in their pharmacokinetics, and adverse effects such as drug interactions. Because of this, some of the newer agents have been considered to be more desirable for clinical use.[3,15] All of these agents are now available without a prescription.

Numerous studies have been undertaken to examine the clinical utility of H_2-antagonists in allergic and immunologic diseases. Although several studies report these agents as having promising immunologic changes in vitro, these findings have not been substantiated clinically.[3,22,113–117] Generally, H_2-antagonists have limited or no use in treating allergen-induced and histamine-mediated diseases in man.[118–121] One notable exception to this rule may be their use in combination with H_1-antagonists in the treatment of chronic idiopathic urticaria.[122] The studies evaluating the H_2-antagonist's clinical efficacy in allergic and immunologic disorders are extensively reviewed elsewhere.[3,117]

H_3-RECEPTOR ANTAGONISTS

The existence of H_3-receptors was first suspected by Arrang and associates[9] in 1983 when they found histamine to inhibit, by negative feedback, its own synthesis and release in the brain. These actions by histamine could not be suppressed by H_1 or H_2 antagonists, leading researchers to theorize the existence of a third class of histamine receptors. Subsequent studies have been directed toward finding a selective H_3-antagonist. Two such agents have been synthesized: (1) (R) α-methylhistamine (α-MeHA), a chiral agonist of histamine; (2) and thioperamide, a derivative of imidazolylpiperidine. Both demonstrate H_3-receptor selectivity but remain strictly for experimental use.[9]

CONCLUSIONS

The discovery of H_1-receptor antagonists has proven to be a significant breakthrough in the treatment of allergic diseases. Chemical modifications of these early agents have yielded the second-generation antihistamines, which are of equal antagonistic efficacy but have fewer side effects because of their lipophobic structures. H_2-receptor antagonists have been found to be extremely useful in treating peptic ulcer disease. However, they have been disappointing in the treatment of allergic and immunologic disorders in humans. It is still unclear whether the newer selective nonsedating H_1-antagonists and dual-action antihistamines will provide therapeutic advantages over currently available agents.

Prescription of H_1-antagonists should follow a practical, stepwise approach. Because dozens of antihistamine preparations are available with or without decongestants, physicians should become familiar with all aspects of only a few of these agents from each structural class. Appropriate selection of one of these antihistaminic agents will satisfy the clinical needs in most instances.

REFERENCES

1. Windaus A, Vogt W. Syntheses des imidazolylathylamines. Ber Dtsch Chem Ges 1907;3:3691.
2. Fried JP. Dorland's illustrated medical dictionary. Philadelphia: WB Saunders, 1974.
3. Middleton E, Reed CE, Ellis EF, et al. Allergy principles and practice. St Louis: CV Mosby, 1988.
4. Dale HH, Laidlaw PP. The physiological action of β-imidazolylethylamine. J Physiol 1953;120:528.
5. Riley JF, West GB. The presence of histamine in tissue mast cells. J Physiol 1953;120:528.
6. Ishizaka T. Analysis of triggering events in mast cells for immunoglobulin E–mediated histamine release. J Allergy Clin Immunol 1981;67:90.
7. Ash ASF, Schild HO. Receptors mediating some actions of histamine. Br J Pharmacol Chemother 1966;27:427.
8. Black JW, Duncan WAM, Durant CJ, et al. Definition and antagonism of histamine H_2 receptors. Nature 1977;236:385.
9. Arrang JM, Garbarg M, Lancelot JC, et al. Highly potent and selective ligands for histamine H_3 receptors. Nature 1987;327:117.
10. Simons FER. H_1 receptor antagonists: clinical pharmacology and therapeutics. J Allergy Clin Immunol 1989;84:845.
11. Kozlowski T, Raymond RM, Kouthuis RJ, et al. Microvascular protein efflux: interaction of histamine and H_1 receptors. Proc Soc Exp Biol Med 1981;166:263.
12. Dobbins DE, Swindall BT, Haddy FJ, Dabney JM. Blockade of histamine-mediated increased in microvascular permeability by H_1- and H_2-receptor antagonists. Microvasc Res 1981;21:343.
13. Duncan WAM, Parsons ME. Reminiscences of the development of cimetidine. Gastroenterology 1980;78:620.
14. Ganellin CR. Medicinal chemistry and dynamic structure-activity analysis in the discovery of drugs acting as histamine H_2-receptors. J Med Chem 1981;24:913.
15. Lipsy RJ, Fennerty B, Fagan TC. Clinical review of histmanine$_2$ receptor antagonists. Arch Intern Med 1990;150:745.
16. Simons FER, Simons KJ. H_1 receptor antagonists: clinical pharmacology and use in allergic disease. Pediatr Clin North Am 1983;30:899.
17. Simons FER, Simons KJ. The pharmacology and use of H_1-receptor-antagonist drugs. N Engl J Med 1994;330:1663.
18. Simons FER, Luciuk GH, Simons KJ. The pharmacokinetics and antihistaminic effects of brompheniraine. J Allergy Clin Immunol 1982;70:458.
19. Simons FER, Frith EM, Simons KJ. The pharmacokinetics and antihistaminic effects of brompheniramine. J Allergy Clin Immunol 1982;70:458.
20. Simons KJ, Singh M, Gillespie CA, Simons FER. An investigation of the H_1-receptor antagonist triprolidine: pharmacokinetics and antihistaminic effects. J Allergy Clin Immunol 1986;77:326.
21. Simons FER, Simons KJ, Frith EM. The pharmacokinetics and antihistaminic of the H_1 receptor antagonist hydroxyzine. J Allergy Clin Immunol 1984;73:69.
22. Simons FER, Simons KJ. H_1 receptor antagonist treatment of chronic rhinitis. J Allergy Clin Immunol 1988;81:975.
23. Church MK, Gradidge CG. Inhibition of histamine release from human lung *in vitro* by antihistamines and related drugs. Br J Pharmacol 1980;69:663.
24. Physicians' desk reference, 49th ed. Oradell, NJ: Medical Economics, 1995.

25. Fowle ASE, Hughes DTD, Knight GJ. The evaluation of histamine antagonists in man. Eur J Clin Pharmacol 1971;3:215.
26. Kotzan JA, Vallner JJ, Stewart JT, et al. Bioavailability of regular and controlled release chlorpheniramine products. J Pharm Sci 1982;71:919.
27. Yacobi A, Stoll RG, Chao GG, et al. Evaluation of sustained-action chlorpheniramine-pseudoephedrine dosage form in humans. J Pharm Sci 1980;69:1077.
28. Brandon ML, Weiner M. Clinical investigation of terfenadine, a non-sedating antihistamine. Ann Allergy 1980;44:71.
29. Laduron PM, Janssen PFM, Gommeren W, Leysen JE. *In vitro* and *in vivo* binding characteristics of a new long-acting histamine H1 antagonist, astemizole. Mol Pharmacol 1982;21:294.
30. Simons FER, Simons KJ. New H_1 receptor antagonists: a review. Am J Rhinol 1988;2:21.
31. Katz RM. The role of antihistamines in asthma therapy. J Respir Dis 1990;11:517.
32. Okerholm RA, Weiner DL, Hook RH, et al. Bioavailability of terfenadine in man. Biopharm Drug Dispos 1981;2:185.
33. Heykants J, Van Peer A, Woestenborghs R, et al. Dose-proportionality, bioavailability and steady-state kinetics of astemizole in man. Drug Develop Res 1986;8:71.
34. Rihoux JP, DeVos C, Baltes E, deLannory J. Pharmacoclinical investigation of cetirizine: a new potent and well tolerated anti-H_1. Ann Allergy 1985;55:392. Abstract.
35. Wood SG, John GA, Chasseaud JF, et al. The metabolism and pharmacokinetics of ^{14}C-cetirizine in humans. Ann Allergy 1987;59:31.
36. Watson WTA, Simons KJ, Chen XY, Simons FER. Cetirizine: a pharmacokinetic and pharmacodynamic evaluation in children with seasonal allergic rhinitis. J Allergy Clin Immunol 1989;84:457.
37. Hilbert J, Radwanski E, Weglein R, et al. Pharmacokinetics and dose proportionality of loratadine. J Clin Pharmacol 1987;27:694.
38. Meltzer EO, Baraniuk, JN, Barbey J, et al. Antihistamine update: consensus conference. Hosp Pract 1995;31:s1.
39. Richards DM, Brogden RN, Heel RC, et al. Astemizole: a review of its pharmacodynamic properties and therapeutic efficacy. Drugs 1984;28:38.
40. Garteiz DA, Hook RH, Walker BJ, Okerholm RA. Pharmacokinetics and biotransformation studies of terfenadine in man. Arzneimittelforschung 1982;32:1185.
41. Simons FER, Watson WTA, Simons KJ. The pharmacokinetics and pharmacodynamics of terfenadine in children. J Allergy Clin Immunol 1987;80:884.
42. Nicholson AN. Antihistaminic activity and central effects of terfenadine: a review of European studies. Arzneimittelforschung 1982;32:1191.
43. Gendreau-Reid L, Simons KJ, Simons FER. Comparison of the suppressive effect of astemizole, terfenadine and hydroxyzine on histamine-induced wheals and flares in humans. J Allergy Clin Immunol 1986;77:335.
44. Simons FER, et al. A double-blind, single-dose, crossover comparison of cetirizine, terfenadine, loratadine, astemizole and chlorpheniramine versus placebo: suppressive effects on histamine-induced wheals and flares during 24 hours in normal subjects. J Allergy Clin Immunol 1990;86:540.
45. Roth T, Roehrs T, Koshorck G, et al. Sedative effects of antihistamines. J Allergy Clin Immunol 1987;80:94.
46. Chu TJ, Yamate M, Biedermann AA, et al. One versus twice daily dosing of terfenadine in the treatment of seasonal allergic rhinitis: US and European studies. Ann Allergy 1989;63:12.
47. Ryan WM. Evaluation of inhibition of wheal response to histamine by multiple doses of terfenadine. Ann Allergy 1989;63:609.
48. Fields DA, Pillar J, Diamantis W, et al. Inhibition by azelastine of nonallergic histamine release from rat peritoneal mast cells. J Allergy Clin Immunol 1984;74:400.
49. Chand N, Pillar J, Diamantis W, Sofia RD. Inhibition of IgE-mediated allergic histamine release from rat peritoneal mast cells by azelastine and selected anti-allergic drugs. Agents Actions 1985;16:318.
50. Tasaka K, Mio M, Okamoto M. Intracellular calcium release induced by histamine releasers and its inhibition by antiallergic drugs. Ann Allergy 1986;56:464.
51. Lowe DA, Richardson BP, Taylor P, et al. Increasing intracellular sodium triggers calcium release from bound pools. Nature 1976;260:337.
52. Busse W, Randlex B, Sedgwick J. The effect of azelastine on neutrophil and eosinophil generation of superoxide. J Allergy Clin Immunol 1989;83:400.
53. Phillips MJ, Meyrick-Thomas RH, Moodley I, Davies RJ. A comparison of the *in vivo* effects of ketotifen, clemastine, chlorpheniramine and sodium cromoglycate on histamine and allergen induced wheals in human skin. Br J Clin Pharmacol 1983;15:277.
54. Armour C, Temple DM. The modification by ketotifen of respiratory responses to histamine and antigen in guinea pigs. Agents Actions 1982;12:285.
55. Chand N, Diamantis W, Sofia RD. Antagonism of leukotrienes, calcium and histamine by azelastine. Pharmacologist 1984;26:152. Abstract.
56. Chand N, Harrison JE, Rooney SM, et al. Inhibition of passive cutaneous anaphylaxis (PCA) by azelastine: dissociation of its antiallergic activities from antihistaminic and antiserotonin properties. Int J Immunopharmacol 1985;7:833.
57. Van Nueten JM, Xhouneux R, Janssen PAJ. Preliminary data on antiserotonin effects of oxatomide, a novel antiallergic compound. Arch Int Pharmacodyn Ther 1978;232:217.

58. Bechel HJ, Broch N, Lenke D, et al. Pharmacologic and toxicological properties of azelastine, a novel antial- lergic agent. Arzneimittelforschung 1981;31:1184.
59. Ney U, Bretz U, Gradwohl P, Martin U. Further characterization of the antianaphylactic action of ketotifen. Allergol Immunopathol (Madr) 1980;8:380.
60. Diamantis W, Chand N, Harrison JE, et al. Inhibition of release of SRS-A and its antagonism by azelastine, an H1 antagonist-antiallergic agent. Pharmacologist 1982;24:200.
61. Ohmori K, Ishii H, Kubota T, et al. Inhibitory effects of oxatomide on several activities of SRS-A and synthetic leukotrienes in guinea pigs and rats. Arch Int Pharmacodyn Ther 1985;275:139.
62. Martin U, Baggiolini M. Dissociation between the antianaphylactic and the antihistaminic actions of ketotifen. Naunyn Schmiedebergs Arch Pharmacol 1981;316:186.
63. Schwartz JC, Garbarg M, Quach TT. Histamine receptors in brain as targets for tricyclic antidepressants. TIPS 1981.
64. Goldsobel AB, Rohr AS, Siegel SC, et al. Efficacy of doxepin in the treatment of chronic idiopathic urticaria. J Allergy Clin Immunol 1986;78:867.
65. Drouin MA. H_1 antihistamines: perspective of the use of the conventional and new agents. Ann Allergy 1985;55:747.
66. Connell JT, Howard JC, Dressler W, Perhach JL. Antihistamines: findings in clinical trials relevant to thera- peutics. Ann J Rhin 1987;1:3.
67. Wong L, Hendeles L, Weinberger M. Pharmacologic prophylaxis of allergic rhinitis: relative efficacy of hydroxyzine and chlorpheniramine. J Allergy Clin Immunol 1981;67:223.
68. Schaaf L, Hendeles L, Weinberger M. Suppression of seasonal allergic rhinitis symptoms with daily hydrox- yzine. J Allergy Clin Immunol 1979;3:129.
69. Empey DW, Bye C, Hodder M, Hughes DTD. A double-blind crossover trial of pseudoephedrine and triproli- dine: alone and in combination, for the treatment of allergic rhinitis. Ann Allergy 1975;34:41.
70. Diamond L, Gerson K, Cato A, et al. An evaluation of triprolidine and pseudoephedrine in the treatment of allergic rhinitis. Ann Allergy 1981;47:87.
71. Guill MF, Buckley RH, Rocha W, et al. Multicenter, double blind, placebo-controlled trial of terfenadine sus- pension in the treatment of fall-allergic rhinitis in children. J Allergy Clin Immunol 1986;78:4.
72. Sooknundun M, Kacker SK, Sundaran KR. Treatment of allergic rhinitis with a new long-acting H_1 receptor antagonist: astemizole. Ann Allergy 1987;58:78.
73. Kreutner W, Chapman RW, Gulbenkian A, Siegel MI. Antiallergic activity of loratadine, a nonsedating anti- histamine. Allergy 1987;42:57.
74. Howarth PH, Holgate ST. Comparative trial of two nonsedative H_1 antihistamines, terfenadine and astemizole, for hay fever. Thorax 1984;39:668.
75. Juniper EF, White J, Dolovich J. Efficacy of continuous treatment with astemizole (Hismanal) and terfenadine (Seldane) in ragweed pollen-induced rhinoconjunctivitis. J Allergy Clin Immunol 1988;82:670.
76. Doland N. A double-blind study of astemizole and terfenadine in the treatment of perennial rhinitis. Ann Allergy 1988;61:18.
77. Dockhorn RJ, Bergner A, Connell JT, et al. Safety and efficacy of loratadine (Sch-29851): a new non-sedating antihistamine in seasonal allergic rhinitis. Ann Allergy 1987;58:407.
78. Bruttman G, Charpin D, Germouty J, et al. Evaluation of the efficacy and safety of loratadine in perennial aller- gic rhinitis. J Allergy Clin Immunol 1989;83:411.
79. Bruno G, D'Amato G, Del Giacco GS, et al. Prolonged treatment with acrivastine for seasonal allergic rhini- tis. J Int Med Res 1989;17:41B.
80. Gervais P, Bruttman G, Pedrali P, et al. French multicentre double-blind study to evaluate the efficacy and safety of acrivastine as compared with terfenadine in seasonal allergic rhinitis. J Int Med Res 1989;17:47B.
81. Grossman J, Ball R, Shulan D, Spickerman V. Cetirizine vs terfenadine in the treatment of seasonal allergic rhinitis. Kansas City, MO: Marion Merrell Dow, Inc. Abstract.
82. Skassa-Brociek W, Bousquet J, Montes F, et al. Double-blind placebo-controlled study of loratadine mequitazine, and placebo in the symptomatic treatment of seasonal allergic rhinitis. J Allergy Clin Immunol 1988;81:725.
83. Gutkowski A, Bedard P, Del Carpio JB, et al. Comparison of the efficacy and safety of loratadine, terfenadine and placebo in the treatment of seasonal allergic rhinitis. J Allergy Clin Immunol 1988;81:902.
84. Zuber P, Pecoud A. Effect of levocabastine, a new H1 antagonist, in a conjunctival provocation test with aller- gens. J Allergy Clin Immunol 1988;82:590.
85. Simons FER, Simons KJ, Becker AB, Haydey RP. Pharmacokinetics and antipruritic effects of hydroxyzine in children with atopic dermatitis. J Pediatr 1984;104:123.
86. Wanderer AA, St. Pierre JP, Ellis EF. Primary acquired cold urticaria: double blind study of treatment with cryproheptadine, chlorpheniramine and placebo. Arch Dermatol 1977;113:1375.
87. Bernstein IL, Bernstein DI. Efficacy and safety of astemizole, a long-acting and nonsedating H1 antagonist for the treatment of chronic idiopathic urticaria. J Allergy Clin Immunol 1986;77:37.
88. Fox RW, Lockey RF, Burkantz SC, Serbousek D. The treatment of mild to severe chronic idiopathic urticaria with astemizole: double-blind and open trials. J Allergy Clin Immunol 1986;78:1159.
89. Sly MR, Kemp JP, Anderson JA, et al. Position statement: the use of antihistamines in patients with asthma. J Allergy Clin Immunol 1988;82:481.
90. Pierson WE, Virant FS. Antihistamines in asthma. Ann Allergy 1989;63:601.

91. Rafferty P. The European experience with antihistamines in asthma. Ann Allergy 1989;63:389.
92. Rafferty P, Holgate ST. Histamine and its antagonists in asthma. J Allergy Clin Immunol 1989;84:144.
93. Ollier S, Gould CAL, Davies RJ. The effect of single and multiple dose therapy with azelastine on the immediate asthmatic response to allergen provocation testing. J Allergy Clin Immunol 1986;78:358.
94. Rafferty P, Harrison J, Aurich R, Holgate ST. The *in vivo* potency and selectivity of azelastine as an H_1 histamine-receptor antagonist in human airways and skin. J Allergy Clin Immunol 1988;82:1113.
95. Cantekin EL, Mandel EM, Bluestone CD, et al. Lack of efficacy of a decongestant-antihistamine combination of otitis media with effusion in children. N Engl J Med 1987;316:432.
96. Mandel EM, Rockette HE, Bluestone CD, et al. Efficacy of amoxicillin with and without decongestant antihistamine for otitis media with effusion in children. N Engl J Med 1987;316:432.
97. Gaffey MJ, Gwaltney JM, Sastre A, et al. Intranasally and orally administered antihistamine treatment of experimental rhinovirus colds. Am Rev Respir Dis 1987;136:556.
98. Schuller DE, Turkewitz D. Adverse effects of antihistamines. Postgrad Med 1986;79:75.
99. Wyngaarden JB, Seevers MH. The toxic effects of antihistaminic drugs. JAMA 1951;145:277.
100. Simons FER, Watson WTA, Chen XY, et al. The pharmacokinetics and pharmacodynamics of hydroxyzine in patients with primary biliary cirrhosis. J Clin Pharmacol 1989;29:809.
101. Nicholson AN. Antihistamines and sedation. Lancet 1982;ii:211.
102. Simons FER, Kesselman MS, Giddens NG, et al. Astemizole-induced torsades de pointes. Lancet 1988;ii:624.
103. Burns JJ, Conney AH, Koster R. Stimulatory effect of chronic drug administration on drug and metabolizing enzymes in liver microsomes. Ann NY Acad Sci 1963;104:881.
104. Simons KJ, Simons FER. The effect of chronic administration of hydroxyzine on hydroxyzine pharmacokinetics in dogs. J Allergy Clin Immunol 1987;79:928.
105. Kemp JB. Tolerance to antihistamines: is it a problem? Ann Allergy 1989;63:621.
106. Taylor RJ, Long WF, Nelson HS. The development of subsensitivity to chlorpheniramine. J Allergy Clin Immunol 1985;76:103.
107. Bantz EW, Dolen WK, Chadwick EW, Nelson HS. Chronic chlorpheniramine therapy: subsensitivity, drug metabolism and compliance. Ann Allergy 1987;59:341.
108. Simons FER, Watson WTA, Simons KJ. Lack of subsensitivity to terfenadine during long-term terfenadine treatment. J Allergy Clin Immunol 1988;82:1068.
109. Roman IJ, Kassem N, Gural RP, Herron J. Suppression of histamine-induced wheal response by loratadine (SCH 29851) over 28 days in man. Ann Allergy 1986;57:253.
110. Paull BR. The role of decongestants in allergic rhinitis management. J Respir Dis 1989;(suppl):S13.
111. Durant GJ, Parsons ME, Black JW. Potential histamine H_2 receptor antagonists: 2N α-guanylhistamine. J Med Chem 1975;18:830.
112. Forest JAH, Shearman DJC, Spence R, Celestin LR. Neupenia associated with metiomide. Lancet 1975;i:392. Letter.
113. Holmberg K, Pipkorn U, Bake B, Blychert LO. Effects of topical treatment H_1 and H_2 antagonists on clinical symptoms and nasal vascular reactions in patients with allergic rhinitis. Allergy 1989;44:281.
114. Norm S, Permin H, Skov PS. H_2 antihistamines (Cimetidine) and allergic-inflammatory reactions. Allergy 1980;35:357.
115. Gonzalez H, Ahmed T. Suppression of gastric H_2-receptor mediated function in patients with bronchial asthma and ragweed allergy. Chest 1986;4:491.
116. Ahmed T, King MM, Krainson JP. Modification of airway histamine-receptor function with methylprednisolone succinate. J Allergy Clin Immunol 1983;71:224.
117. Festen HPM, DePauw BE, Smeulders J, Wagener DJ. Cimetidine does not influence immunological parameters in man. Clin Immunol Immunopathol 1981;21:33.
118. Thomas RHM, Browne PD, Kirby JDT. The effect of ranitidine, alone and in combination with clemastine, on allergen induced cutaneous wheal and flare reactions in human skin. J Allergy Clin Immunol 1985;76:864.
119. Nathan RA, Segall N, Schocket AL. A comparison of the actions of H_1 and H_2 antihistamines on histamine-induced bronchoconstriction and cutaneous wheal response in asthmatic patients. J Allergy Clin Immunol 1981;67:171.
120. Havas TE, Cole P, Parker L, et al. The effects of combined H_1 and H_2 histamine antagonists on alterations in nasal airflow resistance induced by topical histamine provocation. J Allergy Clin Immunol 1986;78:856.
121. Secher C, Kirkegaard J, Borum P, et al. Significance of H_1 and H_2 receptors in the human nose: rationale for topical use if combined antihistamine preparations. J Allergy Clin Immunol 1982;70:211.
122. Harvey RP, Schocket AL. The effect of H_1 and H_2 blockade on cutaneous histamine response in man. J Allergy Clin Immunol 1980;65:136.

Allergic Diseases, 5th Edition,
edited by Roy Patterson, Leslie Carroll Grammer, and
Paul A. Greenberger. Lippincott–Raven Publishers, Philadelphia, © 1997.

6

Allergens and Other Factors Important in Atopic Disease

Randy J. Horwitz and Robert K. Bush

*R.J. Horwitz: Department of Allergy/Immunology,
University of Wisconsin, Madison, WI 53792.
R.K. Bush: Department of Medicine, University of Wisconsin, Madison, WI 53792;
Wm. S. Middleton VA Hospital, Madison, WI 53705.*

Pearls for Practitioners
Roy Patterson

- Avoiding allergens is the first line of defense against allergen attack. It is not possible with some allergens.
- Cats generally cause more severe allergy than dogs.
- There is often greater reluctance to eliminate a cat from the environment than a dog.
- You may hear: "I would rather give up my spouse than my pet." Take this seriously.
- Immunologically, a person who is allergic to a species of animal should be allergic to all animals of that species. Immunogenetically, a person is more allergic to one breed of a species than another. You will see this relative to cats and dogs.
- Know the pollens and their seasons in the geographic area in which you practice.
- No, you don't have to test for dozens of different weed, grass, and trees problems or mold spores.

A knowledge of the pathophysiologic mechanisms of the allergic response is essential to the understanding and proper treatment of allergic diseases. Too often, however, inadequate attention is paid to the nature of the allergen in an allergic response. The first and foremost treatment recommendation for allergies is avoidance of the trigger. Such advice is impossible to render without an intimate familiarity with the nature of common environmental allergens. This chapter presents a comprehensive yet lucid overview of allergen biology for the clinician. It is said that the key to winning a war is to "know thine enemy." Prepare to meet some of the primary perpetrators of allergic disease.

An allergen is an antigen that produces a clinical allergic reaction. In atopic diseases, allergens are antigens that elicit an IgE antibody response. The presence of such an allergen can be demonstrated by a wheal-and-flare reaction to that antigen in a skin test, or by in vitro immunoassays such as the radioallergosorbent test (RAST), which measures antigen-specific IgE in serum. Other methods, usually restricted to research laboratories, also may be used to demonstrate the presence of specific IgE antibody. These include enzyme-linked immunoassay (ELISA), crossed radioimmunoelectrophoresis (CRIE), immunoblotting technique, and leukocyte histamine release assay. When assessing the contribution of a particular antigen to an observed symptom, the nature of the immune response must be clarified. The clinician must differentiate the allergic (or atopic) response from the nonallergic immune response to certain drug or microbial antigens that induce the formation of other antibody isotypes (e.g., IgG or IgA). The allergic response also demonstrates a distinct pathophysiologic mechanism compared with that seen in delayed hypersensitivity reactions, which result from contact antigens.

Allergens most commonly associated with atopic disorders are inhalants or foods, reflecting the most common entry sites into the body. Drugs, biologic products, insect venoms, and certain chemicals also may induce an immediate-type reaction. In practice, however, most atopic reactions involve pollens, fungal spores, house dust mites, animal epithelial materials, and other substances that impinge directly on the respiratory mucosa. The allergenic molecules generally are water soluble and can be easily leached from the airborne particles. They react with IgE antibodies attached to mast cells, initiating a series of pathologic steps that result in allergic symptoms. This chapter is confined to the exploration of these naturally occurring inhalant substances; other kinds of allergens are discussed elsewhere in this text.

The chemical nature of certain allergens has been studied intensively, although the precise composition of many other allergens remains undefined.[1] For an increasing number of allergens, such as the major house dust mite allergen or the fire ant venom, the cDNA sequence has been derived. For others, the physiochemical characteristics or the amino acid sequence is known. Still other allergens are known only as complex mixtures of proteins and polypeptides with varying amounts of carbohydrate. Details of the chemistry of known allergens are described under their appropriate headings.[2]

The methods of purifying and characterizing allergens include biochemical, immunologic, and biologic techniques. The methods of purification involve various column fractionation techniques, newer immunologic techniques such as the purification of allergens by monoclonal antibodies, and the techniques of molecular biology for synthesizing various proteins. All of these purification techniques rely on sensitive and specific assay techniques for the allergen. Specific approaches are discussed in this chapter.

AEROALLERGENS

Aeroallergens are airborne particles that can cause respiratory, cutaneous, or conjunctival allergy (Table 6-1). The water-soluble portion of ragweed pollen, for example, affects the respiratory and conjunctival mucosa, and the lipid-soluble allergens of ragweed pollen may cause a typical contact dermatitis on exposed skin. This ragweed dermatitis is caused by a lymphocyte-mediated immunologic mechanism. Aeroallergens are named using nomenclature established by an International Union of Immunologic Societies subcommittee: the first three letters of the genus, followed by the first letter of the species and an Arabic numeral indicative of the order of discovery.[3] Thus, *Amb a 1* was the first allergen purified from the ragweed plant *Ambrosia artemisifolia*.

For a particle to be clinically significant as an aeroallergen, it must be buoyant, present in significant numbers, and allergenic. Ragweed pollen is a typical example. Pine pollen, by contrast, is abundant in certain regions and is buoyant, but, because it does not readily elicit IgE antibodies, it is not a significant aeroallergen. In general, the insect-pollinated plants do not produce appreciable amounts of airborne pollen, as opposed to wind-pollinated plants, which, by necessity, produce particles that travel for miles. Fungal spores are ubiquitous, highly allergenic, and may be more numerous than pollen grains in the air, even during the height of the pollen season. The omnipresence of house dust mite needs no emphasis. The knowledge of what occurs where and when is essential to treating the allergy. The above aller-

TABLE 6-1. *Commonly encountered allergens*

Source (common name)	Taxonomic name	Purified allergens
Trees		
Birch	*Betula verrucosa*	Bet v 1, Bet v 2, Calmodulin
Alder	*Alnus glutinosa*	Aln g 1
Hazel	*Corylus avellana*	Cor a 1
White oak	*Quercus alba*	Que a 1
Olive	*Olea europa*	Ole e 1
Japanese cedar	*Cryptomeria japonica*	Cry j 1, Cry j 2
Hornbeam	*Carpinus betulus*	Car b 1
Weeds		
Short ragweed	*Ambrosia artemisiifolia*	Amb a 1–7, Cystatin
Giant ragweed	*Ambrosia trifida*	Amb t 5
Western ragweed	*Ambrosia psilostachya*	Amb p 5
Russian thistle	*Salsola pestifer*	Sal p 1
Mugwort	*Artemis vulgaris*	Art v 1–2
Coccharia	*Parietaria judacia*	Par j 1
Grasses		
Ryegrass	*Lolium perene*	Lol p 1–3, 10, 11
Timothy grass	*Phleum pratense*	Phl p 5, Phl p 6
Orchard grass	*Dactylis glomerata*	Dac g 1, Dac g 5
Kentucky bluegrass	*Poa pratensis*	Poa p 10
Bermuda grass	*Cynodon dactylon*	Cyn d 1
Fungi		
—	*Alternaria alternanta*	Alt a 1
—	*Aspergillus fumigatus*	Asp f 1
—	*Cladosporium herbarum*	Cla h 1–6
—	*Trichophyton tonsurans*	Tri t 1
Dust mites		
Dust mite	*Dermatophagoides farinae, pteronyssinus*	Der f 1–2, Der p 1–4
Animals		
Cat	*Felis domesticus*	Fel d 1
Dog	*Canis familiaris*	Can f 1
Horse	*Equus cabalus*	Equ c 1–2
Mouse	*Mus musculus*	Mus m 1
Rat	*Rattus norwegicus*	Rat n 1–2
Insects (excluding venoms)		
Nimitti fly	*Chironimus thummi*	Chi t 1
German cockroach	*Blattella germanica*	Bla g 1–2
American cockroach	*Periplaneta americana*	Per a 1

gens are emphasized because they are the ones most commonly encountered, and they are considered responsible for most of the morbidity among atopic patients.

Certain aeroallergens, such as animal dander, feathers, and epidermal antigens, may be localized to individual homes. Others may be associated with occupational exposures, as is the case in veterinarians who work with certain animals (e.g., cats), in farmers who encounter a variety of pollens and fungi in hay and stored grains, in exterminators who use pyrethrum, in dock workers who unload coffee beans and castor beans from the holds of ships, and in bakers who inhale flour. Some sources of airborne allergens are narrowly confined geographically, such as the mayfly and the caddis fly, whose scales and body parts are a cause of respiratory allergy in the eastern Great Lakes area in the late summer. In addition, endemic asthma has been reported in the vicinity of factories where cottonseed and castor beans are processed.

Aeroallergen particle size is an important element of allergic disease. Airborne pollens are in the range of 20 to 60 μm in diameter; mold spores usually vary between 3 and 30 μm in diameter or longest dimension; dust particles are 1 to 10 μm. Protective mechanisms in the nasal mucosa and upper tracheobronchial passages remove most of the larger particles, so only those 3 μm or smaller reach the alveoli of the lungs. Hence, the conjunctivae and upper respiratory passages receive the largest dose of airborne allergens. These are considerations in the pathogenesis of allergic rhinitis, bronchial asthma, and hypersensitivity pneumonitis as well as the irritant effects of chemical and particulate atmospheric pollutants.

The development of asthma after pollen exposure is enigmatic because pollen grains are deposited in the upper airways as a result of their large particle size. Experimental evidence suggests that rhinitis, but not asthma, is caused by inhalation of whole pollen in amounts encountered naturally.[4] Asthma caused by bronchoprovocation with solutions of pollen extracts is easily achieved in the laboratory, however. Pollen asthma may be cause by the inhalation of pollen debris that is small enough to access the bronchial tree.

Evidence supports this hypothesis. Extracts of materials collected on an 8-μm filter that exclude ragweed pollen grains induced positive skin test results in ragweed-sensitive subjects. These same extracts can specifically inhibit an anti-ragweed IgG–ELISA system.[5] Using an immunochemical method of identifying atmospheric allergens, *Amb a 1* was found to exist in ambient air in the absence of ragweed pollen grains.[6] Positive bronchoprovocation was induced with pollen grains that had been fragmented in a ball mill, but was not induced by inhalation of whole ragweed pollen grains.[7] However, despite the generally accepted limitations previously mentioned, examination of tracheobronchial aspirates and surgical lung specimens has revealed large numbers of whole pollen grains in the lower respiratory tract.[8] Hence, the mechanism of pollen-induced asthma is still an open question.

Another consideration is the rapidity with which various allergens are leached out of the whole pollen grains. The mucous blanket of the respiratory tract has been estimated to transport pollens into the gastrointestinal tract in less than 10 minutes. The allergens of grass pollens and ragweed *Amb a 5* are extracted rapidly from the pollen grains in aqueous solutions and can be absorbed through the respiratory mucosa before the pollen grains are swallowed. Ragweed *Amb a 1*, however, is extracted slowly, and only a small percentage of the total extractable *Amb a 1* is released from the pollen grain in this time frame.[9] This observation has not been reconciled with the presumed importance of *Amb a 1* in clinical allergy, but absorption may be more rapid in the more alkaline mucus found in allergic rhinitis.[10]

Sampling Methods for Airborne Allergens

Increasing attention is being paid to the daily levels of airborne allergen detected in a particular locale. Patients commonly seek out daily reports of ragweed or *Alternaria* levels, frequently reported in newspapers and on television, to correlate and predict their allergy symptoms. The clinician must be acquainted with the various sampling techniques used to accurately assess the validity and accuracy of the readings reported.

Aerobiologic sampling attempts to identify and quantify the allergenic particles in the ambient atmosphere, both outdoors and indoors. Commonly, an adhesive substance is applied to a microscope slide or other transparent surface, and the pollens and spores that stick to the surface are microscopically enumerated. Devices of varying complexity have been used to reduce the most common sampling errors relating to particle size, wind velocity, and rain. Fungi also may be sampled by culture techniques. Excellent resources for these methods are available.[11-13]

Although many laboratories use various immunoassays to identify and quantify airborne allergens, the microscopic examination of captured particles remains the method of choice. Three types of sampling devices are most commonly used: gravitational, impaction, and suction.

Gravitational Samplers

Gravitational settling samplers were the first devices employed to analyze airborne pollen content. They are still occasionally used because they are simple and inexpensive. The Durham sampler is the prototype. It consists of a pair of parallel circular plates 7.5 cm (3 inches) apart. A prepared microscope slide is placed on a holder 2.5 cm (1 inch) above the lower plate and exposed for 24 hours. The slide is stained, usually with an alcoholic solution of basic fuchsin (Calberla's stain), and the pollen grains and fungal spores are counted and identified. The stain both expands the pollens and colors them red, rendering their morphologic features more prominent. Counts usually are expressed as particles per square centimeter after suitable calibration of the microscope stage. Another method is to divide the number of particles found under a 22 × 22 mm cover slip by 4.84, to give the number of particles per square centimeter. This sampling technique is more qualitative than quantitative because it is highly dependent on wind speed and orientation of the samples, and the volume of air sampled over the 24-hour period cannot be ascertained. Although a historical debt is owed to the Durham sampler for most of our knowledge of aerobiology, physicians should realize that this sampling method is considered the most primitive and currently is seldom used.

Impaction Samplers

Impaction samplers currently are the most common types of pollen samplers in use. The principle is that wind speed usually is greater than the rate of gravitational settling. Small particles carried by the wind have an inertial force that causes them to impact on an adhesive surface. If the diameter of the surface is small (e.g., 1 to several millimeters), there is little turbulence to deflect the particles. Thus, the smaller the impacting surface, the higher the rate of impaction. Small surface areas, however, are rapidly overloaded, causing a decrease in the efficiency of capture.

The rotating impaction sampler has two vertical collecting arms mounted on a crossbar, which is rotated by a vertical motor shaft. The speed of rotation is up to several thousand revolutions per minute and is nearly independent of wind velocity. The plastic collecting rods are coated with silicone adhesive. These samplers usually are run intermittently (20 to 60 seconds every 10 minutes) to reduce overloading. In some models, the impacting arms are retracted or otherwise protected while not in use. The Rotorod sampler (Fig. 6-1) is a commercially available impaction sampler and has been shown to be over 90% efficient at capturing pollen particles of approximately 20 μm diameter.

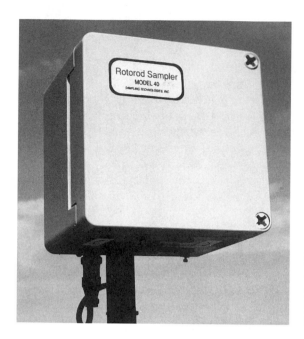

FIG. 6-1. Rotating impaction sampler: Rotorod sampler model 40 (Sampling Technologies, Minnetonka, MN). (Courtesy of Medical Media Service, Wm. Middleton Memorial Veteran's Hospital, Madison, WI.)

Suction Samplers

Suction samplers employ a vacuum pump to draw the air sample into the device. Although suitable for pollens, they are more commonly used to measure smaller particles such as mold spores. Disorientation with wind direction and velocity skews the impaction efficiencies of particles of different sizes. For example, if the wind velocity is less than that generated by the sampler, smaller particles are collected in greater concentrations than exist in the ambient air. The reverse is true for greater wind velocities. The Hirst spore trap is an inertial suction sampler with a clock mechanism that moves a coated slide at a set rate along an intake orifice. This enables discrimination of diurnal variations. A wind vane orients the device to the direction of the wind. The Burkard spore trap collects particles on an adhesive-coated drum that takes 1 week to make a full revolution around an intake orifice. Both of these spore traps are designed to measure nonviable material. Spore traps are the most flexible devices for sampling particles over a wide range of sizes.

The Anderson sampler is another suction device, but it is unique in its adaptability for enumerating viable fungal spores. Air passes through a series of sieve-like plates (either two or six), each containing 400 holes. While the air moves from plate to plate, the diameter of the holes decreases. The larger particles are retained by the upper plates and the smaller ones by successive lower plates. A Petri dish containing growth medium is placed beneath each sieve plate, and the spores that pass through the holes fall onto the agar and form colonies. This method has value for identifying fungi whose spore morphologic features do not permit microscopic identification. In general, however, nonviable volumetric collection techniques more accurately reflect the actual spore prevalence than do volumetric culture methods.[11]

The volume of air sampled is easy to calculate for suction devices because the vacuum pumps may be calibrated. In the case of rotation impaction samplers, there are formulas that depend on the surface area of the exposed bar of slide, the rate of revolution, and the exposure time. After the adherent particles are stained and counted, their numbers can be expressed as particles per cubic meter of air. Gravitational samplers cannot be quantified volumetrically.

The location of samplers is important. Ground level is usually unsatisfactory because of liability, tampering, and similar considerations. Rooftops are used most frequently. The apparatus should be placed at least 6 m (20 ft) away from obstructions and 90 cm (3 ft) higher than the parapet on the roof.

Several adhesives are used in pollen collectors with good results.[14] Silicone stopcock grease (Sampling Technologies, Minnetonka, MN) or petrolatum and Lubriseal stopcock grease (A.H. Thomas, Philadelphia) are used most often. Rubber cement, silicone oil, and glycerin are less reliable because their properties change with desiccation, humidity, and temperature. The methods of staining, enumerating, and calculating are beyond the scope of this discussion but are detailed in the references.

Fungal Culture

Fungi also may be studied by culture techniques. This is often necessary because many spores are not morphologically distinct enough for microscopic identification. In such cases, characteristics of the fungal colonies are required. Most commonly, Petri dishes with appropriate nutrient agar are exposed to the air at a sampling station for 5 to 30 minutes. The plates are incubated at room temperature for about 5 days, then inspected grossly and microscopically for the numbers and types of colonies present. Cotton-blue is a satisfactory stain for fungal morphologic identification. Potato-dextrose agar supports growth of most allergenic fungi, and rose bengal may be added to retard bacterial growth and limit the spread of fungal colonies. Specialized media such as Czapek agar may be used to look for particular organisms (e.g., *Aspergillus* or *Penicillium*).

The chief disadvantage of the culture plate method is a gross underestimation of the spore count. This may be offset by using a suction device such as the Anderson or Burkhard sampler. A microconidium containing many spores still grows only one colony. There may be mutual inhibition or massive overgrowth of a single colony such as *Rhizopus nigricans*. Other disadvantages are short sampling times, as well as the fact that some fungi (rusts and smuts) do not grow on ordinary nutrient media. Furthermore, avoiding massive spore contamination of the laboratory is difficult without precautions such as an isolation chamber and ventilation hood.

Immunologic Methods

Numerous immunologic methods of identifying and quantifying airborne allergens have been developed recently. In general, these methods are too complex to replace the physical pollen count. The immunologic assays do not depend on the morphologic features of the material sampled, but on the ability of eluates of this material collected on filters to interact in immunoassays with human IgE or IgG[15] or with mouse monoclonal antibodies.[16] Studies at the Mayo Clinic have employed a high-volume air sampler that retains 95% of particles larger than 0.3 μm on a fiberglass filter. The antigens, of unknown composition, are eluted from the filter sheet by descending chromatography. The eluate is dialyzed, lyophilized, and reconstituted as needed. This material is analyzed by RAST inhibition for specific allergenic activity or, in the case of antigens that may be involved in hypersensitivity pneumonitis, by interaction with IgG antibodies. The method is extremely sensitive. An eluate equivalent to 0.1 mg of pollen produced 40% to 50% inhibition in the short ragweed RAST. An equivalent amount of 24 µg of short ragweed pollen produced over 40% inhibition in the *Amb a 1* RAST.[17] The allergens identified using this method have correlated with morphologic studies of pollen and fungal spores using traditional methods and with patient symptom scores. The eluates also have produced positive results on prick skin tests in sensitive human subjects.[6] These techniques demonstrate that with short ragweed, different-sized particles from ragweed plant debris can act as a source of allergen in the air before and after the ragweed pollen season. Furthermore, appreciable ragweed allergenic activity has been associated with particles less than 1 µm in diameter.[18]

Use of low-volume air samples that do not disturb the air and development of a sensitive two-site monoclonal antibody immunoassay for the major cat allergen (*Fel d 1*) have made accurate measurements of airborne cat allergen possible.[16] These studies confirm that a high proportion of *Fel d 1* is carried on particles smaller than 2.5 µm. During house cleaning, the amount of the small allergen-containing particles in the air approached that produced by a nebulizer for bronchial provocation (40 ng/m^3). The results indicate that significant airborne *Fel d 1* is associated with small particles that remain airborne for long periods. This is in contrast to prior studies with house dust mites[19] in which the major house dust mite allergen *Der p 1* was collected on large particles with diameters greater than 10 µm. Little of this allergen remained airborne when the room was disturbed.

In other studies, nonparticulate ragweed material collected on 0.8 µm filters inhibited an anti-ragweed IgG–ELISA system and produced positive skin test results in ragweed-sensitive individuals.[11] Liquid impingers that draw air through a liquid system also can be used to recover soluble material.

Many pollen grains may be difficult to distinguish morphologically by normal light microscopic study. Immunochemical methods may permit such distinctions. Grass pollen grains collected from a Burkard trap were blotted onto nitrocellulose; then, by using specific antisera to Bermuda grass, a second antibody with a fluorescent label, and a fluorescent microscope study, Bermuda grass pollen grains could be distinguished from grass pollens of other species.[20] These newer methods show promise because they measure allergenic materials that react in the human IgE system. Currently, immunochemical assays to quantify the major house dust mite allergens *Der p 1* and *Der f 1* and the major cat allergen *Fel d 1* are commercially available (ALK America, Milford, CT). Further studies with these techniques may lead to a better understanding of exposure–symptom relationships.

STANDARDIZATION OF ALLERGENIC EXTRACTS

The need to standardize allergenic extracts has been recognized for many years. Variability in antigen composition and concentration is a major problem in both allergy testing and allergen immunotherapy regimens. Without standardization of extracts, there is no accurate system of quality control. The clinician often is forced to alter immunotherapy schedules with each new vial of extract because of lot-to-lot variability. Each allergen extract supplier uses its own assays and rarely compares specific antigen concentrations with competitors. The result of this disparity is that the clinician must bring more art than science to the field of allergen immunotherapy. Fortunately, this is changing. The development of purified and even cloned allergens that can be expressed in bacteria or yeast hosts have allowed the production of vast quantities of allergen extract with little or no variance between batches.[21–26] With investigators, clinicians, and government agencies that license extracts demanding improved standardization, it is expected that more progress in this area of allergy will be made in the near future.

Quantitation of Allergens

The complexity of biologic material and the extreme sensitivity of the IgE system, which requires only nanogram amounts of allergen, have made standardization of aeroallergens most difficult. The traditional method of standardizing and preparing allergens for clinical use is to extract a known weight of defatted pollen in a specified volume of fluid. For example, 1 g in 100 mL of fluid would yield a 1% (1:100) solution. This weight per volume system still is one of the most commonly used in clinical practice. This solution can be concentrated or diluted as needed. A unit system has been assigned such that 1 mL of a 1:1,000,000 solution contains 1 pollen unit (Noon unit); or 1 Noon pollen unit contains 0.001 mg of extracted pollen.

Another system of measurement, preferred by some allergists and extract manufacturers, is the protein–nitrogen unit (PNU). The basis of the PNU system is the fact that most allergenic moieties of pollens are proteins, and that the ratio of protein to dry weight of pollen varies from plant to plant. In this method, nitrogen is precipitated by phosphotungstic acid and measured by the micro-Kjeldahl technique. Total nitrogen is another method of standardization, but it offers no advantage and is used infrequently.

Both of these methods are used for other inhalant and food allergens, and clinicians generally must communicate in terms of these standards. Unfortunately, neither the weight per volume method nor the protein–nitrogen unit truly measures allergenic activity, because not all measured proteins and extractable components in the solution are allergenic. In addition, many complex allergens are destroyed during the harsh extraction procedure. Such problems have been circumvented through the use of biological assays of "functional" allergen reactivity. Currently, ragweed pollen, grass pollen, house dust mite, and cat allergen extracts are standardized, and their activity is expressed in allergen units (AU) or biological allergenic units (BAU). Other allergen concentrations may be added to this list in the future. It is essential for anyone devising desensitization regimens to have an appreciation for the biological assays of allergenicity. These assays are described later.

Characterization of Allergens

Many methods are available to characterize an allergen. Many of these, such as the determination of protein content, molecular weight, and isoelectric point, are not unique to the study of allergenic compounds. These are simply methods of describing any protein. Several categories of tests, however, are restricted to studying molecules responsible for IgE-mediated symptoms. Both immunologic in vitro methods, such as RAST and Western blotting, as well as in vivo biological assays, such as endpoint dilution skin tests, will be considered here.

Radioallergosorbent Test

The RAST is described elsewhere in this text. Although primarily used in the quantitation of antigen-specific IgE, the test may be adapted to determine antigen concentrations. To measure potency, the unknown allergen is immobilized onto solid-phase supports (cellulose disks or beads) and reacted with a known quantity of antigen-specific IgE in a standard test system. For comparison, the extracts are compared with a reference standard, which should be carefully chosen.[27] The quantity of extract required to obtain a specified degree of reactivity is determined. By definition, in this assay, the greater the binding of IgE to the antigen, the greater the allergenicity.

RAST Inhibition Assay

The most widely used assay for in vitro potency of allergenic extract is the RAST inhibition method. This test is a variation of the direct RAST. Serum from an allergic individual (containing IgE) is first mixed with the soluble unknown allergen. Next, a standard amount of the solid-phase (immobilized) allergen is added. The more "potent" the fluid phase allergen, the less IgE is free to bind to the solid-phase allergen.[28] The technique and its statistical analysis have been standardized. RAST inhibition usually is the key technique to assess total allergenic activity of an extract and is used by manufacturers to calibrate new batches by comparison with the in-house reference preparation. Recently, some workers have raised concern regarding the continued use of RAST inhibition as a standard technique.[29] The arguments concern the fact that the choice of antigen for the solid-phase reaction is variable and may influence results. In addition, the finite supply of allergenic reference sera limits reproducibility: without identical reference sera and immobilized allergen, comparisons are impossible.

Assessment of Allergenicity

Biochemical methods for analyzing allergens, such as protein composition and concentration, are practical but tell nothing about the allergenicity of the extract. Immunologic reactivity with IgE antibodies as assessed in vitro and in vivo provide this information. Preparations of inhalant allergens contain more than one antigen. Of the several antigens in a mixture, usually one or more dominate in both frequency and intensity of skin reactions in sensitive persons. It is inferred from this that these antigens are the most important clinically. Not all persons allergic to a certain pollen allergen react to the same antigens from that pollen allergen extract, however. The antigens of tree, grass, and weed pollens are immunologically distinct, and this agrees with the clinical and skin test data. As more allergens are isolated and purified, it is hoped that correlations between immunogenicity and biochemical structure will emerge.

Marsh[9] proposed that a major allergen be designated when 90% of clinically allergic persons react by skin test to a concentration of 0.001 µg/mL or less of that particular extractable allergen. Others suggest that a component that binds IgE in 50% or more of sensitive patient sera tested by radioimmunoelectrophoresis (another immunologic assay) should be considered a major allergen.[30] This definition currently is widely accepted. A minor allergen would be one that does not meet either of these criteria.

Naturally occurring atopic allergens have few physicochemical characteristics to distinguish them from other antigens. All are proteins or glycoproteins, although high molecular weight polysaccharides that react with IgE have been obtained from *Candida albicans*. Most protein allergens that have been identified are acidic, with molecular weights ranging from 5000 to 60,000 daltons. It has been postulated that larger molecules cannot readily penetrate the mucous membranes. Highly reactive allergens of lower molecular weight are described in conjunction with ragweed and grass pollens. The antigenic determinants that react with IgE antibody molecules have not been clearly identified for most allergens, although it is postulated that there must be at least two such groups on each allergen molecule to trigger the allergic response. The sequence of amino acids in some determinant groups, with less regard for conformation of the protein molecule, is most important for the major codfish antigen *Gad c 1* (codfish antigen M).[31] In other allergens, such as ragweed *Amb a 3* (Ra 3) and *Amb a 5* (Ra 5), the conformation of the native protein is critical for allergenicity.[32]

CLASSIFICATION OF ALLERGENIC PLANTS

The botanical considerations and taxonomic scheme given here are not exhaustive. Individual plants, their common and botanical names, geographical distributions, and relative importance in allergy are considered elsewhere in this book. Excellent sources of information on systematic botany, plant identification, and pollen morphology are listed in the references.[13,33,34]

Anatomy

Seed-bearing plants produce their reproductive structures in cones or flowers. Gymnosperms ("naked seeds") (class Gymnospermae) are trees and shrubs that bear their seeds in cones. Pines, firs, junipers, spruces, yews, hemlocks, savins, cedars, larches, cypresses, retinisporas, and ginkgoes are gymnosperms. Angiosperms produce seeds enclosed in the female reproductive structures of the flower. Angiosperms may be monocotyledons, whose seeds contain one "seed leaf" (cotyledon), or dicotyledons, with two seed leaves. Leaves of monocotyledons have parallel veins, whereas leaves of dicotyledons have branching veins. Grasses are monocotyledons; most other allergenic plants are dicotyledons.

The flower has four fundamental parts:

1. *Pistils* (one or more) are the female portion of the plant and consist of an ovary at the base, a style projecting upward, and a stigma, the sticky portion to which pollen grains adhere.
2. *Stamens*, which are the male portions of the plant, are variable in number and consist of anthers borne on filaments. Pollen grains are produced in the anthers.
3. *Petals*, the colored parts of the flower, vary from three to many in number.
4. *Sepals*, the protective portion of the flower bud, are usually green and three to six in number.

The phylogenetically primitive flower had numerous separate parts, as typified by the magnolia. Fusion of flower parts and reduction of their number is a characteristic of phylogenetic advancement. As a group, dicotyledons are more primitive than monocotyledons.

A "perfect" flower contains both male and female organs; an "imperfect" flower contains only stamens or only pistils. Monoecious ("one house") plants bear both stamens and pistils; the individual flowers may be perfect or imperfect. Dioecious ("two houses") plants have imperfect flowers, and all flowers on a particular plant are the same type (male and female). Ragweed is a monoecious plant with perfect flowers; corn is a monoecious plant with imperfect flowers; willows are dioecious plants. Like the flowering plants, gymnosperms may be either monoecious (pines) or dioecious (cypresses and ginkgoes).

Taxonomy

Plants are classified in a hierarchical system. The principal ranks, their endings, and some examples are as follows:

Class (–ae): Angiospermae, Gymnospermae
Subclass (–ae): Monocotyledonae, Dicotyledonae
Order (–ales): Coniferales, Salicales
Suborder (–ineae)
Family (–aceae): Asteraceae, Poaceae
Subfamily (–oideae)

Tribe (–eae)
Genus (no characteristic ending; italicized): *Acer*
Species (genus name plus "specific epithet"): *Acer rubrum*

Trees Gymnosperms

Trees may be gymnosperms or angiosperms. The gymnosperms include two orders, the Coniferales (conifers) and the Ginkgoales. Neither are of particular importance in allergy, but because of the prevalence of conifers and the incidence of their pollens in surveys, some comments are in order.

Conifers grow mainly in temperate climates. They have needle-shaped leaves. The following three families are germane to this discussion.

Pinaceae (Pines, Spruces, Firs, Hemlocks)

Pines are monoecious evergreens whose leaves are arranged in bundles of two to five and are enclosed at the base by a sheath (all other members of the Pinaceae bear leaves singly, not in bundles). The pollen grains of pines are 45 to 65 μm in diameter and have two bladders (Fig. 6-2). This pollen occasionally has been implicated in allergy.[33] Spruces produce pollen grains morphologically similar to pine pollen but much larger, ranging from 70 to 90 μm exclusive of the bladders. Hemlock pollen grains may have bladders, depending on the species. The firs produce even larger pollen grains, ranging from 80 to 100 μm, not including the two bladders.

Cupressiaceae (Junipers, Cypresses, Cedars, Savins)

Most of these trees are dioecious and produce large quantities of round pollen grains 20 to 30 μm in diameter with a thick intine (internal membrane). The mountain cedar is an important cause of allergic rhinitis in certain parts of Texas and has proliferated where the ecosystem has been disturbed by overgrazing of the grasslands.

Taxodiaceae (Bald Cypress, Redwood)

The bald cypress may be a minor cause of allergic rhinitis in Florida.

Trees: Angiosperms

Most allergenic trees are in this group. The more important orders and families are listed here with relevant notations. Other trees have been implicated in pollen allergy, but most of the tree pollinosis in the United States can be attributed to those mentioned here.

Order Salicales, Family Salicaceae (Willows and Poplars)

Willows are mainly insect-pollinated and are not generally considered allergenic (see Fig. 6-2). Poplars, however, are wind-pollinated, and some (e.g., species of *Populus*) are of considerable

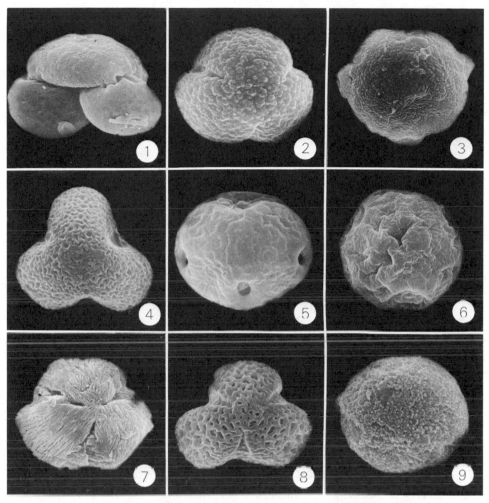

FIG. 6-2. Scanning electron photomicrographs of early spring airborne hayfever-producing pollen grains: 1, pine (*Pinus*); 2, oak (*Quercus*); 3, birch (*Betula*); 4, sycamore (*Platanus*); 5, elm (*Ulmus*); 6, hackberry (*Celtis*); 7, maple (*Acer*); 8, willow (*Salix*); 9, poplar (*Populus*). (Courtesy of Professor James W. Walker.)

allergenic importance. Poplar pollen grains are spherical, 27 to 34 μm in diameter, and characterized by a thick intine (see Fig. 6-2). The genus *Populus* includes poplars, aspens, and cottonwoods. Their seeds are borne on buoyant cotton-like tufts that may fill the air in June like a localized snowstorm. Patients often attribute their symptoms to this "cottonwood," but the true cause usually is grass pollens.

Order Betulales, Family Betulaceae (Birches)

Betula species are widely distributed in North America and produce abundant pollen that is highly allergenic. The pollen grains are 20 to 30 μm and flattened, generally with three pores, although some species have as many as seven (Fig. 6-3; see Fig. 6-2). The pistillate catkins may persist into winter, discharging small winged seeds.

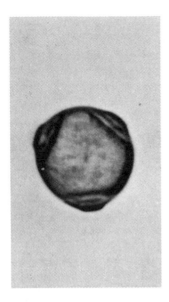

FIG. 6-3. Birch (*Betula nigra*). Average diameter is 24.5 μm. Pollen grains have three pores and a smooth exine. (Courtesy of Center Laboratories, Port Washington, NY.)

Order Fagales, Family Fagaceae (Beeches, Oaks, Chestnuts, Chinquapins)

Five genera of Fagaceae are found in North America, of which only the beeches (*Fagus*) and oaks (*Quercus*) are wind pollinated and of allergenic importance. The pollens of these two genera are morphologically similar but not identical. They are 40 μm in diameter, with an irregular exine (outer covering) and three tapering furrows (Fig. 6-4; see Fig. 6-2). Both produce abundant pollen; oaks in particular cause a great deal of tree pollinosis in areas where they are numerous.

Order Urticales, Family Ulmaceae (Elms, Hackberries)

About 20 species of elms are in the northern hemisphere, mainly distributed east of the Rocky Mountains. They produce large amounts of allergenic pollen and continue to be a major cause

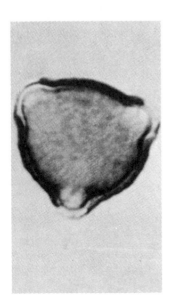

FIG. 6-4. Oak (*Quercus* sp). Average diameter is 32 mm. Pollens of the various species are similar, with three long furrows and a convex, bulging, granular exine. (Courtesy of Center Laboratories, Port Washington, NY.)

of tree pollinosis despite the almost total elimination of the American elm by Dutch elm disease. Elm pollen is 35 to 40 μm in diameter with five pores and a thick, rippled exine (see Fig. 6-2). Hackberries are unimportant for this discussion.

Order Juglandales, Family Juglandaceae (Walnuts)

Walnut trees (*Juglans*) are not important causes of allergy, but their pollen often is found on pollen slides. The pollen grains are 35 to 40 μm in diameter, with about 12 pores predominantly localized in one area and a smooth exine (Fig. 6-5).

The Hickories (Carya)

These trees produce large amounts of highly allergenic pollen. Pecan trees in particular are important in the etiology of allergic rhinitis where they grow or are cultivated. The pollen grains are 40 to 50 μm in diameter and usually contain three germinal pores.

Order Myricales, Family Myricaceae (Bayberries)

Bayberries produce windborne pollen closely resembling the pollen of the *Betulaceae*. The wax myrtles are thought to cause pollinosis in some areas.

Order Urticales, Family Moraceae (Mulberries)

Certain members of the genus *Morus* may be highly allergenic. The pollen grains are small for tree pollens, about 20 μm in diameter, and contain two or three germinal pores arranged with no geometric pattern (neither polar nor meridial).

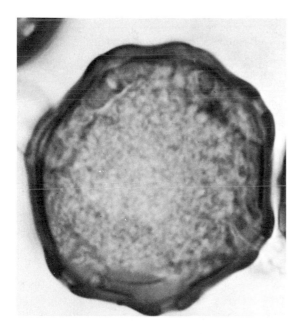

FIG. 6-5. Walnut (*Juglans nigra*). Average diameter is 36 μm. Grains have multiple pores surrounded by thick collars arranged in a nonequatorial band. (Courtesy of William P. Solomon, MD, University of Michigan, Ann Arbor, MI.)

Order Hamamelidales, Family Platanaceae (Sycamores)

These are sometimes called "plane trees." The grains of their plentiful pollen are oblate (flattened at the poles), about 20 μm in diameter, and without pores. There are three or four furrows on the thin, granular exine (see Fig. 6-2). Regionally, sycamores may be of allergenic significance.

Order Rutales, Family Simaroubaceae (Ailanthus)

Only the tree of heaven (*Ailanthus altissima*) is of allergenic importance regionally. Its pollen grains have a diameter of about 25 μm and are characterized by three germinal furrows and three germinal pores.

Order Malvales, Family Malvaceae (Lindens)

One genus, *Tilia* (the linden or basswood tree), is of allergenic importance, although it is insect pollinated. The pollen grains are distinct, 28 to 36 μm, with germ pores sunk in furrows in a thick, reticulate exine.

Order Sapindales, Family Aceraceae (Maples)

There are more than 100 species of maple, many of which are important in allergy. Maple pollen grains have three furrows but no pores (see Fig. 6-2). Box elder, a species of *Acer*, is particularly important because of its wide distribution, its prevalence, and the amount of pollen it sheds.

Order Oleales, Family Oleaceae (Ashes)

This family contains about 65 species, many of which are prominent among the allergenic trees. Pollen grains have a diameter of 20 to 25 μm, are somewhat flattened, and usually have four furrows (Fig. 6-6). The exine is coarsely reticulate.

Grasses (Poaceae)

Grasses are monocotyledons of the family Poaceae (or Gramineae). The flowers usually are perfect (Figs. 6-7 and 6-8). Pollen grains of most allergenic grasses are 20 to 25 μm in diameter, with one germinal pore or furrow and a thick intine (Fig. 6-9). Some grasses are self-pollinated and therefore noncontributory to allergies. The others are wind pollinated, but of the more than 1000 species in North America, only a few are significant in producing allergic symptoms. Those few, however, are important in terms of the numbers of patients affected and the high degree of morbidity produced. Most of the allergenic grasses are cultivated and therefore are prevalent where people live.

The grass family contains several subfamilies and tribes of varying importance to allergists. The most important are listed here.

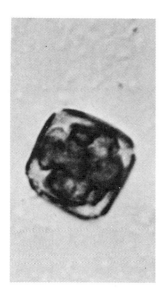

FIG. 6-6. Ash (*Fraxinus americana*). Average diameter is 27 μm. The pollen grains are square or rectangular with four furrows. (Courtesy of Center Laboratories, Port Washington, NY.)

Subfamily Festucoideae—Tribe Festuceae

The tribe Festuceae contains meadow fescue (*Festuca elatior*), Kentucky bluegrass (*Poa pratensis*), and orchard grass (*Dactylis glomerata*) (see Fig. 6-9), which are among the most important allergenic grasses. The pollens are 30 to 40 μm in diameter.

Tribe Argostideae

The Argostideae tribe includes timothy (*Phleum pratense*) (see Fig. 6-8) and redtop (*Agrostis alba*), two particularly significant grasses in terms of the amount of pollen shed,

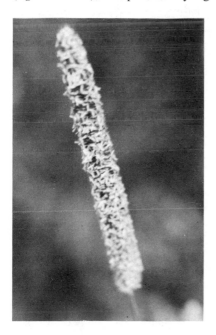

FIG. 6-7. Timothy grass (*Phleum pratense*). Morphologic features of the flowering head. (Courtesy of Arnold A. Gutman, MD, Associated Allergists Ltd., Chicago, IL.)

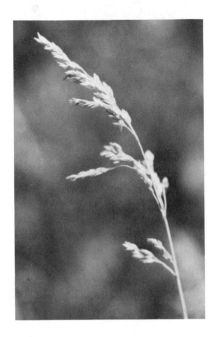

FIG. 6-8. June grass or bluegrass (*Poa pratenesis*). Morphologic features of the flowering head. (Courtesy of Arnold A. Gutman, MD, Associated Allergists Ltd., Chicago, IL.)

their allergenicity, and the intensity of symptoms produced. Both are cultivated as forage, and timothy is used to make hay. Other species of Agrostis immunologically similar to red-top are used for golf course greens. Timothy pollens are 30 to 35 μm in diameter; redtop pollens are 25 to 30 μm.

Tribe Phalarideae

Sweet vernal grass (*Anthoxanthum odoratum*) is an important cause of allergic rhinitis in areas where it is indigenous. In the total picture of grass allergy, however, it is not as important as the species previously mentioned. The pollen grains are 38 to 45 μm in diameter.

Tribes Triticaceae (Wheat and Wheat Grasses), Aveneae (Oats), Zizaneae (Wild Rice)

The Triticaceae, Aveneae, and Zizaneae tribes are of only minor or local importance in allergy because they are self-pollinating or produce pollen that is not abundant or readily airborne.

Subfamily Eragrostoideae—Tribe Chlorideae

Bermuda grass (*Cynodon dactylon*) is abundant in all the southern states. It is cultivated for decorative and forage purposes. It sheds pollen almost year-round and is a major cause of pollen allergy. The pollen grains are 35 μm in diameter.

Weeds

A weed is a plant that grows where people do not intend it to grow. Thus, a rose could be considered a weed if it is growing in a wheat field. What are commonly called weeds are small annual plants that grow wild and have no agricultural or ornamental value. All are angiosperms and most are dicotyledons. Those of interest to allergists are wind pollinated, and thus tend to have relatively inconspicuous flowers.

Family Asteraceae (Compositae)

The composite family is perhaps the most important allergenic weed group. Sometimes called the sunflower family, it is characterized by multiple tiny flowers arranged on a common receptacle and usually surrounded by a ring of colorful bracts. There are many tribes within this family; only those of allergenic or general interest are mentioned.

Tribe Heliantheae. This group includes sunflower, dahlia, zinnia, and black-eyed Susan. The flowers cause pollinosis mainly among those who handle them.

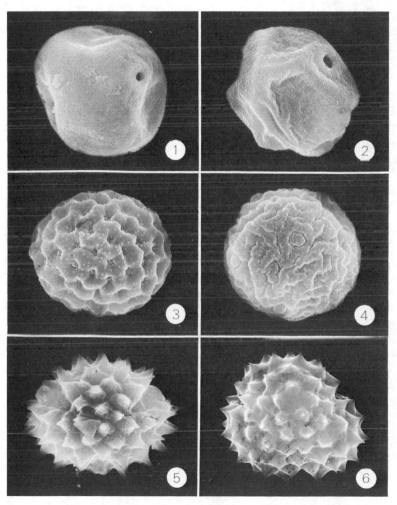

FIG. 6-9. Early and late summer airborne hayfever-producing pollen grains: 1, timothy (*Phleum*); 2, orchard grass (*Dactylis*); 3, lamb's quarter's (*Chenopodium*); 4, plantain (*Plantago*); 5, goldenrod (*Solidago*); 6, ragweed (*Ambrosia*). (Courtesy of Professor James W. Walker.)

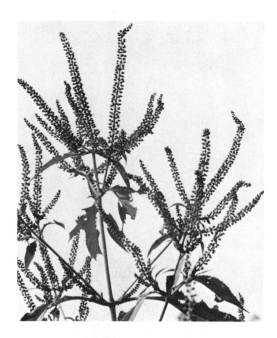

FIG. 6-10. Giant ragweed (*Ambrosia trifida*). Arrangement of staminate heads. (Courtesy of Arnold A. Gutman, MD, Associated Allergists Ltd., Chicago, IL.)

Tribe Ambrosieae. The ragweed tribe is the most important cause of allergic rhinitis and pollen asthma in North America. Other common weeds in this tribe are the cocklebur and marsh elder. *Ambrosia trifida*, giant ragweed, may grow to a height of 4.5 m (15 ft) (Fig. 6-10). The leaves are broad with three to five lobes. The staminate heads are borne on long terminal spikes, and the pistillate heads are borne in clusters at the base of the staminate spikes. The pollen grains, 16 to 19 μm in diameter, are slightly smaller than those of *A artemisifola*, short ragweed. Short ragweed grows to a height of 120 cm (4 ft) (Fig. 6-11). Its leaves are more slender and usually have two pinnae on each side of a central axis. Pollen grains range from 17.5 to 19.2 μm in diameter and are almost indistinguishable from those of giant ragweed (Figs. 6-12 and 6-13; see Fig. 6-9). There is no practical reason, however, for distinguishing between the two. *Ambrosia bidentia,* southern ragweed, is an annual that grows from 30 to 90 cm (1 to 3 ft) tall. The pollen grains are 20 to 21 μm in diameter and resemble those of giant ragweed. *Ambrosia psilostachya,* western ragweed, grows to a height of 30 to 120 (1 to 4 ft). It has the largest pollen grains of all the ragweeds, ranging from 22 to 25 μm in diameter. *Franseria acanthicarpa*, false ragweed, is found mainly in the south and southwest, where it may cause allergic symptoms. *Franseria tenuifolia,* slender ragweed, is another allergenic species of this tribe.

Xanthium (cocklebur) is morphologically distinct from the ragweeds, but its pollen grains are similar. Most species of Xanthium produce scanty pollen and are relatively unimportant causes of allergic rhinitis. Many patients with ragweed sensitivity also give strong skin test reactions to the cockleburs; this is probably a cross-reaction.

Cyclachaerna xanthifolia, burweed marsh elder, is antigenically distinct from ragweed, and the pollen grains are morphologically different from those of ragweed (Fig. 6-14).

Tribe Anthemideae. The mayweed tribe is important to allergy because it contains chrysanthemums. Pyrethrum is an insecticide made from flowers of these plants, and inhalation of this substance may cause allergic symptoms in ragweed-sensitive persons as well as in those who have been sensitized to the pyrethrum itself. The genus *Artemisia* includes the sagebrushes, mugworts, and wormwoods and is one of the most important groups of aller-

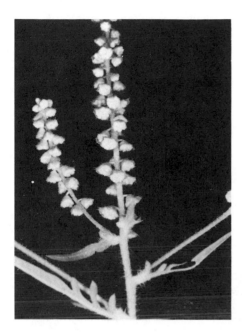

FIG. 6-11. Short ragweed (*Ambrosia artemisi-ifola*). Close-up of staminate head. The anthers are full of pollen just before anthesis. (Courtesy of Arnold A. Gutman, MD, Associated Allergists Ltd., Chicago, IL.)

genic weeds. *Artemisia vulgaris* is the common mugwort, found mainly on the east coast and in the Midwest in the United States. It is indigenous to Europe and Asia. The pollen grains, like those of other *Artemisia* species, are oblately spheroidal, 17 to 28 μm in diameter with three furrows and central pores, a thick exine, and essentially no spines. Other similar species are found on the West Coast and in the Southeast, Great Plains, and Rocky Mountains. *Artemisia tridentata* is common sagebrush, the most important allergenic plant of this tribe. It is most prevalent in the Great Plains and the northwest, where overgrazing of grassland has increased its presence.

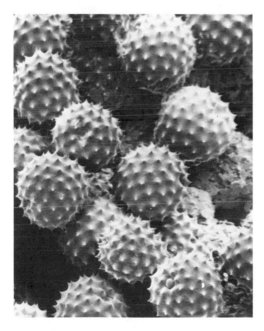

FIG. 6-12. Scanning electron photomicrograph of ragweed pollen. Notice the pore on the pollen grain (*lower right*). (Courtesy of D. Lim, MD, and J.I. Tennenbaum, MD.)

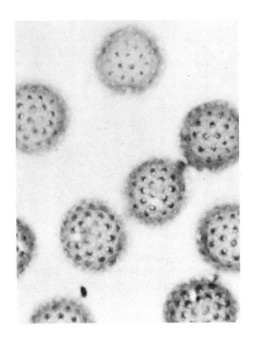

FIG. 6-13. Short ragweed (*Ambrosia artemisiifola*). Average diameter is 20 μm. Pollen grains have spicules on the surface. (Courtesy of Schering Corporation, Kenilworth, NJ.)

Polygonaceae (Buckwheat Family)

The docks, comprising the genus *Rumex*, are the only allergenic members of the buckwheat family. *Rumex acetosella* (sheep sorrel), *Rumex crispus* (curly dock), and *Rumex obtusifolius* (bitter dock) are the most important species. In the whole spectrum of pollen allergy, however, the docks are of minor significance.

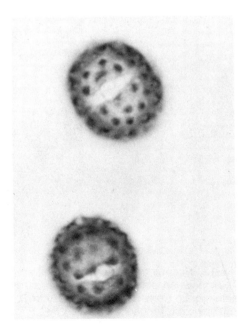

FIG. 6-14. Burweed marsh elder (*Cyclachaerna xanthifolia*). Average diameter is 19.3 μm. Three pores are centered in furrows, distinguishing it from ragweed. (Courtesy of Schering Corporation, Kenilworth, NJ.)

Amaranthaceae (Pigweed and Waterhemp Family)

The best known of the amaranths are *Amaranthus retroflexus* (red-root pigweed), *Amaranthus palmeri* (carelessweed), and *Amaranthus spinosus* (spring amaranth). They are prolific pollen producers and should be considered in the etiology of "hay fever" in the areas where they abound. Western waterhemp (*Amaranthus tamariscinus*), a potent allergen, is most prevalent in the Midwest.

Chenopodiaceae (Goosefoot Family)

The genus *Chenopodium,* "goosefoot," is best represented by *Chenopodium album* (lamb's quarters) (see Fig. 6-9). Each plant produces a relatively small amount of pollen, but in some areas the abundance of plants assures a profusion of pollen in the air. *Salsola pestifer*, Russian thistle, and *Kochia scoparia*, burning bush, are other Chenopodiaceae whose allergenic presence is more significant than that of lamb's quarters. Russian thistle also is known as "tumbleweed" because in the fall the top of the plant separates from its roots and is rolled along the ground by the wind. Burning bush may be recognized easily by the thin wing-like projections along its stems and, in the fall, by the fire engine red color of its leaves. It is often cultivated as an ornamental plant. Indigenous to Europe and Asia, these two weeds first became established in the prairie states but have migrated eastward, and are now important in the pathogenesis of pollinosis. *Atriplex* is the genus of the salt-bushes, wingscale, and shadscale. These are of some allergenic significance in the far west and southwest.

Two crops numbered among the Chenopodiaceae are the sugar beet (*Beta vulgaris*) and spinach (*Spinacea oleracea*). The former has been implicated in allergy where it is cultivated.

Pollens of the Amaranthaceae and Chenopodiaceae are so morphologically similar that they are generally described as "chenopodamaranth" when found in pollen surveys. Although subtle differences exist, it is generally fruitless and impractical to attempt to identify them more pre-

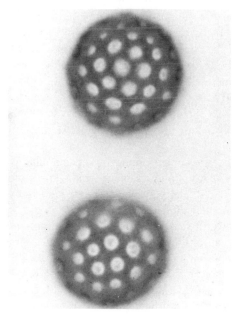

FIG. 6-15. Pigweed (*Amaranthus retroflexus*). Average diameter is 25 μm. The "golf ball" appearance of these grains is characteristic of the chenopod-amaranth group. (Courtesy of Schering Corporation, Kenilworth, NJ.)

cisely. They have the appearance of golf balls, which makes them unique and easy to identify (Fig. 6-15). Multiple pores give this peculiar surface appearance. The grains are 20 to 25 μm in diameter and spheroidal.

Plantaginaceae (Plantain Family)

English plantain (*Plantago lanceolata*) is the only member of this family that is important for allergy. It sheds pollen mainly in May and June, corresponding to the time when grasses pollinate. The pollen grains may be distinguished by their multiple pores (7 to 14) and variable size (25 to 40 μm) (see Fig. 6-9). English plantain may be a potent cause of allergic rhinitis, which may be confused with grass pollinosis.

POLLEN ANTIGENS

Pollen grains are living male gametophytes of higher plants (gymnosperms and angiosperms). Each grain has an internal limiting cellulose membrane, the intine, and a two-layered external covering, the exine, composed of a durable substance called sporopollenin. Sporopollenin is primarily a high molecular weight polymer of fatty acids.

Morphologic studies of pollens using the scanning electron microscope disclose an intricate infrastructure. The morphologic structure varies in relation to size, number of furrows, form and location of pores, thickness of the exine, and other features of the cell wall (spines, reticulations, an operculum in grass pollens, and air sacs [bladders] in certain conifers). Ragweed pollen is about 20 μm in diameter, tree pollens vary from 20 to 60 μm, and grass pollens, which are all morphologically similar, are usually 30 to 40 μm. The identification of pollens important in allergic disease is not difficult and is certainly within the capabilities of the physician with no special expertise in botany.[33,35,36]

Some plants produce prodigious amounts of pollen. A single ragweed plant may expel one million pollen grains in a single day. Trees, especially conifers, may release so much pollen that it is visible as a cloud and may be scooped up by the handful after settling. The seasonal onset of pollination of certain plants (e.g., ragweed) is determined by the duration of light received daily. Pollination occurs earlier in the northern latitudes and demonstrates little year-to-year variation in terms of date. In the belt from the central Atlantic to the north central states, August 15 is a highly predictable date for the onset of ragweed pollination. Most ragweed pollen is released between 6:00 and 8:00 AM, and release is enhanced by high temperature and humidity. Extended dry spells in early summer inhibits flower development, reduces ragweed pollen production, and thus results in lower counts in August and September.

Most brightly colored flowering plants are of little clinical importance in inhalant allergy because their pollen generally is carried by insects (entomophilous plants) rather than the wind (anemophilous plants). Entomophilous plants have relatively scant, heavy, and sticky pollen. Roses and goldenrod are examples of plants that often are erroneously thought to cause pollinosis because of the time they bloom. Nevertheless, in isolated cases, the pollens of most entomophilous plants can sensitize and then cause symptoms if exposure is sufficient. Of the pollens of anemophilous plants, ragweed has a long range, having been detected 400 miles out at sea. The range of tree pollens is much shorter. Thus, an individual living in the center of a city is more likely to be affected by weed and grass pollens than by trees. Local weed eradication programs, more often legislated than accomplished, are futile in light of the forgoing information. Air conditioners significantly reduce indoor particle recovery because windows are shut when they operate and they largely exclude outdoor air.

Ragweed Pollen Antigens

Essentially all of the peptides and proteins in pollen extracts can elicit the formation of IgG antibodies in animals. Therefore, they are antigens. Only some of these antigens, however, are allergens (i.e., stimulate and bind IgE [in humans]). Crossed immunoelectrophoresis shows that short ragweed pollen extract contains at least 52 antigens (as recognized by the rabbit antisera), but only 22 of these are allergens, as shown by their binding of specific IgE from the sera of ragweed-sensitive patients.[37] Use of sophisticated biochemical methods has resulted in the isolation of ragweed fractions of up to 300 times the potency of crude ragweed extracts, as measured by the ability to induce positive skin test results in appropriate subjects and the ability to cause histamine release from their peripheral blood leukocytes in vitro.

Several investigators have studied purified ragweed antigens. The early work of King and Norman[37,38] laid the foundation for the purification and analysis of allergens. Two major allergens, *Amb a 1* (antigen E) and *Amb a 2* (antigen K), have been isolated by gel filtration and ion exchange chromatography. These have certain immunologic and chemical properties in common, but differ in molecular weight and biologic activity. Almost all other "purified" ragweed fractions that have been isolated by other investigators contain large amounts of *Amb a 1*, which constitutes 90% of the allergenic activity of ragweed pollen. Recently, sophisticated molecular biology techniques have enabled workers to isolate and clone DNA sequences (cDNA) for many aeroallergens. This has allowed comparisons of DNA sequences of cross-reacting allergens with subsequent identification of homology that may be related to antigenicity. In addition to the two major ragweed allergens, eight intermediate or minor allergens have been isolated. These are *Amb a 3* through *Amb a 7* and *cystatin*.

Amb a 1 is a protein contained primarily in the intine of the pollen grain.[10] It accounts for about 6% of the total protein of whole ragweed extract. Quantitative studies of ragweed-sensitive patients with *Amb a 1* have shown a positive correlation with skin test reactivity and leukocyte histamine release, but no correlation with protein–nitrogen content in six commercial preparations of ragweed extract.[39] Techniques are available, however, such as radial immunodiffusion, that allow direct quantitation of *Amb a 1* in allergenic extracts, and, by use of RAST inhibition, the potency of ragweed allergenic extracts can be assessed. The Food and Drug Administration (FDA) requires that ragweed allergenic extracts be labeled with their *Amb a 1* content.

Amb a 1 consists of two fragments, named A and B. These fragments are not bound covalently and are dissociated readily, which results in a significant loss of allergenic activity. Recombination of these polypeptide chains does not restore allergenic activity, presumably because the steric conformation is not readily restored. *Amb a 1* is resistant to enzymatic degradation, suggesting that readily accessible amino or carboxyl groups are not the principal immunologic determinants. Interestingly, tenfold more *Amb a 1* is extractable in vitro at the pH of nasal secretions from patients with allergic rhinitis (pH 7 to 8), than at the pH of nasal secretions from nonatopic individuals (pH 6.3).[10]

Four isoallergenic variants have been demonstrated for *Amb a 1*, both by physicochemical studies and recent cDNA analyses.[40] Isoallergens have the same immunologic properties and similar chemical structures, but differ in some way such as isoelectric point, carbohydrate content, or amino acid composition.[9]

It has been calculated that the maximal amount of ragweed *Amb a 1* that a person breathing outdoor air in southeastern Minnesota would inhale is approximately 0.2 μg in a season.[41] The amount of *Amb a 1* produced by an individual ragweed plant appears to be determined genetically. There is considerable variation in the amount extractable by standard methods from pollen from plants grown under identical conditions (59 to 468 μg/mL).[42]

Amb a 2 (antigen K) constitutes about 3% of extractable ragweed pollen protein. Approximately 90% to 95% of ragweed-sensitive subjects show skin reactivity to this antigen. *Amb a 2* may cross-react slightly with *Amb a 1*, a finding reinforced by a 68% sequence homology at a DNA level.[43]

Since the isolation of *Amb a 1* and *2*, additional minor allergens designated *Amb a 3* (Ra 3), *Amb a 4* (Ra 4), *Amb a 5* (Ra 5),[44–46] *Amb a 6* (Ra 6),[47] *Amb a 7* (Ra 7),[48] and *cystatin*[49] have been identified. In contrast to *Amb a 1*, these low molecular weight fractions are rapidly extractable (less than 10 minutes) from pollen and have basic isoelectric points.[51] *Amb a 3* has a relatively high carbohydrate content, making it similar to certain grass pollen antigens. It consists of a single peptide chain of 102 amino acids. Two variants of *Amb a 3* differing by a single amino acid residue have been described; however, this difference does not alter the allergenic specificity.[52] This gene has not been cloned. *Amb a 5* consists of a single polypeptide chain whose 45 amino acids have been sequenced. The two isoallergenic forms differ at the second position by the substitution of leucine for valine in about 25% of samples. The frequency of positive skin test results to these antigens in ragweed-sensitive subjects demonstrates that approximately 90% to 95% react to *Amb a 1* and *Amb a 2*, 20% to 25% react to *Amb a 3*, and *Amb a 6*, and about 10% to *Amb a 5*. The frequency of reaction to *Amb a 4* is not known. A small fraction (10%) of ragweed-sensitive patients are more sensitive to *Amb a 3* and *5* than to *Amb a 1*.

Amb a 6 and *7* show sequence homology to other plant proteins involved in lipid metabolism and electron transport, respectively.[48,50] *Cystatin*, the most recent ragweed allergen to be cloned, shows homology to a family of cysteine protease inhibitors found in other plants.[49]

These various allergens have made it possible to study genetic responses in the ragweed-sensitive population. A complex antigen such as *Amb a 1* appears unrelated to total serum IgE or to any specific HLA phenotype, whereas subjects who respond to the lower molecular weight allergens such as *Amb a 3* have elevated total serum IgE levels.[53] Response to *Amb a 5* requires an immune response (Ir) gene usually associated with HLA DW2.[53] Sensitivity to *Amb a 3* has been associated with increased frequency of the HLA-A2 and HLA-B12 phenotype.[10] When a group of highly pollen-sensitive patients was prick skin tested with individual purified ragweed and ryegrass allergens, each patient reacted a distinctive pattern. This pattern was undoubtedly genetically programmed.[46]

In addition to the short ragweed allergens just described, an allergen from giant ragweed (*A trifida*), *Amb t V* (Ra 5G) has been identified.[54] Other allergens that cause allergic rhinitis have been purified from additional weeds. These include *Sal p 1* from *S pestifer* (Russian thistle),[55] *Par j 1* from *Parietaria judacia* pollen (Coccharia),[56] and *Art v 1* and *2* from *A vulgaris* (mugwort).[57]

Grass Pollen Antigens

Worldwide, grass pollen sensitivity is the most common cause of allergic disease. This is because of the wide distribution of wind-pollinated grasses. Important grass species involved in allergic reactions are *Lolium perenne* (ryegrass), *P pratense* (timothy), *P pratensis* (June grass, Kentucky bluegrass), *Festuca pratensis* (meadow fescue), *D glomerata* (cockfoot, orchard grass), *Agrotis tenuis* (redtop), *A odoratum* (sweet vernal), *Sorghum halepense* (Johnson grass), and *C dactylon* (Bermuda grass). The last two are subtropical grasses, whereas the others are temperate grasses.

Grass pollens differ from ragweed pollen in their allergenic and antigenic properties, and offer additional immunologic perspectives because of their extensive cross-reactivity. In addition, in contrast to ragweed, grasses typically release their pollen grains in the afternoon. Among the grasses, ryegrass and timothy have been most extensively studied.[9,58,59]

Examination of a number of allergenic grass pollen extracts by immunochemical methods has disclosed between 20 and 40 different antigens. Further analysis of these components has shown that some are more able than others to bind IgE from the serum of allergic patients or to produce positive skin test results. Some of these are major allergens in that they produce skin test reactivity or demonstrate IgE binding in more than 50% of grass-sensitive patients.

Several grass pollen allergens have been isolated and categorized into eight groups based on chemical and immunological characteristics. They are as follows: I, II, III, IV, IX (V), X, XI, and the profilins. Within each group, several individual allergens have been identified that are similar immunochemically and are extensively cross-reactive.

The group I allergens are located in the outer wall and cytoplasm of the pollen grains, as well as around the starch granules.[60] These small (3-μm diameter) granules are readily released on contact with water. Two representative members of the group I grass allergens are *Lol p 1* (ryegrass) and *Phl p 1* (timothy). Despite the fact that both of these allergens have been sequenced and cloned, their biochemical identity has not been determined. High cross-reactivity between the group I allergens from different grass species has been observed, including similarities in IgE RAST inhibition, crossed immunoelectrophoresis (CIE), and monoclonal antibody mapping.[61-63] Indeed, amino acid sequences document homologies among these group I members.[64] Other studied group I members include *Poa p 1* (Kentucky bluegrass), *Cyn d 1* (Bermuda), *Dac g 1* (orchard), and *Sor h 1* (Johnson). The group I allergens are of major importance in that by skin testing and histamine release, 90% to 95% of grass pollen-allergic patients react on testing.[65] Groups II and III show significant but lesser degrees of reaction, varying between 60% and 70% of patients.[58]

There is a relative paucity of data regarding the group II, III, and IV grass allergens. Group II allergens include *Lol p 2*, a ryegrass allergen that has been cloned and expressed as a recombinant molecule in a bacterial vector.[66] Forty-five percent of ryegrass allergic patients react to this allergen. Few other group II and III allergens have been sequenced, but thus far similarities to *Lol p 1* have been noted. Group IV allergens from timothy and ryegrass have been described but not characterized. Only about 20% of grass pollen-sensitive patients appear to be skin test reactive to these allergens.

Groups V and IX (now grouped together as IX) are a heterogeneous group of proteins. Group IX allergens from Kentucky bluegrass, ryegrass, and timothy grass all have been sequenced and cloned. Analysis of the cloned Kentucky bluegrass allergen, *Poa p 9*, has suggested the existence of a family of related genes. When compared with the ryegrass allergen, *Lol p 9*, a 44% homology is seen.[67] No other members of group IX show this level of homology. Among the group V allergens, the most work has been done with the timothy grass allergens *Phl p 5a* and *Phl p 5b*. These allergens have been cloned and identified as novel pollen RNases, which may play a role in host-pathogen interactions in the mature plant.[68] Other group V allergens have been isolated from a number of temperate grasses, including *D glomerata* (orchard grass). The *Dac g 5b* allergen also has been cloned and coded for a fusion protein that was recognized by IgE antibodies in six of eight samples of atopic sera tested. This suggests that this may be a major allergen, but it has not been completely characterized.[69]

Profilin, a compound involved in actin polymerization, has been described as a component of several tree pollens.[70] It is allergenic and also has been found to be a minor allergen in the grass allergen group II family, in addition to several weed species.

The most recent major grass pollen to be identified, *Lol p 11*, appears to be a member of a novel allergen family.[71] No sequence homology with known grass pollen allergens was found. This allergen reacted with IgE from over 65% of grass-pollen positive sera tested. *Lol p 11* appears to share some sequences with allergens from olive pollen, as well as tomato pollen. This is the only grass allergen (other than profilin) to have homology with tree pollens.

Tree Pollen Antigens

The allergenic fractions of trees have not been studied as extensively as ragweed or grasses.[72] There seems to be a higher degree of specificity to skin testing with individual tree pollen extracts compared with grass pollens because pollens of individual tree species may contain unique allergens. Despite this observation, several amino acid homologies and antigenic cross-reactivities have been noted. Further efforts to purify major allergens from tree pollens will be useful in confirming this hypothesis. Most tree pollen characterization has been done using birch (*Betula verrucosa*), alder (*Alnus glutinosa*), hazel (*Corylus avellana*), white oak (*Quercus alba*), olive (*Olea europa*), and Japanese cedar (*Cryptomeria japonica*) allergens. The tree pollens have been divided into two groups, I and II. The group I (major) allergens are small, cytoplasmic acidic proteins.[2] Few major allergens have been discovered among tree pollens, and these demonstrate structural and immunochemical cross-reactivity.

A major birch-pollen allergen, *Bet v 1*, has been isolated by a combination chromatographic technique. Monoclonal antibodies directed against this allergen have simplified the purification process.[73] Both amino acid sequence as well as a cDNA clone coding for the *Bet v 1* antigen has been isolated.[74] There is considerable (≥80%) amino acid homology between *Bet v 1* and other group I tree allergens.[2] *Bet v 1* is the birch tree allergen that cross-reacts with a low molecular weight apple allergen, a discovery that helps to explain the association between birch sensitivity and oral apple sensitivity.[75] Further investigations by the same workers extend this cross-reactivity to include pear, celery, carrot, and potato allergens. Most of the 20 patients tested had birch-specific serum IgE (anti-*Bet v 1* and anti-*Bet v 2*) that cross-reacted to these fruits and vegetables. *Bet v 2* and calmodulin are the minor birch allergens that have been isolated. *Bet v 2* has been identified as profilin, a compound responsible for actin polymerization in eukaryotes. There is approximately 33% amino acid homology between the human and birch profilin molecules.[70]

A major allergen has been isolated from the Japanese cedar, which contributes the most important group of pollens causing allergy in Japan. This allergen, designated *Cry j 1*, was separated by a combination of chromatographic techniques. Four subfractions were found to be antigenically and allergenically identical.[76] There is some amino acid homology between *Cry j 1* and *Amb a 1* and 2, but the significance of this is unclear. A second Japanese cedar allergen, *Cry j 2*, also has been described.[77] An allergen from mountain cedar (*Juniperus sabinoides*) has been described and partially sequenced.[78] It is a major allergen as defined by IgE binding in more than 50% of sera tested by CRIE.

FUNGAL ANTIGENS

The role of fungi in producing respiratory allergy is well established. In 1726, Sir John Floyer noted asthma in patients who had just visited a wine cellar; in 1873, Blackley suggested that

Chaetomium and *Penicillium* were associated with asthma attacks; and in 1924, van Leeuwen noted the relationship of climate to asthma and found a correlation between the appearance of fungal spores in the atmosphere and attacks of asthma.[79] Over the next 10 years, case reports appeared attributing the source of fungal allergies to the home or to occupational settings. In the 1930s, Prince and associates[80] and Feinberg[81] reported that outdoor air was a significant source of fungal spores and demonstrated that many of their patients had positive skin test reactivity to fungal extracts. More alarming is the association noted between elevated *Alternaria* airborne spore concentrations and risk of respiratory arrests in *Alternaria*-sensitive individuals.[82]

Initially, fungal sensitivity was equated to skin test reactivity, but more direct evidence for the role of fungal sensitivity in asthma has been presented by inhalation challenge studies by Licorish and coworkers.[83] In addition to IgE-mediated reactions, sensitization to certain fungi, especially *Aspergillus*, can lead to hypersensitivity pneumonitis.[84]

Although fungal spores are thought to be the causative agents in atopic disorders, other particles that become airborne (including mycelial fragments) also may harbor allergenic activity. Most fungal extracts used clinically are extracts of spore and mycelial material. They also may be derived from culture filtrates.

Alternaria is an important allergenic fungus and has been associated with significant episodes of respiratory distress. Among the *Alternaria* species, *A alternata* has been the subject of the most research. The major allergenic fraction, *Alt a 1*, has been obtained by several biochemical methods. In addition, a number of variants have been purified by several laboratories. The *Alt a 1* allergen is rich in carbohydrates, and glycosylation of proteins may be necessary for allergenic activity. *Alt a 1* is heterogeneous by isoelectric focusing and in PAGE.[85] *Alt a 1* can induce positive interdermal test results at extremely low concentrations (6 pg/mL) in *Alternaria*-sensitive subjects. Prick skin test results are positive at concentrations as low as 0.01 mg/mL, but 1.0 mg/mL is the concentration that best identifies patients allergic to *Alternaria*. This allergen is active in RAST, leukocyte histamine release, and bronchial inhalation challenges.[86,87] Interestingly, the fungus *Stemphyllium* shares at least ten antigens with *Alternaria* and an allergen immunochemically identical to *Alt a 1*.[88] Commercial *Alternaria* extracts contain widely varying amounts of *Alt a 1*, underscoring the need for improved methods of standardization.[89]

Although *Alt a 1* is the most completely characterized *Alternaria* allergen, as many as 32 antigens and 19 different allergens have been identified by CRIE and immunoblotting techniques.[90–92] Additional allergens with characteristics differing from *Alt a 1* also have been described.[79]

Cladosporium species are among the most abundant airborne spores in the world.[13] Two species, *Cladosporium cladosporoides* and *Cladosporium herbarum*, have been the focus of intense investigation. Analysis of extracts of *Cladosporium* by CIE and CRIE show complex patterns, revealing as many as 60 discrete antigens. Two major, 10 intermediate, and at least 25 minor allergens have been identified.[93] Allergen content of ten isolates of *Cladosporium* varied from 0% to 100% relative to a reference extract. Two major allergens have been isolated from *Cladosporium herbarum*, *Cla h 1* and *Cla h 2*.[94] *Cla h 1* (Ag-32) was isolated by chromatographic and isoelectric focusing techniques. *Cla h 2* (Ag-54) is a glycoprotein that is reactive in a smaller percentage of patients than *Cla h 1*. Neither allergen is cross-reactive, as determined by passive transfer skin testing. Several cDNA clones of the minor allergens from *C herbarum* have been isolated. The proteins that they code for have been tentatively identified as aldehyde dehydrogenase (*Cla h 3*), ribosomal proteins (*Cla h 4*), and enolase (*Cla h 6*).[95]

In contrast to *Cladosporium* and *Alternaria* extracts, which are prepared by extracting mycelia and spores, *Aspergillus fumigatus* extracts generally are prepared from culture filtrate material. Freshly isolated spores from *A fumigatus* have nearly undetectable levels of the major allergen *Asp f 1*, but begin to produce it within 6 hours of germination. *A fumigatus* and other *Aspergillus* species have been studied with particular reference to allergic bronchopulmonary aspergillosis. This disorder is characterized by the presence of both IgE and IgG antibodies to the offending fungal antigens. Analysis by CRIE has demonstrated some components that bind IgE avidly but bind IgG poorly, whereas other components precipitate strongly (bind IgG) but react poorly with IgE.[96] Another study[97] demonstrated 44 antigens by CIE and 18 allergens by CRIE. The extract used in this study was a ten-strain mixture. When the strains used in the extract were investigated individually, they varied in their quantities of the four most important allergens. Other studies demonstrated that disrupted spore antigens did not cross-react with either mycelial or cultural filtrate allergens.[98]

Unfortunately, *Aspergillus* allergens have not been as well characterized and purified as those of *Cladosporium* and *Alternaria*. Common allergens occur within the *fumigatus* and *niger* groups, which are allergenically distinct from *versicolor*, *nidulans*, and *glaucus* groups.[79] Extracts prepared from cultures grown for 10 and 21 days do not appear to differ significantly, but antigens of *A fumigatus* have been shown to vary with changes in culture technique.[99] Thus far, four allergens have been partially characterized from *A fumigatus*. *Asp f 1* is the major allergen and has been shown to be mitogillin, a fungal cytotoxin.[100] Another interesting *Aspergillus* allergen has been identified as α-amylase, an enzyme often added to bread dough to improve baking characteristics. The role of this molecule in the development of allergic symptoms in bakers has been described.[101]

Spores of the Basidiomycetes are a significant precipitant of allergic disease. Asthma epidemics have been reported in association with elevated Basidiomycetes spore counts.[102] Several species have been shown to be allergenic, and extracts from these species show multiple antigens and allergens.[103] Notice that up to 20% of asthmatic individuals demonstrate positive skin test results to Basidiomycetes species.[104] Despite the progress being made in the isolation and purification of fungal allergens, much work is needed to quantify these important allergens in fungal extracts used to diagnose and treat patients.

C albicans is the most frequently isolated fungal pathogen in humans, yet usually is restricted to immunocompromised individuals. A possible role of this yeast in allergic disease is best appreciated through studies with asthmatic individuals. In studies with 149 asthmatic patients, 48% were positive for *C albicans* on skin tests. Of these, 77% had positive inhalation provocation test results, with most demonstrating positive RAST results to *C albicans*.[105] Two major allergens have been identified and cloned, and one of these has been identified as a subunit of alcohol dehydrogenase.[106,107] The other major allergen has been shown to be enolase. IgE antibodies against *C albicans* enolase cross-react with enolase from *Saccharomyces cerevisiae*, and may represent a cross-allergenicity motif among the yeasts.

Estimating the extent to which a sensitive person's symptoms can be attributed to fungal allergy is a major clinical problem because exposure to fungi, like exposure to house dust mites, is continuous, usually without definite seasonal endpoints. Fungal spores can be roughly quantified in the air by the use of spore traps. Atmospheric fungal spore counts frequently are 1000-fold greater than pollen counts,[79] and exposure to indoor spores can occur throughout the year.[108] This is in contrast to pollens, which have distinct seasons, and to animal dander, for which a definitive history of exposure usually can be obtained. Such a history is sometimes possible for fungal exposure (e.g., raking leaves, or being in a barn with moldy hay), but these exposures are not common for many patients. Some species do show distinctive seasons; nevertheless, during any season, and especially during winter, the number and types of spores a patient inhales on a given day are purely conjectural.

In the natural environment, people are exposed to more than 100 species of airborne or dust-bound microfungi. The variety of fungi is extreme, and dominant types have not been established directly in most areas. The spores produced by fungi vary enormously in size, which makes collection difficult. Moreover, both microscopic evaluation of atmospheric spores and culturing to assess viability are necessary to fully understand the allergenic potential of these organisms. Although most allergenic activity has been associated with the spores, other particles such as mycelial fragments and allergens absorbed onto dust particles may contain relevant activity. Lastly, more than half of the outdoor fungus burden (Ascomycetes and Basidiomycetes) have spores that have not been studied or are practically unobtainable.

Fungi are members of the phylum Thallophyta, plants that lack definite leaf, stem, and root structures. They are separated from the algae in that they do not contain chlorophyll and therefore are saprophytic or parasitic. Almost all allergenic fungi are saprophytes. The mode of spore formation, particularly the sexual spore, is the basis for taxonomic classification of fungi. Many fungi have two names because the sexual and asexual stages initially were described separately. Many fungi produce morphologically different sexual and asexual spores that may become airborne. Thus, describing symptom–exposure relationships becomes difficult. The Deuteromycetes ("Fungi Imperfecti") are an artificial grouping of asexual fungal stages that includes many fungi of allergenic importance (*Aspergillus*, *Penicillium*, and *Alternaria*). These fungi were considered "imperfects," but are now known to be asexual stages (form genera or form species of Ascomycetes). These fungi reproduce asexually by the differentiation of specialized hyphae called conidiophores, which bear the conidia or asexual spore-forming organs. The various species of these fungi are differentiated morphologically by the conidia. Other classes of fungi also can reproduce asexually by means of conidia. Hyphae are filamentous strands that constitute the fundamental anatomic units of fungi. Yeasts are unicellular and do not form hyphae. The mycelium is a mass of hyphae, and the undifferentiated body of a fungus is called a thallus. One taxonomic scheme follows, with annotations of interest to allergists. Additional resources are provided in the references.[13,35,36,79,109]

CLASSES OF ALLERGENIC FUNGI

Oomycetes

This class of fungi is of little allergenic importance, but *Phytophthoria infestans* has been reported to be associated with occupational allergy.[13]

Zygomycetes

The sexual forms of Zygomycetes are characterized by thick-walled spinous zygospores; the asexual forms are characterized by sporangia. Spores of this group generally are not prominent in the air, but can be found in abundance in damp basements and around composting vegetation. The order Mucorales includes the allergenic species *Rhizopus nigricans* and *Mucor racemosus*. *Rhizopus nigricans* is the "black bread mold" whose hyphae are colorless but whose sporangia (visible to the naked eye) are black.

Ascomycetes

The Ascomycetes are the "sac fungi." Their spores are produced in spore sacs called asci. Concentrations of ascospores reaching thousands of particles per cubic meter occur in many areas and are especially numerous during periods of high humidity. Two significant allergenic

Ascomycetes are *S cerevisiae*, a yeast and *Chaetomium indicum*. The former, known as baker's yeast, is seen most commonly in its asexual budding form, but under certain culture conditions it forms hyphae and asci. Skin sensitivity to conidia of a powdery mildew, *Microsphaera alni*, has been reported, but the clinical significance of this is unknown.

The conidial forms of several Ascomycetes may represent the sexual form genera of imperfect fungi. For example, *Leptosphaeria* species are prominent and represent asexual stages of *Alternaria*.

Basidiomycetes

Two major subgroups occur within the class Basidiomycetes. The subclass Homobasidiomycetidae comprises mushrooms, bracket fungi, and puffballs. The spores of these organisms constitute a significant portion of the spores found in the air during nocturnal periods and wet weather. These abundant spores are confirmed to be allergenic[103,110,111] and can provoke bronchoconstriction in sensitive asthmatic subjects.[112] Numerous species, including *Pleurotus ostreatus*, *Cantharellus cibarius*, *Clavata cyanthiformis*, *Geaster saccatum*, *Pisolithus tinctorius*, *Scleroderma areolatum*, *Ganoderma lucidum*, *Psilocybe cubensis*, *Agaricus*, *Armillaria*, and *Hypholoma* sp, and *Merulisus lacrymans* ("dry rot") have been identified as allergens.

The Heterobasidiomycetidae include the rusts (Uredinales), smuts (Ustilaginales), and jelly fungi. The Ustilaginales and Uredinales are plant parasites of enormous agricultural importance and may cause allergy where cereal grains are grown or in the vicinity of granaries. Rust spores are encountered primarily by agricultural workers, whereas smut spores can be identified in urban areas surrounded by areas of extensive cultivation. Among the important allergenic species are *Ustilago*, *Urocystis*, and *Tilletia* sp.

Deuteromycetes (Fungi Imperfecti)

Asexual spores (conidia) rather than sexual spores characterize the reproductive mechanism of Deuteromycetes and are the basis for subclassification into the following orders:

Sphaeropsidales

The conidiospores are grouped in spherical or flask-shaped structures called pycnidia. The genus Phoma is the only common allergenic fungus in this order. It frequently gives positive skin test results in patients sensitive to *Alternaria*.

Melanoconoiales

The order Melanoconoiales is not of allergenic importance.

Moniliales

The conidiophores are spread over the entire colony. Moniliales is by far the largest and most diverse order of the Deuteromycetes and contains most of the recognized and suspected fun-

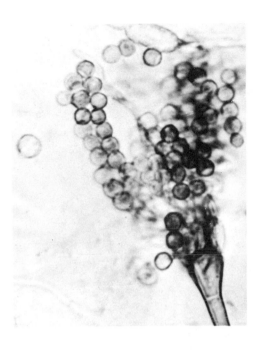

FIG. 6-16. *Aspergillus* sp. Average spore diameter is 4 μm. The spores are borne in chains and have connecting collars. (Courtesy of Bayer Allergy Products [formerly Hollister-Stier Labs], Spokane, WA.)

gus allergens. Three families account for most of the fungi that cause allergy in humans. Moniliaceae, Dematiaceae, and Tuberculariaceae.

The Moniliaceae are characterized by colorless or light-colored hyphae and conidia; the colonies are usually white, green, or yellow. The genera *Aspergillus* (Fig. 6-16), *Penicillium* (Fig. 6-17), *Botrytis, Monilia* and *Trichoderma* are "moniliaceous molds" associated with allergic disease.

The family Dematiaceae, one of the most important from the standpoint of allergy, is characterized by the production of dark pigment in the conidia and often in the mycelia. It contains the genera *Alternaria* (Fig. 6-18), *Cladosporium* (*Hormodendrum*) (Fig. 6-19), *Helminthosporium* (Fig. 6-20), *Stemphyllium* (Fig. 6-21), *Nigrosporia, Curvularia,* and *Aureobasidium* (*Pullularia*). The last is morphologically similar to the yeasts, and is sometimes

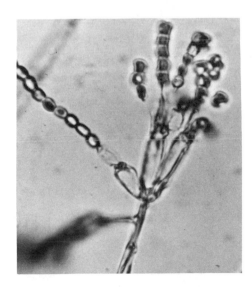

FIG. 6-17. *Penicillium chrysogenum.* Average spore diameter is 2.5 μm. The spores appear in unbranched chains on phialides, the terminal portions of the conidiophores. The phialides and chains of spores resemble a brush. (Courtesy of Bayer Allergy Products [formerly Hollister-Stier Labs], Spokane, WA.)

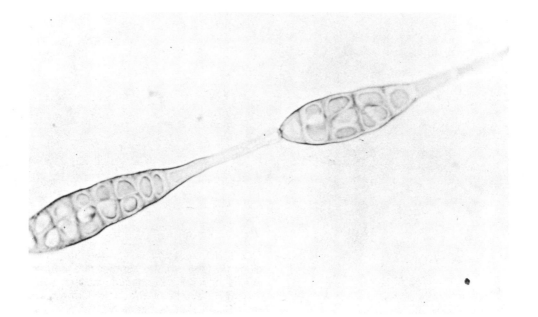

FIG. 6-18. *Alternaria alternata.* Average spore size is 12 × 33 μm. Spores are snowshoe shaped and contain transverse and longitudinal septae with pores. (Courtesy of Schering Corporation, Kenilworth, NJ.)

classified with them and called the "black" yeast. This group often is described as the "dematiaceous molds."

The Tuberculariaceae produce a sporodochium, a round mass of conidiospores containing macroconidia and microconidia in a slimy substrate. The genera *Fusarium* (Fig. 6-22) and *Epicoccum* (Fig. 6-23) are important allergenic fungi in this family.

The family Cryptococcaceae contains the true yeasts, which do not produce hyphae under known cultural or natural circumstances. Allergenic genera within this family include *Rhodotorula* and *Sporobolomyces*.

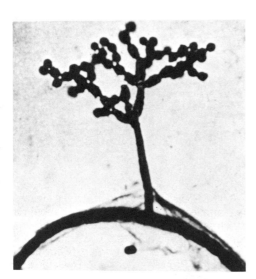

FIG. 6-19. *Cladosporium* sp. Average spore size is 4 × 16 μm. Spores occur in chains and have small attaching collars at one end. The first spore buds off from the conidiophore, then the spore itself buds to form a secondary spore. (Courtesy of Bayer Allergy Products [formerly Hollister-Stier Labs], Spokane, WA.)

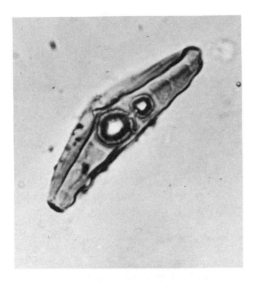

FIG. 6-20. *Helminthsporium* sp. Average spore size is 15 × 75 mm. The spores, which occur in the ends of the conidiophores, are large, brownish, and have transverse septae. (Courtesy of Schering Corporation, Kenilworth, NJ.)

This classification and list of genera are not exhaustive, but do represent most of the important allergenic fungi found in environmental surveys. The fungi listed here are a framework on which an individual allergist can build or make deletions, depending on the region or clinical judgment. Most fungal sensitivity is specific for genus, although species and strain differences have been reported. Where more than one species occurs for a genus, allergenic extracts usually are mixed together, as in "*Aspergillus* mixture" or "*Penicillium* mixture." It should be remembered that extracts prepared from fungi are extremely variable in allergenic content and composition.

Certain data concerning the prevalence and ecology of fungi make the list less formidable in practice. With the exception of the Pacific Northwest, *Alternaria* and *Cladosporium* (*Hormod endrum*) are the most numerous genera encountered in most surveys of outdoor air. These fungi are "field fungi" and thrive best on plants in the field and decaying plant parts in the soil. They

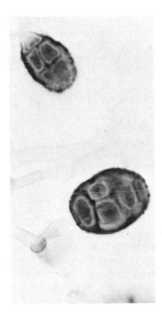

FIG. 6-21. *Stemphyllium* sp. The spores superficially resemble those of *Alternaria* but lack the "tail" appendage. Also, they are borne singly rather than in chains. (Courtesy of Schering Corporation, Kenilworth, NJ.)

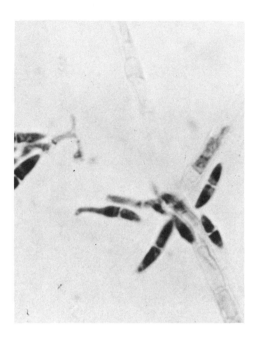

FIG. 6-22. *Fusarium vasinfectum.* Average spore size is 4 × 50 μm. The most prevalent spore type is the macrospore, which is sickle shaped and colorless, and contains transverse septae and a point of attachment at one end. (Courtesy of Bayer Allergy Products [formerly Hollister-Stier Labs], Spokane, WA.)

require a relatively high moisture content (22% to 25%) in their substrate. They are mainly seasonal, from spring to late fall, and diminish markedly with the first hard frost. Their spores generally disappear from air samples during the winter months when snow cover is present. *Helminthosporium* and *Fusarium* are the other common field fungi. These and certain other fungi propagate in the soil, and their spores are released in large numbers when the soil is tilled.

Aspergillus and *Penicillium*, conversely, sometimes are called "storage fungi" because they are common causes of rot in stored grain, fruits, and vegetables. *Aspergillus* in particu-

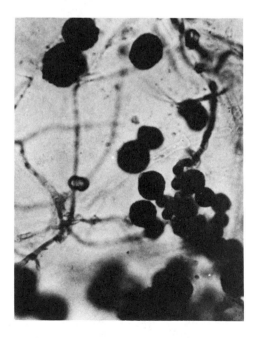

FIG. 6-23. *Epicocccum nigrum.* Average diameter is 20 μm. Large spores are borne singly on the ends of conidiophores. They are yellowish brown and rough, and develop transverse septae when old. (Courtesy of Bayer Allergy Products [formerly Hollister-Stier Labs], Spokane, WA.)

lar thrives on a substrate with low moisture content (12% to 16%). These are the two fungi most commonly cultured from houses, especially from basements, crawl spaces, and bedding. *Penicillium* is the green "mildew" often seen on articles stored in basements. *Rhizopus* causes black moldy bread and proliferates in vegetable bins in homes, especially onions.

The foremost allergenic fungi, based not only on their incidence in atmospheric surveys, but on allergenic skin test reactivity, are *Alternaria, Aspergillus, Cladosporium,* and *Penicillium.* The prevalence of skin test reactivity to fungi in allergic patients is not known but may approach 25% of asthmatics in some surveys.[113] Most patients allergic to fungi typically react on skin testing to one or more of these allergens. Many patients also react to other fungi, however, and some to fungi other than these four.

The designations "field" and "storage" fungi or "indoor" and "outdoor" fungi are not precise because exceptions are common in environmental surveys. Moreover, indoor colonization from molds varies with the season, particularly in homes that are not air conditioned.[114] During the warmer months, *Alternaria* and *Cladosporium* spores are commonly found indoors, having gained entry into the home through open windows.

In contrast to field and storage fungi, yeasts require a high sugar content in their substrates, which limits their habitat. Certain leaves, pasture grasses, and flowers exude a sugary fluid that is a carbon source for the nonfermentative yeasts such as *Aureobasidium* (*Pullularia*) and *Rhodotorula.* Hundreds of millions of yeast colonies may be obtained per gram of leaf tissue. Berries and fruit also are commonly colonized. The soil is not a good habitat for yeasts unless it is in the vicinity of fruit trees. Yeasts are often cultured indoors, however.

The relation of weather to spore dissemination is clinically important, because the symptoms of patients with respiratory allergy are often worse in damp or rainy weather. This has been attributed by some to an increase in the "fungal spore count." Absolute fungal spore counts decrease during and after a rain storm because some spores, like pollen grains, are washed out or made less buoyant. Most of the common allergenic fungi, such as *Aspergillus* and *Cladosporium*, are of the dry spore type, the spores being released by the wind during dry periods. Alternatively, some so called "wet weather spores," including certain yeasts such as *Aureobasidium, Trichoderma,* and *Phoma* and biologically dispersed ascospores, increase. Although these spores are loosened during wet periods and are dispersed by rain droplets, it is unlikely that they are responsible for the mass symptoms that occur during inclement weather. High spore counts are found in clouds and mist, and it is reasonable to attribute some of the symptoms encountered during long periods of high humidity to fungal allergy. Recall that other allergens, such as the house dust mite, also propagate in conditions of high humidity. Snow cover obliterates the outdoor fungal spore count, but the conditions subsequent to thawing predispose to fungal growth and propagation.

The relation of house plants to indoor fungal exposure has been studied. Contrary to common belief, indoor plantings are associated with only a slight increase in the numbers of spores from such genera as *Cladosporium, Penicillium, Alternaria,* and *Epicoccum.* Greenhouses do show an increased number of spores, particularly when plants are agitated by watering or fanning.[115] Similar studies in laboratory animal care units fail to show excessive numbers of fungal spores.[116] Several reviews of fungal sensitivity and the classification of fungi are available.[95,102,103,117]

HOUSE DUST AND DUST MITES

House dust has been recognized as an allergen for many centuries. In 1921, Kern[118] demonstrated that house dust extracts produced positive skin test results in many patients with asthma. In 1964, Voorhorst and co-workers reexamined and subsequently expanded the knowledge of the relationships among house dust, mites, and human allergic disorders.[119] These Dutch workers are to be credited with sparking the worldwide interest in mites as allergens. Miyamoto and associates in Japan[120–124] corroborated and expanded the previous work. They showed that the potency of house dust allergen is related to the number of mites in the dust. Skin tests, RASTs, and bronchoprovocation performed with extracts from pure cultures of mites (*Dermatophagoides pteronyssinus* and *Dermatophagoides farinae*) correlated well with the results obtained using house dust extracts. The equivalent potency of mite extracts was 10 to 100 times that of whole dust. Mites are now accepted as the major source of allergens in house dust. It has been shown that exposure to house dust mite allergen in early childhood is an important determinant in the development of asthma.[125]

Mites are a subclass of arachnids that constitute several orders of Acarina. They are sightless, small (0.33 mm long), eight-legged animals. They may be identified microscopically using a low-power lens or a stereoscope. The family Pyroglyphidae contains most of the mites important in house dust allergy, but Tyroglyphidae are important in storage mite sensitivity. Mites found in houses are called domestic mites, but the term "house dust mite" is reserved for the Pyroglyphidae family of mites.[126] These are free-living organisms whose natural food sources include human skin scales, fungi, and other high-protein substances in the environment. They can be cultured using human skin shavings, dry dog food, or daphnia as substrates, and can be separated from the culture medium by flotation. Mites also can be separated from dust samples by flotation in saturated salt solution, retained by a sieve with 45-μm openings, and differentiated from other retained material by crystal violet staining.[127] The mites do not stain and are seen as white against a purple background.

The numerically dominant mite in European homes is *D pteronyssinus*; in North American homes *D farinae* predominates. There is significant overlap, however.[128,129] Other house dust mite species are *D microceras*, *Euroglyphus maynei*, and the tropical *Blomia tropicalis*.[126,130] Other groups of mites, including *Acarus siro*, *Tyrophagus putresentiae*, *Lepidoglyphus* (*Glycyphagus*) *domesticus*, and *Lepidoglyphus destructor,* which are referred to as "storage mites," are mainly pests of stored grain, but have caused barn allergy in farm workers[131] and occasionally are associated with dust allergy in homes.[132] Some of the 210 residents of London who underwent skin testing for sensitivity to a variety of mites showed strong reactions to *A siro*, *T putresentiae*, *L destructor*, and *L domesticus*. There was some correlation between reactions to these various storage mites, but none to *D pteronyssinus*. The predisposing factors for developing allergic reactions to storage mites were occupation, damp homes, and possibly the type of bedding used for household pets.[133]

Seasonal and geographic variation in the number of house dust mites in house dust have been observed. In North America, sharp peaks of mite growth have been observed in the summer months.[130] The major factors governing mite propagation are temperature and, particularly, humidity. The key determinant for excessive mite growth seems to be an indoor absolute humidity of approximately 7 g/kg. This is equivalent to a relative humidity of 60% at 21°C (70°F) and 75% at 16°C (60°F).[130] When the relative humidity falls below 40% to 50%, mites are unable to survive more than 11 days at temperatures above 25°C (77°F), because increased transpiration of water leads to dehydration.[127] The larval form (protonymph) of *D farinae*, however, may survive the heating season because it is relatively resistant to desiccation. Protonymphs are the likely source of resurgence of mites in the spring. The life cycle from egg to adult is 30 days at 25°C and up to 110 days at 20°C.

Low numbers of mites are found in dust recovered from homes or other buildings at high altitude.[129] At higher altitudes, the absolute humidity of the outdoor air decreases sharply, reducing indoor humidity and therefore mite growth. Environmental conditions influence not only mite growth but also the species of mites found. *D farinae* tend to predominate where there are prolonged periods of dry weather (i.e., more than 3 months with a mean outdoor absolute humidity < 6 g/kg). In humid conditions, *D pteronyssinus* usually predominates. In most areas, it is usual for other species to predominate. *E maynei* has been found as a predominant species in occasional homes in damp conditions. *B tropicalis* is important in the southeastern United States (e.g., Florida) as well as in Central and South America.

Mattress dust usually contains the highest concentration of mites compared with dust from rugs, clothing, closets, automobiles, and other places. Most mites are recovered from areas of the home that are occupied most commonly, including rugs, bedding, and furniture. Fitted bottom sheets may retard the penetration of human dander into mattresses, thus reducing the mite count. Meticulous housekeeping or the presence of household pets does not necessarily influence the mite load. As many as 18,875 mites per gram of dust have been recovered. In Ohio, an annual average heavy density was considered 481±190 mites per gram of dust; a low density was 41±25 mites per gram of dust.[127] Recent efforts to measure dust mite allergen exposure to the major house dust mite antigen, *Der p 1*, have used immunochemical measurements.[134] Based on these measurements, levels of *Der p 1* greater than 10 µg per gram of dust often are associated with allergic and asthmatic symptoms, whereas levels less than 1 µg/g are not associated with allergic symptoms.[134] Although these levels cannot be translated directly into dust mite counts, 10 µg/g of *Der p 1* is approximately equivalent to 200 mites per gram of dust. In some studies, a mite count of more than 100 mites per gram of fine dust has been regarded as a risk factor for development of asthma.[134] The fecal particles of mites contain most of the allergenic activity in mite extracts.[135] Both mite body and feces extracts, however, contain multiple antigens and allergens. A high percentage of dust mite–sensitive patients are skin test positive to both *D farinae* and *D pteronyssinus*. Often, in homes, one or more species may be prevalent. Studies comparing cross-reactivity by CRIE and CIE demonstrate that *D farinae* and *D pteronyssinus* body extracts contain numerous cross-reacting antigens and allergens. Analysis of feces extracts from the two species also demonstrate cross-reactivity. Of significance is the fact that body and fecal extracts of both species contain unique, species specific antigens and allergens.[136]

At least six major groups of house dust mite allergens have been described, with representatives of each isolated, purified, and partially sequenced. The group I allergens are small proteins recognized by most mite-sensitive individuals. These allergens are found in whole-body, fecal, and gut extracts from the various mite species. Examples of group I allergens include *Der p 1*, *Der f 1*, *Der m 1*, and *Eur m 1*. Amino acid sequences of these allergens reveal 80% to 85% homology between the mite species, with moderate levels of antigenic cross-reactivity measured by IgE antibodies.[2] Using sequence data, the group I allergens have tentatively been identified as members of the cysteine protease family, represented in numerous mammalian and plant species.[137] Interestingly, peptides from plant cysteine proteases are potent stimulators of histamine release in allergen-stimulated human basophils.[138]

The group II allergens include *Der p 2* and *Der f 2*. These allergens differ from the group I members in that they are resistant to denaturation by heat and pH variations. Both allergens have been cloned and reveal over 85% sequence homology.[139] The identification of these proteins has not been established, but evidence points to a digestive enzyme or even lysozyme.

The group III allergens, *Der p 3* and *Der f 3*, are found primarily in fecal material from the house dust mites. Thus far, only *Der p 3* has been identified as a major allergen. These allergens are thought to represent trypsin and associated serine proteases. These allergens have yet to be cloned. Groups IV, V, and VI allergens represent minor allergens. They have not yet been extensively studied.

Several monoclonal antibodies have been developed against particular allergens, which has enhanced the investigator's ability to purify these antigens and determine their concentration in the atmosphere. Studies from mite feces show that 90% to 95% of the allergen content is *Der p 1*. The fecal particles have a mean diameter of 24 μm (range, 10 to 40 μm). They are spherical and are surrounded by a peritrophic membrane. The *Der p 1* content is about 0.1 ng per fecal particle.[135] The high concentration of allergen is thought to be clinically significant in that it could cause an intense local inflammatory response when inhaled into the respiratory mucosa.

In the United Kingdom, 10% of the population and 90% of allergic asthmatics have positive skin test results to house dust mite extracts. As many as 75% of the serum antibodies to mites are directed against the *Der p 1* allergen.[135] In some allergic subjects, IgE antibody to *Der p 1* constitutes 9% to 21% of the total IgE, with a mean value of 12%.[140] Removal of allergic children from environmental exposure to house dust mite antigen reduced both specific IgE antibodies to *D pteronyssinus* and total IgE levels.[129] Moreover, another study[141] of prolonged allergen avoidance of house dust mite antigen improved pulmonary function and symptoms, and reduced medication use and bronchial reactivity in a group of children.

In summary, the major allergens in house dust are contained in the fecal particles and bodies of mites that inhabit the dust. Because of the heterogeneous composition of crude house dust mixtures, patients should be tested and treated with house dust mite extracts rather than with crude house dust materials.

EPITHELIAL AND OTHER ANIMAL ALLERGENS

The category of animal allergens includes animal emanations: hair, dander, feathers, saliva, and urine. Because domestic animals are widespread in our society and some of their emanations are potent allergens, the topic is important for the allergist. Occupational exposure of farmers, veterinarians, and laboratory workers has economic importance. Social and family interactions may be strained severely when one person becomes allergic to a beloved family pet. The allergist often is called on to solve these problems.

Hair itself is not an important allergen because it is not buoyant or water soluble. Water-soluble proteins of epidermal or salivary origin that are attached to the hair are important allergens, however. *Dander* is a term used to describe desquamated epithelium. Desquamation is a continuous process for all animals, and the dander materials contain many water-soluble proteins that are highly antigenic and allergenic. Saliva also is rich in proteins such as secretory IgA and enzymes. Persons commonly develop local urticaria at the sites where they have been licked by a cat or dog or where they have been scratched by claws or teeth. Rodents, too, excrete significant amounts of allergenic protein in their urine. All of these substances become part of the amorphous particulate matter of the air and are responsible for allergic morbidity.

Cats seemingly produce the most dramatic symptoms in sensitive individuals, particularly in those who are exposed intermittently. Whether this is caused by the concentration of allergens in the cat's environs or to the potency of the allergens is unknown. Studies with cat pelts have disclosed a substance called *Fel d 1* that appears to be the major allergen, recognized by over 80% of cat-sensitive individuals.[142] *Fel d 1* is produced mainly in cat saliva, but is also in the sebaceous glands of the skin, the sublingual glands, and even in the brain.[143,144] Immunotherapy with cat pelt extract has been associated with decreased bronchial reactivity on inhalation challenge.[145] The *Fel d 1* molecule has been cloned; however, its identity and function are unknown.

Fel d 1 may be detected in the urine of male cats but not of females. Allergens other than *Fel d 1* in some sensitive individuals also have been detected in cat serum and urine, but these are minor allergens.[146] Studies with individual cats show that some cats are high producers of allergen and others are not. Moreover, the rate of allergen production of individual cats varies from hour to hour. Male cats generally produce greater amounts of allergen than females. These factors may explain why some patients are more allergic to certain cats than to others.[143] In addition, there does not appear to be any seasonal variation in *Fel d 1* production.

Air sampling in rooms occupied by cats has shown that the amount of *Fel d 1* allergen required to cause a 20% drop in forced expiratory volume in 1 second (FEV_1) on pulmonary function testing is comparable with the amounts required in conventional bronchoprovocation testing (approximately 0.09 µg/mL). Morphologic room sampling shows abundant squamous cell fragments smaller than 5 µm, enabling these fragments to reach small bronchioles and alveoli.[147] This small particle size also explains why cat allergen can remain airborne in undisturbed conditions for extended periods.

Serial dust samples collected in the study of 15 homes after removal of the family cats were analyzed for *Fel d 1*. Baseline amounts of antigen ranged from 8 to 437 FDA U/g (median, 61 U/g). After removing the cats, the levels decreased to those of control homes in 20 to 24 weeks. However, significant differences occurred in the rate of decline of *Fel d 1* among homes. It might therefore be prudent to advise patients that it might take up to 6 months after removal of a cat for the bulk of the cat allergens to disappear from the home.[148]

Dog allergens have been identified in dander, saliva, urine, and serum, but elegant studies like the ones described for cats have not been published. The major dog allergen, *Can f 1*, has been described and can be assayed, although most skin tests and RASTs use dander as the basis of diagnosing allergy to dogs. Using RAST inhibition, dog sera had little effect on the binding of dog dander.[149] In the same experiments, using dander from 13 breeds of dog and sera of 16 patients with documented dog allergy, the various sera showed significant breed specificity. Danders of all breeds were allergenic, including poodle. However, differences between breeds occur in the number and amount of antigens. Only 20% or fewer of patients clinically allergic to dogs showed positive results on RASTs or prick tests to dog serum albumin.[150] There is individual variation in the positivity of skin test results to different breeds, but in one study these variations did not correlate with the patient's perception of specific breed allergy.[150] The fact that dogs tend to spend more time outdoors and are bathed more frequently may explain their decreased importance as an allergen source relative to cats.

Most patients who are demonstrably sensitive to danders are also sensitive to other perennial allergens. This complicates the determination of which allergen is responsible for the patient's symptoms. The recommendation to eliminate a pet from a home environment places the clinician in a difficult position. Patients do not readily accept the proposition that their pet may be the cause of their allergic problem, even in light of positive skin test results. Positive bronchial provocation might be supportive, but results are not conclusive. Cat allergen is known to persist in the home for up to 24 weeks after removal of the pet, so a trial separation of the patient away from the home environment for several weeks to months is probably the best prognostic indicator at this time.

Horses resemble cats in the explosive symptoms that may occur on exposure to their dander, but this clinical situation is less common and less difficult to manage, primarily because of the absence of horse dander in the home. Horse hair has been used in the manufacture of some mattresses, furniture, and rug pads, but again, the allergenic potential of hair does not approach that of dander. Some antigens are common to horse dander and serum, creating the potential for a serious problem in patients when horse serum (such as an antivenom) may be urgently needed. Tetanus antitoxin currently is available as a human antiserum.

Allergy to cows, goats, and sheep usually is occupational. Rabbits and small rodents such as gerbils, hamsters, guinea pigs, rats, and mice are common household pets, and their danders may induce severe reactions on skin prick testing. Significant skin test reactivity also may be seen to the danders of rats and mice in persons whose homes are infested with these rodents.

Allergic symptoms in laboratory workers exposed to murine allergens have prompted several studies on the nature of these allergens.[151,152] In mouse-sensitive subjects, a major urinary protein, *Mus m 1*, appears to be the primary allergen. It is the prominent member of a family of allergenic murine proteins collectively known as the major urinary proteins.[153] *Mus m 1* protein is synthesized in the liver, and its synthesis is stimulated by androgen, accounting for fourfold higher concentrations in male mice than in females. The urine from both sexes of mice contains ten times more of this allergen than does the serum. *Mus m 1* is also formed in the sebaceous, parotid, and lachrymal glands, which probably explains the small quantities detected in pelt extract. The potency of this allergen in susceptible individuals was illustrated by the finding that intermittent exposure to these allergens of at least 10 days a year produced the same levels of allergy in terms of IgE-related tests as daily exposure.[151]

Rats and other small mammals commonly produce respiratory symptoms in laboratory workers. The airborne level of rat allergens can be high—up to 100 $\mu g/m^3$. Furthermore, urinary allergens are carried in small particles about 7 μm in diameter. Workers with intense exposure to rats develop IgG antibodies to rat urinary protein, but in the absence of IgE to these proteins, these subjects are asymptomatic. The presence of IgE antibodies to rat urinary proteins in laboratory workers usually is associated with asthma or rhinitis. Both atopic and nonatopic individuals are able to make the specific IgE.[154] The two predominant rat urinary allergens are termed *Rat n 1* and *Rat n 2*. Air sampling techniques for rat allergens have shown that feeding and cleaning produce the highest airborne concentrations of the prealbumin protein *Rat n 1* (21 ng/m^3), injection and handling produce exposure to somewhat less allergen, and surgery and killing rats produce only 3.4 ng/m^3. Low concentrations of rat allergens were found outside of the handling rooms.[155] Of the three layers of rat pelt, the outermost fur was most allergenic, probably because of contamination with body fluids. In one study, rat sebaceous glands were not found to be the source of allergenic secretions,[156] but other studies have shown a high molecular weight protein (over 200 kd), which was believed to originate from rat sebaceous glands.[157] *Rat n 2* has been definitively demonstrated demonstrated in liver, lachrymal, and salivary glands.[158]

The question has been raised whether laboratory workers who deal with allergenic rodents should be screened for atopy before employment. Although it was thought initially that workers with seasonal allergic rhinitis are more likely to become allergic to laboratory animals,[159] more recent studies conclude that such screening is not warranted because nonatopic individuals may become allergic when exposed to sufficient allergen loads.[154,160] Of course, a screening test for existing specific animal allergens may be useful, particularly if the worker has a choice of working with different animal species.

MISCELLANEOUS ALLERGENS

Included in this category of miscellaneous allergens are substances that have been shown to be allergenic in selected cases or occupations and some that may be of more general importance but are not yet accepted as such by the allergy community.

Insects

Insects were recognized as inhalant allergens long before mites (which are arachnids, not insects) came to the foreground. Cockroaches have been described as allergens based on skin test data in allergic persons.[161] Kang and associates[162] extended this work to include RASTs and bronchoprovocation studies to further implicate cockroach-associated materials as asthmogenic. It was further pointed out that asthmatics with positive prick test results to cockroach extracts had higher total serum IgE levels than their allergic counterparts with negative skin test results. Bronchoprovocation caused a transient peripheral eosinophilia in those who reacted positively.

Of the over 50 species of cockroach described, only 8 are regarded as "indoor" pests. Allergens from the two most common species, *Blattella germanica* and *Periplaneta americana*, have not been studied in detail. Two allergens from *B germanica*, *Bla g 1* and *Bla g 2*, have been described, but only scant biochemical details have been reported.[163,164] ELISA is available to monitor indoor levels, however. Two allergens from *P americana* have been reported, but these have not been named. Immunoelectrophoretic studies with roach allergens have disclosed multiple antigens, with most allergens residing in the whole-body and cast-skin fractions. Feces and egg casings were less allergenic.[165] Roach hemolymph also may be allergenic.[166]

Outdoor insects such as mayfly and caddis fly have been studied clinically and immunologically.[167] These insects have an aquatic larval stage and therefore are found around large bodies of water such as the Great Lakes, particularly Lake Erie. These flies were reported to cause significant respiratory allergy in the summer months, but their numbers have declined, probably because of pollution of the lakes. Japanese investigators reported that 50% of asthmatics show reaginic sensitivity to the silkworm moth (*Bombyx mori*) caused by antigens found in the wings. These wing allergens cross-react almost completely on RAST inhibition with butterfly allergens, but not at all with mites.[168] Finished silk products are not thought to be allergenic, but contamination of some products, such as silk-filled bed quilts, with waste products of *B mori* and the insect *Antheraea pernyi* can cause asthma and rhinitis.

In the Sudan, during certain seasons, respiratory allergy has been reported from inhalation of allergens of the "green nimmiti midge." These are chironomids, nonbiting members of the order Diptera.[169] Studies of these chironomid antigens by RAST show the allergenic activity of the larvae to be in the hemoglobin molecule.[170] Recent studies on this allergen from *Chironomus thummi* have identified regions of IgE binding and T-cell epitopes.[171]

Outdoor air sampling in Minnesota has disclosed allergens for the moth *Pseudaletia unipuncta* (Haworth). The levels of this moth antigen peaked in June and again in August to September, and the allergen levels were comparable with those of pollen and mold allergens. Furthermore, 45% of patients with positive skin test results to common aeroallergens had positive reactions to whole-body insect extracts. Of 120 patients with ragweed sensitivity, 5% had elevated specific IgE to moths. Hence, Lepidoptera may be considered seasonal allergens.[172]

Occupational exposure to insects may cause respiratory allergy. Chironomid larvae are used as fish food, resulting in symptoms among workers in their production, laboratory personnel, and hobbyists.[171] Similar symptoms, all documented with RAST and inhalation challenge, have been reported in workers handling crickets used for frog food[173] and mealworms (*Tenebrio molitor*) used as fishing bait.[174] Asthma and rhinitis occur in some bee keepers and in workers involved in honey production because of inhalation of honeybee body components. In these individuals, RAST inhibition is not achieved with venom extract.[175] Occupational allergy has been reported in laboratory workers dealing with locusts.[176] In these workers, as in the case of murine allergen–sensitive laboratory workers, atopy was not a prerequisite for sensitization. The primary locust allergen is the peritrophic membrane that surrounds food particles when they pass through the midgut and eventually become feces. In this sense, the locust allergen resembles that of the dust mite. The common housefly (*Musca domestica*) also has been reported as a cause of occupational allergy in laboratory workers,[177] as has the grain beetle *Alphitobius diaperinus*. Larval, pupal, and adult stages of the life cycle of this beetle all are capable of inducing allergy, but pupal extract contains the most significant allergens.[178]

Hypersensitivity to the salivary secretions of biting insects exists. Local immediate and delayed allergy to the bites of mosquitoes, fleas (papular urticaria), sand flies, deer flies, horse flies, and tsetse flies has been reported. Other case reports have described generalized reactions to multiple bites (deer fly) consisting of fever, malaise, and hypotension associated with antibodies to the offending insect. Experimental sensitization in humans with flea bites results first in the induction of delayed, and then in immediate, wheal-and-flare hypersensitivity on skin testing.

Hypersensitivity to the venom of stinging insects (Hymenoptera) is the subject of another chapter and is not discussed here.

Seeds

Seeds may be important causes of asthma and rhinitis. Cottonseed and flaxseed are exceptionally potent antigens and should be used for skin testing only by the epicutaneous method. Deaths have been reported from intradermal tests of both substances. Extreme caution should be used in skin testing.

Cottonseed is the seed of the cotton plant. After extracting the oil, which is not allergenic, the seed is ground into meal, which may be used for animal feeds or fertilizer. Cottonseed meal and flour also are used in the baking industry for certain cakes, cookies, and pan-greasing compounds. Cotton linters are the short cotton fibers that adhere to the seeds after the cotton is ginned. These are separated and used for stuffing mattresses and furniture. Enough of the water-soluble cottonseed allergen adheres to these linters to render them antigenic.[179] Several recent cases of angioedema, urticaria, or anaphylaxis have been reported in individuals who have eaten whole-grain bread or candy containing cottonseed meal.[180,181]

Flaxseed (linseed) has the same properties as cottonseed and has many of the same general uses in industry and agriculture. Additional uses are in hair preparation, poultices, electric wire insulation, and the tough backing material used in the manufacture of rugs. Linseed oil is a common household product and is found in furniture polish and printer's ink. In these forms, it produces contact rather than inhalant allergy.

Coffee bean allergy is largely confined to those who handle the green beans commercially, including longshoremen who unload the sacks of beans from ships. Chlorogenic acid has been considered an allergen in green coffee beans, castor beans, and oranges. It is a simple chemical that was thought to act as a hapten. Its importance is questionable, however, because it is destroyed by roasting and thus cannot account for allergy from drinking coffee. Castor bean (*Ricinus communis*) allergy is mainly from the pulp and hull that remain after castor oil is pressed from the bean. This castor pomace is ground into a meal that is used for fertilizer. Thus castor bean allergy also is largely occupational. Low molecular weight protein fractions have been isolated, as well as a toxic substance, ricin, which is not allergenic. Castor bean allergy also may occur in neighborhoods adjacent to processing plants. Asthma and rhinitis have been reported to be caused by the protein residual in the ambient air. A study from Marseilles, France, reports the incidence of castor bean allergy to be the same in atopic and nonatopic individuals.[182] Three allergenic castor bean proteins have been identified by protein electrophoresis. One of these three, *Ric c 1*, one of the "2S albumins" or storage proteins of the castor bean, has homology to both rice allergens and mustard seed allergens.[183,184] The 2S albumins represent one of two common storage proteins found in a variety of seeds, including sunflower seed, Brazil nut, and rapeseed. In common with other sensitizing allergenic proteins, these have low molecular weights, are highly soluble in water, and generally have no toxicity for nonallergic persons.[185]

Soybean allergy may be more generalized and prevalent because of the increased use of soy flour and meal in commonly encountered products. In addition to use as animal feed, soy products are used for infant formula, bakery goods, Chinese cooking, cereals, fillers in meat and candy products, and in certain topical dermatologic preparations. Occupational asthma caused by soybean flour used as a protein expander in frozen meat patties has been reported. Soybean protein consists of a globulin fraction (85%) and a whey fraction. Nine proteins bound to IgE by immunoblotting have been recognized by an allergic patient's serum.[186] Asthma epidemics have occurred in Barcelona, Spain, in association with unloading soybeans from ships. Case studies of those affected show a high incidence of IgE antibodies to soybean allergens. Subsequent investigations have shown that the major allergens are glycoproteins found in the hulls and dust, with molecular sizes less than 14 kilodaltons.[187–189]

OTHER PLANT AND ANIMAL ALLERGENS

Glues and gums are occasional causes of human allergy. Impure gelatin is the adhesive obtained from the bones and hides of terrestrial animals and fish bones. Other natural glues are made from casein, rubber, and gum arabic. Synthetic adhesives recently have minimized the glue allergy problem, although the amine hardeners used in the manufacture of epoxies have caused asthma and rhinitis in factory workers. In addition to gum arabic, other vegetable gums (acacia, chicle, karaya, and tragacanth) have been reported to cause allergy by inhalation or ingestion. These are used in candies, chewing gum, baked goods, salad dressings, laxatives, and dentifrices. They also are employed as excipients in medications. Guar gum is a vegetable gum that recently has been shown to induce IgE-mediated asthma. This gum is used in the carpet industry and affects about 2% of workers in carpet-manufacturing plants. The gum is used to fix colors to carpeting. It is also used in ice cream and salad dressings and as a hardener in the manufacturing of tablets in the pharmaceutical industry. Guar gum is obtained from *Cyanopsis tetragonolobus*, a vegetable grown in India.[190]

In hair-setting preparations, gums have been largely replaced by polyvinylpyrrolidone, which is not allergenic. Parenthetically, most cases of chronic pulmonary disease attributed to "hair spray allergy" or "hair spray thesaurosis" have turned out to be sarcoidosis, with no basis for attributing the cause to hair spray.

Inhalation of soapbark dust has caused occupational asthma. This wood dust is a product of the Quillaja tree and is used in the manufacture of saponin, a surface-reducing agent. Soapbark is chemically related to acacia and tragacanth, and these gums showed cross-reactivity in the soapbark RAST.[191]

Enzymes used in laundry detergents to enhance cleaning ability may sensitize both the workers where the product is made and the consumer who uses it.[192] The enzyme subtilisin (or subtilin) is proteolytic and is derived from *Bacillus subtilis*, where it plays a role in sporulation. It may produce rhinitis, conjunctivitis, and asthma, associated with IgE antibodies; or it may produce more peripheral alveolar hypersensitivity reactions associated with precipitating antibodies and Arthus-type reactions on skin testing. Many cases reported did not involve atopic individuals. Enzyme-containing detergents currently are not commonly used because of their sensitizing potential. Other enzymes, cellulase and macerozyme, are used to digest cell wall structures of plants. Laboratory workers have been shown to develop IgE-mediated symptoms from inhaling these enzymes.[193] Papain, a sulfhydryl protease, is obtained from the fruit of the papaya tree. It is used as a meat tenderizer, clearing agent in the production of beer, contact lens cleaner, and component of some tooth powders, laxatives, and skin lotions. Asthma has been induced by inhalation of papain, and antipapain IgE and IgG antibodies have been demonstrated in a worker in a meat tenderizer factory. In this case, the IgE–RAST result was not positive until after the other classes of immunoglobulins had been absorbed from the sera.[194] Although papain has been cloned, the mechanism behind its role as an allergen remains unknown.

Grain mill dust and baker's flour have long been recognized as causes of occupational asthma. Positive skin test results to extracts of grain mill dust often are seen in patients who have never worked in granaries. It is generally agreed that allergens are responsible for the symptoms resulting from inhaling these substances, but it is not known if these allergens are primarily from the grains themselves or from organisms that infest them, such as molds, mites, or weevils. Recently, it has been shown that water- and salt-soluble enzymes and enzyme inhibitors in flours may be responsible for most cases of asthma and allergic reactions among bakers. Most data support a role for the α- and β-amylases, the α-amylase inhibitors, and various trypsin inhibitors as the detectable allergens in flours.[195] Cross-reacting species were detected between rye, wheat, and barley flours, but definitive identification of these allergens is pending.[196]

Garlic has caused asthma by inhalation[197] and by inhalation and ingestion.[198] Both cases were documented immunologically, and one was documented by inhalation challenge. In one case,[198] the capacities of onion and asparagus, other members of the Liliaceae family, to inhibit the garlic RAST were two and one half to four times higher than the homologous garlic extract.

INDUSTRIAL AND OCCUPATIONAL CHEMICALS AND AIR POLLUTANTS

Trimellitic anhydride (TMA), a plasticizer and curing agent used in the plastics industry, has been described as a cause of occupational asthma. It is a simple compound that acts as a hapten. Conjugated to human serum albumin (HSA), IgE antibodies to TM-HSA have been demonstrated by Prausnitz-Küstner test reactions in monkeys.[199] Antibodies to the IgE, IgG, and IgA classes have been identified using the technique of solid-phase radioimmunoassay.[200] TMA asthma is associated with IgE, and a late respiratory response similar to symptoms of hypersensitivity pneumonitis correlates with IgG and total antibody measured by ammonium sulfate precipitation. IgA antibody to TM-HSA is found in all workers with high exposure and cannot be used to discriminate those with and without symptoms.[201] An nonallergic, irritative reaction to TMA also may occur. In addition, a pulmonary disease–anemia syndrome, with an immunologic basis, has been described after TMA exposure.[199]

Toluene diisocyanate is an intermediate in the manufacture of polyurethane. It causes asthma in some workers (5% to 10%) in the plastics and electronic industries, but it does not affect the general public who use polyurethane. The mechanism of toluene diisocyanate asthma has been studied extensively, and there is evidence for immunologic mechanisms, although some data point to an autonomic effect, possibly that of beta-adrenergic blockade.[202] Other isocyanates have been associated with pulmonary syndromes of both the immediate and hypersensitivity pneumonitis types. Diphenylmethane diisocyanate is a compound in which both IgE and IgG antibodies have been shown by the polystyrene-tube radioimmunoassay.[203] Hexamethylene diisocyanate in a patient with alveolitis and asthma was associated with IgG antibodies but not IgE antibodies by ammonium sulfate precipitation and an ELISA.[204] All of these immunoassays were done using HSA conjugates of the various isocyanate compounds, which are necessary for antigenic recognition. The specificity, at least for IgE antibodies, lies with both the hapten and specific portions of the carrier protein.[205] Tetrachlorophthalic anhydride is another chemical substance that produces immediate and late asthmatic reactions in a small percentage (fewer than 2%) of exposed workers. Conjugated with HSA, positive skin prick test and RAST results were obtained in the affected workers. Cigarette smoking rather than a history of atopy appeared to be the predisposing factor.[206]

Numerous other chemical and biologic materials, mainly industrial or occupational, have been implicated more recently in human asthma. It is important from practical and heuristic viewpoints to determine if the mechanisms of asthma are caused by IgE-mediation, nonspecific mediator release, or irritative phenomena that are thought to act by nociceptive reflex parasympathetic stimulation. Methods used to study suspected substances include epidemiologic data, bronchoprovocation, and the ability to block bronchoprovocation by disodium cromoglycate or atropine, as well as attempts to identify antigen-specific IgE or IgG by techniques previously described. Detailed reviews have been published.[207–210] Occupational asthma is reviewed in more detail elsewhere in this text.

Some examples of inhalants to which reactions are thought to be immunologically mediated are salts of platinum,[208] chrome, and nickel.[211] Reactions occur mainly in areas where the metals are refined or used in plating. Wood dusts, notably from western red cedar, may cause asthma in woodworkers. Plicatic acid is thought to be the offending component of this wood. Asthma occurs in 5% of sawmill workers and carpenters who handle western cedar. IgE antibodies to conjugates of plicatic acid and HSA are found in 40% of symptomatic workers, but nonspecific bronchial hyperreactivity is the most constant feature of the syndrome.[212] Plicatic acid is able to activate complement and generate chemotactic activity from pooled human serum, but the role of this mechanism, if any, in red cedar asthma has not been determined.[213] Only 50% of those affected eventually recover after terminating exposure to plicatic acid. Hog trypsin, used in the manufacture of plastic resins, and psyllium, a bulk laxative, may be causes of occupational asthma. The latter is related to the weed plantain.

Other examples of occupational asthma occur among snow crab processing workers and individuals who use solder. In the latter case, colophony, a component of flux, is the asthmogenic material.[214] Metabisulfites, sulfiting agents used as preservatives and clearing agents, may act as both allergens and nonspecific irritants.[215]

Byssinosis is an example of bronchoconstriction caused by nonspecific histamine release. Initially reversible, the disorder often leads to chronic obstructive lung disease on prolonged exposure to raw cotton. The pathogenic substance is a proteinaceous dust from the bract of the plant. This dust causes histamine-induced bronchospasm when inhaled, without evidence to support an immunologic basis. Cellulose does not cause the same reaction.

Asthma exacerbated by direct irritation of the bronchi is common in clinical practice. Odors from perfumes and colognes, vapors from petroleum products and organic solvents, and fumes from tobacco and cooking oils cause coughing and wheezing in many patients.

Meat wrapper's asthma is another occupational disorder caused by inhaling the fumes of polyvinyl chloride. The fumes are created when polyvinyl chloride is cut with a hot wire in the process of wrapping cuts of meat.

Air pollution is a prominent current topic and is relevant to the pathogenesis of several disease entities unrelated to asthma and rhinitis. Most pulmonary disease specialists would assign a role to pollutants in producing symptoms in asthmatics (atopic and nonatopic) and patients with rhinitis (allergic and vasomotor), but the primacy, magnitude, and mechanism are still unknown.[216] Epidemic asthma has occurred in Yokohama, Japan, and New Orleans. In Yokohama, pollution has been implicated, but in New Orleans the epidemics have not corresponded with elevated levels of known chemical and particulate pollutants. New Orleans asthma, originally thought to result from air pollution and climatic changes, now seems to be caused by the prevalence of natural inhalant allergens. Hospital admissions for asthma correlate well with high counts of *Ambrosia* pollen and certain fungal spores (possibly Basidiomycetes) obtained by the use of the automatic intermittent rotoslide sampler.[217] Other authors have emphasized the role of allergy in emergency room visits to hospitals. Increased exposure to allergens such as mites, cats, roaches, grass pollens, and ragweed have matched the time of emergency room visits. Authors stress the need for investigation into allergic causative factors in patients who seek emergency treatment for asthma.[218,219]

The United States national ambient air quality standards are as follows for selected pollutants: sulfur dioxide, 0.14 ppm; total particles, 150 μg/mL; carbon monoxide, 35 ppm; ozone, 0.12 ppm; nitrogen dioxide, 0.05 ppm; and lead, 1.5 μg/m^3.[216] Formaldehyde is primarily an indoor pollutant that emanates from particle board, insulation, furnishings, tobacco smoke, and gas stoves. Most formaldehyde symptoms occur in mobile homes, where large amounts of particle board have been used in a relatively small enclosed space. Concentrations of 1 to 3 ppm or higher may cause mucous membrane symptoms in some individuals; atopic persons may react at lower concentrations. This is thought to be largely an irritative phenomenon. Experimentally, formaldehyde can be rendered immunogenic by the formation of formaldehyde–protein complexes. However, it has not been proven that these complexes cause IgE- or IgG-mediated disease, nor has it been proven that inhalation of formaldehyde leads to the formation of formaldehyde–protein complexes.[220]

Sulfur dioxide is a product of soft coal burned for industrial use and is the substance most closely correlated with respiratory and conjunctival symptoms. Sulfur dioxide does not come from automobile exhaust. Incompletely oxidized hydrocarbons from factories and vehicular exhaust make up the "smoke" visible in any highly populated or industrial area. Hydrocarbons, ozone, and nitrates, which are products of photochemical oxidation, may impair pulmonary ventilation. Carbon monoxide impairs oxygen transport, but its concentration in ambient polluted air is probably important only in patients with marginal respiratory reserve. Traces of lead, arsenic, and formaldehyde also are found in polluted air.

Ozone is monitored in many metropolitan areas, but regarding toxic levels there is more a consensus than firm data. At 0.07 ppm of ozone, the warning level, asthma may occur. At 0.30 ppm (red alert), there is a greater incidence of asthma. The emergency level is considered to be 0.50 ppm.[221]

The term *sick building syndrome* refers to outbreaks of acute illness among workers in a particular building or area of a building. Most buildings in which this has been reported have been energy efficient, with little direct outside air exchange. Hence, the term *tight building syndrome* also has been applied. The symptoms most commonly involve the conjunctivae and respiratory tract, with additional nonspecific complaints such as headache, fatigue, and inability to concentrate. Except for unusual instances of contamination with microorganisms (such as *Legionella*) or of hypersensitivity pneumonitis, the outbreaks have not resulted in serious morbidity or permanent disability. The cause in more than half of the instances studied has been inadequate ventilation, and symptoms abated when corrective measures were taken. Specific contamination from inside the building has been observed in 17% of "sick" buildings. Contaminants have included methyl alcohol, butyl methacrylate, ammonia, and acetic acid from various office machines; chlordane (an insecticide); diethyl ethanolamine from boilers; rug shampoos; tobacco smoke; and combustion gases from cafeterias and laboratories. Alkanes, terpenes, benzenes, and chlorinated hydrocarbons also have been identified in investigations of indoor air. In some instances, indoor contamination may occur from outside of the building: for example, the intake of automobile exhaust from an adjacent parking garage.

The role of passive tobacco smoke is one of a respiratory tract irritant. Both allergic and nonallergic persons may be affected. Symptoms range from burning eyes to nasal coryza and coughing or wheezing. Additional ventilation, including outside air, may be required in smoking areas. The role of tobacco alone in the sick building syndrome is not clear when adequate ventilation is present, however. Tobacco smoke contains hundreds of toxic chemicals, including carbon monoxide, hydrogen cyanide, nitrogen dioxide, formaldehyde, acrolein, and ammonia.

Formaldehyde is released as a gas ("off-gassing") from a variety of sources such as foam insulation, new furniture, and carbonless carbon paper. The level in office buildings ranges from 0.01 to 0.30 ppm. In mobile homes, levels up to 0.8 ppm have been recorded in dwellings whose occupants have no physical complaints, but levels up to 3.6 ppm have been measured in mobile homes whose residents do have complaints.

Finally, the role of psychogenic suggestion in the sick building syndrome should be considered. Such instances have been reported, based on a variety of inconsistencies in the affected population and the lack of objective findings in both the patients and the building. The perception of tainted air may be induced by transitory malodors, job dissatisfaction, boredom, frustration, and other considerations.[222]

REFERENCES

1. Marsh DG, Norman PS. Antigens that cause atopic disease. In: Samter M, Talmage DW, Frank MM, Austen KF, Claman HN, eds. Immunological diseases. 4th ed. Vol 2. Boston: Little, Brown, 1988:981.
2. Stewart GA. The molecular biology of allergens. In: Busse WW, Holgate ST, eds. Asthma and rhinitis. Boston: Blackwell Scientific Publications, 1995;898.
3. King TP, Hoffman D, Lowenstein H, et al. Allergen nomenclature. J Allergy Clin Immunol 1995;96:5.
4. Busse WW, Reed CE, Hoehne JH. Where is the allergic reaction in ragweed asthma? II. Demonstration of ragweed antigen in airborne particles smaller than pollen. J Allergy Clin Immunol 1972;50:289.
5. Solomon WR, Burge HA, Muilenberg ML. Allergen carriage by atmospheric aerosol. I. Ragweed pollen determinants in smaller micronic fractions. J Allergy Clin Immunol 1983;72:443.
6. Agarwal MK, Swanson MC, Reed CE, et al. Immunochemical quantitation of airborne short ragweed, *Alternaria,* antigen E, and *Alt-1* allergens: a 2-year prospective study. J Allergy Clin Immunol 1983;72:40.
7. Rosenberg GL, Rosenthal RR, Norman PS. Inhalation challenge with ragweed pollen in ragweed-sensitive asthmatics. J Allergy Clin Immunol 1983;71:302.
8. Michel FB, Marty JP, Quet L, Cour R. Penetration of inhaled pollen into the respiratory tract. Am Rev Respir Dis 1977;115:609.
9. Marsh D. Allergens and the genetics of allergy. In: Sela M, ed. The antigens. Vol 3. New York: Academic Press, 1975:271.
10. Marsh DG, Belin L, Bruce A. Rapidly released allergens from short ragweed pollen. I. Kinetics of release of known allergens in relation to biologic activity. J Allergy Clin Immunol 1981;67:206.
11. Burge HA, Solomon WR. Sampling and analysis of biological aerosols. Atmos Environ 1984;21:451.
12. Solomon WR, Burge HA, Boise JR. Performance of adhesives for rotating arm impactors. J Allergy Clin Immunol 1980;65:467.
13. Solomon WR, Matthews KP. Aerobiology and inhalant allergens. In: Middleton E Jr, Reed CE, Ellis EF, Adkinson NF Jr, Yunginger JW, eds. Allergy principles and practice. 3rd ed. St Louis: CV Mosby, 1988:312.
14. Solomon WR. Aerobiology of pollinosis. J Allergy Clin Immunol 1984;74:449.
15. Reed CE. Measurement of airborne antigens. J Allergy Clin Immunol 1982;70:38.
16. Luczynska CM, Li Y, Chapman MD, Platts-Mills TAE. Airborne concentrations and particle size distribution of allergen derived from domestic cats (*Felis domesticus*): measurements using cascade impactor, liquid impinger, and a two site monoclonal antibody assay for *Fel d I.* Am Rev Respir Dis 1990;141:361.
17. Agarwal MK, Yunginger JW, Swanson BA, et al. An immunochemical method to measure atmospheric allergens. J Allergy Clin Immunol 1981;68:194.
18. Agarwal MK, Swanson MC, Reed CE, et al. Airborne ragweed allergens: association with various particle sizes and short ragweed plant parts. J Allergy Clin Immunol 1984;74:687.
19. Platts-Mills TAE, Heymann PW, Longbottom JL, Wilkins SR. Airborne allergens associated with asthma: particle sizes carrying dust mite and rat allergens measured with a cascade impactor. J Allergy Clin Immunol 1986;77:850.
20. Schumacher MJ, Griffith RD, O'Rourke MK. Recognition of pollen and other particulate aeroantigens by immunoblot microscopy. J Allergy Clin Immunol 1988;82:608.
21. Bousquet J, Guerin B, Michel F-B. Standardization of allergens. In: Spector SL, ed. Provocative challenge procedures: background and methodology. Mount Kisco, NY: Futura Publishing, 1989:85.
22. Bush RK, Kagen SL. Guidelines for the preparation and characterization of high molecular weight allergens used for the diagnosis of occupational lung disease. J Allergy Clin Immunol 1989;84:814.
23. Dreborg S, Belin L, Eriksson NE, et al. Results of biological standardization with standardized allergen preparations. Allergy 1987;42:109.
24. Chua KY, Kehal PK, Thomas WR, et al. High frequency binding of IgE to the *Der p II* allergen expressed in yeast. J Allergy Clin Immunol 1992;89:95.

25. Reed CE, Yunginger JW, Evans R. Quality assurance and standardization of allergy extracts in allergy practices. J Allergy Clin Immunol 1989;84:4.
26. Jeanin P, Didierlaurent A, Gras-Masse H, et al. Specific histamine release capacity of peptides selected from the modelized *Der p I* protein, a major allergen of *Dermatophagoides pteronyssinus*. Mol Immunol 1991;29:739.
27. Schroder H. RAST-based techniques for allergen assay. In: Brede H, Going H, eds. Regulatory control and standardization of allergenic extracts. Stuttgart: Gustav Fisher Verlag, 1980:138.
28. Baer H, Anderson MC. Allergenic extracts. I. Allergenic extracts: sources, preparation and in vitro standardization. In: Middleton E Jr, Ellis EF, Reed CE, et al., eds. Allergy: principles and practice. 3rd ed. St Louis: CV Mosby, 1988:373.
29. Platts-Mills TAE. Allergens. In: Samter M, Talmage DW, Frank MM, Austen KF, Claman HN, eds. Immunological diseases. 5th ed. Vol 2. Boston: Little, Brown, 1993:1231.
30. Løwenstein H. Quantitative immunoelectrophoretic methods as a tool for the analysis and isolation of allergens. Prog Allergy 1978;25:1.
31. Aas K. What makes an allergen an allergen? Allergy 1978;33:3.
32. King TP. Immunochemical properties of some atopic allergens. J Allergy Clin Immunol 1979;64:159.
33. Lewis WR, Vinay P, Zenger VE. Airborne and allergenic pollen of North America. Baltimore: The Johns Hopkins University Press, 1983.
34. Weber RW, Nelson HS. Pollen allergens and their inter-relationships. Clin Rev Allergy 1985;3:291.
35. Smith EG. Sampling and identifying allergenic pollens and molds. Vol. 1. San Antonio: Blewstone Press, 1984.
36. Smith EG. Sampling and identifying allergenic pollens and molds. Vol. 2. San Antonio: Blewstone Press, 1986.
37. King TP, Norman PS. Standardized extracts: weeds. Clin Rev Allergy 1986;4:425.
38. King TP, Norman PS, Lichtenstein LM. Studies on ragweed pollen allergens V. Ann Allergy 1967;25:541.
39. Baer H, Godfrey H, Maloney CJ, Norman PS, Lichtenstein LM. The potency and antigen E content of commercially prepared ragweed extracts. J Allergy 1970;45:347.
40. Rafnar T, Griffith IJ, Kuo MC, et al. Cloning of *Amb a I* (antigen E), the major allergen family of short ragweed pollen. J Biol Chem 1991;266:1229.
41. Gleich GJ, Yunginger JW. Ragweed hay fever: treatment by passive local administration of IgG antibody. Clin Allergy 1975;1:79.
42. Lee YS, Dickinson DB, Schlager D, et al. Antigen E content of pollen from individual plants of short ragweed. J Allergy Clin Immunol 1979;64:173.
43. Rogers BL, Morgenstern JP, Griffith IJ, et al. Complete sequence of the allergen *Amb a II*: recombinant expression and reactivity with T cells from ragweed allergic patients. J Immunol 1991;147:2547.
44. Adolphson C, Goodfriend L, Gleich GJ. Reactivity of ragweed allergens with IgE antibodies. J Allergy Clin Immunol 1978;62:197.
45. Goodfriend L. Toward structure-function studies with ragweed allergens *Ra 3* and *Ra 5*. In: Mathov E, Sindro T, Naranjo P, eds. Allergy and clinical immunology. Amsterdam: Excerpta Medica, 1977:151.
46. Santilli J Jr, Potsus RS, Goodfriend L, et al. Skin reactivity to purified pollen allergens in highly ragweed-sensitive individuals. J Allergy Clin Immunol 1980;65:406.
47. Roebber M, Hussain R, Klapper DG, Marsh DG. Isolation and properties of a new short ragweed pollen allergen, *Ra-6*. J Immunol 1983;131:706.
48. Roebber M, Marsh DG. Isolation and characterization of allergen *Amb a VII* from short ragweed pollen. J Allergy Clin Immunol 1991;87:324.
49. Rogers BL, Pollock J, Klapper DG, et al. Complete sequence of a proteinase inhibitor cystatin homologue from the pollen of *Ambrosia artemisiifolia* (short ragweed). Gene 1993;133:219.
50. Lubahn B, Klapper DG. Cloning and characterization of ragweed allergen *Amb a VI*. J Allergy Clin Immunol 1993;91:338.
51. Hussain R, Norman PS, Marsh DG. Rapidly released allergens from short ragweed pollens. II. Identification and partial purification. J Allergy Clin Immunol 1981;67:217.
52. Goodfriend L, Roebber M, Lundvist U, et al. Two variants of ragweed allergen *Ra 3*. J Allergy Clin Immunol 1981;67:299.
53. Marsh DG, Hsu SH, Hussain R, et al. Genetics of human immune response to allergens. J Allergy Clin Immunol 1980;65:322.
54. Roebber M, Klapper DG, Goodfriend L, Bias WB, Hsu SH, Marsh DG. Immunochemical and genetic studies of *Amb t V* (Ra5G), and Ra5 homologue from giant ragweed pollen. J Immunol 1985;134:3062.
55. Shafiee A, Yunginger JW, Gleich GJ. Isolation and characterization of Russian thistle (*Salsola pestifer*) pollen allergens. J Allergy Clin Immunol 1981;67:472.
56. Cocchiara R, Locorstondo G, Parlato A, et al. Purification of *Par j I*, a major allergen from *Parietara judaica* pollen. Int Arch Allergy Appl Immunol 1990;90:84.
57. Nilsen BM, Grimsen A, Paulsen BS. Identification and characterization of important allergens from mugwort pollen by IEF, SDS-PAGE and immunoblotting. Mol Immunol 1991;28:733.
58. Ford SA, Baldo BA. A re-examination of ryegrass (*Lolium perenne*) pollen allergens. Int Arch Allergy Appl Immunol 1986;81:193.
59. Løwenstein H, Sterballe O. Standardized grass pollen extracts. Clin Rev Allergy 1986;4:405.
60. Staff IA, Taylor PE, Smith P, et al. Cellular localization of water soluble, allergenic proteins in ryegrass (*Lolium perenne*) pollen using monoclonal and specific IgE antibodies with immunogold probes. Histochem J 1990;22:276.

61. van Ree R, Driessen MNBM, van Leeuwen WA, et al. Variability of cross-reactivity of IgE antibodies to group I and V allergens in eight grass pollen species. Clin Exp Allergy 1992;22:611.
62. Matthiesen F, Lowenstein H. Group V allergens in grass pollens. II. Investigation of group V allergen in pollens from ten grasses. Clin Exp Allergy 1991;21:309.
63. Mourad W, Mecheri S, Peltre G, et al. Stusy of the epitope structure of purified *Dac g I* and *Lol p I*, the major allergens of *Dactylis glomerata* and *Lolium perenne* pollens, using monoclonal antibodies. J Immunol 1988;141:3486.
64. Petersen A, Schramm G, Bufe A, et al. Structural investigations of the major allergen *Phl p I* on the complementary DNA and protein level. J Allergy Clin Immunol 1995;95:987.
65. Matthiesen F, Løwenstein H. Gramineae allergens: biochemistry. Horsholm, Denmark: ALK Research, 1990:1.
66. Tamborini E, Brandazza A, De Lalla C, et al. Recombinant allergen *Lol p II*: expression, purification and characterization. Mol Immunol 1995;32:505.
67. Olson, E, Zhang L, Hill RD, et al. Identification and characterization of the *Poa p IX* group of basic allergens of Kentucky bluegrass pollen. J Immunol 1991;147:205.
68. Bufe A, Schramm G, Keown MB, et al. Major allergen *Phl p Vb* in timothy grass is a novel pollen RNase. FEBS Lett 1995;363:6.
69. Walsh DJ, Matthews JA, Denmeade R, Walker MR. Cloning of cDNA coding for an allergen of cocksfoot grass (*Dactylis glomerata*) pollen. Int Arch Allergy Appl Immunol 1989;90:78.
70. Valenta R, Duchene M, Ebner C, et al. Profilins constitute a novel family of functional plant pan-allergens. J Exp Med 1992;175:377.
71. van Ree R, Hoffman DR, van Dijk W, et al. *Lol p XI*, a new major grass pollen allergen, is a member of a family of soybean trypsin inhibitor-related proteins. J Allergy Clin Immunol 1995;95:970.
72. Belin L. Standardized extracts: trees. Clin Rev Allergy 1986;4:189.
73. Jarolim JE, Tejkl M, Rohac M, et al. Monoclonal antibodies against birch pollen allergens: characterization by immunoblotting and use for single-step affinity purification of the major allergen, *Bet v I*. Int Arch Allergy Appl Immunol 1989;90:54.
74. Breiteneder H, Pattenburger K, Bito A, et al. The gene coding for the major birch pollen allergen, *Bet v I*, is highly homologous to a pea disease resistance response gene. EMBO J 1989;8:1935.
75. Valenta R, Duchene M, Vrtala S, et al. Recombinant allergens for immunoblot diagnosis of tree-pollen allergy. J Allergy Clin Immunol 1991;88:889.
76. Yasueda H, Yui Y, Shimizu T, Shida T. Isolation and partial characterization of the major allergen from Japanese cedar (*Cryptomeria japonica*) pollen. J Allergy Clin Immunol 1983;71:77.
77. Sakaguchi M, Inouye S, Taniai M, et al. Identification of the second major allergen of Japenese cedar pollen. Allergy 1990;45:309.
78. Gross GN, Zimburean JM, Capra JD. Isolation and partial characterization of the allergen in mountain cedar pollen. Scand J Immunol 1978;8:436.
79. Bush RK, Yunginger JW. Standardization of fungal allergens. Clin Rev Allergy 1987;5:3.
80. Prince HE, Selle WA, Morrow MB. Molds in the etiology of asthma and hay fever. Tex Med 1934;30:340.
81. Feinberg SM. Mold allergy: its importance in asthma and hay fever. Wis Med J 1935;34:254.
82. O'Hollaren MT, Yunginger JW, Offord KP, et al. Exposure to an aeroallergen as a possible precipitating factor in respiratory arrest in young patients with asthma. N Engl J Med 1991;324:359.
83. Licorish K, Novey HS, Kozak P, et al. Role of *Alternaria* and *Penicillium* spores in the pathogenesis of asthma. J Allergy Clin Immunol 1985;76:819.
84. Pepys J. Hypersensitivity diseases of the lungs due to fungi and organic dusts. Basel: S Karger, 1969.
85. Yunginger JW, Jones RT, Nesheim ME, et al. Studies on *Alternaria* allergens. III. Isolation of a major allergenic fraction (*Alt-1*). J Allergy Clin Immunol 1980;6:138.
86. Miles RM, Parker JL, Jones RT, et al. Studies on *Alternaria* allergens. IV. Biologic activity of a purified fraction (*Alt-1*). J Allergy Clin Immunol 1983;71:36.
87. Nyholm L, Løwenstein H, Yunginger JW. Immunochemical partial identity between two independently identified and isolated major allergens from *Alternaria* (*Alt-1* and *Ag-1*). J Allergy Clin Immunol 1983;71:461.
88. Agarwal MK, Jones RT, Yunginger JW. Shared allergenic and antigenic determinants in *Alternaria* and *Stemphyllium* extracts. J Allergy Clin Immunol 1982;70:437.
89. Helm RM, Squillace DL, Aukrust L, et al. Production of an international reference standard *Alternaria* extract. I. Testing of candidate extracts. Int Arch Allergy Appl Immunol 1987;82:178.
90. Bush RK, Voss MJ, Bashirian S. Detection of *Alternaria* allergens by crossed-radioimmunoelectrophoresis. J Allergy Clin Immunol 1983;71:239.
91. Kroutil LA, Bush RK. Detection of *Alternaria* allergens by Western blotting. J Allergy Clin Immunol 1987;80:170.
92. Steringer I, Aukrust L, Einarsson R. Variability of antigenicity/allergenicity in different strains of *Alternaria alternata*. Int Arch Allergy Appl Immunol 1987;84:190.
93. Aukrust L. Allergens in *Cladosporium herbarum*. In: Oehling A, Glazer J, Mathov E, Arbesman C, eds. Advances in allergology and applied immunology. New York: Pergamon Press, 1980:475.
94. Aukrust L, Borsch SM. Partial purification and characterization of two *Cladosporium herbarum* allergens. Int Arch Allergy Appl Immunol 1979;60:68.
95. Horner WE, Helbling A, Salvaggio JE, et al. Fungal allergens. Clin Microbiol Rev 1995;8:161.

96. Longbottom JL. Allergic bronchopulmonary aspergillosis: reactivity of IgE and IgG antibodies with antigenic components of *Aspergillus fumigatus* (IgE/IgG antigen complexes). J Allergy Clin Immunol 1983;72: 668.
97. Wallenbeck L, Aukrust L, Einarsson R. Antigenic variability of different strains of *Aspergillus fumigatus*. Int Arch Allergy Appl Immunol 1987;73:166.
98. Kauffman HF, van den Heide S, Beaumont F, et al. The allergenic and antigenic properties of spores extracts of *Aspergillus fumigatus*: a comparative study of spore extracts with mycelium and culture filtrate extracts. J Allergy Clin Immunol 1984;73:573.
99. Reed CE. Variability of antigenicity of *Aspergillus fumigatus*. J Allergy Clin Immunol 1978;61:227.
100. Fernandez LJ, Lopez OC, Soriano F, et al. Complete amino acid sequence of the *Aspergillus* cytotoxin mitogillin. Biochemistry 1985;24:861.
101. Baur X, Fruhman G, Haug B, et al. Role of *Aspergillus* amylase in baker's asthma. Lancet 1986;i:43.
102. Salvaggio J, Aukrust L. Mold-induced asthma. J Allergy Clin Immunol 1981;68:327.
103. Koivikko A, Savolainen FJ. Mushroom allergy. Allergy 1988;43:1.
104. Lehrer SB, et al. Basidiomycete mycelia and spore-allergen extracts: skin test reactivity in adults with symptoms of respiratory allergy. J Allergy Clin Immunol 1986;78:478.
105. Akiyama K, Yui Y, Shida T, et al. Relationship between the results of skin, conjunctival, and bronchial tests and RAST with *Candida albicans*. Clin Allergy 1981;11:343.
106. Bennetzen JL, Hall BD. The primary structure of the *Saccharomyces cerevisiae* gene for alcohol dehydrogenase. J Biol Chem 1982;257:3018.
107. Shen HD, Choo KB, Lee HH, et al. The 40-kilodalton allergen of *Candida albicans* is an alcohol dehydrogenase: molecular cloning and immunological analysis using monoclonal antibodies. Clin Exp Allergy 1991;21:675.
108. Solomon WR. Assessing fungus prevalence in domestic interiors. J Allergy Clin Immunol 1975;56:235.
109. Kendrick B. The fifth kingdom. Waterloo, Ontario: Mycologue Publications, 1985.
110. Ibanez MD, Horner WE, Liengsuvangswong V, et al. Identification and analysis of basidiospore allergens from puffballs. J Allergy Clin Immunol 1988;82:787.
111. Weissman DW, Halmepuro L, Salvaggio JE, Lehrer SB. Antigenic/allergenic analysis of basiodiomycete cap, mycelia, and spore extracts. Int Arch Allergy Appl Immunol 1987;84:56.
112. Lopez M, Voigtlander JR, Lehrer SB, Salaggio JE. Broncho-provocation studies in basidiospore-sensitive allergic subjects with asthma. J Allergy Clin Immunol 1989;84:242.
113. Schwartz HJ, Citron KM, Chester EH, et al. A comparison of the prevalence of sensitization to *Aspergillus* antigens among asthmatics in Cleveland and London. J Allergy Clin Immunol 1978;62:9.
114. Hirsch DJ, Hirsch SR, Kalbfleisch JH. Effect of central air conditioning and meteorologic factors on indoor spore counts. J Allergy Clin Immunol 1978;62:22.
115. Burge HA, Solomon WR, Mailenberg ML. Evaluation of indoor plantings as allergen exposure sources. J Allergy Clin Immunol 1982;70:101.
116. Burge HA, Solomon WR, Williams P. Fungus exposure risks associated with animal care units. J Allergy Clin Immunol 1979;64:29.
117. Al-Doory Y, Domson J, eds. Mold allergy. Philadelphia: Lea & Febiger, 1984.
118. Kern RA. Dust sensitization in bronchial asthma. Med Clin North Am 1921;5:751.
119. Voorhorst R, Spieksma-Boezeman MIA, Spieksma FTHM. Is a mite (*Dermatophagoides* sp.) the producer of the house-dust allergen? Aller Asthmaforsch 1964;6:329.
120. Miyamoto T, Oshima S, Domae A, et al. Allergenic potency of different house dusts in relation to contained mites. Ann Allergy 1970;28:405.
121. Miyamoto T, Oshima S, Ishizaki T. Antigenic relation between house dust and a dust mite, *Dermatophagoides farinae*, Hughes, 1961 by a fractionation method. J Allergy 1969;44:282.
122. Miyamoto T, Oshima S, Ishizaki T, et al. Allergenic identity between common flour mite (*Dermatophagoides farinae*, Hughes, 1961) and house dust as a causative antigen in bronchial asthma. J Allergy 1968;42:152.
123. Miyamoto T, Oshima S, Mizunko K, et al. Cross antigenicity among six species of dust mites and house dust antigens. J Allergy 1969;44:228.
124. Morita T, Miyamoto T, Horiuchi T, et al. Further studies in allergenic identity between house dust and house dust mite, *Dermatophagoides farinae*, Hughes, 1961. Ann Allergy 1975;35:361.
125. Sporik R, Holgate ST, Platts-Mills TAE, Cogswell JJ. Exposure to house-dust mite allergen (*Der p I*) and the development of asthma in childhood. N Engl J Med 1990;323:502.
126. Newman LJ, Sporik RB, Platts-Mills TAE. The role of house-dust mite and other allergens in asthma. In: Busse WW, Holgate ST, eds. Asthma and rhinitis. Boston: Blackwell Scientific Publications, 1995;933.
127. Arlian LG, Bernstein IL, Gallagher JS. The prevalence of house dust mites, *Dermatophagoides* spp. and associated environmental conditions in homes in Ohio. J Allergy Clin Immunol 1982;69:527.
128. Murray AB, Zuk P. The seasonal variation in a population of house dust mites in a North American city. J Allergy Clin Immunol 1979;64:266.
129. Vervolet D, Perrand JA, Razzouk H, et al. Altitude and house dust mites. J Allergy Clin Immunol 1982;69:290.
130. Platts-Mills TAE, Chapman MD. Dust mites: Immunology: allergic disease and environmental control. J Allergy Clin Immunol 1987;80:755.

131. Ford AW, Platts-Mills TAE. Standardized extracts, dust mites, and other arthropods (inhalants). Clin Rev Allergy 1987;5:49.
132. Warren CPW, Holford-Strevens V, Sinha RN. Sensitization in a grain handler to the storage mite *Lepidoglyphis destructor* (Schrank). Ann Allergy 1983;50:30.
133. Wraith DC, Cunnington AM, Seymour WM. The role and allergenic importance of storage mites in house dust and other environments. Clin Allergy 1979;9:545.
134. Pollart S, Chapman MD, Platts-Mills TAE. House dust mite and dust control. Clin Rev Allergy 1988;6:23.
135. Tovey ER, Chapman MD, Platts-Mills TAE. Mite faeces are a major source of house dust allergens. Nature 1981;289:592.
136. Arlian LG, Bernstein IL, Vyszenski-Moher DL, Gallagher JS. Investigations of culture medium-free house dust mites. IV. Cross antigenicity and allergenicity between the house dust mites, *Dermatophagoides farinae* and *D. pteronyssinus*. J Allergy Clin Immunol 1987;79:467.
137. Chua KY, Stewart GA, Thomas WR, et al. Sequence analysis of cDNA coding for a major house dust mite allergen, *Der p I*. Homology with cysteine proteases. J Exp Med 1988;167:175.
138. Cardot E, Pestel J, Callebaut I, et al. Specific activation of platelets from patients allergic to *Dermatophagoides pteronyssinus* by synthetic peptides derived from the allergen *Der p I*. Int Arch Allergy Immunol 1992;98:127.
139. Heymann PW, Chapman MD, Aalberse RC, et al. Antigenic and structural analysis of group II allergens (*Der f II* and *Der p II*) from house dust mites (*Dermatophagoides* spp.). J Allergy Clin Immunol 1989;83:1055.
140. Chapman MD, Platts-Mills TAE. Purification and characterization of the major allergen from *Dermatophagoides pteronyssinus* antigen P_1. J Immunol 1980;125:587.
141. Platts-Mills TAE, Tovey ER, Mitchell EB, et al. Reduction of bronchial hyperreactivity during prolonged allergen avoidance. Lancet 1982;ii:675.
142. Ohman JL, Kendall S, Lowell FC. IgE antibody to cat allergens in an allergic population. J Allergy Clin Immunol 1977;60:317.
143. Wentz PE, Swanson MC, Reed CE. Variability of cat-allergen shedding. J Allergy Clin Immunol 1990;85:94.
144. Bartholomé K, Kissler W, Baer H, Kopietz-Schulte E, Wahn U. Where does cat allergen 1 come from? J Allergy Clin Immunol 1985;76:503.
145. Taylor WW, Ohman JL Jr, Lowell FC. Immunotherapy in cat induced asthma: double-blind trial with evaluation of bronchial responses to cat allergen and histamine. J Allergy Clin Immunol 1978;61:283.
146. Anderson MC, Baer H, Ohman JL. A comparative study of the allergens of cat urine, serum, saliva and pelt. J Allergy Clin Immunol 1985;76:563.
147. Van Metre TE Jr, Marsh DG, Adkinson NF, et al. Dose of cat (*Felis domesticus*) allergen 1 (*Fel d I*) that induces asthma. J Allergy Clin Immunol 1986;78:62.
148. Wood RA, Chapman MD, Adkinson NF Jr, Eggleston PA. The effect of cat removal on allergen content in household-dust samples. J Allergy Clin Immunol 1989;83:730.
149. Moore BS, Hyde JS. Breed-specific dog hypersensitivity in humans. J Allergy Clin Immunol 1980;66:198.
150. Lindgren S, Belin L, Dreborg S, Einarsson R, Påhlman I. Breed-specific dog-dandruff allergens. J Allergy Clin Immunol 1988;82:196.
151. Schumacher MJ, Tait BD, Holmes MC. Allergy to murine antigens in a biological research institute. J Allergy Clin Immunol 1981;68:310.
152. Siraganian RP, Sandberg AL. Characterization of mouse allergens. J Allergy Clin Immunol 1979;63:435.
153. Finlayson JS, Asofsky R, Potter M, et al. Major urinary complex of normal mice: origin. Science 1965;49:481.
154. Platts-Mills TAE, Longbottom J, Edward J, Cockroft A, Wilkins S. Occupational asthma and rhinitis related to laboratory rats: serum IgG and IgE antibodies to the rat urinary allergen. J Allergy Clin Immunol 1987;79:505.
155. Eggleston PS, Newill CA, Ansar AA, et al. Task-related variation in airborne concentrations of laboratory animal allergens: studies with *Rat n I*. J Allergy Clin Immunol 1989;84:347.
156. Walls AF, Longbottom JL. Comparison of rat fur, urine, saliva and other rat allergen extracts by skin testing, RAST, and RAST inhibition. J Allergy Clin Immunol 1985;75:242.
157. Longbottom JL, Austwick PKC. Allergy to rats: quantitative immunoelectrophoretic studies of rat dust as a source of inhalant allergen. J Allergy Clin Immunol 1987;80:243.
158. Laperche Y, Lynch KR, Dolan KP, et al. Tissue-specific control of alpha 2μ-globulin gene expression: constitutive synthesis in the submaxillary gland. Cell 1983;32:453.
159. Gross NJ. Allergy to laboratory animals: epidemiologic, clinical and physiologic aspects, and trial of cromolyn in its management. J Allergy Clin Immunol 1980;66:158.
160. Slovak AJM, Hill RN. Does atopy have any predictive value for laboratory animal allergy? A comparison of different concepts of atopy. Br J Ind Med 1987;44:129.
161. Bernton HS, Brown H. Insect allergy: the allergenicity of the excrement of the cockroach. Ann Allergy 1970;28:543.
162. Kang B, Vellody D, Homburger H, et al. Cockroach cause of allergic asthma. Its specificity and immunologic profile. J Allergy Clin Immunol 1979;63:80.
163. Wu CH, Lan JL. Cockroach hypersensitivity: isolation and partial characterization of major allergens. J Allergy Clin Immunol 1988;82:727.
164. Arruda LK, Vailes LD, Chapman MD. Molecular cloning of cockroach (*B. germanica*) allergens. J Allergy Clin Immunol 1993;91:188.

165. Anderson MC, Baer H, Richman P, et al. Immunoelectrophoretic studies of roach allergens. J Allergy Clin Immunol 1983;71:105. Abstract.
166. Steinberg DR, Bernstein DI, Gallagher JS, Arlian L, Bernstein IL. Cockroach sensitization in laboratory workers. J Allergy Clin Immunol 1987;80:586.
167. Shulman S. Insect allergy: biochemical and immunological analysis of allergens. In: Kallós P, Waksman BH, eds. Progress in allergy. Vol 12. Basel: S Karger, 1968:246.
168. Kino T, Oshima S. Allergy to insects in Japan. II. The reaginic sensitivity to silkworm moth in patients with bronchial asthma. J Allergy Clin Immunol 1979;64:131.
169. Gad E, Rab O, Kay AB. Widespread IgE-mediated hypersensitivity in the Sudan to the "green nimitti" midge *Cladotonytarus lewise* (Diptera: Chironidae). I. Diagnosis by RAST. J Allergy Clin Immunol 1980;66:190.
170. Baur X, Dewair M, Fruhmann G, et al. Hypersensitivity to chironomids (non-biting midges): localization of the antigenic determinants within certain polypeptide sequences of hemoglobins (erythrocruorins) of *Chironomus thummi thummi* (Diptera). J Allergy Clin Immunol 1982;69:66.
171. Mazur G, Baur X, Modrow S, et al. A common epitope on major allergens from non-biting midges (Chironomidae). Mol Immunol 1988;25:1005.
172. Wynn SR, Swanson MC, Reed CE, et al. Immunochemical quantitation, size distribution and cross-reactivity of *Lepidoptera* (moth) aeroallergens in southeastern Minnesota. J Allergy Clin Immunol 1988;82:47.
173. Bagenstose AH III, Mathews KP, Homburger HA, et al. Inhalant allergy to crickets. J Allergy Clin Immunol 1980;65:71.
174. Bernstein DI, Gallagher JS, Bernstein IL. Mealworm asthma: clinical and immunological studies. J Allergy Clin Immunol 1983;72:475.
175. Reisman RE, Hale R, Wypych JI. Allergy to honeybee body components: distinction from bee venom sensitivity. J Allergy Clin Immunol 1983;71:302.
176. Tee RD, Gordon DJ, Hawkins ER, et al. Occupational allergy to locusts: an investigation of the sources of the allergen. J Allergy Clin Immunol 1988;81:517.
177. Tee RD, Gordon DJ, Lacey J, et al. Occupational allergy to the common house fly (*Musca domestica*): use of immunologic response to identify atmospheric allergen. J Allergy Clin Immunol 1985;76:826.
178. Schroeckenstein DC, Meier-Davis S, Graziano FM, Falomo A, Bush RK. Occupational sensitivity to *Alphitobius diaperinus* (Panzer) (lesser mealworm). J Allergy Clin Immunol 1988;82:1081.
179. Atkins FM, Wilson M, Bock SA. Cottonseed hypersensitivity: new concerns over an old problem. J Allergy Clin Immunol 1988;82:242.
180. Malanin G, Kalimo K. Angioedema and urticaria caused by cotton seed protein in whole grain bread. J Allergy Clin Immunol 1988;82:261.
181. O'Neil CE, Lehrer SB, Gutman AA. Anaphylaxis apparently caused by a cottonseed-containing candy ingested on a commercial airliner. J Allergy Clin Immunol 1989;84:407. Letter.
182. Thorpe SC, Kemeny DM, Panzani R, Lesoff MH. Allergy to castor bean. I. Its relationship to sensitization to common inhalant allergens (atopy). J Allergy Clin Immunol 1988;82:62.
183. Izumi SD, Adachi T, Fujii N, et al. Nucleotide sequence of a cDNA clone encoding a major allergenic protein in rice seeds: homology of the deduced amino acid sequence with members of the alpha amylase/trypsin inhibitor family. FEBS Lett 1992;302:213.
184. Irwin SD, Lord JM. Nucleotide sequence of a *Ricinus communis* 2S albumin precursor gene. Nucleic Acids Res 1990;18:5890.
185. Thorpe SC, Kemeny DM, Panzani RC, McGurl B, Lord M. Allergy to castor bean. II. Identification of the major allergens in castor bean seed. J Allergy Clin Immunol 1988;82:67.
186. Bush RK, Schroeckenstein D, Meier-Davis S, Balmes J, Rempel D. Soybean flour asthma: detection of allergens by immunoblotting. J Allergy Clin Immunol 1988;82:251.
187. Antó JM, Sunyer J, Rodriguez Roisin R, Suarez M, Vazquez L. Asthma epidemics associated with soybean dust released during harbor unloading activities. N Engl J Med 1989;320:1097.
188. Rodrigo MJ, Morell F, Helm RM, et al. Identification and partial characterization of the soybean dust allergens involved in the Barcelona asthma epidemic. J Allergy Clin Immunol 1990;85:778.
189. Sunyer J, Antó JM, Rodrigo MJ, Morrell F. Epidemic asthma and soybean IgE antibodies. Lancet 1989;i:179.
190. Laglier F, Cartier A, Somer J, Dolovich J, Malo J-L. Occupational asthma caused by guar gum. J Allergy Clin Immunol 1990;85:785.
191. Raghuprasad PK, Brooks SM, Litwin A, et al. *Quillaja* (soap-bark)-induced asthma. J Allergy Clin Immunol 1980;65:285.
192. Belin L, Hoborn J, Falsen E, André J. Enzyme sensitization in consumers of enzyme-containing washing powder. Lancet 1970;ii:1153.
193. Ransom JH, Schuster M. Allergic reactions to enzymes used in plant cloning experiments. J Allergy Clin Immunol 1981;67:412.
194. Novey HS, Marchioli LE, Sokol WN, et al. Papain-induced asthma-physiological and immunological features. J Allergy Clin Immunol 1979;63:103.
195. Sanchez-Monge R, Gomez L, Barber D, et al. Wheat and barley allergens associated with bakers' asthma: glycosylated subunits of the α-amylase inhibitor family have enhanced IgE binding capacity. Biochem J 1992;281:401.

196. Sandiford CP, Tee RD, Newman-Taylor AJ. Identification of crossreacting wheat, rye, barley and soya flour allergens using sera from individuals with wheat-induced asthma. Clin Exper Allergy 1995;25:340.
197. Falleroni AE, Zeiss CR, Levitz D. Occupational asthma secondary to garlic dust. J Allergy Clin Immunol 1981;79:156.
198. Lybarger J, Gallagher JS, Pulver DW, et al. Occupational asthma induced by inhalation and ingestion of garlic. J Allergy Clin Immunol 1982;69:448.
199. Zeiss CR, Wolkonsky B, Pruzansky JJ, Patterson R. Clinical and immunologic evaluation of trimellitic anhydride workers in multiple industrial settings. J Allergy Clin Immunol 1982;70:15.
200. Patterson R. Studies of hypersensitivity lung disease with emphasis on a solid phase radioimmunoassay as a potential diagnostic aid. J Allergy Clin Immunol 1978;61:216.
201. Sale SR, Roach DE, Zeiss CR, et al. Clinical and immunologic correlations in trimellitic anhydride airway syndromes. J Allergy Clin Immunol 1981;68:188.
202. Bernstein IL. Isocyanate-induced pulmonary disease: a current prospective. J Allergy Clin Immunol 1982;70:24.
203. Zeiss CR, Kanellakes TM, Bellone JD, et al. Immunoglobulin E-mediated asthma and hypersensitivity pneumonitis with precipitating anti-hapten antibodies due to diphenylmethane diisocyanate (MDI) exposure. J Allergy Clin Immunol 1980;65:346.
204. Malo JL, Ouimet G, Cartier A, Levitz D, Zeiss CR. Combined alveolitis and asthma due to hexamethylene diisocyanate (HDI) with demonstration of crossed respiratory and immunologic reactivities to diphenylmethane diisocyanate (MDI). J Allergy Clin Immunol 1983;72:413.
205. Baur X. Immunologic cross-reactivity between albumin-bound isocyanates. J Allergy Clin Immunol 1983;71:197.
206. Howe W, Venables KM, Topping MD, et al. Tetrachlorophthlic anhydride asthma: evidence for specific IgE antibody. J Allergy Clin Immunol 1983;71:5.
207. Murphy RLH. Industrial disease with asthma. In: Weiss EB, Segal MS, eds. Bronchial asthma: mechanisms and therapeutics. Boston: Little, Brown, 1976:517.
208. Pepys J. Occupational asthma: review of present clinical and immunologic status. J Allergy Clin Immunol 1980;66:179.
209. Pepys J, Davies RJ. Occupational asthma. In: Middleton E, Reed CE, Ellis CE, eds. Allergy: principles and practice. St Louis: CV Mosby, 1978:812.
210. Salvaggio J. Overview of occupational immunologic lung disease. J Allergy Clin Immunol 1982;70:5.
211. Novey HS, Habib M, Wells ID. Asthma and IgE antibodies induced by chromium and nickel salts. J Allergy Clin Immunol 1983;72:407.
212. Chang-Yeung M. Immunologic and nonimmunologic mechanisms in asthma due to western red cedar (Thuja plicata). J Allergy Clin Immunol 1982;70:32.
213. Chang-Yeung, M, Giclas PC, Henson PM. Activation of complement by plicatic acid, the chemical compound responsible for asthma due to western red cedar. J Allergy Clin Immunol 1980;65:333.
214. Allard C, Cartier A, Ghezzo H, Malo J-L. Occupational asthma due to various agents: absence of clinical and functional improvement at an interval of 4 or more years after cessation of exposure. Chest 1989;96:1046.
215. Yang WH, Purchase ECR, Rivington RN. Positive skin tests and Prausnitz-Küstner reactions in metabisulfite-sensitive subjects. J Allergy Clin Immunol 1986;78:443.
216. Koenig JO. Indoor and outdoor pollutants and the upper respiratory tract. J Allergy Clin Immunol 1988;81:1055.
217. Salvaggio J, Seabury J, Schoenhardt EA. New Orleans asthma V. J Allergy Clin Immunol 1971;48:96.
218. Chapmann D, Pollart SM, Luczynska C, Platts-Mills TAE. Hidden allergic factors in the etiology of asthma. Chest 1988;94:185.
219. Pollart SM, Chapman MD, Fiocco GP, Rose G, Platts-Mills TAE. Epidemiology of acute asthma: IgE antibodies to common inhalant allergens as a risk factor for emergency room visits. J Allergy Clin Immunol 1989;83:875.
220. Patterson R. Formaldehyde reactions and the burden of proof. J Allergy Clin Immunol 1987;79:705. Editorial.
221. Anonymous. We're still in a fog over ozone. Chicago Med 1978;81:759. Editorial.
222. Letz GA. Sick building syndrome: acute illness among office workers. The role of building ventilation, airborne contaminants and work stress. Allergy Proc 1990;11:109.

Allergic Diseases, 5th Edition,
edited by Roy Patterson, Leslie Carroll Grammer, and
Paul A. Greenberger. Lippincott–Raven Publishers, Philadelphia, © 1997.

7

Pollen Survey of the United States

Walter W. Y. Chang

*W.W.Y. Chang: St. Francis Medical Center, Honolulu, HI 96817;
Queens Medical Center, Honolulu, HI 96813.*

Pearls for Practitioners
Roy Patterson

- Know the major aeroallergens for an area about 80 to 160 km (50 to 100 miles) surrounding where you practice.
- Airborne pollens travel for miles. Pollen counts may upset patients because they reflect the pollen where the counts are done, not where the patient is, and symptoms may be severe when counts are low and vice versa.
- Patients have been advised to move geographically to avoid aeroallergens and sometimes move to an area that has greater problems for them.
- Flora with vivid colorful flowers generally have heavy pollen, and transport of pollen occurs by insects. Plants that depend on airborne pollination often are unattractive and are regarded as weeds.

"The physician should know his pollens," as stated by Owen C. Durham, a noted pioneer of aerobiology and pollen survey, emphasizes an important aspect of clinical allergy. Practicing allergists can increase their clinical knowledge and diagnostic acumen by learning about the local and regional common pollen-producing plants. Pollinotic patients have symptoms related to their seasonal pollen exposure, and the diagnosis is partly dependent on this correlation. Daily variations in pollen production and distribution affect patient management, along with other short- and long-term factors. These factors include (1) urbanization and paving over of virgin lands; (2) industrialization and population pollution problems; (3) ethnic and racial differences in skin test reactions; (4) wind, rain, flowering onset, and other meteorologic conditions; (5) geographic and topographic considerations; (6) exotic and other introduced pollinotic species such as baby's breath and *Parietaria judaica*; (7) inherent collection devices differences and height and altitude differences where the collector is placed; and (7) lack of adequate pollen and field surveys. The following pollen survey is a guide and is not an all-encompassing definitive one. Geographic areas are used, including the Northeast, Southeast, Southern, Midwest, and West. The noncontinental areas of Alaska, Hawaii, Puerto Rico, and Virgin Islands are at the end of the chapter, as well as a bibliography of general interest.

Northeastern United States

CONNECTICUT	NEW YORK
DELAWARE	OHIO
DISTRICT OF COLUMBIA AND MARYLAND	PENNSYLVANIA
MAINE	RHODE ISLAND
MASSACHUSETTS	VERMONT
NEW HAMPSHIRE	VIRGINIA
NEW JERSEY	WEST VIRGINIA

Common Name	Botanical Name	Importance	Season
	CONNECTICUT		
Trees			
Elm, American	*Ulmus americana*	High	April
Oak, white	*Quercus alba*	High	May
Birch, red	*Betula nigra*	Secondary	April
Cottonwood	*Populus deltoides*	Secondary	April
Ash, white	*Fraxinus americana*	Secondary	Early May
Hickory, shagbark	*Hicoria ovata*	Secondary	April–May
Grasses			
June/Kentucky blue	*Poa pratensis*	High	Late May–mid-July
Orchard	*Dactylis glomerata*	High	Late May–mid-July
Red top	*Agrostis alba*	High	Late May–mid-July
Timothy	*Phleum pratense*	High	Late May–mid-July
Sweet vernal	*Anthoxanthum* sp	High	Late May–mid-July
Weeds			
Ragweed, giant	*Ambrosia trifida*	High	Mid-August–mid-September
short	*Ambrosia elatior*	High	Mid-August–mid-September
Cocklebur	*Xanthium canadense*	Secondary	Mid-August–mid-September
Lamb's quarters	*Chenopodium alba*	Secondary	August–September
Pigweed, redroot	*Amaranthus retroflexus*	Secondary	August–September
Plantain, English	*Plantago lanceolata*	Secondary	May–July
	DELAWARE		
Trees			
Elm, American	*Ulmus americana*	High	April
Oak, white	*Quercus alba*	High	May
Ash, white	*Fraxinus americana*	Secondary	May
Birch, red	*Betula nigra*	Secondary	April–May
Cottonwood	*Populus deltoides*	Secondary	April–May
Maple, red	*Acer rubrum*	Secondary	April

Northeastern United States (Continued)

Common Name	Botanical Name	Importance	Season
Sycamore	*Platanus occidentalis*	Secondary	April–May
Walnut, black	*Juglans nigra*	Secondary	April–May
Grasses			
June/Kentucky blue	*Poa pratensis*	High	Mid-May–July
Orchard	*Dactylis glomerata*	High	Mid-May–July
Red top	*Agrostis alba*	High	Mid-May–July
Sweet vernal	*Anthoxanthum* sp	High	Mid-May–July
Rye, perennial	*Lolium perenne*	Secondary	Mid-May–July
Timothy	*Phleum pratense*	High	June–July
Bermuda	*Cynodon dactylon*	Secondary	Late spring to early frost
Meadow fescue	*Festuca elatior*	Secondary	Summer
Johnson	*Holcus halepensis*	Secondary	Summer
Velvet	*Holcus lanatus*	Secondary	Summer
Weeds			
Ragweed, giant	*Ambrosia trifida*	High	Mid-August–October
short	*Ambrosia elatior*	High	Mid-August–October
Cocklebur	*Xanthium strumarium*	Secondary	Summer
Dock, yellow	*Rumex crispus*	Secondary	Summer
Lamb's quarters	*Chenopodium alba*	Secondary	Summer
Pigweed, rough	*Amaranthus retroflexus*	Secondary	Summer
Plantain, English	*Plantago lanceolata*	Secondary	Summer

MAINE

Common Name	Botanical Name	Importance	Season
Trees			
Elm, American	*Ulmus americana*	High	April
Oak, white	*Quercus alba*	High	May
Ash, white	*Fraxinus americana*	Secondary	Early May
Beech	*Fagus grandifolia*	Secondary	May
Birch, paper	*Betula papyrifera*	Secondary	April–May
Cottonwood	*Populus deltoides*	Secondary	April–May
Hickory, shagbark	*Hicoria ovata*	Secondary	May
Maple, hard	*Acer saccharum*	Secondary	April–May
Grasses			
June/Kentucky blue	*Poa pratensis*	High	May–June
Orchard	*Dactylis glomerata*	High	May–June
Red top	*Agrostis alba*	High	May–June
Sweet vernal	*Anthoxanthum* sp	High	May–June
Rye, perennial	*Lolium perenne*	High	May–June

continued

Northeastern United States (Continued)

Common Name	Botanical Name	Importance	Season
Timothy	*Phleum pratense*	High	May–July
Weeds			
Ragweed, giant	*Ambrosia trifida*	High	Mid-August–October
short	*Ambrosia elatior*	High	Mid-August–October
Cocklebur	*Xanthium strumarium*	Secondary	Summer
Dock, yellow	*Rumex crispus*	Secondary	Summer
Lamb's quarters	*Chenopodium alba*	Secondary	Summer
Pigweed, rough	*Amaranthus retroflexus*	Secondary	Summer
Plantain, English	*Plantago lanceolata*	Secondary	Summer

MARYLAND AND DISTRICT OF COLUMBIA

Common Name	Botanical Name	Importance	Season
Trees			
Elm, American	*Ulmus americana*	High	March–April
Oak, white	*Quercus alba*	High	April–May
Ash, white	*Fraxinus americana*	Secondary	Late April
Birch, red	*Betula nigra*	Secondary	April–May
Cottonwood	*Populus deltoides*	Secondary	March–April
Hickory, white	*Hicoria alba*	Secondary	April–May
Walnut, black	*Juglans nigra*	Secondary	April–May
Sycamore	*Plantanus occidentalis*	Secondary	April–May
Grasses			
June/Kentucky blue	*Poa pratense*	High	May–July
Orchard	*Dactylis glomerata*	High	May–July
Red top	*Agrostis alba*	High	May–July
Sweet vernal	*Anthoxanthum* sp	High	May–June
Rye, perennial	*Lolium perenne*	High	May–July
Timothy	*Phleum pratense*	High	June–July
Bermuda	*Cynodon dactylon*	Secondary	May–October
Meadow fescue	*Festuca elatior*	Secondary	May–July
Johnson	*Holcus halepensis*	Secondary	May–July
Weeds			
Ragweed, giant	*Ambrosia trifida*	High	Mid-August–mid-September
short	*Ambrosia elatior*	High	Same
Cocklebur	*Xanthium strumarium*	Secondary	August–September
Dock, yellow	*Rumex crispus*	Secondary	May–July
Lamb's quarters	*Chenopodium alba*	Secondary	August–September
Pigweed, rough	*Amaranthus retroflexus*	Secondary	June–August
Plantain, English	*Plantago lanceolata*	Secondary	May–August

Northeastern United States (Continued)

Common Name	Botanical Name	Importance	Season
MASSACHUSETTS			

Trees

Common Name	Botanical Name	Importance	Season
Ash, white	*Fraxinus americana*	High	April
Elm, American	*Ulmus americana*	High	April
Hickory, shagbark	*Hicoria ovata*	High	April
Oak, white	*Quercus alba*	High	May–June
Birch, red	*Betula nigra*	Secondary	April–May
Cottonwood	*Populus deltoides*	Secondary	April
Willow, black	*Salix nigra*	Secondary	April–May

Grasses

Common Name	Botanical Name	Importance	Season
June/Kentucky blue	*Poa pratensis*	High	May–July
Meadow fescue	*Festuca elatior*	High	May–July
Orchard	*Dactylis glomerata*	High	May–July
Red top	*Agrostis alba*	High	May–July
Timothy	*Phleum pratense*	High	May–July
Sweet vernal	*Anthoxanthum* sp	High	May–July
Rye, perennial	*Lolium perenne*	Secondary	May–July

Weeds

Common Name	Botanical Name	Importance	Season
Ragweed, giant	*Ambrosia trifida*	High	Mid-August–late September
short	*Ambrosia elatior*	High	Mid-August late September
Cocklebur	*Xanthium strumarium*	Secondary	August–September
Dock, yellow	*Rumex crispus*	Secondary	August–September
Lamb's quarters	*Chenopodium alba*	Secondary	August–September
Pigweed, redroot	*Amaranthus retroflexus*	Secondary	August–September
Plantain, English	*Plantago lanceolata*	Secondary	May–August
Marsh elder, burweed	*Iva xanthifolia*	Secondary	August–September

NEW HAMPSHIRE

Trees

Common Name	Botanical Name	Importance	Season
Elm, American	*Ulmus americana*	High	April
Oak, white	*Quercus alba*	High	May
Birch, paper	*Betula papyrifera*	Secondary	April
Cottonwood	*Populus deltoides*	Secondary	April
Hickory, shagbark	*Hicoria ovata*	Secondary	April
Maple, hard	*Acer saccharum*	Secondary	Spring

Grasses

Common Name	Botanical Name	Importance	Season
June/Kentucky blue	*Poa pratensis*	High	May–July
Orchard	*Dactylis glomerata*	High	May–July

continued

Northeastern United States (Continued)

Common Name	Botanical Name	Importance	Season
Red top	*Agrostis alba*	High	May–July
Rye, perennial	*Lolium perenne*	High	May–July
Sweet vernal	*Anthoxanthum* sp	High	May–July
Timothy	*Phleum pratense*	High	May–July
Weeds			
Ragweed, giant	*Ambrosia trifida*	High	Mid-August–late September
short	*Ambrosia elatior*	High	Mid-August–late September
Cocklebur	*Xanthium strumarium*	Secondary	August–September
Dock, yellow	*Rumex crispus*	Secondary	August–September
Lamb's quarters	*Chenopodium alba*	Secondary	August–September
Pigweed, redroot	*Amaranthus retroflexus*	Secondary	August–September
Plantain, English	*Plantago lanceolata*	Secondary	May–August
Marsh elder, burweed	*Iva xanthifolia*	Secondary	August–September

NEW JERSEY

Common Name	Botanical Name	Importance	Season
Trees			
Ash, white	*Fraxinus americana*	High	April
Elm, American	*Ulmus americana*	High	March–April
Hickory, shagbark	*Hicoria ovata*	High	April–May
Oak, white	*Quercus alba*	High	May
Birch, red	*Betula nigra*	Secondary	April
Cottonwood	*Populus deltoides*	Secondary	April
Maple, hard	*Acer saccharum*	Secondary	March
Sycamore, eastern	*Platanus occidentalis*	Secondary	April–May
Walnut, black	*Juglans nigra*	Secondary	April–May
Grasses			
June/Kentucky blue	*Poa pratensis*	High	May–July
Orchard	*Dactylis glomerata*	High	May–July
Red top	*Agrostis alba*	High	May–July
Fescue, meadow	*Festuca elatior*	High	May–July
Timothy	*Phleum pratense*	High	May–July
Brome, smooth	*Bromus inermis*	Secondary	May–July
Rye, perennial	*Lolium perenne*	Secondary	May–July
Sweet vernal	*Anthoxanthum* sp	Secondary	May–July
Velvet	*Holcus lanatus*	Secondary	May–July
Weeds			
Ragweed, giant	*Ambrosia trifida*	High	Mid-August–October 1
short	*Ambrosia elatior*	High	Mid-August–October 1
Cocklebur	*Xanthium strumarium*	Secondary	July–August

Northeastern United States (Continued)

Common Name	Botanical Name	Importance	Season
Dock, yellow	*Rumex crispus*	Secondary	July–August
Lamb's quarters	*Chenopodium alba*	Secondary	July–August
Pigweed, rough	*Amaranthus retroflexus*	Secondary	July–August
Plantain, English	*Plantago lanceolata*	Secondary	May–August
Kochia	*Kochia scoparia*	Secondary	July–August

NEW YORK

Trees

Birch, red	*Betula nigra*	High	April–May
Cottonwood	*Populus deltoides*	High	April–May
Elm, American	*Ulmus americana*	High	April
Oak, red	*Quercus rubra*	High	May
Ash, white	*Fraxinus americana*	Secondary	April–May
Maple, hard	*Acer saccharum*	Secondary	March–May

Grasses

Fescue, meadow	*Festuca elatior*	High	May June
June/Kentucky blue	*Poa pratensis*	High	Mid-May–July
Orchard	*Dactylis glomerata*	High	Mid-May–July
Red top	*Agrostis alba*	High	Mid-May–July
Timothy	*Phleum pratense*	High	Mid-May–July

Weeds

Ragweed, giant	*Ambrosia trifida*	High	Mid-August–mid-September
short	*Ambrosia elatior*	High	Mid-August–mid-September
Cocklebur	*Xanthium strumarium*	Secondary	August–September
Lamb's quarters	*Chenopodium alba*	Secondary	August–September
Pigweed, rough	*Amaranthus retroflexus*	Secondary	August–September
Plantain, English	*Plantago lanceolata*	Secondary	May–August

OHIO

Trees

Elm, American	*Ulmus americana*	High	April
Oak, red	*Quercus rubra*	High	May
Sycamore, eastern	*Platanus occidentalis*	High	April
Birch, red	*Betula nigra*	Secondary	April–May
Cottonwood	*Populus deltoides*	Secondary	May
Elder, box	*Acer negundo*	Secondary	April
Hickory, shagbark	*Hicoria ovata*	Secondary	April
Maple, sugar	*Acer saccharum*	Secondary	April–May

continued

Northeastern United States (Continued)

Common Name	Botanical Name	Importance	Season
Grasses			
Fescue, meadow	*Festuca elatior*	High	Mid-May–mid-July
June/Kentucky blue	*Poa pratensis*	High	Mid-May–mid-July
Orchard	*Dactylis glomerata*	High	Mid-May–mid-July
Red top	*Agrostis alba*	High	Mid-May–mid-July
Timothy	*Phleum pratense*	High	Mid-May–mid-July
Sweet vernal	*Anthoxanthum sp*	Secondary	Mid-May–mid-July
Weeds			
Kochia	*Kochia scoparia*	High	August
Ragweed, giant	*Ambrosia trifida*	High	Early August–mid-September
short	*Ambrosia elatior*	High	Early August–mid-September
Cocklebur	*Xanthium strumarium*	Secondary	August
Lamb's quarters	*Chenopodium alba*	Secondary	July–August
Pigweed, rough	*Amaranthus retroflexus*	Secondary	August
Plantain English	*Plantago lanceolata*	Secondary	June–August
Thistle, Russian	*Salsola pestifer*	Local	July–August

PENNSYLVANIA

Common Name	Botanical Name	Importance	Season
Trees			
Elm, American	*Ulmus americana*	High	March–April
Oak, red	*Quercus rubra*	High	April–May
Birch, red	*Betula nigra*	High	April–May
Sycamore, eastern	*Platanus occidentalis*	High	April–May
Ash, white	*Fraxinus americana*	Secondary	April–May
Cottonwood	*Populus deltoides*	Secondary	April–May
Maple, red	*Acer rubrum*	Secondary	March–April
Grasses			
Canadian blue	*Poa compressa*	High	Mid-May–mid-July
June/Kentucky blue	*Poa pratensis*	High	Mid-May–mid-July
Orchard	*Dactylis glomerata*	High	Mid-May–mid-July
Red top	*Agrostis alba*	High	Mid-May–mid-July
Sweet vernal	*Anthoxanthum* sp	High	Mid-May–mid-July
Timothy	*Phleum pratense*	High	Mid-May–mid-July
Weeds			
Ragweed, giant	*Ambrosia trifida*	High	Mid-August–October 1
short	*Ambrosia elatior*	High	Mid-August–October 1
Cocklebur	*Xanthium strumarium*	Secondary	August–September
Lamb's quarters	*Chenopodium alba*	Secondary	July–September
Pigweed, rough	Amaranthus retroflexus	Secondary	July–September
Plantain, English	*Plantago lanceolata*	Secondary	June–September

Northeastern United States (Continued)

Common Name	Botanical Name	Importance	Season
RHODE ISLAND			

Trees

Elm, American	*Ulmus americana*	High	April
Oak, white	*Quercus alba*	High	May
Cottonwood	*Populus deltoides*	Secondary	April
Birch, red	*Betula nigra*	Secondary	April–May
Maple, hard	*Acer saccharum*	Secondary	April
Walnut, black	Juglans nigra	Secondary	May

Grasses

June/Kentucky blue	*Poa pratensis*	High	Mid-May–mid-July
Orchard	*Dactylis glomerata*	High	Mid-May–mid-July
Red top	*Agrostis alba*	High	Mid-May–mid-July
Sweet vernal	*Anthoxanthum* sp	High	Mid-May–mid-July
Timothy	*Phleum pratense*	High	Mid-May–mid-July

Weeds

Ragweed, giant	*Ambrosia trifida*	High	Mid-August–mid-September
short	*Ambrosia elatior*	High	Mid-August–mid-September
Cocklebur	*Xanthium strumarium*	High	July–September
Dock, yellow	*Rumex crispus*	High	May–July
Lamb's quarters	*Chenopodium alba*	High	June–September
Pigweed, redroot	*Amaranthus retroflexus*	Secondary	July–August
Plantain, English	*Plantago lanceolata*	Secondary	May–June

VERMONT			

Trees

Elm, American	*Ulmus americana*	High	April
Oak, white	*Quercus alba*	High	May
Marple, hard	*Acer saccharum*	Secondary	April
Walnut, black	*Juglans nigra*	Local	April–May

Grasses

June/Kentucky blue	*Poa pratensis*	High	May–July
Orchard	*Dactylis glomerata*	High	May–July
Red top	*Agrostis alba*	High	May–July
Rye, perennial	*Lolium perenne*	High	May–July
Timothy	*Phleum pratense*	High	May–July
Sweet vernal	*Anthoxanthum* sp	High	May–July

Weeds

Ragweed, giant	*Ambrosia trifida*	High	Mid-August–mid-September

continued

Northeastern United States (Continued)

Common Name	Botanical Name	Importance	Season
Ragweed, short	*Ambrosia elatior*	High	Mid-August–mid-September
Cocklebur	*Xanthium strumarium*	Secondary	July–August
Lamb's quarter	*Chenopodium alba*	Secondary	July–August
Pigweed, redroot	*Amaranthus retroflexus*	Secondary	July–August
Plantain, English	*Plantago lanceolata*	Secondary	June–August

VIRGINIA

Trees

Common Name	Botanical Name	Importance	Season
Elm, American	*Ulmus americana*	High	February–April
Hickory, white	*Hicoria alba*	High	April–May
Maple, red	*Acer rubrum*	High	February–April
Oak, Virginia live	*Quercus virginiana*	High	April–May
Ash, white	*Fraxinus americana*	Secondary	February–April
Sycamore, eastern	*Platanus occidentalis*	Secondary	April–May

Grasses

Bermuda	Cynodon dactylon	High	May–July
June/Kentucky blue	Poa pratensis	High	May–July
Johnson	*Holcus halepensis*	High	May–July
Orchard	Dactylis glomerata	High	May–July
Red top	Agrostis alba	High	May–July
Rye, Italian	*Lolium multiflorum*	High	May–July
Sweet vernal	*Anthoxanthum* sp	High	May–July
Timothy	*Phleum pratense*	High	May–July
Velvet	*Holcus lanatus*	Secondary	May–July

Weeds

Ragweed, giant	*Ambrosia trifida*	High	Early August–early October
short	*Ambrosia elatior*	High	Early August–early October
Cocklebur	*Xanthium strumarium*	Secondary	August–October
Lamb's quarters	*Chenopodium alba*	Secondary	August–October
Pigweed, rough	*Amaranthus retroflexus*	Secondary	August–October
Plantain, English	*Plantago lanceolata*	Secondary	June–August

WEST VIRGINIA

Trees

Elm, American	*Ulmus americana*	High	April
Oak, red	*Quercus rubra*	High	May
Sycamore, eastern	*Platanus occidentalis*	High	April
Walnut, black	*Juglans nigra*	High	April–May

Northeastern United States (Continued)

Common Name	Botanical Name	Importance	Season
Ash, white	*Fraxinus americana*	Secondary	April
Birch, red	*Betula nigra*	Secondary	April
Cottonwood	*Populus deltoides*	Secondary	April
Grasses			
June/Kentucky blue	*Poa pratensis*	High	May–July
Orchard	*Dactylis glomerata*	High	May–July
Johnson	*Holcus halepensis*	High	May–July
Red top	*Agrostis alba*	High	May–July
Timothy	*Phleum pratense*	High	May–July
Bermuda	*Cynodon dactylon*	Secondary	May–July
Weeds			
Ragweed, giant	*Ambrosia trifida*	High	Mid-August–October 1
short	*Ambrosia elatior*	High	Mid-August–October 1
Plantain, English	*Plantago lanceolata*	High	May–July
Cocklebur	*Xanthium strumarium*	Secondary	July–August
Lamb's quarters	*Chenopodium alba*	Secondary	July–September
Pigweed, rough	*Amaranthus retroflexus*	Secondary	July–September

Southeastern and Southern United States

ALABAMA	NORTH CAROLINA
ARKANSAS	OKLAHOMA
FLORIDA	SOUTH CAROLINA
GEORGIA	TENNESSEE
LOUISIANA	TEXAS
MISSISSIPPI	

ALABAMA

Trees			
Elm, American	*Ulmus americana*	High	February–March
Oak, white	*Quercus alba*	High	April
Pecan	*Hicoria pecan*	High	April–May
Walnut, black	*Juglans nigra*	High	April
Ash, white	*Fraxinus americana*	Secondary	March
Birch, red	*Betula nigra*	Secondary	April
Cedar, red	*Juniperus virginiana*	Secondary	January–February
Grasses			
Bermuda	*Cynodon dactylon*	High	March–November
Blue, annual	*Poa annua*	High	April to frost

continued

Southeastern and Southern United States (Continued)

Common Name	Botanical Name	Importance	Season
June/Kentucky blue	*Poa pratensis*	High	March–November
Johnson	*Holcus halepensis*	High	April–September
Orchard	*Dactylis glomerata*	High	April–September
Red top	*Agrostis alba*	High	April–September
Timothy	*Phleum pratense*	High	May–September
Weeds			
Ragweed, giant	*Ambrosia trifida*	High	Mid-August–late October
short	*Ambrosia elatior*	High	Mid-August–late October
Dock, yellow	*Rumex crispus*	Secondary	April–July
Lamb's quarters	*Chenopodium alba*	Secondary	June–August
Pigweed, rough	*Amaranthus retroflexus*	Secondary	June–August
Plantain, English	*Plantago lanceolata*	Secondary	May–July

ARKANSAS

Common Name	Botanical Name	Importance	Season
Trees			
Elm, American	*Ulmus americana*	High	February–March
Oak, red	*Quercus rubra*	High	March–May
Pecan	*Hicoria pecan*	High	April–May
Cottonwood	*Populus deltoides*	Secondary	March–April
Hickory, white	*Hicoria alba*	Secondary	April–May
Walnut, black	*Quercus nigra*	Secondary	April–May
Grasses			
Bermuda	*Cynodon dactylon*	High	May–November
June/Kentucky blue	*Poa pratensis*	High	March–June
Johnson	*Holcus halepensis*	High	May–November
Orchard	*Dactylis glomerata*	High	March–June
Red top	*Agrostis alba*	High	March–June
Timothy	*Phleum pratense*	High,	March–June
Weeds			
Ragweed, giant	*Ambrosia trifida*	High	Mid-August–mid-October
short	*Ambrosia elatior*	High	Mid-August–mid-October
Marsh elder, burweed	*Iva xanthifolia*	Secondary	Mid-August–mid-October
Hemp, Western water	*Acnida tamarascina*	Secondary	June–September
Kochia	*Kochia scoparia*	Secondary	Mid-August–mid-October
Lambs's quarters	*Chenopodium alba*	Secondary	June–September
Pigweed, rough	*Amaranthus retroflexus*	Secondary	June–September

Southeastern and Southern United States (Continued)

Common Name	Botanical Name	Importance	Season
Ragweed, southern	*Ambrosia bidentata*	Secondary	Mid-August– mid-October
western	*Ambrosia psilostachya*	Secondary	Mid-August– mid-October
Thistle, Russian	*Salsola pestifer*	Secondary	June–September

FLORIDA

Trees

Oak, white	*Quercus alba*	High	February–April
live	*Quercus virginiana*	High	February–April
Pecan (northern Fla)	*Hicoria pecan*	High	December–April
Pine, Australian (south)	*Casuarina* sp	Local	February–April

Grasses

Bermuda	*Cynodon dactylon*	High	April–October
Johnson	*Holcus halepensis*	High	April–October
June/Kentucky blue	*Poa pratensis*	Secondary	April–October
Timothy	*Phleum pratense*	Secondary	April–October
St. Augustine	*Stenolaphrum secundatum*	Local	April–October
Natal	*Rhynechelytrum repens*	Local	April–October
Bahia	*Paspalum notatum*	Local	April–October

Weeds

Ragweed, giant	*Ambrosia trifida*	High	July–October
short	*Ambrosia elatior*	High	July–October
Dock, yellow	*Rumex crispus*	Secondary	May–August
Lamb's quarters	*Chenopodium alba*	Secondary	May–September
Pigweed, spiny	*Amaranthus spinosa*	Secondary	May–September

GEORGIA

Trees

Elm, American	*Ulmus americana*	High	February–March
Oak, live	*Quercus virginiana*	High	March–May
Birch, red	*Betula nigra*	Secondary	March–April
Pine	*Pinus* sp	Local	March–May
Pecan	*Hicoria pecan*	Local	April–May

Grasses

Bermuda	*Cynodon dactylon*	High	May–October
Johnson	*Holcus halepensis*	High	May–October
June/Kentucky blue	*Poa pratensis*	High	March–July
Orchard	*Dactylis glomerata*	Secondary	March–July
Red top	*Agrostis alba*	Secondary	March–July

continued

Southeastern and Southern United States (Continued)

Common Name	Botanical Name	Importance	Season
Rye, Italian	*Lolium multiflorum*	Secondary	March–July
Weeds			
Ragweed, giant	*Ambrosia trifida*	High	August–October
short	*Ambrosia elatior*	High	August–October
Cocklebur	*Xanthium strumarium*	Secondary	August–October
Dock, yellow	*Rumex crispus*	Secondary	April–July
Pigweed, spiny	*Amaranthus spinosa*	Secondary	March–September
Kochia	*Kochia scoparia*	Local	June–August
Plantain, English	*Plantago lanceolata*	Local	May–October

LOUISIANA

Trees			
Elm, American	*Ulmus americana*	High	February–April
Oak, live	*Quercus virginiana*	High	February–April
Pecan	*Hicoria pecan*	High	March–May
Sycamore	*Platanus occidentalis*	Secondary	February–May
Grasses			
Bermuda	*Cynodon dactylon*	High	April–December
Johnson	*Holcus halepensis*	High	April–December
June/Kentucky blue	*Poa pratensis*	Secondary	April–December
Orchard	*Dactylis glomerata*	Secondary	April–December
Rye, Italian	*Lolium multiflorum*	Secondary	April–December
Weeds			
Marsh elder	*Iva ciliata*	High	August–November
Ragweed, giant	*Ambrosia trifida*	High	August–September
, short	*Ambrosia elatior*	High	August–September
Kochia	*Kochia scoparia*	Secondary	June–August
Lamb's quarters	*Chenopodium*	Secondary	June–August
Pigweed, spiny	*Amaranthus spinosa*	Secondary	June–August
Thistle, Russian	*Salsola pestifer*	Secondary	June–August

MISSISSIPPI

Trees			
Elm, American	*Ulmus americana*	High	March–April
Oak, live	*Quercus virginiana*	High	April–May
Pecan	*Hicoria pecan*	High	March–April
Ash, white	*Fraxinus americana*	Secondary	March
Hickory, white	*Hicoria alba*	Secondary	April–May
Grasses			
Bermuda	*Cynodon dactylon*	High	April–October

Southeastern and Southern United States (Continued)

Common Name	Botanical Name	Importance	Season
Johnson	*Holcus halepensis*	High	April–October
June/Kentucky blue	*Poa pratensis*	Secondary	April–October
Orchard	*Dactylis glomerata*	Secondary	April–October
Rye, Italian	*Lolium multiflorum*	Secondary	April–October
Weeds			
Marsh elder	*Iva ciliata*	High	August–October
Ragweed, giant	*Ambrosia trifida*	High	August–October
short	*Ambrosia elatior*	High	August–October
Lamb's quarters	*Chenopodium alba*	Secondary	June–August
Pigweed, rough	*Amaranthus retroflexus*	Secondary	June–August

NORTH CAROLINA

Trees			
Elm, American	*Ulmus americana*	High	February–April
Oak, live	*Quercus virginiana*	High	March–May
Ash, white	*Fraxinus americana*	Secondary	April
Hickory, white	*Hicoria alba*	Secondary	April
Maple, red	*Acer rubrum*	Secondary	February–May
Pecan	*Hicoria pecan*	Secondary	April–May
Sycamore	*Platanus occidentalis*	Secondary	April
Grasses			
Bermuda	*Cynodon dactylon*	High	March–September
Johnson	*Holcus halepensis*	High	March–September
June/Kentucky blue	*Poa pratensis*	High	March–September
Orchard	*Dactylis glomerata*	High	March–September
Red top	*Agrostis alba*	High	March–September
Timothy	*Phleum pratense*	High	March–September
Weeds			
Ragweed, giant	*Ambrosia trifida*	High	Mid-July–early October
short	*Ambrosia elatior*	High	Mid-July–early October
Cocklebur	*Xanthium strumarium*	Secondary	July–August
Lamb's quarters	*Chenopodium alba*	Secondary	July–August
Pigweed, rough	*Amaranthus retroflexus*	Secondary	July–August
Plantain, English	*Plantago lanceolata*	Secondary	July–August

OKLAHOMA

Trees			
Elm, American	*Ulmus americana*	High	March–April
Oak, post	*Quercus stellata*	High	May
Walnut, black	*Juglans nigra*	High	April

continued

Southeastern and Southern United States (Continued)

Common Name	Botanical Name	Importance	Season
Ash, green	*Fraxinus pennsylvanica*	Secondary	March–April
Cottonwood	*Populus deltoides*	Secondary	April
Hickory, shagbark	*Hicoria ovata*	Secondary	April
Sycamore, eastern	*Platanus occidentalis*	Secondary	April
Grasses			
Bermuda	*Cynodon dactylon*	High	May–August
Johnson	*Holcus halepensis*	High	May–August
June/Kentucky blue	*Poa pratensis*	High	May–August
Orchard	*Dactylis glomerata*	Secondary	May–August
Red top	*Agrostis alba*	Secondary	May–August
Rye, Italian	*Lolium multiflorum*	Secondary	May–August
Timothy	*Phleum pratense*	Secondary	May–August
Weeds			
Marsh elder	*Iva ciliata*	High	Late August–October
Ragweed, giant	*Ambrosia trifida*	High	Late August–October
short	*Ambrosia elatior*	High	Late August–October
southern	*Ambrosia bidentata*	High	Late August–October
western	*Ambrosia psilostachya*	High	Late August–October
Cocklebur	*Xanthium strumarium*	Secondary	June–September
Dock, yellow	*Rumex crispus*	Secondary	May–August
Kochia	*Kochia scoparia*	Secondary	June–September
Lamb's quarters	*Chenopodium alba*	Secondary	June–September
Pigweed, rough	*Amaranthus retroflexus*	Secondary	June–September
Plantain, English	*Plantago lanceolata*	Secondary	May–August
Thistle, Russian	*Salsola pestifer*	Secondary	June–September

SOUTH CAROLINA

Trees			
Elm, American	*Ulmus americana*	High	April
Oak, live	*Quercus virginiana*	High	May
Pecan	*Hicoria pecan*	High	April–May
Ash, white	*Fraxinus americana*	Secondary	March–April
Hickory, white	*Hicoria alba*	Secondary	April
Maple, red	*Acer rubrum*	Secondary	April
Sycamore	*Platanus occidentalis*	Secondary	March–April
Grasses			
Bermuda	*Cynodon dactylon*	High	May–September
Johnson	*Holcus halepensis*	High	May–September
June/Kentucky blue	*Poa pratensis*	High	May–September
Orchard	*Dactylis glomerata*	Secondary	May–September

Southeastern and Southern United States (Continued)

Common Name	Botanical Name	Importance	Season
Rye, Italian	*Lolium multiflorum*	Secondary	May–September
Weeds			
Ragweed, giant	*Ambrosia trifida*	High	July–October
short	*Ambrosia elatior*	High	July–October
Cocklebur	*Xanthium canadense*	Secondary	July–October
Marsh elder, seaside	*Iva fructescens*	Secondary	July–September
Lamb's quarters	*Chenopodium alba*	Secondary	July–September
Pigweed, redroot	*Amaranthus retroflexus*	Secondary	July–September
Plantain, English	*Plantago lanceolata*	Secondary	July–September

TENNESSEE

Common Name	Botanical Name	Importance	Season
Trees			
Elm, American	*Ulmus americana*	High	February–April
Oak, red	*Quercus rubra*	High	April–May
Pecan	*Hicoria pecan*	High	April
Ash, white	*Fraxinus americana*	Secondary	March
Maple, red	*Acer rubrum*	Secondary	March
Sycamore	*Platanus occidentalis*	Secondary	April–May
Walnut, black	*Juglans nigra*	Secondary	April–May
Grasses			
Bermuda	*Cynodon dactylon*	High	March–November
Johnson	*Holcus halepensis*	High	March–November
June/Kentucky blue	*Poa pratensis*	High	March–November
Orchard	*Dactylis glomerata*	Secondary	March–November
Red top	*Agrostis alba*	Secondary	March–November
Timothy	*Phleum pratense*	Secondary	March–November
Weeds			
Ragweed, giant	*Ambrosia trifida*	High	Mid-August–late October
short	*Ambrosia elatior*	High	Mid-August–late October
Cocklebur	*Xanthium canadense*	Secondary	June–September
Dock, yellow	*Rumex crispus*	Secondary	April–July
Plaintain, English	*Plantago lanceolata*	Secondary	May–August
Kochia	*Kochia scoparia*	Secondary	June–August
Lamb's quarters	*Chenopodium alba*	Secondary	June–August
Pigweed, redroot	*Amaranthus retroflexus*	Secondary	June–August

TEXAS

Common Name	Botanical Name	Importance	Season
Trees			
Elm, American	*Ulmus americana*	High	February–April
Ash, white	*Fraxinus americana*	Secondary	February–April

continued

Southeastern and Southern United States (Continued)

Common Name	Botanical Name	Importance	Season
Cottonwood	*Populus deltoides*	Secondary	March
Elder, box	*Acer negundo*	Secondary	March
Oak, live	*Quercus virginiana*	Secondary	March–April
Pecan	*Hicoria pecan*	Secondary	April
Willow, black	*Salix nigra*	Secondary	March
Cedar, mountain	*Juniperus sabinoides*	Local	December–February
Mesquite	*Prosopis* sp	Local	February–April
Grasses			
Bermuda	*Cynodon dactylon*	High	February–August
Johnson	*Holcus halepensis*	High	February–August
June/Kentucky blue	*Poa pratensis*	High	February–August
Weeds			
Ragweed, giant	*Ambrosia trifida*	High	End August– early October
short	*Ambrosia elatior*	High	End August– early October
southern	*Ambrosia bidentata*	High	End August– early October
western	*Ambrosia psilostachya*	Secondary	End August– early October
Careless weed	*Amaranthus paleri*	Secondary	June–October
Marsh elder	*Iva ciliata*	Secondary	June–October
Kochia	*Kochia scoparia*	Secondary	June–October
Lamb's quarters	*Chenopodium alba*	Secondary	June–October
Pigweed, redroot	*Amaranthus retroflexus*	Secondary	June–October
Sagebrush, prairie	*Artemisia ludoviciana*	Secondary	June–October
Thistle, Russian	*Salsola pestifer*	Secondary	June–October
Water hemp, western	*Acnida tamarascina*	Secondary	June–October

Midwestern United States

ILLINOIS	MINNESOTA
INDIANA	MISSOURI
IOWA	NEBRASKA
KANSAS	NORTH DAKOTA
KENTUCKY	SOUTH DAKOTA
MICHIGAN	WISCONSIN

ILLINOIS

Trees

Elm, American	*Ulmus americana*	High	February–April
Oak, white	*Quercus alba*	High	May
Ash, white	*Fraxinus americana*	Secondary	April–May
Cottonwood	*Populus deltoides*	Secondary	April–May
Maple, hard	*Acer saccharum*	Secondary	March–April
Walnut, black	Juglans nigra	Secondary	March–April

Grasses

June/Kentucky blue	*Poa pratensis*	High	Mid-May–mid-July
Orchard	*Dactylis glomerata*	High	Mid-May–mid-July
Red top	*Agrostis alba*	High	Mid-May–mid-July
Timothy	*Phleum pratense*	High	Mid-May–mid July

Weeds

Ragweed, giant	*Ambrosia trifida*	High	Early August–late September
short	*Ambrosia elatior*	High	Early August–late September
Kochia	*Kochia scoparia*	Secondary	July–October
Lamb's quarters	*Chenopodium alba*	Secondary	July–October
Pigweed, rough	*Amaranthus retroflexus*	Secondary	July–October
Plantain, English	*Plantago lanceolata*	Secondary	June–August
Thistle, Russian	*Salsola pestifer*	Secondary	July–October
Cocklebur	*Xanthium strumarium*	Local	August–September
Marsh elder, burweed	*Iva xanthifolia*	Local	August–September
Ragweed, southern	*Ambrosia bidentata*	Local	August–September
western	*Ambrosia psilostachya*	Local	August–September

INDIANA

Trees

Elm, American	*Ulmus americana*	High	February–March
Oak, red	*Quercus rubra*	High	April–May
Ash, white	*Fraxinus americana*	Secondary	April–May

continued

Midwestern United States (Continued)

Common Name	Botanical Name	Importance	Season
Cottonwood	*Populus deltoides*	Secondary	April–May
Hickory, shagbark	*Hicoria ovata*	Secondary	May–June
Sycamore, eastern	*Platanus occidentalis*	Secondary	April
Walnut, black	*Juglans nigra*	Secondary	March–April
Grasses			
June/Kentucky blue	*Poa pratensis*	High	May–June
Orchard	*Dactylis glomerata*	High	May–June
Red top	Agrostis alba	High	May–June
Timothy	Phleum pratense	High	May–June
Weeds			
Ragweed, giant	Ambrosia trifida	High	August–September
short	Ambrosia elatior	High	August–September
Cocklebur	Xanthium strumarium	Secondary	August–September
Lamb's quarters	Chenopodium alba	Secondary	August–September
Pigweed, rough	Amaranthus retroflexus	Secondary	August–September
Kochia	Kochia scoparia	Local	August–September
Sagebrush, annual	Artemisia annua	Local	August–September
Thistle, Russian	Salsola pestifer	Local	August–September

IOWA

Common Name	Botanical Name	Importance	Season
Trees			
Elm, American	Ulmus americana	High	March–April
Oak, red	Quercus rubra	High	April–May
Walnut, black	Juglans nigra	High	March–April
Cottonwood	Populus deltoides	Secondary	March–April
Elder, box	Acer negundo	Secondary	March–April
Sycamore, eastern	Platanus occidentalis	Secondary	April–May
Grasses			
June/Kentucky blue	*Poa pratensis*	High	May–June
Orchard	*Dactylis glomerata*	High	May–June
Red top	*Agrostis alba*	High	May–June
Timothy	*Phleum pratense*	High	May–June
Brome, smooth	*Bromus inermis*	Secondary	May–June
Weeds			
Marsh elder, burweed	*Iva xanthifolia*	High	Mid-August–late September
Ragweed, giant	*Ambrosia trifida*	High	Mid-August–late September
short	*Ambrosia elatior*	High	Mid-August–late September
Cocklebur	*Xanthium strumarium*	Secondary	July–August

Midwestern United States (Continued)

Common Name	Botanical Name	Importance	Season
Hemp, western water	*Acnida tamarascina*	Secondary	July–August
Kochia	*Kochia scoparia*	Secondary	July–August
Plaintain, English	*Plantago lanceolata*	Secondary	July–August
Thistle, Russian	*Salsola pestifer*	Secondary	July–August
Hemp	Cannabis sativa	Local	July–September
Lamb's quarters	*Chenopodium alba*	Local	July–August
Pigweed, rough	Amaranthus retroflexus	Local	July–August

KANSAS

Trees			
Elm, American	*Ulmus americana*	High	March
Oak, post	*Quercus stellata*	High	May
Ash, white	*Fraxinus americana*	Secondary	April–May
Cottonwood	*Populus deltoides*	Secondary	March–April
Elder, box	*Acer negundo*	Secondary	March–April
Hickory, shagbark	*Hicoria ovata*	Secondary	April–May
Walnut, black	*Juglans nigra*	Secondary	April–May
Grasses			
June/Kentucky blue	*Poa pratensis*	High	May–July
Orchard	*Dactylis glomerata*	High	May–July
Red top	*Agrostis alba*	High	May–July
Timothy	*Phleum pratense*	High	May–July
Bermuda	*Cynodon dactylon*	Secondary	May–July
Fescue, meadow	*Festuca elatior*	Secondary	May–July
Johnson	*Holcus halepensis*	Secondary	May–July
Weeds			
Kochia	*Kochia scoparia*	High	July–October
Ragweed, giant	*Ambrosia trifida*	High	Mid-August–mid-October
short	*Ambrosia elatior*	High	Mid-August–mid-October
western	*Ambrosia psilostachya*	High	Mid-August–mid-October
Thistle, Russian	*Salsola pestifer*	High	July–October
Marsh elder, burweed	*Iva xanthifolia*	Secondary	August–October
Hemp, western water	*Acnida tamarascina*	Secondary	July–September
Lamb's quarters	*Chenopodium alba*	Secondary	July–September
Pigweed, rough	*Amaranthus retroflexus*	Secondary	July–September
Ragweed, Southern	*Ambrosia bidentata*	Secondary	Mid-August–mid-October

KENTUCKY

Trees			
Elm, American	*Ulmus americana*	High	February–March
Oak, red	*Quercus rubra*	High	April–May

continued

Midwestern United States (Continued)

Common Name	Botanical Name	Importance	Season
Hickory, white	*Hicoria alba*	Secondary	April–May
Maple, hard	*Acer saccharum*	Secondary	April–March
Sycamore	*Platanus occidentalis*	Secondary	April–May
Walnut, black	*Juglans nigra*	Secondary	April–May
Grasses			
June/Kentucky blue	*Poa pratensis*	High	May–July
Timothy	*Phleum pratense*	High	May–July
Bermuda	*Cynodon dactylon*	Secondary	May–August
Fescue, meadow	*Festuca elatior*	Secondary	May–August
Orchard	*Dactylis glomerata*	Secondary	May–August
Red top	*Agrostis alba*	Secondary	May–August
Weeds			
Ragweed, giant	*Ambrosia trifida*	High	Mid-August–early October
short	*Ambrosia elatior*	High	Mid-August–early October
Amaranth, spiny	*Amaranthus spinosus*	Secondary	July–September
Cocklebur	*Xanthium canadense*	Secondary	Mid-August–early October
Lamb's quarters	*Chenopodium alba*	Secondary	July–September
Marsh elder, burweed	*Iva xanthifolia*	Secondary	Mid-August–early October
Plantain, English	*Plantago lanceolata*	Secondary	June–July
Dock, yellow	*Rumex crispus*	Local	July–September
Kochia	*Kochia scoparia*	Local	July–September
Ragweed, southern	*Ambrosia bidentata*	Local	Mid-August–early October

MICHIGAN

Trees			
Elm, American	*Ulmus americana*	High	April
Oak, red	*Quercus rubra*	High	May
Cottonwood	*Populus deltoides*	Secondary	April
Hickory, shagbark	*Hicoria ovata*	Secondary	May–June
Maple, red	*Acer saccharum*	Secondary	April
Sycamore	*Platanus occidentalis*	Secondary	April
Walnut, black	*Juglans nigra*	Secondary	May–June
Grasses			
June/Kentucky blue	*Poa pratensis*	High	May–July
Orchard	*Dactylis glomerata*	High	May–July
Red top	*Agrostis alba*	High	May–July
Timothy	*Phleum pratense*	High	May–July

Midwestern United States (Continued)

Common Name	Botanical Name	Importance	Season
Weeds			
Ragweed, giant	*Ambrosia trifida*	High	Mid-August–mid-September
short	*Ambrosia elatior*	High	Mid-August–mid-September
Cocklebur	*Xanthium canadense*	Secondary	July–August
Dock, yellow	*Rumex crispus*	Secondary	May–July
Lamb's quarters	*Chenopodium alba*	Secondary	July–September
Pigweed, redroot	*Amaranthus retroflexus*	Secondary	July–September
Plantain, English	*Plantago lanceolata*	Secondary	June–August

MINNESOTA

Common Name	Botanical Name	Importance	Season
Trees			
Elm, American	*Ulmus americana*	High	April–May
Oak, red	*Quercus rubra*	High	May
Ash, white	*Fraxinus americana*	Secondary	April–May
Birch, paper	*Betula papyrifera*	Secondary	April–May
Hickory, shagbark	*Hicoria ovata*	Secondary	May
Maple, hard	*Acer saccharum*	Secondary	March–April
Walnut, black	*Juglans nigra*	Secondary	May
Grasses			
June/Kentucky blue	*Poa pratensis*	High	May–August
Orchard	*Dactylis glomerata*	High	May–August
Red top	*Agrostis alba*	High	May–August
Timothy	*Phleum pratense*	High	May–August
Weeds			
Ragweed, giant	*Ambrosia trifida*	High	August–September
short	*Ambrosia elatior*	High	August–September
Cocklebur	*Xanthium canadense*	Secondary	August–September
Marsh elder, burweed	*Iva xanthifolia*	Secondary	August–September
Hemp, western water	*Acnida tamarascina*	Secondary	July–August
Lamb's quarters	*Chenopodium alba*	Secondary	July–September
Pigweed, redroot	*Amaranthus retroflexus*	Secondary	July–September
Plantain, English	*Plantago lanceolata*	Secondary	June–July
Sagebrush	*Artemisia* sp	Secondary	July–September

MISSOURI

Common Name	Botanical Name	Importance	Season
Trees			
Elm, American	*Ulmus americana*	High	March
Oak, red	*Quercus rubra*	High	May
Ash, white	*Fraxinus americana*	Secondary	April

continued

Midwestern United States (Continued)

Common Name	Botanical Name	Importance	Season
Cottonwood	Populus deltoides	Secondary	March–April
Hickory, shagbark	Hicoria ovata	Secondary	May
Sycamore, eastern	Platanus occidentalis	Secondary	April–May
Walnut, black	Juglans nigra	Secondary	April–May
Grasses			
June/Kentucky blue	Poa pratensis	High	May–August
Orchard	Dactylis glomerata	High	May–August
Red top	Agrostis alba	High	May–August
Timothy	Phleum pratense	High	May–August
Blue, Canadian	Poa compressa	Secondary	May–August
Weeds			
Ragweed, giant	Ambrosia trifida	High	August–early October
short	Ambrosia elatior	High	August–early October
southern	Ambrosia bidentata	High	August–early October
Hemp, western water	Acnida tamarascina	Secondary	July–August
Kochia	Kochia scoparia	Secondary	July–September
Lamb's quarters	Chenopodium alba	Secondary	July–September
Pigweed, redroot	Amaranthus retroflexus	Secondary	July–August
Platain English	Plantago lanceolata	Secondary	June–July
Thistle, Russian	Salsola pestifer	Secondary	July–August

NEBRASKA

Trees			
Elm, American	Ulmus americana	High	March
Oak, burr	Quercus macrocarpa	High	May
Ash, white	Fraxinus americana	Secondary	April–May
Cottonwood	Populus deltoides	Secondary	April
Elder, box	Acer segundo	Secondary	April–May
Hickory, shagbark	Hicoria ovata	Secondary	April–May
Walnut, black	Juglans nigra	Secondary	April–May
Grasses			
June/Kentucky blue	Poa pratensis	High	May–July
Orchard	Dactylis glomerata	High	May–July
Red top	Agrostis alba	High	May–July
Timothy	Phleum pratense	High	May–July
Wheat, western	Agropyron Smithii	Secondary	May–July
Weeds			
Ragweed, giant	Ambrosia trifida	High	Mid August–October
short	Ambrosia elatior	High	Mid August–October
Marsh elder, burweed	Iva xanthifolia	High	Mid August–October

Midwestern United States (Continued)

Common Name	Botanical Name	Importance	Season
Hemp, western water	*Acnida tamarascina*	Secondary	July–August
Kochia	*Kochia scoparia*	Secondary	July–August
Lamb's quarters	*Chenopodium alba*	Secondary	July–August
Pigweed, redroot	*Amaranthus retroflexus*	Secondary	July–August
Plantain, English	*Plantago lanceolata*	Secondary	June–July
Sagebrush	*Artemisia* sp	Secondary	July–September
Thistle, Russian	*Salsola pestifer*	Secondary	July–August

NORTH AND SOUTH DAKOTA

Trees

Elm, American	*Ulmus americana*	Secondary	April
Elder, box	*Acer negundo*	Secondary	April–May
Willow, pussy	*Salix discolor*	Secondary	April–May
Aspen	*Populus tremuloides*	Secondary	April–May
Birch, paper	*Betula papyrifera*	Secondary	April–May

Grasses

June/Kentucky Blue	*Poa pratensis*	High	May–July
Timothy	*Phleum pratense*	Secondary	May–July
Brome, smooth	*Bromus inermis*	Secondary	May–July
Wheat, crested	*Agropyron cristatum*	Secondary	May–July
western	*Agropyron smithii*	Secondary	May–July

Weeds

Ragweed, giant	*Ambrosia trifida*	High	July–September
short	*Ambrosia elatior*	High	July–September
Marsh elder, burweed	*Iva xanthifolia*	High	July–September
Kochia	*Kochia scoparia*	High	July–August
Thistle, Russian	*Salsola pestifer*	High	July–August
Hemp, Western water	*Acnida tamarascina*	Secondary	July–August
Lamb's quarters	*Chenopodium alba*	Secondary	July–August
Pigweed, redroot	*Amaranthus retroflexus*	Secondary	July–August
Plantain, English	*Plantago lanceolata*	Secondary	June–August
Sagebrush	*Artemisia* sp	Secondary	September

WISCONSIN

Trees

Elm, American	*Ulmus americana*	High	April
Oak, red	*Quercus rubra*	High	May
Ash, white	*Fraxinus americana*	Secondary	April
Birch, red	*Betula nigra*	Secondary	April–May
Cottonwood	*Populus deltoides*	Secondary	April

continued

Midwestern United States (Continued)

Common Name	Botanical Name	Importance	Season
Maple, hard	*Acer saccharum*	Secondary	April
Grasses			
June/Kentucky blue	*Poa pratensis*	High	June–July
Orchard	*Dactylis glomerata*	High	June–July
Red top	*Agrostis alba*	High	June–July
Timothy	*Phleum pratense*	High	June–July
Weeds			
Ragweed, giant	*Ambrosia trifida*	High	Early August– late September
short	*Ambrosia elatior*	High	Early August– late September
Cocklebur	*Xanthium canadense*	Secondary	Same
Marsh elder, burweed	*Iva xanthifolia*	Secondary	Same
Lamb's quarters	*Chenopodium alba*	Secondary	July–August
Pigweed, redroot	*Amaranthus retroflexus*	Secondary	July–August
Plaintain, English	*Plantago lanceolata*	Secondary	June–July
Kochia	*Kochia scoparia*	Local	July–August
Thistle, Russian	*Salsola pestifer*	Local	July–August

Western and Non Continental United States

ARIZONA	UTAH
CALIFORNIA	WASHINGTON
COLORADO	WYOMING
IDAHO	ALASKA
MONTANA	HAWAII
NEVADA	PUERTO RICO
NEW MEXICO	VIRGIN ISLANDS
OREGON	

Common Name	Botanical Name	Importance	Season
		ARIZONA	
Trees			
Ash, Arizona	*Fraxinus velutina*	Secondary	February–April
Cottonwood	*Populus deltoides*	Secondary	January–April
Juniper	*Juniperus* sp	Secondary	December–April
Mesquite	*Prosopis* sp	Secondary	April–June
Olive	*Olea europaea*	Secondary	March–May
Mulberry	*Morus* sp	Local	March–April

Western and Non Continental United States (Continued)

Common Name	Botanical Name	Importance	Season
Grasses			
Bermuda	*Cynodon dactylon*	High	February–November
Johnson	*Holcus halepensis*	Secondary	February–November
June/Kentucky blue	*Poa pratensis*	Secondary	February–November
Rye, perennial	*Lolium perenne*	Secondary	February–November
Weeds			
Careless weed	*Amaranthus palmeri*	High	May–September
Ragweed, false	*Franseria* sp	Secondary	March–May
slender	*Franseria tenuifolia*	Secondary	August–October
western	*Ambrosia psilostachya*	Secondary	August–October
Atriplex-scale	*Atriplex* sp	Secondary	April–October
Pigweed, redroot	*Amaranthus retroflexus*	Secondary	May–November
Plantain, English	*Plantago lanceolata*	Secondary	April–Ootober
Sagebrush	*Artemisia* sp	Secondary	April–October
Thistle, Russian	*Salsola pestifer*	Secondary	May–October
Sugarbeet	*Beta vulgaris*	Local	April–June

CALIFORNIA (NORTHERN)

Common Name	Botanical Name	Importance	Season
Trees			
Elm, American	*Ulmus americana*	High	February–March
Oak	*Quercus* sp	High	February–May
Birch	*Detula* sp	High	February–May
Cottonwood	*Populus* sp	High	March–April
Olive	*Olea europaea*	High	April–June
Walnut, black	*Juglans nigra*	High	April–June
Acacia	*Acacia* sp	Secondary	January–December
Alder	*Alnus* sp	Secondary	March–June
Elder, box	*Acer negundo*	Secondary	February–April
Sycamore	*Platanus* sp	Secondary	March–April
Grasses			
Bermuda	*Cynodon dactylon*	High	April–September
Brome	*Bromus* sp	High	April–September
Oat, wild	*Avena fatua*	High	April–September
Red top	*Agrostis alba*	High	April–September
Rye	*Lolium* sp	High	April–September
Fescue, meadow	*Festuca elatior*	Secondary	April–September
Orchard	*Dactylis glomerata*	Secondary	April–September
Timothy	*Phleum pratense*	Secondary	April–September

continued

Western and Non Continental United States (Continued)

Common Name	Botanical Name	Importance	Season
Weeds			
Pigweed, redroot	*Amaranthus retroflexus*	High	May–October
Sagebrush	*Artemisia* sp	High	July–October
Cocklebur	*Xanthium canadense*	Secondary	July–November
Lamb's quarters	*Chenopodium alba*	Secondary	April–September
Atriplex-scale	*Atriplex* sp	Secondary	June–September
Ragweed, false western	*Franseria acanthicarpa*	Secondary	June–October
Sheep sorrel	*Rumex acetosella*	Secondary	March–September
Plantain, English	*Plantago lanceolata*	Secondary	April–August
Ragweed, western	*Ambrosia psilostachya*	Local	July–November

CALIFORNIA, SOUTHERN

Common Name	Botanical Name	Importance	Season
Trees			
Cottonwood, Fremont	*Populus fremontii*	High	February–March
Oak	*Quercus* sp	High	March–May
Walnut, black	*Juglans nigra*	High	March–May
Sycamore, western	*Platanus racemosa*	High	March–May
Cypress, Arizona	*Cupressus arizonica*	Secondary	February–March
Maple, big leaf	*Acer macrophyllum*	Secondary	March–April
Olive	*Olea europaea*	Secondary	April–June
Mesquite	*Prosopis* sp	Local	Spring–summer
Grasses			
Bermuda	*Cynodon dactylon*	High	April–October
Oats, wild	*Avena fatua*	High	April–June
Brome	*Bromus* sp	Secondary	April–June
June/Kentucky blue	*Poa pratensis*	Secondary	April–June
Johnson	*Holcus halepensis*	Secondary	April–October
Rye	*Lolium* sp	Secondary	April–October
Salt	*Distichlis spicata*	Secondary	April–September
Weeds			
Ragweed, false	*Franseria acanthicarpa*	High	July–September
Sagebrush	*Artemisia* sp	High	July–October
Atriplex-scale	*Atriplex* sp	Secondary	June–September
Cocklebur	*Xanthium canadense*	Secondary	June–October
Lamb's quarters	*Chenopodium alba*	Secondary	June–October
Ragweed, Western	*Ambrosia psilostachya*	Secondary	July–September
Thistle, Russian	*Salsola pestifer*	Secondary	June–September

COLORADO

Common Name	Botanical Name	Importance	Season
Trees			
Cottonwood	*Populus deltoides*	High	April–May
Elm, American	*Ulmus americana*	High	February–May

Western and Non Continental United States (Continued)

Common Name	Botanical Name	Importance	Season
Cedar	*Juniperus* sp	Secondary	March–May
Maple	*Acer saccharum*	Secondary	March–May
Oak, scrub	*Quercus gambelii*	Secondary	May–June
Grasses			
June/Kentucky blue	*Poa pratensis*	High	May–September
Fescue, meadow	*Festuca elatior*	Secondary	May–September
Orchard	*Dactylis glomerata*	Secondary	May–September
Red top	*Agrostis alba*	Secondary	May–September
Timothy	*Phleum pratense*	Secondary	May–September
Weeds			
Kochia	*Kochia scoparia*	High	July–September
Thistle, Russian	*Salsola pestifer*	High	July–September
Marsh elder, burweed	*Iva xanthifolia*	Secondary	August–September
Lamb's quarters	*Chenopodium alba*	Secondary	July–September
Pigweed, redroot	*Amaranthus retroflexus*	Secondary	July–September
Plantain, English	*Plantago lanceolata*	Secondary	June–August
Ragweed, giant	*Ambrosia trifida*	Secondary	August–September
short	*Ambrosia elatior*	Secondary	August–September
Sagebrush	*Artemisia* sp	Secondary	August–September
Ragweed, western	*Ambrosia psilostachya*	Local	August–September

IDAHO

Trees			
Alder	*Alnus tenuifolia*	Secondary	March–April
Aspen	*Populus tremuloides*	Secondary	April
Birch, spring	*Betula* sp	Secondary	May
Cottonwood, black	*Populus trichocarpa*	Secondary	April–May
Grasses			
June/Kentucky blue	*Poa pratensis*	High	May–September
Red top	*Agrostis alba*	High	May–September
Brome, smooth	*Bromus Inermis*	Secondary	May–September
Orchard	*Dactylis glomerata*	Secondary	May–September
Timothy	*Phleum pratense*	Secondary	May–September
Weeds			
Thistle, Russian	*Salsola pestifer*	High	June–September
Atriplex-scale	*Atriplex* sp	Secondary	August–September
Marsh elder, burweed	*Iva xanthifolia*	Secondary	August–September
Lamb's quarters	*Chenopodium alba*	Secondary	July–September
Pigweed, rough	*Amaranthus retroflexus*	Secondary	July–September
Plantain, English	*Plantago lanceolata*	Secondary	June–September

continued

Western and Non Continental United States (Continued)

Common Name	Botanical Name	Importance	Season
Ragweed, false	*Franseria acanthicarpa*	Secondary	August–September
Sagebrush	*Artemisia* sp	Secondary	July–August
Sheep sorrel	*Rumex acetosella*	Secondary	May–October

MONTANA

Trees

Aspen	*Populus tremuloides*	Secondary	May
Cottonwood	*Populus trichocarpa*	Secondary	April–May
Willow	*Salix lasiandracaudata*	Secondary	March–April
Elder, box	*Acer negundo*	Local	April
Pine	*Pinus* sp	Local	June

Grasses

June/Kentucky blue	*Poa pratensis*	High	May–June
Red top	*Agrostis alba*	High	May–June
Brome, smooth	*Bromus inermis*	Secondary	May–June
Orchard	*Dactylis glomerata*	Secondary	May–June
Timothy	*Phleum pratense*	Secondary	May–June

Weeds

Thistle, Russian	*Salsola pestifer*	High	July–September
Atriplex-scale	*Atriplex* sp	Secondary	June
Marsh elder, burweed	*Iva xanthifolia*	Secondary	August–September
Lamb's quarters	*Chenopodium alba*	Secondary	July–September
Pigweed, rough	*Amaranthus retroflexus*	Secondary	July–August
Ragweed, giant	*Ambrosia trifida*	Secondary	August–September
short	*Ambrosia elatior*	Secondary	August–September
Sagebrush	*Artemisia* sp	Secondary	September–October
Sheep sorrel	*Rumex acetosella*	Secondary	May–October
Kochia	*Kochia scoparia*	Local	July–September
Ragweed, western	*Ambrosia psilostachya*	Local	August–September

NEVADA

Trees

Ash	*Fraxinus* sp	Secondary	February–May
Cottonwood	*Populus* sp	Secondary	February–April
Elm	*Ulmus* sp	Secondary	February–April
Sycamore, maple leaf	*Platanus acerifolia*	Secondary	April
Willow, narrow leaf	*Salix exigua*	Secondary	April–May
Elder, box	*Acer negundo*	Local	April–May
Juniper, Utah	*Juniperus utahensis*	Local	March–May
Mesquite	*Prosopis* sp	Local	April–July

Western and Non Continental United States (Continued)

Common Name	Botanical Name	Importance	Season
Grasses			
Bermuda	*Cynodon dactylon*	High	March–October
June/Kentucky blue	*Poa pratensis*	High	May–July
Salt	*Distichlis stricata*	High	May–July
Rye	*Lolium* sp	Secondary	May–July
Timothy	*Phleum pratense*	Secondary	May–July
Quack	*Agropyron repens*	Local	May–July
Orchard	*Dactylis glomerata*	Local	May–July
Red top	*Agrostis alba*	Local	May–July
Weeds			
Sagebrush	*Artemisia* sp	High	August–September
Thistle, Russian	*Salsola pestifer*	High	July–September
Atriplex-scale	*Atriplex* sp	Secondary	July–September
Kochia	*Kochia scoparia*	Secondary	July–September
Lamb's quarters	*Chenopodium alba*	Secondary	July–September
Pigweed, rough	*Amaranthus retroflexus*	Secondary	July–September
Plantain, English	*Plantago lanceolata*	Secondary	April–August
Ragweed, false	*Franseria acanthicarpa*	Secondary	August–September
Dock, yellow	*Rumex crispus*	Local	May–July

NEW MEXICO

Common Name	Botanical Name	Importance	Season
Trees			
Cottonwood	*Populus deltoides*	Secondary	March
Elder, box	*Acer negundo*	Secondary	April–May
Elm	*Ulmus* sp	Secondary	February–March
Juniper, cherrystone	*Juniperus monosperma*	Secondary	March
Oak, scrub	*Quercus gambelii*	Secondary	May
Grasses			
Bermuda	*Cynodon dactylon*	High	April–August
Fescue, meadow	*Festuca elatior*	Secondary	April–August
Johnson	*Holcus halepensis*	Secondary	April–August
June/Kentucky blue	*Poa pratensis*	Secondary	April–August
Rye, perennial	*Lolium perenne*	Secondary	April–August
Weeds			
Kochia	*Kochia scoparia*	High	June–September
Thistle, Russian	*Salsola pestifer*	High	June–September
Atriplex-scale	*Atriplex* sp	Secondary	June–September
Careless weed	*Amaranthus palmeri*	Secondary	June–September
Pigweed, rough	*Amaranthus retroflexus*	Secondary	June–September

continued

Western and Non Continental United States (Continued)

Common Name	Botanical Name	Importance	Season
Plantain, English	*Plantago lanceolata*	Secondary	June–September
Ragweed, false	*Franseria acanthicarpa*	Secondary	August–October
Sagebrush	*Artemisia* sp	Local	August–October

OREGON

Trees

Alder	*Alnus* sp	High	March–April
Birch	*Betula* sp	High	March–April
Walnut, English	*Juglans* regia	High	May–June
Elder, box	*Acer negundo*	Secondary	March–April
Poplar	*Populus* sp	Secondary	March–April
Willow	*Salix* sp	Local	February–March

Grasses

June/Kentucky blue	*Poa pratensis*	High	May–September
Timothy	*Phleum pratensis*	High	May–September
Orchard	*Dactylis glomerata*	Secondary	May–September
Red top	*Agrostis alba*	Secondary	May–September
Rye, perennial	*Lolium perenne*	Secondary	May–September
Velvet	*Holcus lanatus*	Secondary	May–September

Weeds

Dock, yellow	*Rumex crispus*	High	May–September
Lamb's quarters	*Chenopodium alba*	High	June–September
Pigweed, redroot	*Amaranthus retroflexus*	High	June–September
Plantain, English	*Plantago lanceolata*	High	May–September
Thistle, Russian	*Salsola pestifer*	High	July–September
Atriplex-scale	*Atriplex* sp	Secondary	July–September
Sagebrush	*Artemisia* sp	Secondary	August–September

UTAH

Trees

Elder, box	*Acer negundo*	High	April–May
Alder, mountain	*Alnus tenuifolia*	Secondary	April–May
Cottonwood	*Populus deltoides*	Secondary	April–May
Elm	*Ulmus* sp	Secondary	March
Juniper	*Juniperus* sp	Secondary	March–May

Grasses

June/Kentucky blue	*Poa pratensis*	High	May–July
Koelers	*Koeleria cristata*	Secondary	May–July
Orchard	*Dactylis glomerata*	Secondary	May–July
Red top	*Agrostis alba*	Secondary	May–July
Timothy	*Phleum pratense*	Secondary	May–July

Western and Non Continental United States (Continued)

Common Name	Botanical Name	Importance	Season
Weeds			
Kochia	*Kochia scoparia*	High	July–September
Thistle, Russian	*Salsola pestifer*	High	July–September
Atriplex-scale	*Atriplex* sp	Secondary	June–September
Cocklebur	*Xanthium canadense*	Secondary	August–September
Lamb's quarters	*Chenopodium alba*	Secondary	June–September
Pigweed, redroot	*Amaranthus retroflexus*	Secondary	June–September
Plantain, English	*Plantago lanceolata*	Secondary	May–August
Ragweed, false	*Franseria acanthicarpa*	Secondary	August–September
short	*Ambrosia elatior*	Local	August–September
western	*Ambrosia psilostachya*	Local	August–September
Sagebrush	*Artemisia* sp	Secondary	August–September

WASHINGTON

Common Name	Botanical Name	Importance	Season
Trees			
Aspen	*Populus tremuloides*	Secondary	April
Birch	*Betula* sp	Secondary	April–May
Cottonwood	*Populus trichocarpa*	Secondary	April
Elder, box	*Acer negundo*	Secondary	April
Willow	*Salix lasiandracaudata*	Secondary	March–April
Elm	*Ulmus* sp	Local	March
Grasses			
June/Kentucky blue	*Poa pratensis*	High	May–September
Timothy	*Phleum pratense*	High	June–July
June, annual	*Poa annua*	Secondary	April–October
Orchard	*Dactylis glomerata*	Secondary	June–July
Red top	*Agrostis alba*	Secondary	June–July
Rye	*Lolium* sp	Secondary	June–July
Brome	*Bromus* sp	Local	June–July
Weeds			
Plantain, English	*Plantago lanceolata*	High	June–September
Ragweed, short	*Ambrosia elatior*	High	August–September
false	*Franseria acanthicarpa*	High	August–September
Thistle, Russian	*Salsola pestifer*	High	June–September
Dock, yellow	*Rumex crispus*	Secondary	June–July
Marsh elder, burweed	*Iva xanthifolia*	High	August–September
Lamb's quarters	*Chenopodium alba*	Secondary	July–September
Pigweed, redroot	*Amaranthus retroflexus*	Secondary	June–September
Ragweed, western	*Ambrosia psilostachya*	Secondary	August–September

continued

Western and Non Continental United States (Continued)

Common Name	Botanical Name	Importance	Season
Sagebrush	*Artemisia* sp	Secondary	August–September

WYOMING

Trees

Alder	*Almus tenuifolia*	Secondary	April
Birch	*Betula* sp	Secondary	April–May
Cottonwood	*Populus trichocarpus*	Secondary	April–May
Willow	*Salix lasiandracaudata*	Secondary	February–March

Grasses

June/Kentucky blue	*Poa pratensis*	High	May–July
Fescue, meadow	*Festuca elatior*	Secondary	May–July
Orchard	*Dactylis glomerata*	Secondary	May–July
Red top	*Agrostis alba*	Secondary	May–July
Timothy	*Phleum pratense*	Secondary	May–July

Weeds

Kochia	*Kochia scoparia*	High	July–September
Thistle, Russian	*Salsola pestifer*	High	July–September
Ragweed, giant	*Ambrosia trifida*	Secondary	August–September
short	*Ambrosia elatior*	Secondary	August–September
false	*Franseria acanthicarpa*	Local	August–September
western	*Ambrosia psilostachya*	Local	August–September
Atriplex-scale	*Atriplex* sp	Secondary	May–July
Marsh elder, burweed	*Iva xanthifolia*	Secondary	August–September
Lamb's quarters	*Chenopodium alba*	Secondary	August–September
Pigweed, redroot	*Amaranthus retroflexus*	Secondary	August–September
Sagebrush	*Artemisia* sp	Secondary	August–September

ALASKA

Durham in 1939 found no ragweed pollen in Fairbanks, Nome, or Juneau. A 1984 study by Anderson of the Anchorage area found birch to be the most important tree pollen, followed by alder, spruce, and poplar. Grasses and sedge also were important, along with sheep sorrel, lamb's quarters, wormwood, and plantain. Fairbanks to the north also showed birch as a major allergen.

HAWAII

Roth and Shira believe that frequent rains, tradewinds, mountain barriers, and insect pollination partially explain the low pollen counts obtained in Hawaii. Olive, mesquite, and Australian pine (*Casuarina*) are occasional windborne tree pollen offenders, and insect-pollinated trees of local importance include hibiscus, mango, eucalyptus, acacia, and mimosa. Grasses pollinate almost year long, and important grasses include Bermuda, red top, Johnson, sugar cane, panicum, and pennisetum. False ragweed is located in the western Oahu area but causes little difficulty. Other local important weeds are lamb's quarters, pigweed redroot, and English plantain. Vu, in 1977, found low levels of pollens in the Honolulu southwestern Oahu area using rotorod samplers. These included, besides the predominant grasses, breadfruit, fern, mesquite, haole koa (*Leucaena lucocephala*), and spiny amaranth.

Western and Non Continental United States (Continued)

PUERTO RICO

Trees are a minor cause of inhalant allergy and include Australian pine (*Casuarina*), pines, mango, acacia, and the mimosa family. Bermuda grass is the primary grass offender, followed by sugar cane, panicum, pennisetum, and chloris grasses. False western ragweed, chenopods, amaranths, and English plantain are the locally important weeds.

VIRGIN ISLANDS

Durham and Fafalla found no ragweed in the National Park area in 1961. Mango and coconut were the local tree pollens noted, but the coconut trees were located close to the sampler. Bermuda grass, pennisetum, and chloris were the grasses found to be of local importance.

BIBLIOGRAPHY

Al Doory Y, Domson J, Best J. Airbourne fungi and pollens of the metropolitan District of Columbia area. Ann Allergy 1982;49:265.

Anderson JH. Allergenic airborne pollens of Anchorage, Alaska. Ann Allergy 1985;54:390.

Anderson EF, Dorsett CS, Fleming EO. Airbourne pollens of Walla Walla, Washington. Ann Allergy 1978;41;232.

Armentia A, Quintero A, Fernandez-Garcia A, Salvador J, Martin-Santos JM. Allergy to pine pollen and pinon nuts. Ann Allergy 1990;64:49.

Bucholtz GA, Hensel AE III, Lockey RF, Serbusek D. Australian pine pollen as an aeroallergen. Ann Allergy 1987;59:52.

Bucholtz GA, Lockey RF, Serbousek D. Bald cypress tree pollen, an allergen. Ann Allergy 1985;55:805.

Bucholtz GA, Lockey RF, Wunderlin RP, et al. A three year aerobiologic pollen survey of the Tampa Bay area, Florida. Ann Allergy 1991;67:534.

Buck P, Levetin E. Airborne pollens and mold spores in a subalpine environment. Ann Allergy 1985;55:794.

Buck P, Levetin E. Weather patterns and ragweed production in Tulsa, Oklahoma. Ann Allergy 1982;49:272.

Dungy CL, Kozak PP, Gallup J, Galant SP. Aeroallergen exposure in the elementary school setting. Ann Allergy 1986;56:218.

Durham OC, Fafalla H. A pollen survey at the national park and St. John's Island, Virgin Islands. Ann Allergy 1961;32:23

Enberg RN, Leickly FE, McCullough J, Bailey J, Ownby DR. Watermellon and ragweed share allergens. J Allergy Clin Immunol 1987;79:867.

Fairley D, Batchelder GL. A study of oak pollen production and phenology in northern California: prediction of annual variation in pollen counts based on geographic and meteorologic factors. J Allergy Clin Immunol 1986;78:300.

Feinbold I. A two year pollen and spore survey of southeast Florida. Ann Allergy 1975;35:37.

Freeman GL. Pine pollen allergy in northern Arizona. Ann Allergy 1993;70:491.

Gergen PJ, Turkeltaub PC, Kovar MG. The prevalence of allergenic skin test reactivity to eight common aero allergens in the US population: results from the second national Health and Nutritional Examination Survey. J Allergy Clin Immunol 1987;80:669.

Girsh L. Ragweed pollen distribution in the United States with graphic maps. Ann Allergy 1982;49:1.

Kaufman HS. Parietaria: an unrecognized cause of respiratory allergy in the United States. Ann Allergy 1990;64:293.

Kaufman HS, Ranck K. Antigen recognition in Filipinos, Japanese, Chinese, and Caucasians. Ann Allergy 1988;60:53.

Keynan N, Waisel Y, Shomer-Ilan A, Tamir R. Forecasting pollen pollution: correlation with floral development. Ann Allergy 1989;63:417.

Larson JB, Gleich GJ. Changes in the antigenic composition of the short ragweed plant during maturation. J Allergy 1975;56:112.

Leavengood DC, Renard RL, Martin BG, Nelson HS. Cross allergenicity among grasses determined by tissue threshold changes. J Allergy Clin Immunol 1986;76:789.

Levetin E, Puck P. Evidence of mountain cedar pollen in Tulsa, Oklahoma. Ann Allergy 1986;56:295.

Lewis WH, Dixit AB, Wedner HJ. Asteraceae aeropollen of the western United States Gulf Coast. Ann Allergy 1991;67:37.

Lewis WH, Imber WE. Allergy epidemiology in the St. Louis, Missouri area. II. Grasses. Ann Allergy 1975;35:42.

Lewis WH, Imber WE. Allergy epidemiology in the St. Louis, Missouri area. III. Trees. Ann Allergy 1975;35:113.

Lewis WH, Imber WE. Allergy epidemiology in the St. Louis, Missouri area. IV. Weeds. Ann Allergy 1975;35:180.

Lewis WH, Vinay P. The unique role of pollen in relation to allergy. In: Johnson F, Spencer JT (eds). Allergy, immunology & medical treatment. Miami: Symposia Specialists, 1980:101.

Mansfield LE, Harris NS, Rael E, Goldstein P, Acosta T. Regional individual allergen based miniscreen to predict IgE mediated airborne allergy. Ann Allergy 1988;61:259.

Martin BG, Mansfield LE, Nelson HA. Cross-allergenicity among grasses. Ann Allergy 1985;54:99.

McLean AC, Parker L, von Reis J, von Reis J. Airborne pollen and fungal spore sampling on the central California coast: the San Luis Obispo pollen project. Ann Allergy;.1991;67:441.

Nelson R. Pollen guide. Spokane, WA: Hollister-Stier Laboratories.

Newark FM. The hayfever plants of Colorado. Ann Allergy 1978;40:18.

Novey HS, Roth M, Wells ID. Mesquite pollen: an aero allergen in asthma and allergic rhinitis. Ann Allergy 1977;59:359.

Pence HL, Mitchell DQ, Greely RL, et al. Immunotherapy for mountain cedar pollinosis. Ann Allergy 1976;58:39.

Phillips JW, Bucholtz GA, Fernandez-Caldas E, Bukantz SC, Lockey RF. Bahia grass pollen, a significant aeroallergen: evidence for the lack of clinical cross reactivity with timothy grass pollen. Ann Allergy 1989;63:503.

Prince HE, Meyers GH. Hayfever from the southern wax myrtle (*Myrica cerifera*): a case report. Ann Allergy 1977;38:252.

Raynor GS, Hayes JV. Experimental prediction of daily ragweed concentration. Ann Allergy 1970;28:580.

Raynor GS, Ogden EC, Hayes JV. Spatial variability in airborne pollen concentrations. Ann Allergy 1975;55:195.

Raynor GS, Ogden EC, Hayves JV. Temporal variability in airborne pollen concentration. Ann Allergy 1976;36:386.

Raynor GS, Ogden EC, Hayes JV. Variations in ragweed pollen concentration to a height of 108 meters. Ann Allergy 1973;51:199.

Reid MJ, Moss RB, Hsu YP, Kwasnicki JM, Commerford TM, Nelson BL. Seasonal asthma in northern California: allergic causes and the efficacy of immunotherapy. J Allergy Clin Immunol 1986;78:590.

Reiss N, Kostic SR. Pollen season severity and meteorologic parameters in New Jersey. J Allergy 1976;57:609.

Roth A, Shira J. Allergy in Hawaii. Ann Allergy 1966;24:76.

Samter M, Durham OC. Regional allergy of the United States, Canada, Mexico, and Cuba. Springfield, IL: Charles C Thomas, 1955.

Schroeckenstein DC, Meier-Davis S, Yunginger JW, Bush RK. Allergy involved in occupational asthma caused by baby's breath (*Gypsophila paniculata*). J Allergy Clin Immunol 1990;86:189.

Sheldon JA, Lovell RG, Matthew KP. A manual of clinical allergy. Philadelphia: WB Saunders, 1967.

Sherman WB. Hypersensitivity: mechanics and management. Philadelphia: WB Saunders, 1968.

Silvers WS, Ledoux RA, Dolen WK, Morrison MR, Nelson HS, Weber RW. Aerobiology of the Colorado Rockies: pollen count comparisons between Vail and Denver, Colorado. Ann Allergy 1992;69:421.

Smith EG. Sampling and identifying allergenic pollens and molds. San Antonio, TX: Blewstone Press, 1984.

Smith EC. Sampling and identifying allergenic pollens and molds. Vol 2. San Antonio, TX: Blewstone Press, 1986.

Sneller MR, Hayes HD, Pinnas JL. Pollen changes during five decades of urbanization in Tucson, Arizona. Ann Allergy 1993;71:519.

Solomon WR. Volumetric studies of aeroallergen prevalence. I. Pollens of weedy forbs at a Midwestern station. J Allergy 1976;57:318.

Statistical report of the pollen and mold committee. Milwaukee, WI: American Academy of Allergy, Asthma & Immunology, 1994.

Street DH, Hamburger RN. Atmospheric pollen and spore sampling in San Diego, California: meteorological correlations and potential clinical relevance. Ann Allergy 1976;37:32.

Vaughan WT, Black JH. Practice of allergy. St Louis: CV Mosby, 1954.

Vu DD. Respiratory allergic diseases and their association with aeropollens in an Hawaiian community. PhD dissertation. Honolulu, Hawaii, University of Hawaii, 1977.

Weber R. Cross reactivity among pollens. Ann Allergy 1981;46:208.

Wodehouse RP. Hayfever plants. Waltham, MA: Chronica Botanica, 1945.

Wodehouse RP. Pollen grains. New York: McGraw Hill, 1935.

Yoo T, Spitz E, McGerrity JL. Conifer pollen allergy: studies of immunogenicity and cross antigenicity of conifer pollens in rabbits and man. Ann Allergy 1975;34:87.

Allergic Diseases, 5th Edition,
edited by Roy Patterson, Leslie Carroll Grammer, and
Paul A. Greenberger. Lippincott–Raven Publishers, Philadelphia, © 1997.

8

Diagnosis of Immediate Hypersensitivity

Bernard H. Booth

B.H. Booth: Mississippi Asthma and Allergy Clinic, Oxford, MS 38655.

Pearls for Practitioners
Roy Patterson

- The diagnosis of allergy is made by correlating the type of symptoms and time of their occurrence with a demonstrated presence of IgE antibody. Successfully managing a patient, however, is dependent on determining the patient's response to the initial trial of therapy. This response tells the physician whether the selected drugs and doses are appropriate or if modifications should be made.
- Allergic disease is so common, written about so much, and discussed so much that occasionally patients with nonallergic rhinitis have a history compatible with seasonal allergic rhinitis. They have read about pollen seasons and correlate their symptoms with the seasons.
- If lesions appear on a patient's hands while wearing latex gloves, latex anaphylaxis may occur in the future.

Immediate hypersensitivity is one of the explanations for conjunctivitis, rhinitis, and wheezing dyspnea. In addition, it may be responsible for some cases of eczema and some cases of urticaria. Many other causative explanations are possible for each of these conditions. Consequently, when a patient has been troubled enough with one of these conditions to consult a physician, it is necessary to perform a complete medical evaluation.

First, the clinician must determine if the symptoms are allergic in origin or if they have another cause. If the symptoms are considered to be allergic in origin, a more specific diagnostic evaluation must be completed by identifying the antigen or antigens responsible for producing the symptoms. In addition, other variable factors must be evaluated. The degree of sensitivity to an antigen may vary, as may the degree of exposure to a clinically significant antigen. Many patients are sensitive to multiple antigens, and cumulative effects of exposure to several antigens may be important. The influence of nonimmunologic phenomena on symptoms also must be evaluated. Infections, inhaled irritants, fatigue, and emotional problems may be significant factors independently or cumulatively, and may fluctuate widely in degree of significance. Considering the large number of variables, it is not surprising that the most important portion of any clinical evaluation is the expertly taken history.

PATIENT HISTORY

Many techniques have been used in obtaining a history, and these include completion of forms by the patient or the interviewer (Fig. 8-1). These may be useful, but they only facilitate and do not replace the careful inquiries of a skilled historian. The significant information can be obtained in some cases with relative ease, but adequate information usually can be obtained only after investing considerable time and energy.

The history not only provides most of the information necessary for diagnosis, but it is necessary before further diagnostic tests can be selected that will confirm the diagnosis and not be dangerous to a patient with an extreme degree of sensitivity.

History to Establish Presence of Immediate Hypersensitivity

The history of the patient is taken in the same way as an ordinary medical history. The patient is asked to state the major complaint and to describe the symptoms. During the history, the presence or absence of symptoms of nonallergic conditions must be determined and evaluated. Certain details of the allergic history are so characteristic that they should be always be specifically asked and noted:

1. *Are there other symptoms in addition to the presenting complaint that may be allergic in origin?* The presence of urticaria, other skin eruptions, sneezing, nasal obstruction and itching, eye irritation, intermittent hearing loss, wheezing dyspnea, or cough should be determined. Often, several allergic symptoms exist simultaneously, although the patient has not associated them with a common cause. If several of these symptoms are present, they are more likely to all have an allergic origin. Conversely, a single symptom in a single system such as isolated nasal obstruction probably is not allergic.
2. *Are the symptoms bilateral?* Unilateral symptoms, whether ocular, nasal, or pulmonary, suggest the presence of nonallergic conditions.
3. *Is there a family history of atopic disease?* Most allergic patients have a positive history in this respect. Specifically ask about allergic diseases in parents, grandparents, siblings, aunts, uncles, cousins, and children.
4. *How has the patient responded to previous treatment?* Information about previous therapy is useful. A good response to antihistamines increases the likelihood that the symptoms have an allergic origin. Response to bronchodilator or steroid therapy, either systemically or by inhalation, gives valuable information regarding the presence or absence of reversible airway obstruction. Previously used nasal sprays must be identified and their results assessed. Sympathomimetic nasal sprays may be the primary cause of nasal obstruction. Failure to respond to cromolyn or steroid nasal sprays makes an allergic cause seem less likely.

   All medications taken for any reason should be elicited and their role evaluated. In addition to nasal sprays, rauwolfia and other medications can cause nasal obstruction. Beta-blockers can be responsible for wheezing and dyspnea. Angiotensin-converting enzyme inhibitors can produce a severe persistent cough. Awareness of these reactions can prevent unnecessary and expensive allergic evaluations. Conversely, a prior good response to immunotherapy strongly implicates an allergic problem.
5. *Are symptoms continuous or intermittent?* Allergic symptoms often are intermittent, and even in the cases in which they are continuous, intermittent exacerbations may occur.

text continues

Allergy Survey Sheet

Name _____ Age _____ Sex _____ Date _____

I. Chief complaint:

II. Present illness:

III. Collateral allergic symptoms

Eyes:	Pruritus _____	Burning _____	Lacrimation _____
	Swelling _____	Infection _____	Discharge _____
Ears:	Pruritus _____	Fullness _____	Popping _____
	Frequent infections _____		
Nose:	Sneezing _____	Rhinorrhea _____	Obstruction _____
	Pruritus _____	Mouth breathing _____	
	Purulent discharge _____		
Throat:	Soreness _____	Postnasal discharge _____	
	Palatal pruritus _____	Mucus in the morning _____	
Chest:	Cough _____	Pain _____	Wheezing _____
	Sputum _____	Dyspnea _____	
	Color _____	Rest _____	
	Amount _____	Exertion _____	
Skin:	Dermatitis _____	Eczema _____	Urticaria _____

IV. Family allergies:

V. Previous allergic treatment or testing:

Prior skin test:

Drugs:

Antihistamines	Improved _____	Unimproved _____
Bronchodilators	Improved _____	Unimproved _____
Nose drops	Improved _____	Unimproved _____
Hyposensitization	Improved _____	Unimproved _____
Duration _____		
Antigens _____		
Reactions _____		
Antibiotics	Improved _____	Unimproved _____
Steroids	Improved _____	Unimproved _____

VI. Physical agents and habits: Bothered by:

Tobacco for _____ years	Alcohol _____	Air cond. _____
Cigarettes _____ packs/day	Heat _____	Muggy weather _____
Cigars _____ per day	Cold _____	Weather changes _____
Pipe _____ per day	Perfumes _____	
Never smoked _____	Paints _____	Chemicals _____
Bothered by smoke _____	Insecticides _____	Hair spray _____
	Cosmetics _____	Newspapers _____

FIG. 8-1. Allergy survey sheet. *(Continued.)*

Time and circumstances of 1st episode:

Prior health:

Course of illness over decades: progressing _____ regressing _____

Time of year: Exact dates

  Perennial _____

  Seasonal _____

  Seasonally exacerbated _____

Monthly variations (menses, occupation): _____

Time of week (weekends vs weekdays): _____

Time of day or night: _____

After insect stings: _____

VIII. Where symptoms occur:

Living where at onset: _____

Living where since onset: _____

Effect of vacation or major geographic change: _____

Symptoms better indoors or outdoors: _____

Effect of school or work: _____

Effect of staying elsewhere nearby: _____

Effect of hospitalization: _____

Effect of specific environments: _____

Do symptoms occur around: _____

old leaves _____ hay _____ lakeside _____ barns _____

summer homes _____ damp basement _____ dry attic _____

lawnmowing _____ animals _____ other _____

Do symptoms occur after eating:

cheese _____ mushrooms _____ beer _____ melons _____

bananas _____ fish _____ nuts _____ citrus fruits _____

other foods (list) _____

Home: city _____ rural _____ house _____ age _____

  apartment _____ basement _____ damp _____ dry _____

  heating system _____

  pets (how long) _____ dog _____ cat _____ other _____

Bedroom:	Type	Age	**Living Room:**	Type	Age
Pillow	_____	_____	Rug	_____	_____
Mattress	_____	_____	Matting	_____	_____
Blankets	_____	_____	Furniture	_____	_____
Quilts	_____	_____			
Furniture	_____	_____			

Anywhere in home symptoms are worse: _____

IX. What does patient think makes symptoms worse: _____

X. Under what circumstances is he or she free of symptoms:

_____

XI. Summary and additional comments:

History to Identify Specific Causative Agents

The general practitioner usually can determine if an allergic disease is present and initiate appropriate therapy. For a more specific diagnosis of the antigens responsible for the illness, a detailed allergic history is essential. Its purpose is to obtain the information necessary to allow a correlation of symptoms with the known time and place of occurrence of various antigens.

The decision to pursue a more specific diagnosis depends on several factors. If the disease is mild, produces no disability, and responds to symptomatic therapy, an elaborate investigation may not be indicated. Conversely, severe discomfort or disability makes a complete evaluation necessary. Because asthma is a potentially lethal illness, most asthmatic patients should have an allergic evaluation.

Whether the general practitioner performs the more detailed evaluation or consults an allergist for this depends on the physician's interest, training, and experience; the severity of the patient's illness; and the availability of competent consultants.

Characteristics of Antigens

Table 8-1 provides a review of the antigens. Some general characteristics of the antigens responsible for allergic illnesses must be appreciated before an adequate clinical history can be obtain or interpreted. Although foods may be important in cases of infantile eczema, urticaria, angioedema, or anaphylaxis, they are seldom important in cases of allergic conjunctivitis, allergic rhinitis, or allergic asthma. The antigens most important in those conditions usually are airborne. Several different groups of these aeroallergens are of major clinical significance, including pollens, fungi, house dust mites, and animal dander.

Pollens

The grains of pollen from plants are among the most important antigens that cause clinical sensitization.

Most plants produce pollen that is rich in protein and consequently is potentially antigenic. Whether a specific pollen regularly causes symptoms depends on several factors. The pollens that routinely cause illness usually fulfill three criteria: (1) they are produced in large quantity by a plant that is common; (2) they depend primarily on the wind for their dispersal; (3) and the pollen itself is antigenic.

Many plants produce pollens that are large, thick, and waxy. Under natural conditions, transfer of the pollen between flowering plants is accomplished chiefly by insects. These pollens are not widely dispersed in the air; therefore, they are rarely clinically significant. Goldenrod, which is popularly considered to cause hay fever, has little significance because its pollen rapidly falls from the air before it can be dispersed widely and reach the hay fever patient. In contrast, the ragweed plant pollinates at the same time, and its pollen is small, light, widely dispersed by the wind, and highly antigenic. Ragweed plants also grow abundantly in many geographic areas.

In the United States, many trees, grasses, and some weeds produce large quantities of highly antigenic, windborne pollen. The seasonal occurrence of tree, grass, and weed pollens varies with the geographic location. Although many factors alter the total amount of pollen produced in any year, the season of pollination of a plant remains remarkably constant in any area from year to year. The physician treating allergies must know which windborne pollens

TABLE 8-1. *Symptoms characteristically produced by common antigens*

Antigen	Symptoms
Pollens	Seasonal symptoms or seasonal exacerbation of symptoms
Mold spores	Perennial symptoms in warm climates
	Seasonal exacerbations in some moderate climates
	Reduced symptoms when living or vacationing in dry climates
	Symptoms that decrease with snowfall
	Sudden increase in symptoms if exposed to basements, moldy hay or leaves, barns or silos, dairies, breweries, food storage areas, buildings with contaminated air conditioning systems, rotting wood, or any location that might have high humidity
	Symptoms are rarely exacerbated after ingesting mold products
House dust	Characteristically perennial symptoms
	Exacerbations when making beds, cleaning, or dusting the home
	Occasional exacerbations when entering older homes with older furnishings
Animal dander	Perennial symptoms
	Marked improvement in symptoms when leaving home, if animal lives in the home
	Sudden exacerbations of symptoms after a new pet has been introduced to the home
	Sudden increase in symptoms when visiting a home where animals live
	Less frequently, sudden increase in symptoms when playing with an animal
	Worsening of symptoms at work and clearing of symptoms on weekends or vacations if exposure is occupational

are abundant in the area and their seasons of pollination. The major clinically significant pollens vary with geographic location and are discussed elsewhere in this text.

Fungi and Molds

Many thousands of different fungi exist. The role of many of them in producing allergic symptoms is speculative, but some species have been definitely implicated. Because fungi can colonize almost every possible habitat and reproduce spores prolifically, the air is seldom free of spores. Consequently, they are important in some patients with perennial symptoms. However, seasonal or local influences greatly alter the number of airborne spores.

Periods of warm weather with relatively high humidity allow optimal growth of molds. If this period is followed by hot, dry, windy weather, the spores often become airborne in large concentration. In large portions of the United States, there may be a maximal peak between late June and early September. Therefore, mold-sensitive patients may have great difficulty between the grass and weed pollen seasons. A frost may produce a large amount of dying vegetation, but the decreased temperature may reduce the growth rate of fungi. In contrast, spring may provide the relative warmth, humidity, and adequate substrate necessary for the growth of fungi.

High local concentrations of mold spores also are encountered frequently. Deep shade may produce high humidity because of water condensing on cool surfaces. High humidity may occur in areas of water seepage such as basements, refrigerator drip trays, or garbage pails. Food storage areas, dairies, breweries, air conditioning systems, piles of fallen leaves or rotting wood, and barns or silos containing hay or other grains may provide nutrients as well as a high humidity, and therefore may have high concentrations of mold spores.

Persons who have symptoms when molds are inhaled also may have occasional difficulty after ingesting foods that contain molds or their products. Cheeses and fermented drinks, usually beer or wine, are the most common offenders. Occasionally, other foods may be implicated, such as those prepared with a large amount of yeast, buttermilk, mushrooms, dried fruits, or vinegar.

House Dust

The content of house dust usually is heterogenous, containing bacteria, fungi, insect debris, debris from small mammals and humans, food remnants, fibrous materials from plants, and inorganic substances. Many of these are potential antigens, but the role of insects, fungi, and mammals in indoor antigens has been more definitely established.[1,2]

House dust mites (*Dermatophagoides* sp) are recognized as the major source of antigen in house dust.[3,4] They are discussed in another chapter.

Dust-sensitive patients have perennial symptoms, although these may improve outdoors or during summer months. They may have a history of sneezing, lacrimation, rhinorrhea, or mild asthma whenever the house is cleaned or the beds are made. In many dust-sensitive patients, the history is not so obvious, and the presence of perennial symptoms is the only suggestive feature.

Animal Dander

Particles of skin and the dried saliva of animals can act as potent antigens. When pets live inside a home, these products can reach high concentrations and completely permeate the furniture, bedding, rugs, and air. Household pets often are entirely responsible for severe disabling asthma. A short-haired pet does not eliminate this hazard. Although cats and dogs are involved most frequently, many other animals occasionally are responsible. A remarkable number of homes have hamsters, gerbils, rabbits, parakeets, parrots, or mice. Certain occupational groups (e.g., laboratory worker, veterinarians, ranchers, farmers) may be exposed to an unusual variety of animal danders.

A patient with clinical sensitivity to a household pet may have a history similar to that of dust-sensitive patients. In addition, they may have rapid, marked symptomatic improvement when leaving home or being hospitalized. Symptoms may persist outside of the home, however, and patients may use this as inappropriate evidence that animals that they do not wish to eliminate from the environment are not a cause of their problem. Many patients may give a history of a wheal-or-erythema at a skin site that was scratched or bitten by the animal. Sensitivity to animals always should be suspected when a patient develops fairly severe asthma as an adult.

A patient with an inhalant allergy may respond well to treatment for many months, only to have a sudden increase in symptoms. Frequently, this increase may be caused by the introduction of a pet into the home. If unaware of the presence of a new pet, the physician may completely misinterpret the symptoms and embark on incorrect therapy.

Type and Sequence of Clinical Manifestations

Knowledge of the commonly significant allergens allows the physician to use the detailed history to confirm the differential diagnosis of allergic disease and to provide clues to the specific diagnosis. The course of the disease over decades should be determined. Age of onset, geographic location of the patient throughout life, health during school years, the nature and place of employment, and any change in symptoms with puberty or pregnancy should be recorded. It should be determined if the disease has improved or worsened progressively over the years.

It is critical to establish when the patient does and does not have symptoms. The yearly seasonal variations are significant. Even if perennial symptoms are present, a seasonal variation may be superimposed. The date of symptoms should be determined as exactly as possible. Significant differences may occur between springtime symptoms that occur in early March and those that arise in late May.

Fluctuations in symptoms during the week sometimes is common and suggests the importance of antigens encountered in the home, school, or work environment. Variation in symptoms during the day is far less helpful, because nasal congestion increases during recumbency and asthma tends to occur at night. This does not necessarily indicate a reaction to something in the bedroom.

Are any places regularly associated with an increase in symptoms, such as barns, damp basements, a weekend or summer home, fields, or factories?

Next, determine where the patient does not have symptoms. Did the symptoms change when the patient moved from one place to another? Are symptoms lessened indoors or outdoors? Was the patient better when on vacation in other places? Does the patient improve rapidly in the hospital or at the homes of friends?

Often it is helpful to ask what agents the patient believes to be causing the difficulty.

Environmental Survey

A detailed survey of the patient's home, work, or school environment may be useful. Are there pets in the house? What are the ages of the mattress, pillows, and carpets? What type of heating, air conditioning, and air filters are in the home? When and how is the home cleaned? A detailed survey of the work environment also is necessary. Specific information is needed, and general information may be worthless. An accountant may sit in an air-conditioned office or may take inventory in damp, dusty warehouses. Many antigenic substances have been identified that are encountered only in specific work places.

Nonimmunologic Factors

Certain nonimmunologic factors so frequently make allergic persons worse that they should always be evaluated. Primary irritants should be identified such as tobacco smoke, paint, hair spray, perfumes, colognes, or other strong odors or more generalized air pollution. The effects of infection on the disease should be noted, and the effects of weather, psychological conflicts, and exercise must be evaluated.

While the history is being taken, it is also appropriate to evaluate in detail the severity of the illness. The severity of the symptoms not only determines the extent of the diagnostic evaluation, but dictates the intensity of the therapy. This also later allows an objective evaluation of the results of therapy. Whether the symptoms are nasal, ocular, dermatologic, or pulmonary, it is necessary to judge the degree of discomfort that they cause. This judgment is subjective and depends on the personalities of the patient and the physician. More objective evaluation can determine the frequency of the symptom. Define the number of days that symptoms occur, the number of hours that they persist, and the number of days lost from work or school. In severe cases, also note the number of days hospitalized or if the illness has ever been life-threatening.

Physical Examination

Every patient should have a complete physical examination. Particular attention must be paid to sites affected by the common allergic diseases (e.g., eyes, nose, chest, skin).

Conjunctivitis

Physical findings of allergic conjunctivitis are hyperemia and edema of the conjunctiva. Occasionally, a pronounced chemosis occurs associated with clear, watery discharge. Periorbital edema may be present, and rarely a bluish discoloration about the eyes may occur. If chemosis is severe, acute allergic conjunctivitis may be confused with epidemic keratoconjunctivitis.

Rhinitis

The examination of the nose requires good exposure and adequate light. In a patient with allergic rhinitis, the inferior turbinates usually appear to be swollen and actually may meet the nasal septum. They may have a uniform bluish or pearly gray discoloration, but more frequently there may be adjacent areas where the membrane is red, giving a mottled appearance. Polyps may be seen within the nose. The skin of the nose, and particularly of the upper lip, may show irritation and excoriation produced by the nasal discharge and continuous nose wiping. Tenderness over the paranasal sinuses may be present if concomitant infection is present. In patients with nasal allergic disease, the ears should be examined for evidence of acute or chronic otitis media, either serous or infectious. Nasal secretions also may be observed draining into the posterior pharynx.

Asthma

Physical findings in asthmatic patients are highly variable, not only between patients, but in the same patient at different times. The rapidity with which symptoms and physical findings appear or disappear is one of the characteristic features of the illness.

During an acute attack of asthma, the patient usually uses the accessory muscles of respiration. Mechanically, these muscles are more effective if the patient stands or sits and leans slightly forward. During an acute attack, the patient rarely lies down unless severely exhausted. Intercostal, subcostal, and supraclavicular retraction, as well as flaring of the alae nasi, may be present with inspiratory effort.

Physical findings attributable to hyperinflation of the chest may be present. The chest may be held continuously in the midinspiratory position, and there may be increased resonance to percussion. In addition, percussion may disclose that the diaphragms are in a low position and have limited respiratory excursion.

On auscultation, musical wheezes may be heard during both inspiration and expiration, and the expiratory phase of respiration may be prolonged. In uncomplicated asthma, these auscultatory findings tend to be present uniformly throughout the lungs. Asymmetry of auscultory findings might be caused by concomitant disease such as pneumonia, or by a complication of the asthma itself, such as plugging of a large bronchus with a mucous plug. In severely ill patients, extreme bronchial plugging and loss of effective mechanical ventilation may be associated with a disappearance of wheezing and a marked decrease in all audible breath sounds. In these patients, alveolar ventilation has almost disappeared and they may be cyanotic.

In less severe, uncomplicated, acute cases, cyanosis seldom occurs and the patient is afebrile. Tachycardia is regularly present during acute attacks.

When the asthmatic patient is not having an acute attack, there may be no demonstrable abnormalities on auscultation, even when evidence of reversible airway obstruction can be demonstrated with pulmonary function studies. In many instances, asthma is chronic, and wheezes may be heard even while the patient is feeling subjectively well. In some cases, wheezes are not heard during normal respiration but can be heard if the patient exhales forcefully.

Atopic Dermatitis

The findings on physical examination of a patient with atopic dermatitis also vary widely. The findings depend on the stage of the disease. In an infant 4 to 6 months of age, the initial manifestation usually is erythema and edema. Initial lesions are most likely to occur on the cheeks, in the antecubital fossa, the popliteal spaces, or about the neck and ears. Generalized skin involvement then may occur, involving any area of the body. After the initial erythema, a finely papular rash may appear. The papules then may form small vesicles, and when these vesicles rupture there may be oozing and crusting. Different areas of the skin may show erythema, papules, vesicles, or oozing and crusting, indicating that there are multiple lesions in varying stages of development. Secondary bacterial infection frequently is present.

In the chronic form, lichenification of the skin is the predominant lesion. The skin appears thickened, coarse, and dry. There may be moderate scaling and alteration in pigmentation. Pruritus may not be as severe as during the acute phases but is still present. The cosmetic effects of the chronic form often are disturbing to the patient.

Other Examinations

Abnormalities of red cells or of the sedimentation rate are not associated with atopic disease. If such abnormalities are present, other illnesses or complications should be suspected. The differential white blood cell count usually is normal, with the frequent exception of eosinophilia, which may range from 3% to 10%. Eosinophilia of 12% to 20% seldom is present in allergies to extrinsic antigens unless there is also an infection. Higher eosinophil counts are not ordinarily seen in atopic diseases. This unusual condition requires an entirely different clinical approach.

The urine examination may rule out nonallergic disease. Stool examination of patients with peripheral blood eosinophilia may help to exclude parasitic infestations.

Chest x-rays may be necessary to rule out concomitant disease or complications of extreme asthma. X-ray examination or computed tomographic scans of the paranasal sinuses frequently are useful. Gross and microscopic changes in nasal secretions and in sputum have been described in allergic patients. These changes include eosinophilia, Curschmann's spirals, Charcot-Leyden crystals, and Creola bodies. Although interesting findings, their presence or absence is seldom of diagnostic value.

Sputum Gram stains, cultures, and cytologic study, rhinoscopy, bronchoscopy, bronchial lavage, electrocardiograms, and computed tomographic and magnetic resonance imaging scans of the chest and head aid in diagnosing nonatopic disease. All or some of these procedures may be necessary to establish the correct diagnosis in some patients.

Evaluation of Respiratory Function

Quantitative tests of ventilation can be of great value. They may yield some insight into the type and severity of the functional defect, and more importantly, may provide an objective means for assessing changes that may occur with time or may be induced by treatment. These tests are described in detail elsewhere. Remember that single sets of values describe conditions at designated points in time, and conditions such as asthma have rapid pathophysiologic changes.

SKIN TESTS

Most testing depends on producing an allergic reaction on a small scale by intentionally exposing the patient to a minute amount of antigen. Clinically, the organ tested usually is the skin. The skin must be free of lesions, and antihistamines should be eliminated for at least 24 hours and preferably 48 hours before testing. One long-acting antihistamine, astemizole, may interfere for as long as 6 weeks. Furthermore, terfenadine, hydroxyzine, chlorpromazine, and tricyclic antidepressants should be avoided at least 5 days before testing.[5]

Two types of direct skin tests are recommended for clinical practice, and each has its relative merits. Both involve the production of the immediate wheal-and-erythema reaction that is characteristic of atopic sensitization.

The prick test is performed by pricking the skin with a needle through a drop of the antigen solution. These tests can be performed with a minimum of equipment. The insensitivity of this method as compared with intracutaneous testing accounts for its major value and its major limitation. There is relatively little risk of anaphylaxis, and even extreme sensitivity to an antigen can be determined without significant hazard to the patient. However, prick tests may not be sufficiently sensitive to demonstrate significant atopic sensitization unless concentrated antigens are used.

Intracutaneous testing is performed by injecting a small amount of antigen into the superficial layers of the skin. Because there is a risk of a systemic reaction, preliminary prick tests with the same antigen are advisable, or else the initial intracutaneous tests must be performed with dilute solutions of antigen. In the same patient, the concentration of an antigen solution required to elicit a positive reaction with a prick test may be 100 times as great as that needed in the intracutaneous test. If the prick test shows a reaction, intracutaneous testing is not needed and should be avoided.

The number and variety of prick tests performed depend on clinical aspects of the particular case. The antigens used may vary because of the prevalence of particular antigens in any geographic location. Satisfactory information usually can be obtained with a small number of tests if they are carefully chosen.

Intracutaneous tests are chosen from the list of antigens giving negative or equivocal results on scratch testing. Most allergists believe that intracutaneous testing with foods produces so many nonspecific reactions that it has no value and therefore the risk to patients is not justified.

Prick Test

The prick test may be performed on the back or on the volar surface of the forearms. The patient should be placed in a comfortable position before the testing is begun. The skin should be cleaned properly with alcohol and air dried. Small drops of the test antigens then are placed on the skin. A drop of saline can be a negative control, and histamine or codeine may be the positive control. (Antigen extracts can be obtained commercially from various pharmaceutical houses.) Several rows of antigens may be used. Because large reactions at adjacent test sites might coalesce, the test sites should be at least 4 or 5 cm apart. It is useful to mark the location of the drops with a marking pencil. Various scarifying instruments are available, but a sharp darning needle is adequate. After the antigen has been placed, the needle can be used to puncture the skin. This procedure should lightly abrade the skin but should not draw blood. The needle should be wiped free of antigen after each test with an alcohol sponge.

The tests should be read in 20 minutes to 30 minutes, but if a large wheal reaction occurs before that time, the test site should be wiped free of antigen to reduce the possibility of a systemic reaction.

Intracutaneous Tests

For intracutaneous testing, 1-mL tuberculin syringes with 26-gauge needles are adequate. Disposable syringes are recommended.

The test sites are marked and are cleaned with an alcohol sponge. The skin is held tense and the needle is inserted almost parallel to its surface, just far enough to cover the beveled portion. The injection of 0.02 mL of antigen extract is then performed as superficially as possible.

Because of the increased sensitivity of this method, more dilute solutions of the antigens are employed than are used for prick testing. For example, 1:1000 or 1:5000 dilutions are used only if the results of preliminary prick tests are negative. The patient should be kept under observation until the tests are read after 20 minutes.

Many systems for grading positive reactions have been devised. A simple, adequate system involves grading the reactions from negative to 4+. A 4+ reaction consists of erythema and a wheal with pseudopod formation. A 3+ reaction shows erythema and wheal formation without pseudopod formation. A 2+ reaction consists of an area of erythema larger than a nickel in diameter (21 mm). A 1+ reaction is characterized by an area of erythema smaller than a nickel in diameter and definitely larger than the control site. A negative skin test result (–) has no reaction or has a reaction that is no different from the control.

In cases of dermographism, there may be reactivity at the control site. This should be noted when the results of the tests are recorded. Interpretation of the tests is then more difficult. Test results that do not clearly have a greater reaction than the negative control must be considered negative.

Occasionally, delayed reaction occurs at the site of skin tests. They become apparent 1 to 2 hours after application, peak between 6 to 12 hours, and usually disappear after 24 to 48 hours. They have been designated as late-phase cutaneous reactions (LPCRs). In contrast to the immediate reactions, they are inhibited by conventional doses of corticosteroids but not by H_1 antihistamines.[6,7] Whether a LPCR indicates that a similar reaction will occur in the nose or lung of the same patient is uncertain. Some investigators believe that a correlation exists and others do not.[8–12] The recommendation has been made that they be quantified between 6 and 8 hours by measuring the mean diameter of the area of induration and edema.[5]

Interpreting Skin Test Results

Table 8-2 reviews the interpretation of skin test results. Both false-negative and false-positive skin test results may occur because of improper technique or material. Improperly prepared or outdated extracts may contain nonspecific irritants or may not be physiologic with

TABLE 8-2. *Interpretation of skin test results*

If:	And:	Then:
History suggests sensitivity,	Skin test results are positive,	Strong possibility that antigen is responsible
History does not suggest sensitivity,	Skin test results are positive,	May want to observe patient during time of high natural exposure
History suggests sensitivity,	Skin test results are negative,	1. Review medications the patient has taken: antihistamines, antidepressants
		2. Review other reasons for false-negative test results, such as poor quality of testing materials or poor technique
		3. Observe patient during a period of high natural exposure
		4. Perform provocative challenge (rarely)

respect to pH or osmolarity, and therefore produce false-positive test results. Injecting an excessive volume can result in mechanical irritation of the skin and false-positive results.

Antihistamines, chlorpromazine, hydroxyzine, and tricyclic antidepressants interfere with skin testing, and if not omitted may yield false-negative results. In these cases, the positive controls (histamine or codeine) also should give negative results. The skin of young infants or the elderly may give smaller reactions than those seen in older children or adults of comparable sensitivity.

Even after false-positive and false-negative test results have been eliminated, the proper interpretation of results requires a thorough knowledge of the history. A positive skin test result only demonstrates the presence of IgE antibody that is specifically directed against the test antigen. A positive skin test result does not mean that a person has an allergic disease, or that an allergic person has ever had a clinically significant reaction to the specific antigen. *With inhalant antigens, correlating positive skin test results with a history that suggests clinical sensitivity may strongly incriminate an antigen. Conversely, a negative skin test result and a negative history exclude the antigen as being clinically significant.*

Interpretation of skin tests that do not correlate with the clinical history or physical findings, or the interpretation of LPCRs, is much more difficult. If there is no history suggesting sensitivity to an antigen, and the skin test result is positive, the patient should be seen again during a period of maximal exposure to the antigen. At that time, if there are no symptoms or physical findings of sensitivity, skin test results may be ignored.

Patients with a history that strongly suggests an allergic disease or clinical sensitivity to specific antigens may have negative skin test results to the suspected antigens. It is difficult to make an allergic diagnosis in these cases because, when properly done, negative skin test findings indicate that no specific IgE antibody is present. These patients may be requestioned and reexamined, and the possibility of false-negative skin test results must be excluded.

IN VITRO MEASUREMENT OF IgE ANTIBODIES

In vitro procedures have been devised that detect antigen-specific IgE. These are considered to be in vitro analogues of the allergy tests. Most of these tests use an allergosorbent technique. The same clinical problems are present when the results are interpreted. In addition, there are several technical problems over which the clinician has no control that can influence the test results. Unfortunately, test results from different commercial sources have been impossible to compare.[13]

Comparisons of results from in vitro and skin tests have been performed by numerous investigators.[14–23] Several extensive reviews have been published.[5,24–29]

Both in vitro and skin testing can give false-negative, false-positive, or equivocal results, depending on several variables. If performed optimally, both methods detect specific IgE antibody accurately and reproducibly.

Because the results are immediately available and they are the more cost effective procedure per allergen tested, skin tests clearly remain the choice in most clinical situations.[5,22,25]

In vitro testing may be indicated in some circumstances:

1. Some patients may not be able to omit medications that interfere with skin testing. Since no medications interfere with in vitro testing, it may be useful in these patients.
2. Some patients may have a history of extreme sensitivity to allergens. In vitro tests avoid the possibility of anaphylaxis or even uncomfortable local reactions.
3. In contrast to skin testing, dermographism and widespread skin diseases do not interfere with in vitro testing and therefore may be useful in patients with these problems.

Irresponsible promotion of any testing method has been condemned. Commercial firms and individual physicians may misrepresent the value of either testing method. The results of any tests must correlate with the production of allergic symptoms and signs by a specific antigen to have any meaning. Consequently, the history and physical examination personally performed by the physician remain the fundamental investigative procedures for diagnosing allergic disease.[26]

REFERENCES

1. Bronswijk JEMH, Sinha RN. Role of fungi in the survival of *Dermatophagoides* in house dust environment. Environ Entol 1973:2:142.
2. Bronswijk JEMH. House dust biology for allergists, acarologists, and mycologists. Zeist, The Netherlands: NIB Publishers, 1981.
3. Platts-Mills TAE, Chapman MD. Dust mites: immunology, allergic disease, and environmental control. J Allergy Clin Immunol 1987;80:755.
4. Platts-Mills TAE, de Weck, AL, et al. Dust mite allergens and asthma: a worldwide problem. J Allergy Clin Immunol 1989;83:416.
5. Bernstein IL. Proceedings of the Task Force on Guidelines for Standardizing Old and New Technologies Used for the Diagnosis and Treatment of Allergic Diseases. J Allergy Clin Immunol 1988;82:487.
6. Umemoto L, Poothullil J, Dolovich J, et al. Factors which influence late cutaneous allergic responses. J Allergy Clin Immunol 1976;58:60.
7. Poothullil J, Umemoto L, Dolovich J, et al. Inhibition by prednisone of late cutaneous allergic response induced by antiserum to human IgE. J Allergy Clin Immunol 1976;57:164.
8. Atkins PC, Martin GL, Yost R, Zweiman B. Late onset reactions in humans: correlation between skin and bronchial reactivity. Ann Allergy 1988;60:27.
9. Price KF, Hey EN, Soothill JF. Antigen provocation to the skin, nose, and lung in children with asthma: immediate and dual hypersensitivity reactions. Clin Exp Immunol 1982;47:587.
10. Warner JO. Significance of late reactions after bronchial challenge with house dust mite. Arch Dis Child 1976;51:905.
11. Boulet LP, Robert RS, Dolovich JE, et al. Prediction of late asthmatic responses to inhaled allergen. Clin Allergy 1984;14:379.
12. Taylor G, Shivalkor PR. Arthus-type reactivity in the nasal airways and skin in pollen sensitive subjects. Clin Allergy 1971;1:407.
13. Przybyszewski VA, Taylor RN. Allergen-specific immunoglobulin E performance evaluation results. Atlanta: Centers for Disease Control, 1983.

14. Aas K, Johansson SGO. The radioallergosorbent test in the in vitro diagnosis of multiple reaginic allergy: a comparison of diagnostic approaches. J Allergy Clin Immunol 1971;48:134.
15. Aas K, Lundkvist U. The radioallergosorbent test with a purified allergen from codfish. Clin Allergy 1973;3:255.
16. Bert TLO, Johansson SGO. Allergy diagnosis with the radioallergosorbent test: a comparison with the results of skin and provocation tests in an unselected group of children with asthma and hayfever. J Allergy Clin Immunol 1974;54:209.
17. Bryant DH, Burns MW, Lazarus L. The correlation between skin tests, bronchial provocation tests and serum level of IgE specific for common allergens in patients with asthma. Clin Allergy 1975;1975;5:145.
18. Collins-Williams C, Bremmer K. Comparison of skin tests and RAST in the diagnosis of atopic hypersensitivity. Ann Allergy 1976;36:161.
19. Fourcard T, Aas K, Johansson SGO. Concentration of IgE antibodies, PK titers and chopped lung titers in sera from children with hypersensitivity to cod. J Allergy Clin Immunol 1973:51:39.
20. Van der Zee JS, de Groot H, van Swieten P, et al. Discrepancies between the skin test and IgE antibody assays: study of mediator release, complement activation *in vitro*, and occurrence of allergen-specific IgE. J Allergy Clin Immunol 1988;82:270.
21. Kelso JM, Sodhi N, Gosselin VA, Yunginger JW. Diagnostic performance characteristics of the standard Phadebas RAST, modified RAST, and Pharmacia CAP system versus skin testing. Ann Allergy 1991;67:511.
22. Williams PB, Dolen WK, Koepke JW, Selner JC. Comparison of skin testing and three *in vitro* assays for specific IgE in the clinical evaluation of immediate hypersensitivity. Ann Allergy 1992;68:35.
23. Plebani M, Borghesian F, Faggian D. Clinical efficiency of *in vitro* and *in vivo* tests for allergic diseases. Ann Allergy 1994;74:21.
24. Aas K. The radioallergosorbent test (RAST): diagnostic significance. Ann Allergy 1974;33:251.
25. American Academy of Allergy. Position statements: controversial techniques. J Allergy Clin Immunol 1981;67:333.
26. American Academy of Allergy. Position statement: skin testing and radioallergosorbent testing (RAST) for diagnosis of specific allergens responsible for IgE mediated diseases. J Allerg Clin Immunol 1983;72:515.
27. Baer H. In vitro methods in allergy. Med Clin North Am 1974;58:85.
28. Yunginger JW, Gleich GJ. The impact of the discovery of IgE on the practice of allergy. Pediatr Clin North Am 1975;22:3.
29. O'Connell EJ, Heilman DK, Sachs MI, Yunginger MD. Selecting the right test for presumed allergy. J Respir Dis 1995;16:476.

Allergic Diseases, 5th Edition,
edited by Roy Patterson, Leslie Carroll Grammer, and
Paul A. Greenberger. Lippincott–Raven Publishers, Philadelphia, © 1997.

9

Allergic Rhinitis

Anthony J. Ricketti

*A.J. Ricketti: Section of Allergy/Immunology and Pulmonary Medicine,
St. Francis Medical Center, Trenton, NJ 08629.*

Pearls for Practitioners
Roy Patterson

- Allergic rhinitis of moderate severity may be a problem of major significance for performing artists, including singers, actors, and public speakers. This results when vocal changes occur or hearing is altered because of eustachian tube obstruction. Intense therapy is warranted.
- A patient with nonallergic (vasomotor rhinitis) may test positive test for IgE antibody. Immunologic management does not alter the course of these patients. This problem is uncommon, but the differential diagnosis is difficult.
- Rarely a patient has *nasal neurosis*. Examination results are negative, all therapies fail, and psychological therapy, when recommended, generally is not accepted.
- A physician who has no allergic rhinitis should consider how an allergic patient feels when the physician has a viral upper respiratory infection.

The term rhinitis is used to describe disease that involves inflammation of the nasal membrane and is characterized by periods of nasal discharge, sneezing, and congestion that persist at least 1 hour per day. It is also considered pathologic when a person occasionally has symptoms of such intensity to require therapy or when an individual's nasal reaction to certain stimuli differs fundamentally from that of other persons. Rhinitis may be classified into two types, infectious and noninfectious (Table 9-1). Infectious rhinitis is characterized predominantly by cloudy (white, yellow, or green) nasal secretions with many neutrophils, and, less commonly, bacteria.[1] Noninfectious rhinitis is characterized by clear (watery or mucoid) discharge that often contains eosinophils. The noninfectious group can be subdivided into seasonal allergic rhinitis, perennial allergic rhinitis, and perennial nonallergic rhinitis.

Perennial nonallergic rhinitis is a heterogenous group consisting of at least two subgroups.[2] One subgroup is characterized by nasal eosinophilia, frequent occurrence of polyps, abnormal sinus radiographs, concurrent asthma, and good response to therapy, whereas these characteristics usually are lacking in the other subgroup. This subdivision of patients with nonallergic rhinitis may not be possible in a particular case, and therefore may not be an entirely suitable system for routine clinical use.

TABLE 9-1. *Classification of rhinitis*

Type	Skin Test Findings	Predominant Cells in Secretions
Infectious (purulent)	−	
Common cold		Neutrophils
Rhinosinusitis (various organisms)	−	Neutrophils
Noninfectious (nonpurulent)		
Seasonal allergic rhinitis	+	Eosinophils
Perennial allergic rhinitis	+	Eosinophils
Perennial nonallergic rhinitis		
Eosinophilic subgroup	−	Eosinophils
Noneosinophilic	−	Few cells
Nasal polyps	+/−	Eosinophils
Atrophic rhinitis	−	Few cells

SEASONAL ALLERGIC RHINITIS

Definition

Seasonal allergic rhinitis is a specific allergic reaction of the a nasal mucosa to allergens and is characterized mainly by watery rhinorrhea, nasal congestion, sneezing, and pruritus of the eyes, nose, ears, and throat. These symptoms are periodic, occurring during the pollination season of the plants to which the patient is sensitive.

Incidence

Although allergic rhinitis may have its onset at any age, the incidence of onset is greatest in children at adolescence, with a decrease in incidence seen in advancing age. Occasionally, however, symptoms may appear first in middle or advanced age. Although it has been reported in infants as young as 6 months of age,[3] in most cases an individual requires two or more seasons of exposure to a new antigen before exhibiting the clinical manifestations of allergic rhinitis.[4] Allergic rhinitis is more prevalent in urban than rural areas. A community study of allergic rhinitis reveals that 75% of patients resided inside the city compared with 25% who lived in the surrounding rural area.[5] Allergic rhinitis is more common in nonwhites than whites and in upper than lower social classes.[6] Boys tend to have an increased incidence of allergic rhinitis in childhood, but the sex ratio becomes even in adulthood. Seasonal and perennial allergic rhinitis account for the loss of 1.5 million school days per year. Although some studies report that as many as 10% of children and 20% to 30% of adolescents[7-9] have allergic rhinitis, an accurate estimate of the incidence rate of allergic rhinitis is difficult to obtain. Some obstacles in obtaining accurate estimates of allergic disease include variability in geographic pollen counts, misinterpretation of symptoms by patients, or inability of the physician to recognize the disorder. Regardless of the exact incidence, allergic rhinitis is an important disorder, and the suffering and annoyance that many experience should not be underestimated. Considerable expenditures are involved in medication, physician fees, and economic loss secondary to absenteeism and inefficient performance at work. In 1990, annual illness costs for hay fever patients were conservatively estimated to total $1.8 billion. This figure includes an estimated $881 million for physician office visits, $276 million for medications, and $639 million for effects on productivity (work loss and decreased performance caused by the illness itself or sedative effects of drugs used for treatment).[10] The disease tends to persist indefinitely after clinical symptoms appear. The severity of symptoms, however, may vary from year to year, depending on the quality of pollen released and patient exposure during the specific pollinating seasons. Occasionally, the disease undergoes a spontaneous remission without specific therapy.

Etiology

Pollen and mold spores are the allergens responsible for seasonal allergic rhinitis (Table 9-2).

The pollens important in causing allergic rhinitis are from plants that depend on the wind for cross-pollination. Many grasses, trees, and weeds produce lightweight pollen in sufficient quantities to sensitize individuals with genetic susceptibility. Plants that depend on insect pollinations, such as goldenrod, dandelions, and most flowers, do not cause allergic rhinitis symptoms.

The pollination season of the various plants depends on the individual plant and on the various geographic locations. For a particular plant in a given locale, however, the pollinating season is constant from year to year. Weather conditions, such as temperature and rainfall, influence the amount of pollen produced but not the actual onset or termination of a specific season.

Ragweed pollen, a significant cause of allergic rhinitis, produces the most severe and longest seasonal rhinitis in the eastern and midwestern portions of the United States. In those areas, ragweed pollen appears in significant amounts from the second or third week of August through September. Occasionally, sensitive patients may exhibit symptoms as early as the

TABLE 9-2. *Major aeroallergens in allergic rhinitis*

Outdoor (generally seasonal)

Pollens

   Weeds (ragweed)

   Grasses (rye, timothy, orchard)

   Trees (oak, elm, birch, alder, hazel)

Molds (*Alternaria, Cladosporium*)

Indoor (generally perennial)

House dust mites

   Dermatophagoides farinae

   Dermatophagoides pteronyssinus

Warm-blooded pets

Pests

   Mice

   Cockroaches

   Rats

Molds

   Aspergillus

   Penicillium

Occupational allergens

   Laboratory animals

first few days of August, when smaller quantities of pollen first appear. Western ragweed and marsh elder in the western states, sagebrush and franseria in the Pacific areas, and careless weed, pigweed, and franseria in the southwestern United States all are important allergens in the late summer and early fall. In the northern and eastern United States, the earliest pollens to appear are tree pollens, usually in March, April, or May. Late spring and early summer allergic rhinitis in this locale is caused by grass pollens, which appear from May to late June or early July. During this season patients complain of "rose fever," which, like "hay fever" is a misnomer. Roses coincidentally are in full bloom during the grass pollinating season, and this accounts for the misconception. Approximately 75% of pollinosis patients in the United States experience ragweed allergic rhinitis: 40% from grass allergic rhinitis, and 9% from tree rhinitis.[11] Approximately 25% of pollinosis patients have both grass and ragweed allergic rhinitis, and about 5% have all three allergies. In other geographic locations, these generalizations are not correct, because of the particular climate and because some less common plants may predominate. For example, grass pollinates from early spring through late fall in the southwestern regions, and accounts for allergic rhinitis that is almost perennial.

Airborne mold spores, the most important of which throughout the United States are *Alternaria* and *Hormodendrum*, also cause seasonal allergic rhinitis. Warm, damp weather favors the growth of molds and thereby influences the severity of the season. Generally, molds first appear in the air in the spring, become most significant during the warmer months, and usually disappear with the first frost. Thus, patients with marked hypersensitivity to molds may exhibit symptoms from early spring through the first frost, whereas those with a lesser degree of hypersensitivity may have symptoms from early summer through late fall only.

Clinical Features

The major symptoms of allergic rhinitis are sneezing, rhinorrhea, nasal pruritus, and nasal congestion, although patients may not have the entire symptom complex. When taking the patient's history, record the specific characteristics of symptoms:

1. Define onset and duration of symptoms and emphasize any relation to seasons or life events such as changing residence or occupation, or acquiring a new pet.
2. Define current symptoms including secretions, degree of congestion, sneezing, nasal itching, and sinus pressure and pain. Obtain a history regarding ocular symptoms, such as itching, lacrimation, puffiness, and chemosis; pharyngeal symptoms of mild sore throat, throat clearing, and itching of the palate and throat; and associated systemic symptoms of malaise, fatigue, or sleep disturbances.
3. Identify exacerbating factors such as seasonal or perennial allergens and nonspecific irritants (cigarette smoke, chemical fumes, cold air).
4. Identify other associated allergic diseases such as asthma or atopic dermatitis, or a family history of allergic diathesis.
5. Obtain a complete medication history, including both prescription and over-the-counter medications.

Sneezing is the most characteristic symptom, and occasionally a patient may have paroxysms of 10 to 20 sneezes in rapid succession. Sneezing episodes may arise without warning, or they may be preceded by an uncomfortable itching or irritated feeling in the nose. Sneezing attacks result in tearing of the eyes because of activation of the nasal lacrimal reflex, which, when combined with closing the eyelids at the apex of the sneeze, may create a significant hazard during driving. During the pollinating season, nonspecific factors such as dust exposure, sudden drafts, air pollutants, or noxious irritants also may trigger violent sneezing episodes.

The rhinorrhea is typically a thin discharge that may be profuse and continuous. Because of the copious nature of the rhinorrhea, the skin covering the external nose and the upper lip may become irritated and tender. Purulent discharge is never seen in uncomplicated allergic rhinitis, and its presence usually indicates secondary infection. Nasal congestion resulting from swollen turbinates is a frequent complaint. Early in the season, the nasal obstruction may be intermittent or more troublesome in the evening and at night, only to become almost continuous as the season progresses. If the nasal obstruction is severe, interference with aeration and drainage of the paranasal sinus or the eustachian tube may occur, resulting in complaints of headache or earache. The headache is of the so-called vacuum type, presumed to be caused by the development of negative pressure when air is absorbed from the obstructive sinus or middle ear. Patients also complain that their hearing is decreased and that sounds seem muffled. Patients also may notice a crackling sensation in the ears, especially when swallowing. Nasal congestion alone, particularly in children, occasionally may be the major or sole complaint. With continuous severe nasal congestion, the senses of smell and taste may be lost. Itching of the nose also may be a prominent feature, inducing frequent rubbing of the nose, particularly in children. Eye symptoms (pruritus and lacrimation) often accompany the nasal symptoms. Patients with severe eye symptoms often complain of photophobia and sore, "tired" eyes. Scleral and conjunctival injection and chemosis often occur. Occasionally, there may be marked itching of the ears, palate, throat, or face, which may be extremely annoying. Because of irritating sensations in the throat and the posterior drainage of the nasal secretions, a hacking, nonproductive cough may be present. A constricted feeling in the chest, sometimes severe enough to cause the patient to complain of shortness of breath, may accompany the cough. This sensation of tightness in the chest is particularly bothersome to the patients with severe nighttime cough. The diagnosis of coexisting asthma should be considered in such patients. Some patients have systemic symptoms of seasonal allergic rhinitis. Complaints may include weakness, malaise, irritability, fatigue, and anorexia. Certain patients relate that nausea, abdominal discomfort, and poor appetite occur with swallowing excess mucous.

A characteristic feature of the symptom complex is the periodicity of its appearance. Symptoms usually recur each year for many years in relation to the duration of the pollinating season of the causative plant. The most sensitive patients exhibit symptoms early in the season, almost as soon as the pollen appears in the air. The intensity of the symptoms tends to follow the course of pollination, becoming more severe when the pollen concentration is highest and waning as the season comes to an end, when the amount of pollen in the air decreases. In some patients, symptoms disappear suddenly when the pollination season is over, whereas in others, symptoms may disappear gradually over a period of 2 or 3 weeks after the pollination season is completed. There may be an increased reactivity of the nasal mucosa after repeated exposure to the pollen.[11] This local and nonspecific increased reactivity has been termed the *priming effect*. The nonspecificity of this effect was suggested by demonstration under experimental conditions that a patient may respond to an allergen not otherwise considered clinically significant if the patient had been exposed or primed to a clinically significant allergen. This effect may account for the presence of symptoms in some patients beyond the termination of the pollinating season, because an allergen not important clinically by itself may induce symptoms in the "primed nose." For example, a patient with positive skin test results to mold antigens and ragweed, and no symptoms until August, may have symptoms until late October, after the ragweed pollinating season is over. The symptoms persist because of the presence of molds in the air, which affect the primed mucous membrane. In most patients, however, this does not occur.[12] The presence of a secondary infection, or the effects of nonspecific irritants on inflamed nasal membranes, also may prolong rhinitis symptoms beyond a specific pollinating season.

To a lesser degree, the symptoms of allergic rhinitis may exhibit periodicity within the season. Many patients have more intense symptoms in the morning because most windborne pollens are released in greatest numbers between sunrise and 9:00 AM. Other specific factors modify the intensity of rhinitis symptoms. These symptoms may diminish while it is raining because of the clearing of the pollen from the air. Dry, windy days aggravate the symptoms because a higher concentration of pollen may be distributed over larger areas.

In addition to specific factors, nonspecific factors also may influence the degree of rhinitis symptoms. Some of these include tobacco smoke, paints, newspaper ink, and soap powders. Rapid atmospheric changes may aggravate symptoms in predisposed patients. Nonspecific air pollutants also may potentiate the symptoms of allergic rhinitis, such as sulfur dioxide, ozone, carbon monoxide, and nitrogen dioxide.

Overall, allergic rhinitis tends to increase in severity for 2 or 3 years until a stabilized condition is reached. Symptoms then recur year after year. Occasionally, patients spontaneously lose their hypersensitivity for reasons that are not well understood.

Physical Examination

The most abnormal physical findings are present during the acute stages of the patient's seasonal complaints. The following common physical findings appear in allergic rhinitis patients during a seasonal exacerbation:

Nasal obstruction, associated mouth breathing
Pale to bluish nasal mucosa and enlarged (boggy) inferior turbinates
Clear nasal secretions; whitish secretions may be seen in patients experiencing severe
    allergic rhinitis
Clear or white secretions along the posterior wall of the nasopharynx
Conjunctival erythema, lacrimation, puffiness of the eyes.

The physical findings, usually confined to the nose, ears, and eyes, aid in the diagnosis. Rubbing of the nose and mouth breathing are common findings in children. Some children rub the nose in an upward and outward fashion, which has been termed the allergic salute. The eyes may exhibit excessive lacrimation, the sclera and conjunctiva may be reddened, and chemosis often may be present. The conjunctive may be swollen and may appear granular in nature. In addition, the eyelids often are swollen. The skin above the nose may be reddened and irritated because of the continuous rubbing and blowing of the nose. Examination of the nasal cavity discloses a pale, wet, edematous, mucosa, frequently bluish in color. A clear, thin nasal secretion may be seen within the nasal cavity. Swollen turbinates may completely occlude the nasal passageway and severely affect the patient. Nasal polyps may be present in individuals with allergic rhinitis. Occasionally, there is fluid in the middle ear, resulting in decreased hearing. The pharynx is usually normal. The nose and eye examinations give normal results during asymptomatic intervals.

Pathophysiology

The nose has five major functions. It is:

1. An olfactory organ
2. A resonator for phonation

3. A passageway for air flow in and out of the lungs
4. A means of humidifying and warming inspired air
5. A filter of noxious particles from inspired air

Allergic reactions occurring in the nasal mucous membranes markedly effect the nose's major functions. The nose can initiate immune mechanisms, and the significance of mediator release from nasal mast cells and basophils in immediate-type allergic reactions is well established. Patients with allergic rhinitis have IgE antibodies that bind to high-affinity receptors on mast cells, basophils, and eosinophils, and to low-affinity receptors on cells such as monocytes, eosinophils, and platelets.[13–16] On nasal reexposure to antigen, the mast cells degranulate, releasing several mediators of inflammation. Mediators that are released include histamine, leukotrienes, prostaglandins, platelet-activating factor, and bradykinin. These mediators are responsible for the vasodilation, increased vascular permeability, increased glandular secretion, and stimulation of afferent nerves,[17–19] which culminate in the immediate-type rhinitis symptoms. Stimulation of the afferent nerves also promotes an axon reflex with local release of the neuropeptides substance P and bradykinins, which have the potential to promote further mast cell degranulation.

With continuation of allergic inflammation, there is an accumulation of CD4 T lymphocytes, eosinophils, neutrophils, and basophils.[20,21] Eosinophils release major basic protein, which may further disrupt the respiratory epithelium and promote further mast cell mediator release. There are strong correlations between the number of basophils and the level of histamine in the late reaction, and between the number of eosinophils and the amount of eosinophil major basic protein,[22] which suggest that these cells may participate in allergic inflammation by not only entering the nose but also degranulating. Other evidence for the participation of eosinophils in allergic inflammation is that eosinophils increase during the seasonal exposure,[23,24] and the number of eosinophil progenitors in nasal scrapings increases after exposure to allergens and correlates with the severity of seasonal disease.[25] Basophils also may participate in the late-phase allergic response since cell counts have confirmed increases of basophils from nasal lavage fluids. Recent studies involving nasal mucosal biopsy confirm an increase in CD4+ T lymphocytes in addition to neutrophils and eosinophils during late responses.[26] Although neutrophils enter the nose in large numbers when compared with eosinophils, their role in allergic inflammation is undetermined. In situ hybridization studies[27] using gene probes directed against specific cytokines confirm an increase in messenger RNA expression of the so-called "Th2 type" cytokines with known eosinophil modifying properties closely correlating with the allergen-induced local increases in eosinophil numbers in the nasal mucosa during late responses.

The heating and humidification of inspired air is an important function of the nasal mucosa. The highly vascularized mucosa of the turbinates in the septum provides an effective structure to heat and humidify air as it passes over them. The blood vessels are under the direction of the autonomic nervous system, which controls reflex adjustments for efficient performance of this function. The sympathetic nervous system provides for vascular constriction with a reduction of secretions. The parasympathetic nervous system enables vascular dilatation and an increase in secretions. These two systems are in a constant state of balance to meet any specific demand.

The protecting and cleansing role of the nasal mucosa also is an important function. Relatively large particles are filtered out of the inspired air by the hairs within the nostrils. The nasal secretions contain an enzyme, lysozyme, which is bacteriostatic. The pH of the nasal secretions remains relatively constant at pH 7. Lysozyme activity and ciliary action are optimal at this pH. The major portions of the nose, septum, and paranasal sinuses are lined by ciliated cells.

The cilia beat at a frequency of 10 to 15 beats per minute, producing a streaming mucus blanket at an approximate rate of 2.5 to 7.5 mm/minute. The mucus is produced by mucous and serous glands and epithelial goblet cells in the mucosa. The mucus blanket containing the filtered materials is moved toward the pharynx to be expectorated or swallowed.

Laboratory Findings

The only characteristic laboratory finding in allergic rhinitis is the presence of many eosinophils in a Hansel-stained smear of the nasal secretions obtained during a period of symptoms. In classic seasonal allergic rhinitis, this test usually is not necessary to make a diagnosis. Its use is limited to questionable cases and more often in defining chronic allergic rhinitis. Peripheral blood eosinophilia of 4% to 12% may be present in active seasonal allergic rhinitis. The clinician should not rely on the presence or absence of eosinophilia when making the diagnosis of seasonal allergic rhinitis. A significantly elevated level of serum IgE may occur in the serum of some patients with allergic rhinitis,[28] but is not a prerequisite for this diagnosis.

Diagnosis

The diagnosis of seasonal allergic rhinitis usually presents no difficulty by the time the patient has had symptoms severe enough to seek medical attention. The seasonal nature of the condition, the characteristic symptom complex, and the physical findings should establish a diagnosis in almost all cases. If the patient is first seen during the initial or second season, or if the major symptom is conjunctivitis, there may be a delay in making the diagnosis from the history alone.

Additional supporting evidence is a positive history of allergic disorders in the immediate family, and a collateral history of other allergic disorders in the patient. After the history and physical examination are performed, skin tests should be done to determine the reactivity of the patient against the suspected allergens. For the proper interpretation of a positive skin test result, remember that patients with allergic rhinitis may exhibit positivity on skin tests to allergens other than those that are clinically important. The radioallergosorbent test (RAST), an in vitro procedure for assessing the presence of specific IgE antibodies to various allergens, has been employed as a diagnostic aid in some allergic diseases. RAST determination of circulating IgE antibodies can be used instead of skin testing when high-quality extracts are not available, when a control skin test with the diluent consistently gives positive findings, when antihistamine therapy cannot be discontinued, or in the presence of a widespread skin disease such as atopic dermatitis. The serum RAST correlates well with other measures of sensitivity such as skin tests, endpoint titration, histamine release, and provocation tests.[29–32] Although occasional patients may have an elevated nasal secretion with RAST (relative to serum RAST levels), usually a good correlation exists between specific IgE measurements of skin tests, nasal secretion with RAST, and serum RAST levels. These findings usually reflect the fact that specific IgE, regardless of where it is synthesized, is in equilibrium with the skin, nose, and serum of allergic rhinitis patients.[33] Clinical symptoms usually correlate well with findings on skin tests, nasal RASTs, and serum RASTs. The frequency of positive reactions obtained from skin testing usually is greater than that found on serum or nasal RAST.

In view of these findings, the serum or nasal RAST may be used as a supplement to skin testing, but skin testing is the diagnostic method of choice to demonstrate IgE antibodies. When the skin test result is positive, there is little need for other tests. When the skin test result is dubiously positive, the RAST result will, as a rule, be negative. Therefore, the information obtained by examining serum IgE antibody by RAST usually adds little to the information obtained by critical evaluation of skin testing with high-quality extracts.

Another procedure used as a diagnostic aid is nasal provocation. When possible, however, skin testing should be performed, because in contrast to the nasal test, the skin test is quick, inexpensive, safe, and without discomfort to the patient, and it has the additional advantage of possessing better reproducibility.

The major clinical entity that enters into the differential diagnosis of allergic rhinitis is that of infectious rhinitis. Fever, sore throat, thick purulent rhinorrhea, erythematous nasal mucosa, and the presence of cervical lymphadenopathy are helpful differential findings in infectious rhinitis. Stained smears of the nasal secretions usually show a predominance of polymorphonuclear neutrophils. The total duration of symptoms—4 to 10 days—is another helpful sign, because pollination seasons usually are much longer.

PERENNIAL ALLERGIC RHINITIS

Definition

Perennial allergic rhinitis is characterized by intermittent or continuous nasal symptoms resulting from an allergic reaction without seasonal variation. The symptoms generally persist throughout the year. Some clinicians have used the term perennial allergic rhinitis to include both allergic and nonallergic forms of nonseasonal rhinitis, but it should be applied to the cases in which an allergic etiology is known to exist. The term *allergic* in this book is used only for the responses mediated by, or presumed to be mediated by an immunologic reaction. Although many aspects related to the etiology, pathophysiology, symptomatology, and diagnosis have been discussed in the preceding section, separate consideration of perennial allergic rhinitis is warranted because of certain complexities of the disease with particular reference to the diagnosis, management, and complications.

Etiology

Perennial allergic rhinitis has the same mechanisms as seasonal allergic rhinitis. The only difference is that chronic antigen challenge results in recurring, almost continuous, symptoms throughout the year. Inhalant allergens are the most important cause of perennial allergic rhinitis. The major perennial allergens are house dust mites, mold antigens, feather pillows, animal dander, and cockroaches (see Table 9-2). Pollen allergy may contribute to seasonal exacerbations of rhinitis in patients with perennial symptoms. Occasionally, perennial allergic rhinitis may be the result of exposure to an occupational allergen. Symptoms are perennial but not constant in such cases because there is a clear, temporal association with workplace exposure. Occupational allergic rhinitis has been described in flower industry workers,[34] detergent workers,[35] and woodworkers.[36].

Although some clinicians believe that food allergens may be significant factors in the cause of perennial allergic rhinitis, a direct immunologic relation between ingested foods and persistent rhinitis symptoms has been difficult to establish. Rarely does hypersensitivity to dietary proteins induce the symptoms of nonseasonal allergic rhinitis. Such reactions usually are confirmed by double-blind food challenges.[37] Cow's milk, both on an allergic and non-immunolgic basis, has been the food most associated with precipitating or aggravating upper respiratory symptoms.[38] Usually, however, most patients with proven food allergies exhibit other symptoms, including gastrointestinal disturbances, urticaria, angioedema, asthma, and anaphylaxis in addition to rhinitis after ingesting the specific food.

Nonspecific irritants and infections may influence the course of perennial allergic rhinitis. Children with this condition have a higher incidence of respiratory infections that tend to aggravate the condition and often lead to the development of complications.[8,39] Irritants such as tobacco smoke, air pollutants, and chemical fumes can aggravate the symptoms. Drafts, chilling, and sudden changes in temperature also tend to do so, and in this event also may indicate that the patient has nonallergic vasomotor rhinitis.

Pathophysiology

The alterations of normal physiologic mechanisms that have been described for seasonal allergic rhinitis are present to a lesser degree in the perennial form of the disease but are more persistent. These changes are more chronic and permanent, and are significant factors in the development of many of the complications associated with nonseasonal allergic rhinitis. The histopathologic changes that occur are initially identical to those found in seasonal allergic rhinitis. With persistent disease, more chronic and irreversible changes may be noted, such as thickening and hyperplasia of the mucosal epithelium, more intense mononuclear cellular infiltration, connective tissue proliferation, and hyperplasia of adjacent periosteum.

Clinical Features

The symptoms of perennial allergic rhinitis are similar to those of seasonal allergic rhinitis, although they frequently are less severe. This is because of the constant exposure to low concentrations of an allergen such as the house dust mite. The decreased severity of symptoms seen in these patients may lead them to interpret their symptoms as resulting from "sinus trouble" or "frequent colds." Nasal obstruction may be the major or sole complaint, particularly in children, in whom the passageways are relatively small. Sneezing, clear rhinorrhea, itching of the nose, eyes, ears, and throat, and lacrimation also may occur. The presence of itching in the nasopharyngeal and ocular areas is consistent with an allergic cause of the chronic rhinitis. The chronic nasal obstruction may cause mouth breathing, snoring, almost constant sniffling, and a nasal twang to the speech. The obstruction has been reported to be severe enough to cause a form of sleep apnea in children. Because of the constant mouth breathing, patients may complain of a dry, irritated, or sore throat. Loss of the sense of smell may occur in patients with marked chronic nasal obstruction. In some patients, the nasal obstruction is worse at night and may interfere with sleep. Sneezing episodes on awakening or in the early morning hours are a complaint. Because the chronic edema involves the opening of the eustachian tube and the paranasal sinuses, dull frontal headaches and ear complaints, such as decreased hearing, fullness in the ears, or popping in the ears, are common. Children may experience recurrent episodes of serous otitis media. In addition, chronic nasal obstruction may lead to eustachian tube dysfunction. Persistent, low-grade nasal pruritus leads to almost constant rubbing of the nose and nasal twitching. In children, recurrent epistaxis may occur because of the friability of the mucous membranes, sneezing episodes, forceful nose blowing, or nose picking. After exposure to significant levels of an allergen, such as close contact with a pet or when dusting the house, the symptoms may be as severe as in the acute stages of seasonal allergic rhinitis. Constant, excessive post-nasal drainage of secretions may be associated with a chronic cough or a continual clearing of the throat.

Physical Examination

Physical examination of the patient with perennial allergic rhinitis aids in diagnosis, particularly in a child who may constantly rub the nose or eyes. A child may have certain facial characteristics that have been associated with chronic allergic disease.[40] These include a gaping appearance caused by the constant mouth breathing and a broadening of the midsection of the nose. In addition, there may be a transverse nasal crease across the lower third of the nose where the soft cartilaginous portion meets the rigid bony bridge. This is a result of the continual rubbing and pushing of the nose to relieve itching. The mucous membranes are pale, moist, and boggy, and may have a bluish tinge. Polyps may be present in cases of chronic perennial allergic rhinitis of long duration. Their characteristic appearance is smooth, glistening, and white. They may take the form of grape-like masses. Polyps also may occur in patients without allergic rhinitis, and thus causality cannot be inferred. The nasal secretions are usually clear and watery, but may be more mucoid and may show large numbers of eosinophils when examined microscopically.

Dark circles under the eyes, known as allergic shiners, appear in some children. These are presumed to be caused by venous stasis secondary to constant nasal congestion. The conjunctiva may be injected or may appear granular. In children affected with perennial allergic rhinitis early in life, narrowing of the arch of the palate may occur, leading to the Gothic arch. In addition, these children may develop facial deformities such as dental malocclusion or gingival hypertrophy. The throat usually is normal on examination, although the posterior pharyngeal wall may exhibit prominent lymphoid follicles.

Laboratory Findings

A nasal smear examined for eosinophils may be of value when diagnosing perennial allergic rhinitis. It is particularly useful in cases in which there is no clear clinical relation of symptoms to positive skin test results. The presence of large numbers of eosinophils suggests an allergic cause for the chronic rhinitis, although nonallergic rhinitis with eosinophilia syndrome certainly occurs. Their absence does not exclude an allergic cause, especially if the test is done during a relatively quiescent period of the disease, or in the presence of bacterial infection, when large numbers of polymorphonuclear neutrophils obscure the eosinophils. There is no particular diagnostic relation between the presence or absence of low-grade peripheral blood eosinophilia and the presence of the disease, although eosinophilia is suggestive evidence. An elevated level of serum IgE also supports the diagnosis.

Diagnosis

Positive skin test results to aeroallergens are important confirmatory findings in patients whose history and physical examinations suggest chronic allergic rhinitis. The RAST may be a useful diagnostic aid in conjunction with an appropriate history when skin testing cannot be performed. In rare patients in whom food allergy might play a significant role, a food elimination diet is indicated, although food allergy as a hidden cause of allergic rhinitis seldom is seen. Only by avoiding suspected food substances, and a consequent reduction or complete abatement of the symptoms, which then recur with reintroduction of the food, can the clinician be assured of a specific food allergy. Food allergy rarely is an important factor in perennial allergic rhinitis, particularly in adults. Therefore, good medical judgment must be used to avoid the over diagnosis of food allergy.

Differential Diagnosis

Incorrect diagnosis may result in expensive treatments and alterations of the patient's environment; therefore, the diagnosis must be established carefully. Major disease entities that may be confused with perennial allergic rhinitis are chronic sinusitis; recurrent infectious rhinitis; abnormalities of nasal structures; and nonseasonal, nonallergic, noninfectious rhinitis (Table 9-3). In addition, skin tests in these conditions usually yield negative results or do not correlate clinically with the symptoms. In infectious rhinitis and chronic rhinitis, eosinophilia is not common in nasal secretions. The predominant cell found in the nasal secretions in these conditions is the neutrophil, unless there is a coexistent allergic rhinitis. These entities are discussed in greater detail in the last section of this chapter.

Causes of chronic nasal congestion and discharge include rhinitis medicamentosa, drugs, pregnancy, nasal foreign bodies, other bony abnormalities of the lateral nasal wall, concha bulbosa (air cell within the middle turbinate), enlarged adenoids, nasal polyps, cerebral spinal fluid rhinorrhea, tumors, hypothyroidism, ciliary dyskinesia from cystic fibrosis, primary ciliary dyskinesia or Kartagener's syndrome, granulomatous diseases (e.g., sarcoidosis, Wegener's granulomatosis, or midline granuloma), nasal mastocytosis, congenital syphilis, or atrophic rhinitis.

TABLE 9-3. *Known causes of nonallergic rhinitis*

Associated Drugs	**Structural Abnormalities**
Topical alpha-adrenergic agonists	Marked septal deviation
Alpha-adrenergic blockers	Concha bullosa
Oral estrogens	Nasal polyps
Ophthalmic and oral beta-blockers	Adenoidal hypertrophy
Infections	Foreign body
Chronic sinusitis	**Neoplasms**
Tuberculosis	Squamous cell carcinoma
Syphilis	Nasopharyngeal carcinoma
Fungal infection	**Granulomatous Diseases**
Systemic Conditions	Wegener's granulomatosis
Cystic fibrosis	Sarcoidosis
Immunodeficiencies	Midline granuloma
Immotile cilia syndrome	**Other**
Hypothyroidism	Atrophic rhinitis
Rhinitis of pregnancy	

Rhinitis Medicamentosa

A condition that may enter into the differential diagnosis is rhinitis medicamentosa, which results from the overuse of vasoconstricting nose drops. Every patient who presents with the complaint of chronic nasal congestion should be questioned carefully as to the amount and frequency of the use of nose drops.

Drugs

Patients taking antihypertensive agents such as propranolol, clonidine, alpha-blockers such as terazosin and prazosin, alpha-methyldopa, reserpine, quanabenz, hydralazine, and certain psychoactive drugs may complain of marked nasal congestion, which is a common side effect of these drugs. A medical history of current drug therapy suggests a diagnosis. Discontinuing these drugs for a few days results in marked symptomatic improvement. Contraceptives have been incriminated as a cause of perennial rhinitis,[41,42] but the evidence for this is meager, except in cases in which other history factors strongly implicate causality. It is not currently recommended that women with rhinitis stop using oral contraceptives. Cocaine sniffing also can produce rhinorrhea.

Pregnancy

Congestion of the nasal mucosa is a normal physiologic change in pregnancy. This is presumably a major factor in the development in some women of "rhinitis of pregnancy," a syndrome of nasal congestion and vasomotor instability limited to the gestational period.[43] The rhinitis characteristically begins at the end of the first trimester and then disappears immediately after delivery. Patients with or without a history of chronic nasal symptoms may develop rhinitis medicamentosa or acute pharyngitis–sinusitis during pregnancy. In one series, 32% of 79 pregnant women surveyed reported frequent or constant nasal problems during pregnancy.[44]

Foreign Body

On rare occasions, a patient with a foreign body in the nose may be thought to have chronic allergic rhinitis. Foreign bodies usually present as unilateral nasal obstruction accompanied by a foul, purulent nasal discharge. Children often put foreign bodies into the nose, most commonly peas, beans, buttons, and erasers. Sinusitis often is diagnosed if the nose is not examined properly. Examination is best done after secretions are removed so that the foreign body may be visualized.

Physical Obstruction

Careful physical examination of the nasal cavity should be performed to exclude septal deviation, enlarged adenoids, choanal atresia, and nasal polyps as the cause of nasal congestion.

Cerebral Spinal Fluid Rhinorrhea

Cerebral spinal fluid (CSF) rhinorrhea may follow a head injury. Cerebral spinal fluid is clear and watery, simulating that seen in allergic rhinitis. In most cases, the CSF rhinorrhea is unilateral. Because spinal fluid contains sugar and mucus does not, testing for the presence of glucose should be done to make the diagnosis. CSF rhinorrhea results from a defect in the cribriform plate that requires surgical repair.

Tumor

Several tumors and neoplasms occur in the nasopharyngeal area. The most important are encephalocele, inverting papilloma, squamous cell carcinoma, sarcoma, and angiofibroma. Encephaloceles generally are unilateral. They usually occur high in the nose and occasionally within the nasopharynx. They increase in size with straining, lifting, or crying. They may have a pulsating quality. If a biopsy is done, a CSF rhinorrhea and meningitis may ensue.

Inverting papillomas have a somewhat papillary appearance. They are friable and more vascular than nasal polyps, and they bleed more readily. They occur either unilaterally or bilaterally and frequently involve the nasal septum, as well the lateral wall of the nose. A biopsy is necessary to confirm the diagnosis.

Angiofibromas are the most common in preadolescent boys. They arise in the posterior choana of the nasopharynx. They have a polypoid appearance but usually are reddish blue. They do not pit on palpation. Angiofibromas are highly vascular tumors that bleed excessively when injured or when a biopsy is done. Larger tumors may invade bone and extend into adjacent structures.[45]

Carcinomas and sarcomas may stimulate nasal polyps. They generally occur unilaterally, at any site within the nasal chamber, are firm, and usually bleed with manipulation. While the disease progresses, adjacent structures are involved.

Hypothyroidism

A careful review of systems is important to exclude hypothyroidism as a cause of nasal congestion.

Syphilis

Congenital syphilis can cause rhinitis in infancy.

Ciliary Disorders

With the dyskinetic cilia syndrome, patients may experience rhinitis symptoms secondary to abnormalities of mucociliary transport. The criteria for diagnosis include the following: (1) absence or near absence of tracheobronchial or nasal mucociliary transport; (2) total or near-total absence of dynein arms of the cilia in nasal or bronchial mucosa, or, rarely, defective radial spokes or transposition of a peripheral microtubular doublet to the center of the axoneme; and (3) clinical manifestations of chronic upper and lower respiratory tract infections such as sinusitis, bronchitis, and bronchiectasis.[46] Occasionally, the clinician may see the triad of bronchiectasis, sinusitis, and situs inversus known as Kartagener's syndrome.[47] In some patients, cilia, although abnormal in structure, may be motile. The cilia in patients with this syndrome can be distinguished from those of patient with asthma, sinusitis, chronic bronchitis, and emphysema, who may have nonspecific abnormalities in cilia structure.[48]

Course and Complications

Allergic rhinitis accounts for most of the patients with respiratory allergy. Most patients develop symptoms before 20 years of age, with the highest rate of increase of onset of symptoms occurring between the ages of 12 and 15 years.[8] Because of a variety of factors, including geographic location, allergen load, weather conditions, and emotions, the course and prognosis for any single patient cannot be predicted. One study suggests that over one third of patients with allergic rhinitis were better over a 10-year period, but most were worse.[49] In another study, 8% of those with allergic rhinitis had remissions for at least 2 years' duration. A chance for remission was better in those with seasonal allergic rhinitis and if the disease was present for less than 5 years.[50]

The possibility of developing asthma as a sequela to allergic rhinitis may worry the patient, or the parents if the patient is a child. Generally, approximately 30% of patient with allergic rhinitis not treated with specific immunotherapy eventually develop allergic asthma. A survey of an entire city, however, showed that only 7% of those with allergic rhinitis developed asthma as a late sequela.[51] In most patients with both allergic rhinitis and asthma, the asthmatic condition develops before the onset of allergic rhinitis, or the two conditions appear almost simultaneously. If asthma develops, the patient's concern for the symptoms of asthma usually overshadows those of allergic rhinitis. It is frequently stated that the individual with more severe allergic rhinitis has a greater risk of developing asthma, but clear evidence for this is lacking.

Patients with allergic rhinitis may develop complications because of chronic nasal inflammation, including recurrent otitis media with hearing loss, sinusitis, and nasal or sinus polyps. It is apparent, therefore, that allergic rhinitis is a significant problem. For these reasons, early diagnosis and treatment of chronic or seasonal allergic rhinitis is recommended.

TREATMENT

There are three types of management of seasonal allergic or perennial allergic rhinitis: avoidance therapy, pharmacologic therapy, and immunotherapy.

Avoidance Therapy

Complete avoidance of an allergen results in a cure when there is only a single allergen. For this reason, attempts should be made to minimize contact with any important allergen, regardless of what other mode of treatment is instituted.

Allergic rhinitis because of a household pet can be controlled completely by removing the pet from the home. If the patient is allergic to feathers, pillows should be changed from feather to Dacron, or should be covered with plastic. Mold-sensitive patients occasionally notice the precipitation or aggravation of symptoms after ingesting certain foods having a high mold content. Avoiding beer, wine, cantaloupe, melons, mushrooms, and various cheeses may be helpful. Tips for controlling allergic rhinitis are listed in Table 9-4.

TABLE 9-4. *Tips for patients with allergic rhinitis*

1. Keep pets out of the bedroom and preferably outside of the house.

2. Avoid smoking or secondhand smoke.

3. Routinely clean areas of the home that promote mold growth such as shower stalls, basements, and window sills (mold sensitivity).

4. Have cooking systems in the home checked periodically for mold growth.

5. Avoid locations that promote the growth of molds such as damp, poorly ventilated areas. Avoid sleeping in a bedroom located in a basement or attic.

6. Use air conditioning to reduce humidity and decrease temperature. Keep windows closed to avoid contact with outdoor allergens (house dust mite and pollen sensitivity).

7. Encase pillows, mattresses, and box springs in zippered protective plastic or vinyl covers (house dust mite sensitivity).

8. Replace heavily mite-infected mattresses and pillows. Use foam pillows instead of down or feather pillows (house dust mite sensitivity).

9. Launder bedding regularly, including mattress pads and blankets in hot water (60°C [140°F]) (house dust mite sensitivity).

10. Vacuum carpets and clean floors regularly. If possible, remove carpeting from bedroom (house dust mite sensitivity).

11. Minimize dust-collecting reservoirs such as stuffed animals, books, stored blankets, and woolens.

In most cases of allergic rhinitis, complete avoidance therapy is difficult, if not impossible, because aeroallergens are so widely distributed. Attempts to eradicate sources of pollen or molds have not proven to be significantly effective. Mold-sensitive patients should avoid damp, musty basements, raked or burning leaves, barns, moldy hay, and straw, and they should disinfect or destroy moldy articles.

In the case of house dust mite allergy, complete avoidance is not possible, but certain measures decrease the exposure to antigen. Instructions for a dust-control program also should be given to the patient with house dust mite sensitivity. At least one room in the house should be relatively dust-free. The most practical program is to make the bedroom as dust-free as possible, so that the patient may have the sleeping area as a controlled environment. Certain measures to decrease house dust mite exposure are relatively easy to perform. Bed linens should be washed in hot water (54°C [130°F]). Both the mattress and box spring should be encased in plastic covers. Upholstered furniture, wall-to-wall carpeting, chenille spreads, bed pads, and stuffed toys can be eliminated from the bedroom for more complete control. These simple measures often are enough to enable the patient to have fewer and milder symptoms.

Pharmacologic Therapy

Antihistamines

Antihistamines are the foundation of symptomatic therapy for allergic rhinitis, and are most useful in controlling the sneezing, rhinorrhea, and pruritus that occur in allergic rhinitis. They are less effective, however, against the nasal obstruction and ocular symptoms in these patients. Antihistamines are compounds of varied chemical structures that have the property of antagonizing some of the actions of histamine.[52] Histamine acts through three receptors: H_1, H_2, and H_3. Activation of H_1 receptors causes smooth-muscle contraction, increases vascular permeability, increases the production of mucus, and activates sensory nerves to induce pruritus and reflexes such as sneezing.[53] Activation of H_2 receptors primarily causes gastric acid secretion and some vascular dilatation and cutaneous flushing. The more recently discovered H_3 receptors on histaminergic nerve endings in brain tissue control the synthesis and release of histamine.[54] The antihistamines used in treating allergic rhinitis are directed against the H_1 receptors, and thus are most effective in preventing histamine-induced capillary permeability. They also inhibit mediator release (azatadine, terfenadine, ketotifen),[55] inhibit tissue eosinophil influx (cetirizine),[56] and act as a mild bronchodilator (terfenadine, astemizole, cetirizine).[57] In clinical use, these drugs are most effective when given early, at the first appearance of symptoms, because they do not abolish existing effects of histamine, but rather prevent the development of new symptoms caused by further histamine release. The antihistamines also may exhibit sedative, antiemetic, or local anesthetic effects, depending on the particular antihistamine, route of administration, and dosage used. Many of them also possess atropine-like effects, which accounts for side effects such as blurred vision or dry mouth.

All of the antihistamines are readily absorbed after oral administration. They vary in speed, intensity, and duration of effect. Because so many are available, the clinician should become familiar with selected antihistamines for use. In practice, clinical choice should be based on effectiveness of antihistaminic activity and the limitation of side effects. However, contrary to previous belief, pharmacologic tolerance to antihistamines does not occur, and poor compliance is a major factor in treatment failures.[58] Thus, there is no rationale for the practice of rotating patients through the various pharmacologic classes of antihistamines. In general, children have shorter elimination half-life values of antihistamines than older adults. Dryness of the mouth, vertigo, gastrointestinal upset, irritability in children, and drowsiness account for over 90% of the side effects seen with these drugs. The depressed effect on the CNS is the major limiting side effect. Drowsiness in some patients with antihistamines is mild and temporary, and may disappear after a few doses of the drug. Because patients exhibit marked variability in response to various antihistamines, individualization of dosage and frequency of administration is important. Recent studies indicate that these drugs may be administered less frequently than previously recommended because of the prolonged biologic actions of these medications in tissues.[59]

Because the newer antihistamines do not appreciably penetrate the CNS, most studies show that the incidence of sedation and other abnormal measures of CNS function are minimal with astemizole,[60] terfenadine,[61] loratadine,[62] and cetirizine.[63] The other major advantage of the nonsedating antihistamines is that these medications usually are free of anticholinergic side effects such as dry mouth, constipation, difficulty voiding, and blurry vision. These drugs are usually tolerated by older patients who may have benign prostatic hypertrophy or xerostomia as complicating medical problems. Terfenadine usually is well absorbed from the gastrointestinal tract and usually has a short onset of action and short half-life,[61] but the antihistaminic activity is prolonged secondary to active metabolism.[64,65] Loratadine has a metabolic profile similar to terfenadine.[66] Astemizole has a slower onset of action but has a half-life of 18 days. This must be noted in skin testing, because astemizole may suppress allergy skin tests for 6 to 8 weeks.[67] Astemizole also may cause significant weight gain in a small percentage of patients. Caution should be exercised when prescribing astemizole or terfenadine to patients with serious hepatic impairment or for patients who are concurrently taking drugs that undergo significant hepatic metabolism such as ketoconazole, itraconazole, clarithromycin, erythromycin, cimetidine, and disulfiram because of the potential risk for fatal cardiac arrhythmias. This side effect has not been reported with loratadine or cetirizine.[68]

In contrast to its parent compound hydroxyzine, the carboxylic acid metabolite of hydroxyzine, cetirizine, has poor penetration into the CNS, and therefore is relatively nonsedating.

Cetirizine is highly selective for H_1 receptors in the brain and does not bind to serotonin, dopamine, or alpha-adrenergic and calcium antagonists receptors in the brain.[69] The drug is not metabolized by the hepatic cytochrome system and is excreted unchanged in the urine,[70] and, therefore, the half-life of cetirizine may be prolonged in patients with renal failure.

Topical intranasal antihistamines (azelastine and levocabastine) have been shown to be useful for treating allergic rhinitis in preliminary studies. Currently, these agents are investigational.

Sympathomimetic Agents

Sympathomimetic drugs are used as vasoconstrictors for the nasal mucous membranes. The current concept regarding the mechanism of action of these includes two types of adrenergic receptors called alpha- and beta-receptors. Activation of the alpha-receptors results in constriction of smooth muscle in the vessels of the skin, viscera, and mucous membranes, whereas activation of beta-receptors induces dilation of vascular smooth muscle, relaxation of bronchial smooth muscle, and cardiac stimulation. By taking advantage of drugs that stimulate alpha-receptors, the edema of the nasal mucous membranes in allergic rhinitis can be reduced by topical or systemic administration. In large doses, these drugs induce elevated blood pressure, nervousness, and insomnia. Although differences occur in blood pressure response to the various preparations,[71,72] these agents should be used with caution in patients who have hypertension, organic heart disease, angina pectoris, and hyperthyroidism. In addition to their use as decongestants, the sympathomimetic drugs also are combined with antihistamines in many oral preparations to decrease the drowsiness that often accompanies antihistamine therapy.

Nose drops or nasal sprays containing sympathomimetic agents may be overused. The topical application of these drugs often is followed by a "rebound" phenomenon in which the nasal mucous membranes become even more congested and edematous as a result of the use of the drugs. This leads the patient to use the drops or spray more frequently and in higher doses to obtain relief from nasal obstruction. The condition resulting from the overuse of topical sympathomimetics is called rhinitis medicamentosa. The patient must abruptly discontinue their use to alleviate the condition. Other measures, including a course of topical corticosteroids for a few weeks, are needed to decrease the nasal congestion until this distressing side effect disappears. Because of the duration of seasonal or perennial allergic rhinitis, topical vasoconstrictors should not be used in the allergic patient, except temporarily during periods of infectious rhinitis. The systemic use of sympathomimetic drugs has not been associated with rhinitis medicamentosa. Phenylephrine, ephedrine, isoephedrine, phenylpropanolamine, and cyclopentamine are some of the more common vasoconstricting agents used in association with various antihistamines in oral preparations.

Topical Corticosteroids

Cortisone and its derivatives have marked beneficial effects in managing various allergic processes. The mechanism of their therapeutic effect is not understood completely, but it appears to involve regulation of the formation and action of transcription modifying factors such as AP-1.[73] Intranasal steroids suppress neutrophil chemotaxis and decrease late responses to nasal allergen challenge.[74] The number of eosinophils, the presence of eosinophils and cationic protein, and the number of mast cell progenitors are also reduced by topical steroids during seasonal exposure to allergen. Topical corticosteroids can be highly effective in allergic rhinitis and also in many patients with nonallergic rhinitis. Although topical dexamethasone phosphate treatment may be associated with significant suppression of adrenal function and other side effects, this is not the case with more recently developed corticosteroid nasal sprays. Beclomethasone dipropionate and flunisolide have been used for several years as treatment for allergic rhinitis. Triamcinolone, budesonide, and fluticasone are newer topical corticosteroids that have been released for clinical use.

Both beclomethasone and flunisolide are rapidly absorbed from the nasal mucosa and the gastrointestinal tract after intranasal administration and partial swallowing of the dose. A drug that is swallowed undergoes a rapid first-pass hepatic metabolism to relatively inactive metabolites. A drug absorbed from the nasal mucosa initially avoids the first-pass metabolism but is ultimately metabolized in the liver. This first-pass metabolism of these medications prevents systemic side effects, but the topical efficacy is maintained. In fact, the antiinflammatory activity of beclomethasone and flunisolide are, respectively, 5000 and 3000 times greater than hydrocortisone.[75]

Intranasal steroids have been helpful in relieving the common allergic symptoms of the upper airway such as sneezing, congestion, and rhinorrhea. In addition, they may be of value in relieving throat pruritus and cough associated with allergic rhinitis, and one study suggests an improvement in seasonal allergic asthma symptoms with the use of these agents.[76]

The major side effects of intranasal steroids include local dryness or irritation in the form of stinging, burning, or sneezing[77] (Table 9-5). With prolonged administration of intranasal steroids, the risk of nasal septal perforation increases, and therefore periodic examination of the nasal cavity while patients are on these medications is warranted, especially in patients who experience nasal crusting or bleeding.[78,79] Hemorrhagic crusting and perforation of the nasal septum is more common in patients who improperly point the spray toward the septal wall, and this complication can be reduced by (1) careful education, (2) using a mirror when spraying into the nose, and (3) the new actuators used for beclomethasone sprays. Generally, stinging and burning are more common with flunisolide. These side effects are secondary to

TABLE 9-5. *Complications of topical steroids sprays*

Systemic Reactions

    Common (>5% incidence rate)

        Headaches

    Uncommon (<5% incidence rate)

        Nausea and vomiting

        Loss of senses of taste and smell

        Dizziness and light-headedness

    Rare

        Increased intraocular pressure

        Anaphylaxis, urticaria, angioedema, bronchospasm

Local Reactions

    Nasal burning and stinging

    Sneezing, sinus congestion, watery eyes, throat irritation, bad taste in mouth

    Drying of the mucous membranes with epistaxis or bloody discharge

    Perforation of nasal septum (rare)

the acidic pH and high propylene glycol content of the pump spray system. Beclomethasone has Freon as an aerosol propellant, which predisposes to the excessive dryness, crusting, and bleeding with scab formation. Recently, aqueous formulations of beclomethasone have been released for clinical use that have a pump spray delivery system with an acceptable pH and therefore are better tolerated and preferred by some patients.

Initially, some patients may require topical decongestants before administering intranasal steroids. In some patients, the congestion is so severe that a 3- to 5-day course of oral corticosteroids is required to allow delivery of the intranasal steroids. In contrast to decongestant nasal sprays, patients should be informed that intranasal steroids should be used prophylactically, and that maximum benefit is not immediate and may take weeks. Treatment with these medications is usually started at the first sign of clinical symptoms and continued for the duration of the pollination season. The education of patients regarding the use of these medications regularly is critical because patients are inclined to forgo these medications in the absence of symptoms.[77]

Although triamcinolone, budesonide, and fluticasone are more expensive than beclomethasone, these drugs can be prescribed on a once daily schedule with consistent relief of rhinitis symptoms, similar to beclomethasone prescribed on a twice or three times daily schedule.[80,81]

Intranasal Corticosteroid Injection

Intranasal corticosteroid injections have been commonly used for clinical practice in management of patients with common allergic and nonallergic nasal conditions such as nasal polyposis. With the advent of newer and safer intranasal steroids, the use of this technique has decreased. Turbinate injections have two major sides effects that are not seen with intranasal corticosteroid sprays: (1) adrenal suppression secondary to absorption of the steroid, and (2) absorption of steroid emboli, which may lead to transient or permanent loss of vision.[82]

Systemic Corticosteroids

Systemic corticosteroids are regarded by many allergists as inappropriate therapy for patients with mild to moderate allergic rhinitis. Although rhinitis is not a threat to life, it can seriously impair its quality, and some patients respond only to corticosteroids. Also, when the topical steroid cannot be adequately distributed in the nose because of marked obstruction, it will not be effective. In such cases, the blocked nose can be opened by giving a systemic corticosteroid for 3 to 5 days, and the improvement then can be maintained by the topical corticosteroid spray. The clinician should always relate the risk of side effects to the dosage given, and especially to the length of the treatment period. When short-term systemic steroid treatment is given for 1 to 2 weeks, it can be a valuable and safe supplement to topical treatments in the management of severe allergic rhinitis or nasal polyposis. As in the use of topical corticosteroids, however, systemic steroids should be reserved for severe cases that cannot be controlled by routine measures and they should only be used for a limited period and never on a chronic basis.

Anticholinergics

Ipratropium is an anticholinergic drug that was released in for treating chronic bronchitis and chronic obstructive lung disease. It has a quaternary ammonia structure, which gives this medication high topical activity; but, because of its structure, there is no appreciable absorption of this medication across mucosal barriers. Therefore, the unpleasant anticholinergic side effects commonly associated with atropine are not experienced with this medication.

Because cholinergic mechanisms in the nose may lead to hypersecretion and blood vessel dilation, interest in this medication has increased. Ipratropium decreases the watery rhinorrhea in patients with perennial rhinitis[83] and reduces nasal drainage in patients with the common cold.[84] Unfortunately, it has no appreciable effect on obstruction or sneezing in patients with rhinitis, and therefore has a limited role in treatment.

Intranasal Cromolyn

Cromolyn sodium is a derivative of the natural product khellin. The proposed mechanism of action of cromolyn in allergic rhinitis is to stabilize mast cell membranes, apparently by inhibiting calcium transmembrane flux and thereby preventing antigen-induced degranulation. It has been shown to be effective in the management of seasonal and perennial allergic rhinitis.[85,86] Cromolyn can be effective in reducing sneezing, rhinorrhea, and nasal pruritus,[87,88] but is minimally useful in nonallergic types of rhinitis and nasal polyps,[89] and has little effect on mucociliary transport. Cromolyn often prevents the symptoms of both seasonal and perennial allergic rhinitis, and diligent prophylaxis significantly reduces both immediate and late symptoms after allergen exposures.[90]

Adverse effects occur in fewer than 10% of patients, and most commonly include sneezing, nasal stinging, nasal burning, transient headache, and an unpleasant aftertaste. Patients also may experience mucosal irritation from the preservatives benzalkonium chloride and ethylenediaminetetraacetic acid. For managing seasonal rhinitis, treatment should begin 2 to 4 weeks before contact with offending allergens and should be continued throughout the period of exposure. The patient must understand the rate and extent of response to be expected from intranasal cromolyn, and, because the product is prophylactic, it must be used on a regular basis for maximum benefit.

Several studies compare the therapeutic efficacy of cromolyn nasal solution with that of the intranasal corticosteroids in allergic rhinitis. In both perennial[91,92] and seasonal allergic rhinitis,[93,94] intranasal steroids have been shown to be more effective than cromolyn. Nedocromil sodium is a new pyranoquinolone dicarboxylic acid derivative that is reported to be effective against both mucosal and connective tissue-type mast cells. In contrast, cromolyn sodium appears to be effective only against connective tissue-type mast cells. Nedocromil has been shown to be effective in seasonal and perennial allergic rhinitis.[95] Like cromolyn, nedocromil is recommended primarily for prophylactic use, and therapy should be instituted 2 to 4 weeks before the allergy season.

IMMUNOTHERAPY

Immunotherapy is a treatment that attempts to increase the threshold level for symptom appearance after exposure to the aeroallergen. This altered degree of sensitivity may be the result of either the induction of a new antibody, the so-called "blocking" antibody, a decrease in allergic antibody, a change in the cellular histamine release phenomenon, or an interplay of all three possibilities. Other immunologic changes seen with immunotherapy include induction of the generation of antigen-specific suppressor cells, reduction of the production of lymphokines, and reduction in the production of a mononuclear cell-derived histamine releasing factor. (See Chap. 10.)

The severity of allergic rhinitis and its complications is a spectrum varying from minimal to marked symptoms, and from short to prolonged duration. The indications for the type of intensity of therapy vary depending on the clinical situation. Therefore, the indications for immunotherapy, a fairly long-term treatment modality, are relative rather than absolute. For example, a patient who has mild grass pollinosis for only a few weeks in June may be managed well by symptomatic therapy alone.

Those with perennial allergic rhinitis or allergic rhinitis in multiple pollen seasons who require almost daily symptomatic treatment for long periods also may be considered as candidates for specific therapy. The advantages of long-term relief of such therapy, which is relatively expensive, should be considered in relation to the cost and potential side effects of daily medication. In addition, specific therapy may help to deter the development of some of the complications of chronic rhinitis. Antigens used for immunotherapy should be those that cannot be avoided such as pollens, molds, and the house dust mite. Animal dander injection therapy should be restricted to veterinarians and laboratory personnel whose occupation makes avoidance practically and financially impossible. Patients are generally not cured of their disease, but rather have fewer symptoms that are more easily controlled by symptomatic medication.

A frequent cause of treatment failure is that a patient expects too much, too soon, and thus prematurely discontinues the injection program because of dissatisfaction. Another important cause of failure is seen in patients with nonallergic rhinitis who have positive but clinically insignificant skin test or RAST results, and have received immunotherapy based on those tests. Immunotherapy based on positive findings on skin tests or RASTs alone should not be expected to be beneficial.

There is no adequate laboratory method of indicating to a patient how long immunotherapy must be continued. There are no long-term clinical studies of how patients fare after variable years of therapy. Therefore, the clinical response to therapy dictates that decision concerning the duration of specific treatment. A minimum of 3 years of immunotherapy should be given to avoid the rapid recurrence of symptoms in uncomplicated allergic rhinitis.

REFERENCES

1. Pederson N, Mygind N. Rhinitis, sinusitis and otitis media in Kartagener's syndrome. Clin Otolaryngol 1982;52:189.
2. Mygind N. Nasal allergy. 2nd ed. Oxford: Blackwell, 1979.
3. Hill LW. Certain aspects of allergy in children. N Engl J Med 1961;265:1194.
4. Phillips EW. Time required for production of hayfever by a newly encountered pollen. J Allergy 1939;11:28.
5. Broder I, Higgins MW, Matthews KP, Keller JB. Epidemiology of asthma and allergic rhinitis in a total community, Tecumseh, Michigan. III. Second Survey of the community. J Allergy Clin Immunol 1974;53:127.
6. Sibbald B. Epidemiology of allergic rhinitis: epidemiology of clinical allergy. Monogr Allergy 1993;31:61.
7. Haahtela R, Heiskala M, Suonemi I. Allergic disorders and immediate skin test reactivity in Finnish adolescents. Allergy 1980;35:433.
8. Hagy GW, Settipane GA. Bronchial asthma, allergic rhinitis and allergy skin tests among college students. J Allergy Clin Immunol 1969;44:323.
9. Malmberg H. Symptoms of chronic and allergic rhinitis and occurrence of nasal secretion granulocytes in university students, school children and infants. Allergy 1981;36:209.
10. McMenamin P. Costs of hayfever in the United States in 1990. Ann Allergy 1994;73:35.
11. Connell JT. Quantitative intranasal pollen challenges. III. The priming effect in allergic rhinitis. J Allergy 1969;43:33.
12. Grammer L, Wiggins C, Shaughnessy MA, Chmiel J. Absence of nasal priming as measured by rhinitis symptom scores of ragweed allergic patient during seasonal exposure to ragweed pollen. Allergy Proc 1990;11:243.
13. Tada T, Ishizaka K. Distribution of gamma E-forming cells in lymphoid tissues of the human and monkey. J Immunol 1970;104:377.
14. Grangette C, Grunt V, Ouaissi MA et al. IgE receptor on human eosinophils: comparison with B cell CD23 and association with the adhesion molecule. J Immunol 1989;143:3580.

15. Melewicz FM, Spiegelberg HL. Fc receptors for IgE on a subpopulation of human peripheral blood monocytes. J Immunol 1980;125:1026.
16. Clines DB, Vander Keyl H, Levinson AI. In vitro binding of an IgE protein to human platelets. J Immunol 1986;136:3433.
17. Proud D, Reynolds CH, Lacapra S, Kagey-Sobotka A, Lichtenstein L, Naclerio RM. Nasal provocation with bradykinin induces symptoms of rhinitis and sore throat. Am Rev Resp Dis 1988;187:613.
18. Karim SMM, Adaikian PG, Kumaratnam N. Effects of topical prostaglandins on nasal potency in man. Prostaglandins 1978;15:457.
19. Okuda M, Watase T, Mezawa A, Lire CM. The role of leukotriene D_4 in allergic rhinitis. Ann Allergy 1988;39:537.
20. Bascom R, Wachs M, Naderio RM, Pipkonn U, Galli SJ, Lichtenstein LM. Basophil influx occurs after nasal antigen challenge: effects of topical corticosteroid pretreat ment. J Allergy Clin Immunol 1988;81:580.
21. Bascom R, Pipkorn U, Lichtenstein LM, Naderio RM. The influx of inflammatory cells into nasal washings during the late response to antigen challenge: effect of systemic steroid pretreatment. Annu Rev Respir Dis 1988;138:406.
22. Linder A, Venge P, Deusch LH. Eosinophil cationic protein and myeloperoxidase in nasal secretion as markers of inflammation in allergic rhinitis. Allergy 1987;42:583.
23. Svensson C, Andersson M, Persson CGA, Venge P, Alkner U, Pipkorn U. Albumin, bradykinins, and eosinophil cationic protein on the nasal mucosa surface in patients with hay fever during natural allergen exposure. J Allergy Clin Immunol 1990;85:828.
24. Furin MJ, Norman PS, Creticos PS, et al. Immunotherapy decreases antigen-induced eosinophil migration into the nasal cavity. J Allergy Clin Immunol 1991;88:27.
25. Denburg JA, Dolovich J, Harnish D. Basophil mast cell and eosinophil growth and differentiation factors in human allergic disease. Clin Exp Allergy 1989;19:249.
26. Varney VA, Jacobson MR, Robinson DS, et al. Immunohistology of the nasal mucosa following allergen-induced rhinitis. Am Rev Respir Dis 1992;146:170.
27. Durham SR, Sun Ying, Varney VA, et al. Cytokine messenger RNA expression for IL-3, IL-4, IL-5 and granulocyte macrophage colony stimulating factor in the nasal mucosa after local allergen provocation: relationship to tissue eosinophilia. J Immunol 1992;148:2390.
28. Ishizaka T, Ishizaka K. Biology and immunoglobulin E: molecular basis of reaginic hypersensitivity. Prog Allergy 1976;19:60.
29. Berg T, Bennich H, Johansson SGO. In vitro diagnosis of atopic allergy. I. A comparison between provocation tests and the RAST test. Int Arch Allergy 1971;40:770.
30. Fouchard T, Aas K, Johansson SGO. Concentration IgE antibodies, P-K titers and chopped lung titers in sera from children with hypersensitivity to cod. J Allergy Clin Immunol 1973;51:39.
31. Norman P. RAST. In: Evans R, ed. Advances in the diagnosis of allergy. Miami: Symposia Specialists, 1970:45.
32. Reddy PM, Nagaga H, Pascual HE, et al. Reappraisal of intracutaneous tests in diagnosis of reaginic allergy. J Allergy Clin Immunol 1978;61:36.
33. Schatz M, Incaudo F, Yamamoto F, et al. Nasal serum, and skin-fixed IgE in perennial rhinitis patients treated with flunisolide. J Allergy Clin Immunol 1978;61:150.
34. Streseman E. Results of bronchial testing in bakers. Acta Allergol 1967;22(Suppl 8):99.
35. Newhouse M, Tagg B, Polock S, et al. An epidemiological study of workers producing enzyme washing powders. Lancet 1970;i:689.
36. Sosman AJ, Schleuter DP, Fink JN, et al. Hypersensitivity to wood dust. N Engl J Med 1969;281:977.
37. Bock SA. Prospective appraisal of complaints of adverse reaction to foods in children during the first three years of life. Pediatrics 1987;79:683.
38. Perlman DS. Chronic rhinitis in children. Clin Rev Allergy 1984;2:197.
39. Siegel SC, Goldstein JD, Swyer WA, et al. Incidence of allergy in persons who have many common colds. Ann Allergy 1952;10:24.
40. Marks MB. Physical signs of allergy on the respiratory tract in children. Ann Allergy 1969;25:310.
41. Ammat-Kohja A. Influence des contraceptifs oranux sur las muquenuse nasal. Rev Laryngol Otol Rhinol (Board) 1971;92:40.
42. Chilla R, Haubrich J. Vasomotorische rhinitis: Eine nebenwirkung homonaler kontrazeption. HNO 1975;23:202.
43. Sorri M, Hortikamen-Sorri AL, Karja J. Rhinitis during pregnancy. Rhinology 1980;18:83.
44. Mabry RL. Intranasal steroid injection during pregnancy. South Med J 1980;73:1176.
45. English GM, Henenway WG, Cundy RI. Surgical treatment of invasive angiofibroma. Arch Otolaryngol 1972;96:312.
46. Rossman CM, Lee RM, Forrest JB, Newhouse M. Nasal ciliary ultrastructure and function in patient with primary ciliary dyskinesia compared with that in normal subjects and in subjects with various respiratory diseases. Annu Rev Respir Dis 984;129:161.
47. Eliasson R, Mossberg B, Cammer P, Afzelius BA. The immotilecilia syndrome: a congenital ciliary abnormality as an etiologic factor in chronic airway infections and male sterility. N Engl J Med 1977;197:1.
48. Afzelius BA. Immotile-cilia syndrome and ciliary abnormalities induced by infection and injury. Am Rev Respir Dis 1981;124:107.
49. McKnee WD. The incidence and familial occurrence of allergy. J Allergy 1966;38:226.

50. Broder I, Higgings MN, Matthews KP, et al. Epidemiology of asthma and allergic rhinitis in a total community, Tecumseh, Michigan. IV. Natural history. J Allergy Clin Immunol 1974;54:10.
51. Broder I, Barlow PP, Horton RJM. The epidemiology of asthma and hayfever in a total community, Tecumseh, Michigan. II. The relationship between asthma and hayfever. J Allergy 1962;33:524.
52. Goodman LS, Gilman A. The pharmacological basis of therapeutics. 6th ed. New York: Macmillan, 1980.
53. Douglus WW. Histamine and serotonin and their antagonists. In: Gilman Ag, Goodman LS, Rall TW, Murad F, eds. Goodman and Gilman's the pharmacological basis of therapeutics. 7th ed. New York: Macmillan, 1985:605.
54. Arrang J, Garbarg M, Lancelot J, et al. Highly potent and selective ligands for histamine H_3 receptors. Nature 1987;327:117.
55. Togias AG, Naclerio RM, Warner J, et al. Demonstration of inhibition of mediator release from human mast cells by azatadine base. JAMA 1986;255:225.
56. Massey WA, Lichtenstein LM. The effects of antihistamines beyond H_1 antagonism in allergic inflammation. J Allergy Clin Immunol 1990;86:1019.
57. Gong H Jr, Lashkin DP, Dauphinee B, et al. Effects of oral cetirizine, a selective H_1 antagonist on allergen and exercise induced bronchoconstriction in subjects with asthma. J Allergy Clin Immunol 1990;85:632.
58. Kemp JP, Buckley CE, Gershwin ME, et al. Multicenter, double-blind placebo controlled trial of terfenadine in seasonal allergic rhinitis and conjunctivitis. Ann Allergy 1985;54:502.
59. Simmons FER. H_1 receptor antagonists: clinical pharmacology and therapeutics. J Allergy Clin Immunol 1989;84:845.
60. Richards DM, Brogden RN, Heel RC, Speight TM, Avery BG. Astemizole: a review of its pharmacodynamic properties and therapeutic efficacy. Drugs 1984;28:38.
61. Surkin EM, Heel RC: Terfenadine: a review of its pharmacodynamic properties and therapeutic efficacy. Drugs 1985;29:34.
62. Loratadine: a new antihistamine. Med Lett 1993;35:71.
63. Barnes CL, McKenzi CA, Webster KD, Poinset-Holmes K. Cetirizine: a new nonsedating antihistamine. Ann Pharmacother 1993;27:464.
64. Cheng HC, Woodward JK. Antihistamine effect of terfenadine, a new piperidine type antihistamine. Drug Dev Res 1982;2:181.
65. Ganteiz DA, Hook RH, Walker BJ, Okerolm RA. Pharmacokinetics and biotransformation studies of terfenadine in man. Arznermittelforshung 1982;32:1185.
66. Simons FE, Simmons KJ. Use of nonsedating antihistamines. In: Lichenstein LM, Fauci AS, eds. Current therapy in allergy, immunology, and rheumatology. 4th ed. Philadelphia: BC Decker 1992:17.
67. Lantin JP, Huguenot C, Perond AR. Effect of astemizole on skin tests with histamine, codeine and allergens. J Allergy Clin Immunol 1988;81:312.
68. Woosley RL, Barby JT, Yeh J, et al. Lack of electrocardiographic effects of cetirizine in healthy humans. J Allergy Clin Immunol 1993;91:258. Abstract.
69. Synder, Solomon H, Snowman AM. Receptor effects of cetirizine. Ann Allergy 1987;59:4.
70. Wood SG, John BA, Chasseared LF, Yeh J, Chung M. The metabolism and pharmaco kinetics of cetirizine in humans. Ann Allergy 1987;59:31.
71. Orr TSG, Jackson DM, Greenwood B, et al. In: Kay AB, ed. Asthma: clinical pharmacology and therapeutic progress. Oxford: Blackwell Scientific Publications, 1986:265.
72. Horowitz JD, Howes LD, Christophilis N, et al. Hypertensive responses induced by phenylpropanolamine in anorectic and decongestant preparations. Lancet 1980;1:60.
73. Schule R, Rangarajan P, Kliewer S, et al. Functional antagonism between oncoprotein c-Jun and the glucocorticoid receptor. Cell 1990;62:1217.
74. Pipkorn U, Proud D, Lichtenstein LM, et al. Inhibition of mediator release in allergic patients by pretreatment with topical glucocorticoids. N Engl J Med 1987;316:1506.
75. Siegel SC. Topical intranasal corticosteroid therapy in asthma. J Allergy Clin Immunol 1987;81:964.
76. Welsh PW, Strickwe WE, Chu CP, et al. Efficacy of beclomethasone nasal solution, flunisolide, and cromolyn in relieving symptoms of ragweed allergy. Mayo Clinic Proc 1987;62:125.
77. Mygind N. Topical steroid treatment for allergic rhinitis and allied conditions. Clin Otolaryngol 1982;7:343.
78. Soderberg-Warner ML. Nasal septal perforation associated with topical corticosteroid spray. J Pediatr 1984;105:840.
79. Schoelzl EP, Menzel ML. Nasal sprays and perforation of the nasal septum. JAMA 1985;253:2046.
80. Spector S, Broncky EA, Grossman J, et al. Clinical evaluation of triamcinolone acetonide nasal aerosol in children with perennial allergic rhinitis. Ann Allergy 1990;64:300.
81. Shaw RJ. Pharmacology of fluticasone propionate. Respir Med 1994;88(Suppl A):5.
82. Mabry RL. Practical applications of intranasal corticosteroid injection. Ear Nose Throat J 1981;60:23.
83. Sjogren I, Johasz J. Ipratropium in the treatment of patients with perennial rhinitis. Allergy 1984;39:457.
84. Borum P, Olsen L, Winther B, Myrind N. Ipratropium nasal spray: a new treatment for rhinorrhea in the common cold. Am Rev Respir Dis 1981;123:418.
85. Pelikan Z, Pelikan-Filipek M. The effect of disodiumcromoglycate and beclomethasone diproprionate on the immediate response of the nasal mucosa to allergic challenge. Ann Allergy 1982;49:283.
86. Coffman DA. A controlled trial of disodium cromoglycate in seasonal allergic rhinitis. Br J Clin Pract 1971;25:403.

87. Jenssen AO. Measurement of resistance to airflow in the nose in a trial with sodium cromoglycate (BP) solution in allergen-induced nasal stenosis. Clin Allergy 1983;3:277.

88. Hasegawa M, Watanabe K. The effect of sodium cromoglycate on the antigen-induced nasal reaction in allergic rhinitis as measured by rhinomanometry and symptomatology. Clin Allergy 1976:6:359.

89. Nelson BL, Jacobs RL. Responses of the nonallergic rhinitis with eosinophilia syndrome to 4% cromolyn sodium nasal solution. J Allergy Clin Immunol 1982;70:125.

90. Okunda M, Ohnishi M, Ohstuka H. The effects of cromolyn sodium on the nasal mast cells. Ann Allergy 1985;55:721.

91. Hillas J, Booth RJ, Somerfield S, et al. A comparative trial of intranasal beclomethasone diproprionate and sodium cromoglycate in patients with chronic perennial rhinitis. Clin Allergy 1980;10:53.

92. Tanilon MK, Strahan EG. Double-blind cross-over trial comparing beclomethasone diproprionate and sodium cromoglycate in perennial allergic rhinitis. Clin Allergy 1980;10:450.

93. Brown HM, Engler C, English JR. A comparative trial of flunisolide and sodium cromoglycate nasal sprays in the treatment of seasonal allergic rhinitis. Clin Allergy 1981;11:169.

94. Pelikan Z, Pelikan EM. The effect of disodium cromoglycate and beclomethasone diproprionate on the immediate response of the nasal mucosa to allergen challenge. Ann Allergy 1982;49:283.

95. Ruhno J, Derburg J, Dolovich J. Intranasal nedocromil sodium in the treatment of ragweed-allergic rhinitis. J Allergy Clin Immunol 1988;81:571.

Allergic Diseases, 5th Edition,
edited by Roy Patterson, Leslie Carroll Grammer, and
Paul A. Greenberger. Lippincott–Raven Publishers, Philadelphia, © 1997.

10

Principles of Immunologic Management of Allergic Diseases Due to Extrinsic Antigens

Leslie C. Grammer and Martha A. Shaughnessy

L.C. Grammer and M. A. Shaughnessy: Division of Allergy-Immunology, Northwestern University Medical School, Chicago, IL 60611.

Pearls for Practitioners
Roy Patterson

- If you are going to use allergen immunotherapy, use it correctly:
   No low-dose therapy
   Proper diagnosis
   No prolonged unnecessary therapy
   No remote therapy
   Use appropriate allergens
- When comparing the cost effectiveness of allergen immunotherapy, consider the months per year of symptoms, the duration of symptoms (which may be for decades), and the continuing cost of medications over the years if immunotherapy is not used.
- Allergen immunotherapy is the only method available now, or in the foreseeable future, of altering the immunologic reactivity of the patient to the allergen.

Three principal modalities are available to treat allergic diseases: avoidance of allergens, pharmacologic intervention, and immunotherapy. Pharmacologic intervention is discussed in the chapters relating to specific allergic diseases. The immunologic interventions—avoidance of allergens and immunotherapy—are the subjects of this chapter.

AVOIDANCE OF ANTIGENS

Allergic diseases result from antigen–antibody interaction that subsequently releases mediators and cytokines that affect target organs. If exposure to the antigen or allergen can be avoided, no antigen–antibody interaction takes place, and thus no allergic disease manifestations occur. Consequently, the first tenet of allergic management is to remove the allergen if possible.

In the case of certain allergens, removal can be accomplished readily. For instance, an individual who is sensitive to cat or dog dander or other animal protein should not have the animal in the home if complete control of symptoms is the goal of management. Another example is an individual who is sensitive to certain foods or drugs. That individual should avoid ingesting those agents.

House Dust Mite

In the case of house dust mite allergy, complete avoidance is not possible in most climates, but the degree of exposure to this allergen can be diminished. The following is a list of measures to control exposure to house dust mites[1–3]:

Encase the mattress, box springs, and pillow in allergen-nonpermeable cover.
Wash bed linens in water that is 54°C (130°F) or hotter.
Reduce indoor humidity to 50% or less.
Replace carpets with polished floors such as linoleum, hardwood, and terrazzo (since carpets are reservoirs for mites). This is especially important in the bedroom.
Do not sleep on upholstered furniture.

Mold Spores

Exposure to mold spores also may be reduced by environmental precautions.[3] The patient should avoid entering barns, mowing grass, or raking leaves to avoid exposure to the the high concentrations of mold spores associated with these places and activities. Indoor molds are particularly prominent in humid environments. Bathrooms, kitchens, and basements require adequate ventilation and frequent cleaning. If the patient's home has a humidifier, it should be cleaned regularly so that mold does not have an opportunity to grow. Humidity should ideally be 25% to 50%. Certain foods and beverages such as aged cheese, canned tomatoes, and beer may produce symptoms in some mold-sensitive patients. These foods and beverages should be avoided in highly sensitive persons.

Other Inhalant Allergens

Other airborne allergens such as tree, grass, and ragweed pollens cannot be avoided except by staying out of geographic areas where these plants pollinate. For most individuals, this is impractical socially and economically. Air conditioning and air-filtration systems reduce but do not eliminate exposure to these pollens and to dust and mold spores.

IMMUNOTHERAPY

Immunotherapy is known by various other names: "allergy shots" to the lay public, and hyposensitization or desensitization in older medical literature. These terms are not strictly correct in that they imply a mechanism that has not been proven. Desensitization applies in clinical situations in which antigens are administered in a few hours in sufficient quantity to rapidly neutralize available IgE antibody.[4] This type of true desensitization may be necessary in treating patients with allergy to an antibiotic. It is not the operative mechanism in immunotherapy.

Immunotherapy, a term introduced by Norman and coworkers,[5] does not imply a mechanism. It consists of injections of increasing amounts of allergen to which the patient has type I immediate hypersensitivity. As a result of these injections, the patient is able to tolerate exposure to the allergen with fewer symptoms. The mechanism by which this improvement occurs has not been definitely established. However, over the years, several mechanisms have been postulated to account for the improvement. Immunotherapy was first used by Noon and Freeman,[6] who observed that pollen was the etiologic agent of seasonal rhinitis and that immunization was effective in treating various infectious diseases, including tetanus and diphtheria.

Immunotherapy was used empirically by physicians over the ensuing 40 years. Cooke[7] observed that cutaneous reactivity was not obliterated by allergy injections. Cooke also discovered a serum factor, which he called *blocking antibody*, in the serum of patients receiving immunotherapy.[8] This serum factor could inhibit the passive transfer of allergic antibody described by Prausnitz and Küstner. However, there was not a constant relation between blocking antibody titers and symptom relief.

The first controlled study of the efficacy of immunotherapy was published in 1949.[9] Within a short time, in vitro techniques were developed to objectively assess the immunologic results of immunotherapy. Many immunologic changes occur as a result of immunotherapy[10,11]:

Increase in allergen-specific IgG
Decrease in allergen-specific IgE after prolonged therapy
Decrease in seasonal rise of specific IgE
Increase in antiidiotypic antibodies
Decrease in allergen-induced basophil histamine release
Increase in T-suppressor cells
Decrease in histamine-releasing factors
Change of CD4+ cells from the Th2 to the Th1 phenotype

Which changes are responsible for the efficacy of immunotherapy is unknown.

In general, immunotherapy is indicated for clinically significant disease when the usual methods of avoidance and medication are inadequate to control symptoms.[3,10] Specific indications for allergen immunotherapy are as follows:

IgE mediated disease (allergic rhinitis or extrinsic asthma)
Significant symptomatology in terms of duration and severity
Avoidance is not possible
Pharmacologic therapy yields unsatisfactory results
High-potency extract and appropriate dosage schedule are available.

Immunotherapy is considered to be effective in ameliorating symptoms of allergic rhinitis, *Hymenoptera* sensitivity, and extrinsic asthma. These topics are discussed in Chapters 9, 12, and 22, respectively. Many studies report the efficacy of immunotherapy in treating allergic rhinitis or extrinsic asthma caused by various inhalants, including ragweed, grass, and tree pollens, mold spores, and house dust mites[12–20] (Table 10-1). Assessment of efficacy in these studies is difficult because the diseases being treated are chronic and have variations based on geography, climate, and individuals. Assessments generally are made from subjective daily symptom and medication reports by the patient. In some studies, objective clinical eval-

TABLE 10-1. Double-blind placebo-controlled allergen immunotherapy studies reporting efficacy

Study	Allergen	No. of patients	No. of controls
Allergen Rhinitis			
Norman et al.[12] 1968	Ragweed	29	27
Ortolani et al.[13] 1984	Grass	8	7
Pence et al.[14] 1976	Mountain cedar	17	15
McHugh et al.[15] 1990	House dust mite	20	30
Horst et al.[16] 1990	*Alternaria*	13	11
Asthma			
Reid et al.[17] 1986	Grass	9	9
Rak et al.[18] 1990	Birch	20	20
Bousquet et al.[19] 1988	House dust mite	171	44
Malling et al.[20] 1986	*Cladosporium*	11	11

uation by physicians, by nasal or bronchial challenge, or both also were a part of the assessment. A metaanalysis of immunotherapy studies in asthma concluded that immunotherapy was efficacious.[21]

Immunotherapy is not indicated in food allergy or chronic urticaria, nor is evidence sufficient to support using a bacterial vaccine.[3,22]

Choice of Allergens

The aeroallergens that are commonly used in immunotherapy of allergic rhinitis or extrinsic asthma include extracts of house dust mites, mold spores, and pollen from trees, grasses, and weeds. The pollen species vary to some extent with geographic location, and this information can be obtained from Chapter 7. Because the population is mobile, it is usual practice to skin test and treat with common, important allergens outside of a physician's geographic location.[23] For instance, there is no Bermuda grass in Chicago. However, it is a potent allergen in the southern United States. Thus, it is used in skin testing and treating patients in Chicago. In the allergic evaluation, a patient undergoes skin testing with various allergens. Radioallergosorbent tests and other in vitro assays are less sensitive and more expensive than skin testing, and therefore should be reserved for situations in which skin testing is unsatisfactory.[24] If the patient's history of exacerbations temporally corresponds to the skin test reactivity, the patient probably will benefit from immunotherapy. For example, a patient having a positive reaction on the grass skin test, rhinorrhea, and palatal itching in May and June in the Midwest will benefit from grass pollen immunotherapy. In contrast, a patient with an isolated positive grass skin test result and with perennial symptoms of rhinorrhea and nasal congestion probably has vasomotor rhinitis, and will not benefit from immunotherapy.

Many patients have allergic rhinitis or extrinsic asthma from various animal danders. Avoidance is the most appropriate therapeutic maneuver for such patients. In rare instances, avoidance is unacceptable; for example, a blind person with a seeing eye dog, or a veterinarian whose livelihood depends on animal exposure. In these rare instances, immunotherapy with animal dander may be given.[25,26] Patients who are sensitive to dander extracts may have difficulties with local or systemic reactions, so that it is difficult to attain clinically efficacious doses.[27]

Technical Aspects

Allergen Extract Potency and Dosage Schedules

With some exceptions, the contents of currently available allergenic extracts are not standardized and their potency is not established. In general, they are simply identified by the taxonomic classification of the source material. There are few reference preparations available, and they are not routinely used by manufacturers to produce consistent extracts.[28] However, the Food and Drug Administration has reference preparations available for eight common grasses and is moving toward requiring extract manufacturers to standardize commercial preparations. Allergen extracts are quantified in several ways using different unitage systems (Table 10-2).

Notice that neither of the common unitages, protein nitrogen unit (PNU), or weight per volume (W/V) are necessarily indicators of potency.[28] Potency can be measured practically in various ways: cutaneous endpoint titration,[28] radioimmunoassay inhibition,[29] or content of a known major allergen like antigen E (*Amb a* I) in ragweed,[30] *Rye* I in certain grasses,[31] *Der p* I in mite extracts,[32] or *Fel d* I in cat extracts.[33] Characterizing extracts by crossed immuno-electrophoresis or isoelectric focusing is useful for standardization.[34] Standard extracts such as short ragweed[35] and *Dermatophagoides pteronyssinus*[36] have been developed by the Allergen Standardization Subcommittee of the International Union of Immunologic Societies. These extracts have been extensively tested for allergen content and immunologic properties and have been assigned an arbitrary unitage, international units (IUs). Until reference standards and exact quantification of potency can be established for all extracts, such less exact methods as W/V will continue to be used.

Allergen extracts may be given individually or may be mixed in one vial. That is, a patient receiving immunotherapy to grass pollen and tree pollen could receive two injections, one of grass and one of tree, or could receive one injection containing both grass and tree pollens. The latter usually is preferable for patient comfort.

Three forms of immunotherapy have been used: coseasonal, preseasonal, and perennial. Coseasonal therapy is the least satisfactory of the three. It is sometimes used when the patient first presents during the season in which the allergic symptoms occur. There is no current indication for this type of therapy.

Preseasonal treatment is begun 3 to 6 months before the season during which the patient has allergic symptoms. Injections are given every 4 to 7 days, before the onset of the season, until the dose of maximum tolerance is reached. Immunotherapy is then resumed the following year at the same time. Coseasonal and preseasonal therapies are mentioned for historical perspective; they are not recommended forms of immunotherapy.

TABLE 10-2. Allergy extract unitage

Unitage	Derivation of unit
Weight-to-volume ratio (W/V)	Weight (g) extracted per volume (mL)
Protein nitrogen unit (PNU)	0.01 µg of protein nitrogen
Biologic allergy unit (BAU)	Based on average skin test endpoint of allergic individuals
RAST allergy unit (RAU)	Based on RAST inhibition using pooled allergic sera
Biologic unit (BU)	Based on skin test endpoint relative to histamine
International unit (IU)	Based on in vitro assays relative to WHO standard allergenic preparations

RAST, radioallergosorbent test; WHO, World Health Organization.

Perennial therapy is the recommended form. It consists of year-round injection of antigens to which the patient is sensitive. Treatment with higher doses of pollen extracts results in better long-term reduction of clinical symptoms and greater immunologic changes than low-dose therapy. Perennial treatment produces a higher cumulative dose of antigen than that achieved with preseasonal or coseasonal therapy, and appears to be responsible for a longer and more significant clinical response. Dosage based on the Rinkel technique, a low-dose protocol, is not effective.[37]

There are no clear data as to the optimal length of time immunotherapy should be continued. If patients are maintained on immunotherapy and show improvement through three annual pollen seasons, most will continue to maintain improvement even when their injections are discontinued.

The most common method of administering perennial immunotherapy is by using a dose schedule similar to that in Table 10-3. Rarely, sensitive patients must begin at 1:100,000 W/V. The injections are given weekly until the patient reaches the maintenance dose of 0.50 mL of 1:100 W/V. At that point, the interval between injections may be gradually increased to 2

TABLE 10-3. Allergy treatment tentative dosage schedule

Date	Extract concentration (W/V)	Extract concentration (PNU/mL)	Volume	Remarks
–	1:10,000	100 PNU/mL	0.05	–
			0.10	–
			0.15	–
			0.20	–
			0.30	–
			0.40	–
			0.50	–
–	1:1000	1000 PNU/mL	0.05	–
			0.10	–
			0.20	–
			0.30	–
			0.40	–
			0.50	–
–	1:100	10,000 PNU/mL	0.05	–
			0.10	–
			0.15	–
			0.20	–
			0.25	–
			0.30	–
			0.35	–
			0.40	–
			0.45	–
			0.50	–

PNU, protein nitrogen unit; W/V, weight-to-volume ratio.

weeks, 3 weeks, and ultimately 4 weeks. When a new vial of extract is given to a patient on a maintenance dose of 0.50 mL of 1:100 W/V, the volume should be reduced to about 0.35 mL and increased by 0.05 mL each injection to 0.50 mL. The reason for this is that the new vial may be more potent. Some patients have an achievable maintenance dose lower than the standard shown in Table 10-3. Other types of dosage schedules have been published. In rush immunotherapy schedules, the starting doses are similar to those in Table 10-3, but patients receive injections more frequently, at least twice a week. In cluster immunotherapy schedules, the initial dosages are similar to Table 10-3 and the visit frequency usually is weekly; however, at each visit more than one injection is administered, with the interval between injections varying from 30 minutes to 2 hours. The advantage of both rush and cluster regimens is that the maintenance dose can be achieved more quickly; the cluster regimen is especially useful in treating a patient who resides at a significant distance from the physician's office. The disadvantage of both cluster and rush regimens is that the reaction rate is probably higher than with more conventional schedules.[38] For patients on those regimens, initial doses from new vials should also be reduced. Allergen extracts should be kept refrigerated at 4°C for retention of maximum potency. If a vial freezes or heats above 4°C, it should be discarded because the allergen may be altered.

A radioallergosorbent test–based method for determining patient sensitivity and first injection doses has been proposed.[39] However, evidence does not support the use of this expensive technique instead of history and properly interpreted results from skin tests.[40] In a position statement, the American Academy of Allergy and Immunology notes that in vitro tests may be abused.[41] Abuses of particular concern included the screening of unselected populations and the use of in vitro test results for translation into immunotherapy prescriptions without an appropriate clinical evaluation.[41]

Procedures for Injections

Immunotherapy injections should be given only after the patient, the patient's dose schedule, and the patient's vial have been carefully identified, because improper dosing is a common cause of allergic reactions to immunotherapy. Injections should be given with a 1-mL syringe so that the appropriate dose can be given accurately. The injection should be subcutaneous with a 26-gauge needle. Before injecting material, the plunger of the syringe should be withdrawn; if blood appears, the needle and syringe should be withdrawn and discarded. Another needle and syringe should be used for the injection. Patients should be observed at least 20 minutes after their injections for evidence of reactions.

Reactions

Small local reactions with erythema and induration less than 20 mm are common and are of no consequence. Large local reactions and generalized reactions —rhinitis, conjunctivitis, urticaria, angioedema, bronchospasm, and hypotension—are cause for concern. Large local reactions generally can be treated with antihistamines and local application of ice. Rarely, significant swelling occurs such that 2 days of oral steroids are indicated. Generalized reactions consisting of bronchospasm, angioedema, or urticaria usually respond to 0.3 mL of 1:1000 epinephrine subcutaneously. The dose for children weighing up to 30 kg is 0.01 mL/kg. This may be repeated every 10 or 15 minutes for up to three doses. If the patient has laryngeal edema and is unresponsive to epinephrine, intubation or tracheostomy is necessary. If the patient has hypotension unresponsive to epinephrine, intravenous fluids and pressors are necessary. Physicians who administer allergen injections must be prepared to treat serious anaphylactic reactions. If a patient has a large local reaction, the dose should be reduced or repeated, depending on clinical judgment. If a systemic reaction occurs, the dose should be reduced to approximately one tenth the dose at which the reaction occurred before subsequent slow increase. The management of local and systemic reactions is outlined in Table 10-4.

Because of local or systemic reactions, some patients are unable to tolerate the usual maintenance doses and must be maintained on a smaller dose, for instance, 0.20 mL of 1:100 W/V.

The safety of immunotherapy has been questioned. In one report, five of nine patients who developed polyarteritis nodosa had received immunotherapy.[42] However, asthma may be the first symptom of polyarteritis nodosa, and the latter disease may have been present subclinically before the start of the injection therapy. If the polyarteritis nodosa was directly related to immunotherapy, an immunologic mechanism must be postulated, the likely one being antigen–antibody complex damage. However, the amount of antigen used in standard immunotherapy is far less than that producing antigen–antibody complex damage in experimental animals.

Another study compares a group of atopic patients who received immunotherapy for at least 5 years with a group of atopic patients who did not have injection therapy.[43] The treated group did not show an increased incidence of autoimmune, collagen vascular, or lymphoproliferative disease. There were no adverse effects on immunologic reactivity as measured by several laboratory immunologic tests. Appropriate immunotherapy is accepted as a safe therapy.

TABLE 10-4. Management of reactions to immunotherapy

Local Reactions

1. Oral antihistamine

2. Local application of cold

3. Review of dosage schedule

Systemic Reactions*

1. 0.01 mL/kg up to 0.2 mL aqueous adrenalin, 1:1000 SQ, at site of immunotherapy injection to slow absorption of antigen

2. 0.01 mL/kg up to 0.3 mL aqueous adrenalin, 1:1000 SQ, at another site

3. Diphenhydramine IV or IM, 1.25 mg/kg to 50 mg

4. Tourniquet above the site of injection of allergen

5. Specific reaction

   Bronchospasm: intravenous aminophylline 4 mg/kg up to 500 mg given over 20 min, aqueous hydrocortisone 5 mg/kg up to 200 mg, oxygen

   Laryngeal edema: oxygen, intubation, tracheostomy

   Hypotension: vasopressors, fluids, corticosteroids

   Cardiac arrest: resuscitation, sodium bicarbonate, defibrillation, antiarrhythmia medications

6. Review of dosage schedule

SQ, subcutaneously; IV, intravenously; IM, intramuscularly.
*Includes generalized erythema, urticaria, angioedema, bronchospasm, laryngeal edema, shock, and cardiac arrest.

Special Considerations

Pregnancy

Patients doing well on maintenance doses of immunotherapy who become pregnant can be continued on immunotherapy.[44] However, if a pregnant patient is not on immunotherapy, therapy may be started with due caution.

Other Drugs

Because patients who receive immunotherapy may require treatment with epinephrine, the risks and benefits of concomitant drug therapy must be considered. For example, the *Physicians' Desk Reference* cautions that monoamine oxidase inhibitors should not be administered in conjunction with sympathomimetics.[45] Also, beta-blocking agents may make the treatment of anaphylaxis more difficult in some cases.[46]

Failure

If a patient has been on maintenance doses of immunotherapy for 12 months and has no improvement, the clinical allergy problem should be reassessed. Perhaps a new allergen such as an animal has been introduced into the environment. Perhaps the patient has developed new sensitivities that are not being treated with immunotherapy. Perhaps the patient's disease is not allergic in origin but is nonallergic rhinitis or nonallergic asthma, neither of which is altered by immunotherapy. Or, the patient may have misunderstood the benefits of immunotherapy. That is, symptom reduction, not symptom eradication, is all that can be expected from immunotherapy. The patient must understand this at the initiation of therapy.

Alternate Administration Routes

Besides using the subcutaneous route to administer allergen, several other routes have been suggested. Local nasal immunotherapy consists of extracts that are sprayed into the nasal cavity by the patient at specified dosages at specified time intervals. Clinical successes have been reported, but local side effects may be bothersome, making local nasal immunotherapy relatively unpalatable.[47]

Oral immunotherapy with birch pollen in capsules has been reported.[48] Sublingual immunotherapy in a trial of low-dose house dust mite extract has been reported to be efficacious.[49] In a trial of sublingual immunotherapy with a standardized cat extract, efficacy was not demonstrated.[50] International consensus is that no convincing controlled studies show effectiveness in asthma.[3]

Modified Allergens

Although immunotherapy has demonstrated efficacy, it is still a long, expensive process and there is a risk of severe systemic reactions. Administration of purified antigens, for instance antigen E of short ragweed,[12] was tried as a possible improvement of immunotherapy.

Improvements similar to those obtained with whole extracts but with fewer reactions and injections were found with antigen E. The expense of the antigen E purification process has made this sort of administration impractical. Recombinant allergens have also been produced.[51] At present there are two basic avenues of research to improve immunotherapy. The first is to attempt to inhibit IgE antibody production to a given allergen. There are several compounds devised individually by Katz,[52] Sehon and Lee,[53] and Takatsu and colleagues[54] that have been successful in animal models, but not in humans. Immunotherapy with T cell epitope containing peptides has been reported to induce T cell anergy and clinical efficacy.[55,56]

Administration of a neuropeptide, substance P with allergens, has reduced immediate cutaneous and airway responses in a subhuman primate model.[1,57] Human studies are underway to assess this promising therapy.

The other avenue is to reduce allergenicity of allergens while maintaining immunogenicity.

Alum Precipitation

The absorption of the antigen from the injection site can be slowed by using an aluminum-precipitated, buffered, aqueous extract of pollen antigen. Patients receiving this extract have shown significant clinical response and immunologic changes with fewer injections and reactions.[58]

Alum-Precipitated, Pyridine-Extracted Pollen Extracts (Allpyral)

This material is prepared by using pyridine to extract the pollen antigen before alum precipitation. However, several reports have questioned its antigenicity.[59]

Repository Therapy

Aqueous antigens were used in a mineral oil emulsion to delay the absorption of antigen from the injection site.[60] Problems with this method of treatment include persistent nodules, sterile abscesses, and granulomas. The induction of tumors in animals by the mineral oil has contraindicated this program, and mineral oil emulsions are not licensed in the United States for human use. Use of liposomes as a form of repository therapy has been considered.[61]

Allergoids

Marsh and coworkers[62] treated allergens with formalin to alter antigenic determinants. This reduced the allergenicity of the original extract and the skin test reactivity. Data demonstrate efficacy of grass allergens equivalent to that of standard allergy therapy in grass hay fever.[63]

Glutaraldehyde-Modified–Tyrosine-Adsorbed Extracts

Glutaraldehyde-modified–tyrosine-adsorbed short ragweed extracts have been reported to result in only a modest reduction in symptoms.[64]

Polymerized Allergens

Patterson and coworkers[65] have polymerized ragweed and other pollen proteins with glutaraldehyde. Because there are fewer molecules of polymer on a weight basis compared with monomer allergens, there are fewer molecules to react with histamine-containing cells. There are data that demonstrate efficacy of polymer equivalent to monomer with fewer injections and fewer systemic reactions. There are also data demonstrating efficacy and safety in a multiinstitutional trial[66] comparing polymerized ragweed with no treatment and in two double-blind histamine placebo-controlled trials.[67,68]

REFERENCES

1. Platts-Mills TAE, Chapman M. Dust mites: immunology, allergic disease, and environmental control. J Allergy Clin Immunol 1987;80:755.
2. Dorward AJ, Colloff MJ, McKay NS, McSharry C, Thomson NC. Effect of house dust mite avoidance measures on adult atopic asthma. Thorax 1988;43:98.
3. NHLBI 1992 international consensus report on diagnosis and management of asthma. NIH publ no. 92-3091. Bethesda, MD: NHLBI.
4. Patterson R, Mellies CJ, Roberts M. Immunologic reactions against insulin. II. IgE anti-insulin, insulin allergy and combined IgE and IgG immunologic insulin resistance. J Immunol 1973;110:1135.
5. Norman P. The clinical significance of IgE. Hosp Pract 1975;10:41.
6. Freeman J, Noon L. Further observations on the treatment of hayfever by hypodermic inoculations of pollen vaccine. Lancet 1911;ii:814.
7. Cooke RA. Studies in specific hypersensitiveness. IX. On the phenomenon of hyposensitization (the clinically lessened sensitiveness of allergy). J Immunol 1922;7:219.
8. Cooke RA, Barnard JH, Hebald S, et al. Serologic evidence of immunity with coexisting sensitization in a type of human allergy (hayfever). J Exp Med 1935;62:733.
9. Bruun E. Control examination of the specificity of specific desensitization in asthma. Acta Allergol 1949;2:122.
10. Immunotherapy Subcommittee of the European Academy of Allergology and Clinical Immunology. Immunotherapy. Allergy 1988;43(Suppl 6):292.
11. Secrist H, Cheben CJ, Wen Y, Marshall JD, Umetsu DT. Allergen immunotherapy decreases interleukin 4 production in CD4+ T cells from allergic individuals. J Exp Med 1993;178:2123.
12. Norman PS, Winkenwerder WL, Lichtenstein LM. Immunotherapy of hay fever with ragweed antigen E: comparison with whole pollen extract and placebos. J Allergy 1968;42:93.
13. Ortolani C, Pestorello E, Moss RB. Grass pollen immunotherapy: a single year double blind placebo controlled study in patients with grass pollen induced asthma and rhinitis. J Allergy Clin Immunol 1984;73:283.
14. Ponce HL, Mitchell DQ, Greely RL, Updegraff BR, Selfridge HA. Immunotherapy for mountain cedar pollinosis: a double-blind controlled study. J Allergy Clin Immunol 1976;58:39.
15. McHugh SM, Lavelle B, Kemeny DM, Patel S, Ewan PW. A placebo controlled trial of immunotherapy with two extracts of *Dermatophagoides pteronyssinus* in allergic rhinitis, comparing clinical outcome with antigen specific IgE, IgG, and IgG subclasses. J Allergy Clin Immunol 1990;86:521.
16. Horst M, Hejjaoui A, Horst V, Michel FB, Bousquet J. Double-blind placebo controlled rush immunotherapy with a standardized *Alternaria* extract. J Allergy Clin Immunol 1990;85:460.
17. Reid MJ, Moss RB, Hsu YP, Kwasnicki JM, Commerford TM, Nelson BL. Seasonal asthma in northern California: allergic causes and efficacy of immunotherapy. J Allergy Clin Immunol 1986;78:590.
18. Rak S, Hakanson L, Venge P. Immunotherapy abrogates the generation of eosinophil and neutrophil chemotactic activity during pollen season. J Allergy Clin Immunol 1990;86:706.
19. Bousquet J, Hejjaoui A, Clauzel A-M, et al. Specific immunotherapy with a standardized *Dermatophagoides pteronyssinus* extract. II. Prediction of efficacy of immunotherapy. J Allergy Clin Immunol 1988;82:971.
20. Malling HJ, Dreborg S, Weeke B. Diagnosis and immunotherapy of mould allergy. V. Clinical efficacy and side effects of immunotherapy with *Cladosporium herbarum*. Allergy 1986;41:507.
21. Abramson MJ, Puy RM, Weiner JM. Is allergen immunotherapy effective in asthma? A meta-analysis of randomized controlled trials. Am J Respir Crit Care Med 1995;151:969.
22. Bukantz SC, Lockey RF. Diagnostic tests and hyposensitization therapy in asthma. In: Weiss EB, Segal MS, eds. Bronchial asthma. Boston: Little, Brown, 1975:613.
23. Schatz M. An approach to diagnosis and treatment in the migrant allergic population. J Allergy Clin Immunol 1977;59:254.
24. American Academy of Allergy. Statement by executive committee. J Allergy Clin Immunol 1980;66:431.
25. Sundin B, Lilja G, Graff-Lonnevig V, et al. Immunotherapy with partially purified and standardized animal dander extracts. I. Clinical results from double-blind study on patients with animal dander asthma. J Allergy Clin Immunol 1986;77:478.

26. Van Metre TE Jr, Marsh DG, Adkinson NF Jr, et al. Immunotherapy for cat asthma. J Allergy Clin Immunol 1988;82:1055.

27. Ohman JL, Findlay SR, Leitermann KM. Immunotherapy in cat induced asthma: double blind trial with evaluation of both *in vivo* and *in vitro* responses. J Allergy Clin Immunol 1984;74:230.

28. Adolphson CR, Gleich GJ, Yunginger JW. Standardization of allergens. In: Rose NR, Friedman H, eds. Manual of clinical immunology. Washington, DC: American Society for Microbiology, 1986:652.

29. Gleich GJ, Larson JB, Jones RT, Baer H. Measurement of the potency of allergy extracts by their inhibitory capacities in the radioallergosorbent test. J Allergy Clin Immunol 1974;53:158.

30. Baer H, Godfrey H, Maloney CJ, Norman PS, Lichtenstein LM. The potency and antigen E content of commercially prepared ragweed extracts. J Allergy 1970;45:347.

31. Baer H, Maloney CJ, Norman PS, Marsh DG. The potency and group I antigen content of six commercially prepared grass pollen extracts. J Allergy Clin Immunol 1974;54:157.

32. Bousquet J, Calvayrac P, Guerin B, et al. Immunotherapy with a standardized *Dermatophagoides pteronyssinus* extract. J Allergy Clin Immunol 1985;76:734.

33. Van Metre TE Jr, Marsh DG, Adkinson NF Jr, et al. Immunotherapy decreases skin sensitivity to cat extract. J Allergy Clin Immunol 1989;83:888.

34. Lowenstein H. Quantitative immunoelectrophoretic methods as a tool for the analysis and isolation of allergens. Prog Allergy 1978;25:1.

35. Helm RM, Gauerke MB, Baer H, et al. Production and testing of an international reference standard of short ragweed pollen extract. J Allergy Clin Immunol 1984;73:790.

36. Ford A, Seagroatt V, Platts-Mills TAE, Lowenstein H. A collaborative study on the first international standard of *Dermatophagoides pteronyssinus* (house-dust mite) extract. J Allergy Clin Immunol 1985;75:676.

37. Hirsch SR, Kalbfleisch JH, Golbert TM, et al. Rinkel injection therapy: a multicenter controlled study. J Allergy Clin Immunol 1981;68:133.

38. Van Metre TE Jr, Adkinson NF Jr, Amodio FJ, et al. A comparison of immunotherapy schedules for injection treatment of ragweed hay fever. J Allergy Clin Immunol 1982;69:181.

39. Fadal RG, Nalebuff DJ. A study of optimum dose immunotherapy in pharmacological treatment failures. Arch Otolaryngol 1980;106:38.

40. Adkinson NR Jr. The radioallergosorbent test: uses and abuses. J Allergy Clin Immunol 1980;65:1.

41. Position Statement. The use of in vitro tests for IgE antibody in the specific diagnosis of IgE mediated disorders and in the formulation of allergen immunotherapy. J Allergy Clin Immunol 1992;90:263.

42. Phanupak P, Kohler PF. Recent advances in allergic vasculitis. Adv Allergy Pulmon Dis 1978;5:19.

43. Levinson AI, Summers RJ, Lawley TJ, Evans R III, Frank MM. Evaluation of the adverse effects of long term hyposensitization. J Allergy Clin Immunol 1978;62:109.

44. Metzger WJ, Turner E, Patterson R. The safety of immunotherapy during pregnancy. J Allergy Clin Immunol 1978;61:268.

45. Physicians' desk reference. 50th ed. Oradell, NJ: Medical Economics Data, 1996.

46. American Academy of Allergy. Position statement: beta-adrenergic blockers, immunotherapy, and skin testing. J Allergy Clin Immunol 1989;84:129.

47. Georgitis JW, Nickelsen JA, Wypych JI, Kane JH, Reisman RE. Local nasal immunotherapy: efficacy of low-dose aqueous ragweed extract. J Allergy Clin Immunol 1985;75:496.

48. Taudorf E, Laursen LC, Lanner A, et al. Oral immunotherapy in birch pollen hay fever. J Allergy Clin Immunol 1987;80:153.

49. Scadding GK, Brostoff J. Low dose sublingual therapy in patients with allergic rhinitis due to house dust mite. Clin Allergy 1986;16:483.

50. Nelson HS, Opperheimer J, Vatsio GA, Buchmeier A. A double-blind, placebo-controlled evaluation of sublingual immunotherapy with standardized cat extract. J Allergy Clin Immunol 1993;92:229.

51. Roberts AM, Van Ree R, Cardy SM, Bevan LJ, Walker MR. Recombinant pollen allergens from *Dactylis glomerata*. Immunology 1992;76:389.

52. Katz DH. Lymphocyte differentiation, recognition and regulation. New York: Academic Press, 1977:648.

53. Sehon AH, Lee WY: Suppression of immunoglobulin E antibodies with modified allergens. J Allergy Clin Immunol 1979;64:242.

54. Takatsu K, Ishizaka K, King TP. Immunogenic properties of modified antigen E. J Immunol 1975;115:1469.

55. Schad VC, Garman RD, Greenstein JL. The potential use of T cell epitopes to alter the immune response. Semin Immunol 1991;3:217.

56. O'Hehir RE, Hoyne GF, Thomas WR, Lamb JR. House dust mite allergy: from T cell epitopes to immunotherapy. Eur J Clin Invest 1993;23:763.

57. Patterson R, Harris KE. Substance P and IgE-mediated allergy: reduction of rhesus IgE antibody after aerosol exposure to substance P and allergen. Allergy Proc 1993;14:53.

58. Norman PS, Lichtenstein LM. Comparisons of alum-precipitated and unprecipitated aqueous ragweed pollen extracts in the treatment of hayfever. J Allergy Clin Immunol 1978;61:384.

59. Reisman RE, Arbesman CE. Clinical studies of two ragweed preparations: "purified" delta and Allpyral. Int Arch Allergy Appl Immunol 1965;28:353.

60. Loveless MH. Repository immunization in pollen allergy. J Immunol 1957;79:68.

61. Walls AF. Liposomes for allergy immunotherapy? Clin Exp Allergy 1992;22:1.

62. Marsh DG, Lichtenstein LM, Campbell DH. Studies on allergoids prepared from naturally occurring allergens. I. Assay of allergenicity and antigenicity of formalinized rye group I component. Immunology 1970;18:705.

63. Bousquet J, Hejjaoui A, Soussana M, Michel FB. Double-blind placebo controlled immunotherapy with mixed grass-pollen allergoids. J Allergy Clin Immunol 1990;85:490.

64. Metzger WJ, Dorminey HC, Richerson HB, Weiler JM, Donnelly A, Moran D. Clinical and immunologic evaluation of glutaraldehyde-modified, tyrosine-adsorbed short ragweed extract: a double-blind, placebo controlled trial. J Allergy Clin Immunol 1981;68:442.

65. Patterson R, Suszko IM, McIntyre FC. Polymerized ragweed antigen E. J Immunol 1973;110:1402.

66. Hendrix SG, Patterson R, Zeiss CR, et al. A multi-institutional trial of polymerized whole ragweed for immunotherapy of ragweed allergy. J Allergy Clin Immunol 1980;66:486.

67. Grammer LC, Zeiss CR, Suszko, Shaughnessy MA, Patterson R. A double-blind placebo-controlled trial of polymerized whole ragweed for immunotherapy of ragweed allergy. J Allergy Clin Immunol 1982;69:494.

68. Grammer LC, Shaughnessy MA, Bernhard MI, et al. The safety and activity of polymerized ragweed: a double-blind, placebo-controlled trial in 81 patients with ragweed rhinitis. J Allergy Clin Immunol 1977;80:177.

Allergic Diseases, 5th Edition,
edited by Roy Patterson, Leslie Carroll Grammer, and
Paul A. Greenberger. Lippincott–Raven Publishers, Philadelphia, © 1997.

11

Allergic Diseases of the Eye and Ear

Phillip L. Lieberman and Michael S. Blaiss

*P.L. Lieberman: Division of Allergy and Immunology,
University of Tennessee College of Medicine, Cordova, TN 38018.
M.S. Blaiss: Department of Pediatrics,
University of Tennessee, Memphis, TN 38105.*

Pearls for Practitioners
Roy Patterson

- Ocular allergy may be made worse by wearing contact lenses.
- Allergic conjunctivitis may be markedly improved by treating the associated allergic rhinitis with topical nasal corticosteroids. This may result from improved tear flow through the nasal lacrimal duct.
- Professional singers who have intermittent or chronic eustachian tube obstruction may have serious interference with their professional career. Treating allergic rhinitis in these patients should be intense.
- People who must be in committee meetings, courtrooms, or classrooms also require intensive treatment.
- Dermatitis around the eyes is not caused by aeroallergens. Look for contact allergens, especially nail polish.
- Bilateral, persistent, symmetric puffiness beneath the eyes in middle-aged women is not caused by allergy, but is part of the normal aging process. If the patient is unhappy, refer her for cosmetic surgery.

THE EYE

The allergic eye diseases are contact dermatoconjunctivitis, acute allergic conjunctivitis, vernal conjunctivitis, and atopic keratoconjunctivitis (allergic eye diseases associated with atopic dermatitis). Several other conditions mimic allergic disease and should be considered in any patient presenting with conjunctivitis. These include the blepharoconjunctivitis associated with staphylococcal infection, seborrhea and rosacea, acute viral conjunctivitis, chlamydial conjunctivitis, keratoconjunctivitis sicca, herpes simplex keratitis, giant papillary conjunctivitis, and the floppy eye syndrome. Each of these entities is discussed in relation to the differential diagnosis of allergic conjunctivitis. The allergic conditions themselves are emphasized.

In addition to the systematic discussion of these diseases, because the chapter is written for the nonophthalmologist, an anatomic sketch of the eye (Fig. 11-1) is included.

Diseases Involving the External Eye Surfaces

Contact Dermatitis and Dermatoconjunctivitis

Because the skin of the eyelid is thin (0.55 mm), it is particularly prone to develop both immune and irritant contact dermatitis. When the causative agent has contact with the conjunctiva and the lid, a dermatoconjunctivitis occurs.

Clinical Presentation

Contact dermatitis and dermatoconjunctivitis affect women more commonly than men because women use cosmetics more frequently. Vesiculation may occur early, but by the time the patient seeks care the lids usually appear thickened, red, and chronically inflamed. If the conjunctiva is involved, there is erythema and tearing. A papillary response with vasodilation and chemosis occurs. Pruritus is the cardinal symptom; a burning sensation also may be present. Rubbing the eyes intensifies the itching. Tearing can occur. An erythematous blepharitis is common, and in severe cases keratitis can result.

Causative Agents

Contact dermatitis and dermatoconjunctivitis can be caused by agents directly applied to the lid or conjunctiva, aerosolized or airborne agents contacted by chance, and cosmetics applied to other areas of the body. In fact, eyelid dermatitis occurs frequently because of cosmetics (e.g., nail polish, hair spray) applied to other areas of the body.[1] Agents applied directly to the eye are probably the most common causes. Contact dermatitis can be caused by eye makeup, including eyebrow pencil and eyebrow brush-on products, eye shadow, eye liner, mascara, artificial lashes, and lash extender. These products contain coloring agents, lanolin, paraben, sorbitol, paraffin, petrolatum, and other substances such as vehicles and perfumes.[1] Brushes and pads used to apply these cosmetics also can produce a dermatitis. In addition to agents applied directly only to the eye, soaps and face creams also can produce a selective dermatitis of the lid because of the thin skin in this area. Cosmetic formulations are frequently altered.[1] Therefore, a cosmetic previously used without ill effect can become a sensitizing agent.

Any medication applied to the eye can produce a contact dermatitis or dermatoconjunctivitis. Ophthalmic preparations contain several sensitizing agents including benzalkonium chloride, chlorobutanol, chlorhexidine, ethylenediaminetetra-acetate (EDTA), and phenylmercuric salts. EDTA cross-reacts with ethylenediamine, so that patients sensitive to this agent are subject to develop dermatitis to several other medications. Today, neomycin and idoxuridine are probably the major cause of iatrogenic contact dermatoconjunctivitis. Several other topically applied medications, however, have been shown to cause dermatoconjunctivitis. These include antihistamines such as antazoline, as well as atropine, chloramphenicol (Chloromycetin), pilocarpine, gentamycin, phenylephrine, epinephrine, and topical anesthetics.[2]

Of increasing importance is the conjunctivitis associated with the wearing of contact lenses, especially soft lenses. Reactions can occur to the lenses themselves or to the chemicals used to treat them. Both toxic and immune reactions can occur to contact lens solutions. Thimerosal, a preservative used in contact lens solutions, has been shown to produce classic, cell-mediated contact dermatitis.[3] Other substances found in lens solutions that might cause

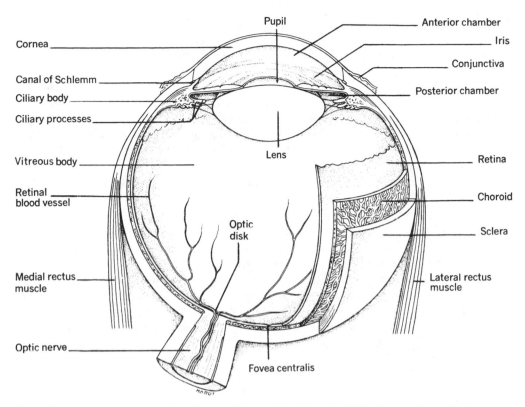

FIG. 11-1. Transverse section of eye. (Brunner L, Suddarth D. Textbook of medical-surgical nursing. 4th ed. Philadelphia: JB Lippincott, 1980.)

either toxic or immune reactions are the bacteriostatic agents (methylparaben, chlorobutanol, and chlorhexidine) and EDTA, which is used to chelate lens deposits.

Dermatitis of the lid and conjunctiva also can result from exposure to airborne agents. Hair spray, volatile substances contacted at work, and the oleoresin moieties of airborne pollens all have been reported to produce contact dermatitis and dermatoconjunctivitis. Hair preparations and nail enamel frequently cause problems around the eye while sparing the scalp and the hands.

Finally, rhus dermatitis can affect the eye, producing unilateral periorbital edema, which can be confused with angioedema.

Diagnosis and Identification of Causative Agents

The differential diagnosis includes seborrheic dermatitis and blepharitis, infectious eczematous dermatitis, especially chronic staphylococcal blepharitis, and rosacea. Seborrheic dermatitis usually can be differentiated from contact dermatitis on the basis of seborrheic lesions elsewhere and the lack or pruritus. Also, pruritus does not occur in staphylococcal blepharitis or rosacea. If the diagnosis is in doubt, an ophthalmology consultation should be obtained.

In some instances, the etiologic agents may be readily apparent. This is usually the case in dermatitis caused by the application of topical medications. However, many cases present as chronic dermatitis, and the cause is not readily apparent. In such instances, an elimination–

provocation procedure and patch tests can identify the offending substance. The elimination–provocation procedure requires the patient to remove all substances under suspicion from the environment. This is often difficult because it requires the complete removal of all cosmetics, hair sprays, spray deodorants, and any other topically applied substances. It should also include the cessation of visits to hair stylists and beauty parlors during the course of the elimination procedure. The soaps and shampoo should be changed. A bland soap (Basis) and shampoo free of formalin (e.g., Neutrogena, Ionil) should be employed. In recalcitrant cases, the detergent used to wash the pillowcases also should be changed. The elimination phase of the procedure should continue until the dermatitis subsides, or for a maximum of 1 month. When the illness has cleared, cosmetics and other substances can be returned at a rate of one every week. On occasion, the offending substances can be identified by the recurrence of symptoms on the reintroduction of the substance in question.

Patch tests can be helpful in establishing a diagnosis. However, the skin of the lid is markedly different from that of the back and forearm, and drugs repeatedly applied to the conjunctival sac concentrate there, producing high local concentrations of the drug. Thus, false-negative results from patch tests are common.[1] Testing should be performed not only to substances in standard patch test kits, but also to the patient's own cosmetics. In addition to the cosmetics themselves, tests can be performed to applying agents such as sponges and brushes. Both open and closed patch tests are indicated when testing with cosmetics.[1] Fisher[1] describes a simple test consisting of rubbing the substances into the forearm three times daily for 4 to 5 days, and then examining the sites.

Therapy

The treatment of choice is removal of the offending agent. On occasion, this can be easily accomplished. An example of this is the switch from chemically preserved to heat-sterilized systems in patients with contact lens–associated contact conjunctivitis. The offending agent, however, frequently cannot be identified, regardless of the diagnostic procedures applied. In these instances, chronic symptomatic therapy, possibly in conjunction with an ophthalmologist, is all that can be offered to the patient.

Symptomatic relief can be obtained with topical corticosteroid creams, ointments, and drops. Corticosteroid drops should be employed only under the direction of the ophthalmologist. Cool tap water soaks and boric acid eye baths may help.

Acute Allergic Conjunctivitis

Pathophysiology

Acute allergic conjunctivitis is the most common form of allergic eye disease.[4] It is produced by IgE-induced mast cell and basophil degranulation. As a result of this reaction, histamine, kinins, leukotrienes, prostaglandins, and other mediators are liberated.[5,6] Patients with allergic conjunctivitis have elevated amounts of total IgE in their tears,[7,8] and tear fluid also contains IgE specific for seasonal allergens.[9] Eosinophils are found in ocular scrapings.[10–12] These eosinophils are activated, releasing contents such as eosinophil cationic protein from their granules. These contents appear in tear fluid.[12] Ocular challenge with pollen produces both an early- and a late-phase ocular response.[13] In humans, the early phase begins approximately 20 minutes after challenge. The late phase is dose dependent, and large doses of allergen cause the initial inflammation to persist and progress.[13] The late phase differs from that which occurs in the nose and lungs in that it usually is continuous and progressive rather than biphasic.[13] It is characterized by the infiltration of inflammatory cells including neutrophils, eosinophils, and lymphocytes. The eosinophil is the predominant cell.[13] In addition, during the late-phase reaction, mediators are continually released, including histamine, leukotrienes, and eosinophil contents.[14]

Subjects with allergic conjunctivitis have an increased number of mast cells in their conjunctivae,[15] and they are hyperresponsive to intraocular histamine challenge.[16] Of interest is the fact that there is evidence of complement activation. Elevated levels of C3a des-Arg appear in tear fluid.[5]

The consequence of this immune reaction is conjunctival vasodilation and edema. The clinical reproducibility of the reaction is dependable. Instillation of allergen into the conjunctival sac was once used as a diagnostic test.[17]

Clinical Presentation

Acute allergic conjunctivitis usually is recognized easily. Itching is always a prominent feature. Rubbing the eyes intensifies the symptoms. The illness usually is bilateral. However, unilateral acute allergic conjunctivitis can occur secondary to manual contamination of the conjunctiva with allergens such as foods and animal dander. Ocular signs usually are minimal despite significant symptoms. The conjunctiva may be injected and edematous. In severe cases, the eye may be swollen shut. These symptoms of allergic conjunctivitis may be so severe as to interfere with the patient's sleep and work.

Allergic conjunctivitis rarely occurs without accompanying allergic rhinitis. Occasionally, the eye symptoms may be more prominent than nasal symptoms and can be the patient's major complaint. However, if symptoms or signs of allergic rhinitis are totally absent, the diagnosis of allergic conjunctivitis is doubtful. Allergic conjunctivitis also exists in a chronic form. Symptoms usually are less intense. As in acute allergic conjunctivitis, ocular findings may not be impressive.[7]

Diagnosis and Treatment

The diagnosis of allergic conjunctivitis usually can be made on the basis of history. There is an atopic personal or family history; the disease usually is seasonal. At times the patient may be able to define the offending allergen accurately. Skin tests are confirmatory. Stain of the conjunctival secretions may show numerous eosinophils, but the absence of eosinophils does not rule out the condition.[18] Normal individuals do not have eosinophils in conjunctival scrapings, and the presence of one eosinophil therefore is consistent with the diagnosis.[18] The differential diagnosis should include other forms of acute conjunctivitis, including viral and bacterial conjunctivitis, contact dermatoconjunctivitis, conjunctivitis sicca, and vernal conjunctivitis.

Treating allergic conjunctivitis is the same as for other atopic illness: avoidance, symptomatic relief, and immunotherapy, in that order. When allergic conjunctivitis is associated with respiratory allergic disease, the course of treatment usually is dictated by the more debilitating respiratory disorder. Avoiding ubiquitous aeroallergens is impractical, but avoidance measures outlined elsewhere in this text can be employed in the treatment of allergic conjunctivitis.

Effective symptomatic therapy for allergic conjunctivitis usually can be achieved with topical medications. Five classes of topical drugs (Table 11-1) are available: vasoconstrictors,

TABLE 11-1. *Topical agents used in the treatment of allergic eye disease*

Trade Name	Manufacturer	Drug	Dosage	Comments
Combination products				
Vasocon	Iolab	Antazoline phosphate Naphazoline HCl	1–2 drops, q 4 h, prn (no more than qid)	These agents do not require a prescription. Other similar preparations also are available. Examples: AK-CON-A, Opcon-A
Naphcon A	Alcon	Pheniramine maleate Naphazoline HCl	1–2 drops, q 4 h, prn (no more than qid)	
Prefrin A	Allergen	Pyrilamine maleate Phenylephrine HCl	1–2 drops, q 4 h, prn (no more than qid)	
Antihistamines— single drug				
Livostin	Iolab	Levocabastine HCl	1 drop qid	Officially indicated only for acute allergic conjunctivitis for up to 2 wk
Mast cell stabilizers				
Crolom	Bausch & Lomb	Cromolyn NA	1–2 drops, q 4–6 h/d at regular intervals	This drug has an official indication for vernal conjunctivitis; however, it has been used extensively for acute allergic conjunctivitis in the past.
Alomide	Alcon	Lodoxamide tromethamine	1–2 drops, qid for up to 3 mo	The only official indication for this drug is vernal conjunctivitis
Nonsteroidal antiinflammatory drugs				
Acular	Allergen	Ketorolac tromethamine	1 drop qid	The only official indication for this drug is for acute seasonal allergic rhinitis. It is also officially indicated only for itching, and its efficacy (according to its package insert) has not been established beyond 1 wk of therapy.

q, every; prn, as needed; qid, four times daily.

antihistamines, mast cell stabilizers, nonsteroidal antiinflammatory agents, and cortico-steroids. Corticosteroids are not discussed here since, because of their well-known side effects, patients should use them only when prescribed by the ophthalmologist.

Several preparations contain a mixture of a vasoconstrictor combined with an antihista-mine (see Table 11-1). These drugs can be purchased over the counter. The antihistamine is most useful for itching but can reduces vasodilation. Vasoconstrictors only diminish vasodi-lation and have little effect on pruritus. The two most frequently employed decongestants are naphazoline and phenylephrine. The two most common antihistamines available in combina-tion products are antazoline and pheniramine maleate.

A recently released antihistamine, levocabastine (Livostin) is available only by prescrip-tion. Levocabastine was specifically designed for topical application. In animal studies, it is 1500 times more potent than chlorpheniramine on a molar basis.[19] It has a rapid onset of action,[20] is effective in blocking intraocular allergen challenge,[21] and appears to be as effec-tive as other agents, including sodium cromoglycate[22] and terfenadine.[23]

As a rule, vasoconstrictors and antihistamines are well tolerated. However, antihistamines may be sensitizing. In addition, each preparation contains several different vehicles that may produce transient irritation or sensitization.[11] As a rule, however, these drugs are effective and well tolerated.[24]

Two mast cell stabilizers have been shown to be effective in the treatment of allergic con-junctivitis. These are nedocromil sodium and cromolyn sodium. Nedocromil is not available in this country, but cromolyn has been rereleased and is available as Crolom. Both are effi cacious and well tolerated.[25-27] Ideally, cromolyn should be started before the beginning of the allergy season. It is more effective when used regularly, four times a day,[28] but has been shown to relieve symptoms within 2 minutes after administration after ocular allergen chal-lenge.[29] It is also useful in preventing symptoms caused by isolated allergen exposure, such as when it is necessary to visit a home with a pet to whom the patient is allergic. In this situ-ation, it should be administered immediately before exposure.

Ketorolac tromethamine is the first nonsteroidal antiinflammatory drug to be used in this country for the therapy of allergic conjunctivitis. It is available as Acular. It is most effective in controlling itching but also ameliorates other symptoms.[30] Its effect results from its ability to inhibit the formation of prostaglandins, which cause itching when applied to the conjunc-tiva.[31] The dosages of each topical agent are noted in Table 11-1.

Allergen immunotherapy can be helpful in treating allergic conjunctivitis. A study designed to assess the effect of immunotherapy on allergic rhinitis has demonstrated improve-ment in ocular symptoms as well.[32] In addition, immunotherapy to grass pollen has been shown to reduce conjunctival sensitivity to intraocular grass pollen challenge.[33]

Finally, another mast cell stabilizer, lodoxamide (Alomide), also is available but has not been approved for use in the United States for allergic conjunctivitis. It has, however, been approved for use in vernal conjunctivitis (see later).

Vernal Conjunctivitis

Clinical Presentation

Vernal conjunctivitis is a chronic, bilateral, catarrhal inflammation of the conjunctiva, most commonly arising in children during the spring and summer. It can be perennial in severely affected patients. It is characterized by an intense itching. Burning and photophobia can occur.

The illness usually is seen during the preadolescent years and often resolves at puberty. Male patients are affected approximately three times more often than female patients. The incidence is increased in warmer climates.

Vernal conjunctivitis presents in palpebral and limbal forms. In the palpebral variety, which is more common, the tarsal conjunctiva of the upper lid is deformed by thickened, gelatinous vegetations produced by marked papillary hypertrophy. This hypertrophy imparts a cobblestone appearance to the conjunctiva. The "cobblestoning" results from intense proliferation of collagen and ground substance along with a cellular infiltrate.[34] The papillae are easily seen when the upper lid is everted. In severe cases, the lower palpebral conjunctiva may be similarly involved. In the limbal form, a similar gelatinous cobblestoning occurs at the corneal–scleral junction. Trantas' dots—small white dots composed of eosinophils— often are present. Usually, there is a thick, stringy exudate full of eosinophils. This thick, ropey, white or yellow mucus discharge has highly elastic properties and produces a foreign body sensation. It is pathognomonic for vernal conjunctivitis.[34] It is usually easily distinguished from the globular mucus seen in seasonal allergic conjunctivitis or the crusting of infectious conjunctivitis. The patient may be particularly troubled by this discharge, which can string out for more than 2.5 cm (1 inch) when it is removed from the eye. Widespread punctate keratitis may be present. Severe cases can result in epithelial ulceration with scar formation.

Pathophysiology and Cause

The cause and pathophysiologic mechanisms of vernal conjunctivitis remain obscure. Several features of the disease, however, suggest that the atopic state is related to its pathogenesis. The seasonal occurrence, the presence of eosinophils, and the fact that most of the patients have other atopic disease[35] are circumstantial evidence supporting this hypothesis. In addition, several different immunologic and histologic findings are consistent with an allergic etiology. Patients with vernal conjunctivitis have elevated levels of total IgE,[36] allergen-specific IgE,[37] histamine,[36] and tryptase[38] in the tear film. In addition, the histologic study supports an immune origin. Patients with vernal conjunctivitis have markedly increased numbers of eosinophils, basophils, mast cells, and plasma cells in biopsy specimens taken from the conjunctiva.[39] The mast cells often are totally degranulated.[36] Elevated levels of major basic protein are found in biopsy specimens of the conjunctiva.[40] Finally, ocular shields, designed to prevent pollen exposure, have been reported to be therapeutically effective.[41,42]

Also of interest is the hypothesis that complement, perhaps activated by IgG–allergen immune complexes, plays a role in producing vernal conjunctivitis. Pollen-specific IgG antibodies[43] and complement activation products (C3 des-Arg) occur in tears of patients with vernal conjunctivitis.[44] The specific IgG antipollen found in the tear film may not be acting through the complement system, however, since much of it appears to be IgG4,[43] a noncomplement-fixing subclass with putative reaginic activity.

Also, patients with vernal conjunctivitis have decreased tear lactoferrin, an inhibitor of the complement system.[45]

Diagnosis and Treatment

Vernal conjunctivitis must be distinguished from other conjunctival diseases that present with pruritus or follicular hypertrophy. These include acute allergic conjunctivitis, conjunctivitis and keratoconjunctivitis associated with atopic dermatitis, the giant papillary conjunctivitis associated with soft contact lenses and other foreign bodies, the follicular conjunctivitis of viral infections, and trachoma (rarely found in the United States).

In most instances, the distinction between acute allergic conjunctivitis and vernal conjunctivitis is not difficult. However, in the early phases of vernal conjunctivitis or in mild vernal conjunctivitis, giant papillae may be absent. In such instances, the distinction may be more difficult because both conditions occur in atopic individuals, and pruritus is a hallmark of each. However, in vernal conjunctivitis, the pruritus is more intense, the tear film contains a significantly greater concentration of histamine and greater amounts of eosinophils, and the conjunctival epithelium has more abundant mast cells.[36] Also, the cornea is not involved in acute allergic conjunctivitis.

The conjunctivitis and keratoconjunctivitis associated with atopic dermatitis can be similar to vernal conjunctivitis. In atopic dermatitis, the conjunctivitis can produce hypertrophy and opacity of the tarsal conjunctiva.[46,47] A form of keratoconjunctivitis with papillary hypertrophy and punctate keratitis can occur.[48] Many of these patients have signs and symptoms typical of vernal conjunctivitis, including giant follicles and pruritus. In addition, vernal conjunctivitis and atopic dermatitis can occur together in the same patient. However, because the treatment of both conditions is similar, the distinction, except for its prognostic value, may not be essential.

The giant papillary conjunctivitis caused by wearing of soft contact lenses is similar to vernal conjunctivitis. Patients complain of itching, mucous discharge, and a decreasing tolerance to the lens. Symptoms usually begin 3 to 36 months after lenses are prescribed.[49] The syndrome can occur with hard and soft lenses, and can be seen with exposed sutures[49] and plastic prostheses.[50] Thus, chronic trauma to the lid appears to be the common inciting agent. Several features distinguish this entity from vernal conjunctivitis. Lens-associated papillary conjunctivitis causes less intense itching and shows no seasonal variation. It resolves with discontinuation of lens use.

Viral infections can be distinguished from vernal conjunctivitis by their frequent association with systemic symptoms and the absence of pruritus. A slit-lamp examination can produce a definitive distinction between these two entities.

Patients with mild vernal conjunctivitis can be treated with cold compresses and topical vasoconstrictor-antihistamine preparations. Levocabastine has been shown to be effective in a double-blind, placebo-controlled trial of 46 patients over a period of 4 weeks.[51] Oral antihistamines may be of modest help. Cromolyn sodium has been used effectively not only for milder but for more recalcitrant, chronic forms of the condition.[52-55] Cromolyn has been shown to decrease conjunctival injection, punctate keratitis, itching, limbal edema, and tearing when administered regularly. It may be more effective in patients who are atopic.[54] In a multicenter, double-blind 28-day study, another mast cell stabilizer, lodoxamide, was found to be more effective than cromolyn sodium.[56]

Aspirin[57,58] has been found to be helpful in a dose of 0.5 to 1.5 g daily. Ketorolac tromethamine has not been approved for use in vernal conjunctivitis, but based on the studies of aspirin, might be an effective agent in this regard. Acetylcysteine 10% (Mucomyst) has been suggested as a means of counteracting viscous secretions. In severe cases, cyclosporine has been used.[59]

None of the above medications are universally effective, however, and topical corticosteroids often are necessary. If topical corticosteroids are needed, the patient should be under the care of an ophthalmologist. A sustained-release, hydrocortisone epiocular depository also has been successfully employed.[60] Fortunately, spontaneous remission usually occurs at puberty.

Eye Manifestation Associated With Atopic Dermatitis

Atopic dermatitis is associated with several manifestations of eye disease. These include lid dermatitis, blepharititis, conjunctivitis, keratoconjunctivitis, keratoconus, cataracts, and a predisposition to develop ocular infections, especially with herpes simplex and vaccinia viruses.[61]

Lid involvement can resemble contact dermatitis. The lids become thickened, edematous, and coarse. They may be pruritic.

Conjunctivitis may vary in intensity with the degree of skin involvement of the face.[46] It resembles acute allergic conjunctivitis, and to some extent resembles vernal conjunctivitis. It actually may be allergic conjunctivitis occurring with atopic dermatitis.

Atopic keratoconjunctivitis usually does not appear until the late teenage years. The peak incidence is between 30 and 50 years of age. Male patients are affected in greater numbers than female patients.

Atopic keratoconjunctivitis is bilateral. The major symptoms are itching, tearing, and burning. The eyelids may be red, thickened, and macerated. There is usually erythema of the lid margin and crusting around the eyelashes. The palpebral conjunctiva may show papillary hypertrophy. The lower lid is usually more severely afflicted and more often involved. Punctate keratitis can occur and the bulbar conjunctiva is chemotic.

Atopic keratoconjunctivitis must be differentiated from blepharitis and vernal conjunctivitis. This may be difficult in the case of blepharitis. Indeed, staphylococcal blepharitis often complicates this disorder. Vernal conjunctivitis usually is distinguished from atopic keratoconjunctivitis by the fact that it most often involves the upper rather than lower lids and is more seasonal. It also occurs in a younger age group. The papillae in vernal conjunctivitis also are larger.

Cromolyn sodium is helpful in treating atopic keratoconjunctivitis.[62] Topical corticosteroids often are needed, however. Their use should be under the direction of the ophthalmologist.

Keratoconus occurs less frequently than conjunctival involvement. The cause of the association between atopic dermatitis and keratoconus is unknown, but there appears to be no HLA haplotype that distinguishes atopic dermatitis patients with keratoconjunctivitis from patients without it or from controls.[47]

The incidence rate of cataract formation in atopic dermatitis has been reported to range from 0.4% to 25%.[47] These cataracts may be anterior or posterior in location as opposed to those caused by administering corticosteroids, which are usually posterior. They have been observed in both children and adults. They may be unilateral or bilateral. Their presence cannot be correlated with the age of onset of the disease, its severity, or its duration.[63]

Eyelid disorders may be the most common ocular complaint in patients with atopic dermatitis.[64] Dermatitis of the lid produces itching with lid inversion. The skin becomes scaly, and the skin of the eyes around the lid may become more wrinkled. The skin is extremely dry. The lesion is pruritic and can be confused with contact dermatitis of the lid.

Herpes keratitis is more common in patients with atopic dermatitis. This condition may be recurrent, and recalcitrant epithelial defects can occur.[65]

Blepharoconjunctivitis (Marginal Blepharitis)

Blepharoconjunctivitis (marginal blepharitis) refers to any condition where inflammation of the lid margin is a prominent feature of the disease. A conjunctivitis usually occurs in conjunction with the blepharitis. Three illnesses are commonly considered under the generic heading of blepharoconjunctivitis: staphylococcal blepharoconjunctivitis, seborrheic blepharoconjunctivitis, and rosacea. They often occur together.

Staphylococcal Blepharoconjunctivitis

The staphylococcal organism probably is the most common cause of conjunctivitis and ble-pharoconjunctivitis. The acute bacterial conjunctivitis is characterized by irritation, redness, and mucopurulent discharge with matting of the eyelids. Frequently, the conjunctivitis is present in a person with low-grade inflammation of the eyelid margins.

In the chronic form, symptoms of staphylococcal blepharoconjunctivitis include erythema of the lid margins, matting of the eyelids on awakening, and discomfort, which is usually worse in the morning. Examination frequently shows yellow crusting of the margin of the eyelids, with collarette formation at the base of the cilia, and disorganized or missing cilia. If the exudates are removed, ulceration of the lid margin may be visible. Fluorescein staining of the cornea may show small areas of dye uptake in the inferior portion. It is believed that exotoxin elaborated by *Staphylococcus* organisms is responsible for the symptoms and signs. Because of the chronicity of the disease and the subtle findings, the entity of chronic blepharoconjunctivitis of staphylococcal origin can be con-fused with contact dermatitis of the eyelids and contact dermatoconjunctivitis. The absence of pruritus is the most important feature distinguishing staphylococcal from contact dermatoconjunctivitis.

Seborrheic Dermatitis of the Lids

Staphylococcal blepharitis also can be confused with seborrheic blepharitis. Seborrheic blepharitis occurs as part of seborrheic dermatitis. It is associated with oily skin, seborrhea of the brows, and usually scalp involvement The scales, which occur at the base of the cilia, tend to be greasy, and if these are removed, no ulceration is seen. There is no pruritus.

Rosacea

The blepharoconjunctivitis of rosacea often occurs in combination with seborrhea. Patients with blepharoconjunctivitis exhibit the classic hyperemia with telangiectasia over the malar area. Symp-toms often are worsened by the ingestion of spicy foods

Diagnosis and Treatment of Blepharoconjunctivitis

In all three forms of blepharoconjunctivitis, the cardinal symptoms are burning, redness, and irrita-tion. True pruritus usually is absent or minimal The inflammation of the lid margin is prominent. The discharge usually is mucopurulent, and matting in the early morning may be an annoying fea-ture. In the seborrheic and rosacea forms, cutaneous involvement elsewhere is present.

All three forms usually are chronic and often difficult to manage. In staphylococcal blepharo-conjunctivitis, lid scrubs using a cotton-tipped applicator soaked with baby shampoo and followed by the application of a steroid ointment may be helpful. Control of other areas of seborrhea is nec-essary. Tetracycline can be beneficial in the therapy of rosacea. Ophthalmologic and dermatologic consultation may be needed.

Viral Conjunctivitis

Viral conjunctivitis usually is of abrupt onset, frequently beginning unilaterally and involving the second eye within a few days. Conjunctival injection, slight chemosis, watery discharge, and enlargement of a preauricular lymph node help to distinguish viral infection from other entities. Clinically, lymphoid follicles appear on the conjunctiva as elevated avascular areas, which usually are grayish. These correspond to the histologic picture of lymphoid germinal centers.

Viral conjunctivitis usually is of adenoviral origin, and is frequently associated with a pharyngitis and low-grade fever in pharyngoconjunctival fever.

Epidemic keratoconjunctivitis presents as an acute follicular conjunctivitis, with a watery discharge and preauricular adenopathy. This conjunctivitis usually runs a 7- to 14-day course and frequently is accompanied by small corneal opacities. Epidemic keratoconjunctivitis can be differentiated from allergic conjunctivitis by the absence of pruritus, the presence of a mononuclear cellular response, and a follicular conjunctival response.

The treatment of viral conjunctivitis usually is supportive, although prophylactic antibiotics frequently are used. If significant corneal opacities are present, the application of topical steroid preparations has been suggested.

Chlamydial (Inclusion) Conjunctivitis

In adults, inclusion conjunctivitis presents as an acute conjunctivitis with prominent conjunctival follicles and a mucopurulent discharge. There is usually no preceding upper respiratory infection or fever. This process occurs in adults who may harbor the chlamydial agent in the genital tract, but with no symptoms referable to this system. A nonspecific urethritis in men and a chronic vaginal discharge in women are common. The presence of a mucopurulent discharge and follicular conjunctivitis, which lasts more than 2 weeks, certainly suggest inclusion conjunctivitis. A Giemsa stain of conjunctival scraping specimen may reveal intracytoplasmic inclusion bodies and helps to confirm the diagnosis. The treatment of choice is systemic tetracycline for 10 days.

Keratoconjunctivitis Sicca

Keratoconjunctivitis sicca is a condition characterized by a diminished tear production. This is predominately a disorder of menopausal or postmenopausal women and may present in patients with connective tissue disease, particularly rheumatoid arthritis. Although keratoconjunctivitis sicca may present as an isolated condition affecting the eyes only, it also may be associated with xerostomia or Sjögren's syndrome.

Symptoms may begin insidiously and frequently are confused with a mild infectious or allergic process. Mild conjunctival injection, irritation, photophobia, and mucoid discharge are present. Corneal epithelial damage can be demonstrated by fluorescein or rose Bengal staining, and hypolacrimation can be confirmed by inadequate wetting of the Schirmer test strip. Frequent application of artificial tears usually provides relief.

Herpes Simplex Keratitis

A primary herpetic infection occurs subclinically in many patients. However, acute primary keratoconjunctivitis may occur with or without skin involvement. The recurrent form of the disease is seen most commonly. Patients usually complain of tearing, ocular irritation, blurred vision, and occasionally photophobia. Fluorescein staining of the typical linear branching ulcer (dendrite) of the cornea confirms the diagnosis. Herpetic keratitis is treated with antiviral compounds, or by debridement. After the infectious keratitis has healed, the patient may return with a geographic erosion of the cornea, which is known as metaherpetic (trophic) keratitis. In this stage, the virus is not replicating, and antiviral therapy usually is not indicated. If the inflammation involves the deep corneal stroma, a disciform keratitis may result and may run a protracted course, leaving a corneal scar. The exact cause of disciform keratitis is unknown, but it is thought that immune mechanisms play an important role in its production.[66,67] It is important to distinguish herpetic keratitis from allergic conjunctivitis. The absence of pruritus and the presence of photophobia, blurred vision, and a corneal staining area should alert the clinician to the presence of herpetic infection. Using corticosteroids in herpetic disease only spreads the ulceration and prolongs the infectious phase of the disease process.

Giant Papillary Conjunctivitis

Giant papillary conjunctivitis, which is characterized by the formation of large papillae (larger than 0.33 mm in diameter) on the upper tarsal conjunctiva, has been associated with the wearing of contact lenses, prostheses, and sutures.[68,69] Although it is most commonly cause by soft contact lenses,[70] it can also occur with gas permeable and rigid lenses. Patients experience pruritus, excess mucus production, and discomfort when wearing their lenses. There is decreased lens tolerance, blurred vision, and excessive lens movement (frequently with lens displacement). Burning and tearing also are noted.

The patient develops papillae on the upper tarsal conjunctiva. These range from 0.3 to greater than 1 mm in diameter. The area involved correlates with the type of contact lens worn by the patient.[34]

The mechanism of production of giant papillary conjunctivitis is unknown. One hypothesis is that the reaction is caused by an immunologic response to deposits on the lens surface. Deposits consist not only of exogenous airborne antigens but also of products in the tear film such as lysozyme, IgA, lactoferrin, and IgG.[71,72] More than two thirds of soft lens wearers develop deposits within 1 year of wear. Evidence suggesting an immune mechanism in the production of giant papillary conjunctivitis is based on several observations. The condition is more common in atopic subjects. Patients with giant papillary conjunctivitis have elevated, locally produced tear IgE.[73] Eosinophils, basophils, and mast cells are found in giant papillary conjunctivitis in greater amounts than in acute allergic conjunctivitis.[34] Finally, there are elevated levels of major basic protein in conjunctival tissues of patients with giant papillary conjunctivitis[40] and elevated levels of tryptase in their tears.[34]

Non–IgE-mediated immune mechanisms also have been incriminated in the production of this disorder. IgG levels are elevated, but the IgG is blood-borne rather than locally produced.[73] There is also evidence for complement activation, and there is decreased lactoferrin in the tears of patients with giant papillary conjunctivitis.[44,45] Neutrophil chemotactic factor is present in tear fluids in amounts exceeding levels found in nonaffected soft contact lens wearers.[74]

Treatment of giant papillary conjunctivitis usually is carried out by the ophthalmologist. Early recognition is important since discontinuation of lens wear early in the stage of the disease and prescription of appropriate lens type and edge design can prevent recurrence. It is also important to adhere to a strict regimen for lens cleaning and use preservative-free saline. Enzymatic cleaning with papain preparations is useful to reduce the coating of the lenses by antigens. Disposable lenses also may be beneficial. Both cromolyn sodium and nedocromil sodium have been found to be helpful.[75]

Floppy Eye Syndrome

Floppy eye syndrome is a condition characterized by lax upper lids and a papillary conjunctivitis resembling giant papillary conjunctivitis. Men older than 30 years of age constitute the majority of patients. The condition is thought to result from chronic traction on the lax lid produced by the pillow at sleep. It may be unilateral or bilateral.[69]

Approach to the Patient With an Inflamed Eye

The physician seeing a patient with acute or chronic conjunctivitis should first rule out diseases (not discussed in this chapter) that may be acutely threatening to the patient's vision. These include conditions such as acute keratitis, uveitis, acute angle–closure glaucoma, and endophthalmitis. The two most important symptoms pointing to a threatening condition are a loss in visual acuity and pain. These are signs that the patient could have an elevated intraocular pressure, keratitis, endophthalmitis, or uveitis. On physical examination the presence of circumcorneal hyperemia (dilation of the vessels adjacent to the corneal edge limbus) is present in four threatening conditions, including keratitis, uveitis, acute angle–closure glaucoma, and endophthalmitis. This contrasts with the pattern of vasodilation seen in acute allergic conjunctivitis, which produces erythema that is more pronounced in the periphery and decreases as it approaches the cornea.

If the physician believes that the patient does not have a threatening eye disease, the next step is to differentiate between allergic and nonallergic diseases of the eye (Table 11-2). Five cardinal questions should to be asked in this regard:

The differential diagnosis between allergic and nonallergic diseases of the eye can usually be made by focusing on a few key features:

1. *Does the eye itch?* This is the most important distinguishing feature between allergic and nonallergic eye disorders. All allergic conditions are pruritic. Nonallergic conditions usually do not itch. The physician must be certain that the patient understands what is meant by itching, since burning, scratching, sandy eyes are often described as "itchy" by the patient.
2. *What type of discharge, if any, is present?* A purulent discharge with early morning matting is not a feature of allergic disease and points toward infection.
3. *Is the lid involved?* Lid involvement indicates the presence of atopic dermatitis, contact dermatitis, or occasionally seborrhea or rosacea. Often the patient complains of "eye irritation," which may mean the lid, conjunctiva, or both. The physician should be careful to ascertain which area of the eye is involved.
4. *Are other allergic manifestations present?* Examples include atopic dermatitis, asthma, and rhinitis.
5. *Are there other associated nonallergic conditions?* Nonallergic conditions include dandruff and rosacea.

THE EAR: OTIC MANIFESTATIONS OF ALLERGY

The most common otologic problem seen by the allergist–immunologist is otitis media with effusion (OME). In the following discussion, the potential role of allergic disease in the pathogenesis of OME is evaluated.

TABLE 11-2. *Differential features to be considered in diagnosing allergic eye disease*

	Seasonal	Itching	Scratchy (sandy) irritation	Skin of lids and/or margin involved	Bilateral	Tearing	Discharge	Remarks
Acute allergic conjunctivitis	Yes	Prominent	Not usual	No	Yes	Increased	Mucoid	Itching is cardinal feature; rhinitis is present
Vernal conjunctivitis	Yes	Prominent	Not usual	No	Yes	Slightly increased	Stringy and tenacious	Seasonal—spring and summer; more common in children
Conjunctivitis sicca	No	No	Prominent	No	Yes	Markedly decreased	Slight mucoid	Dry mouth, associated with autoimmune disease, especially Sjögren's syndrome
Acute viral conjunctivitis	Variable; usually is not	No	Variable	No	Variable	Normal to slightly increased	Watery	Follicular conjunctivitis, prominent injection, may have preauricular node enlargement
Acute bacterial conjunctivitis	No	No	Variable	Matting	Variable	Normal to increased	Mucopurulent	Exudate most prominent feature
Dermato-conjunctivitis	No	Yes	No	Variable	Usually	Normal to increased	Variable	Itching usually is a helpful diagnostic feature
Chronic staphylococcal blepharo-conjunctivitis	No	No	No	Yes	Usually	Normal	Early morning matting	Crusting of lids, loss of cilia
Seborrheic dermatitis	No	No	No	Yes	Yes	Normal	None	Signs of seborrheic dermatitis elsewhere

Otitis media is a general term defined as any inflammation of the middle ear with or without symptoms and usually associated with an effusion. It is one of the most common medical condition seen in children by primary care physicians. Close to $2 billion a year is spent on treating this condition in the United States.[76] The classification of otitis media can be confusing. The First International Symposium on Recent Advances in Middle Ear Effusions[77] includes the following types of otitis media: (1) acute purulent otitis media, (2) serous otitis media, and (3) mucoid or secretory otitis media. Chronic otitis media is a condition displaying a pronounced, retracted tympanic membrane with pathologic changes in the middle ear such as cholesteatoma or granulation tissue. The acute phase of otitis media occurs during the first 3 weeks of the illness, the subacute phase from the fourth through the eighth week, and the chronic phase begins after the eighth week. For this review, acute otitis media (AOM) applies to the classic ear infection that is rapid in onset and associated with a red, bulging, and painful tympanic membrane. The presence of middle ear fluid without signs or symptoms of infection is OME. Other commonly used names for OME are serous otitis media and secretory otitis media.

In the United States, approximately 10 million children are treated for OME annually,[78] and this condition results in the one of the most commonly performed surgeries in the United States, tympanostomy tubes.[79] OME is of major importance in children since the effusion can lead to a mild to moderate conductive hearing loss of 20 dB or more.[80] Chronic conductive hearing loss in the child may lead to poor language development and learning disorders. There are many epidemiologic factors for the development of recurrent and chronic OME in children, with age being a major risk (Table 11-3). A study of 2565 children by Teele and coworkers[81] found that 50% of all infants have had one or more episodes of OME in the first year of life, with 75% having at least one episode of OME by 6 years of age. One third had three or more episodes of OME by 3 years of age. The study further showed that after the first episode, 40% of the children had middle ear effusion that persisted for 4 weeks, and 10% had effusions that were still present after 3 months. Bluestone and Shuring[82] showed that 20% of American children in their study had middle ear effusion by 5 years of age, but the incidence

TABLE 11-3. *Risk factors for chronic and recurrent otitis media with effusion*

1. Age: children with OME in the first year of life have increased incidence of recurrence
2. Males > females
3. Bottle-fed infants
4. Passive smoking exposure
5. Allergy
6. Lower socioeconomic status
7. Race: Native Americans and Eskimos > Whites > African Americans
8. Day care centers
9. Season: winter > summer
10. Genetic predisposition: if sibs have OME, higher risk
11. Down's syndrome
12. Primary immunodeficiency disorders
13. Primary and secondary ciliary dysfunction
14. Craniofacial abnormalities

OM, otitis media with effusion; sibs, siblings.

rate in this study dropped dramatically to 3% by 10 years of age. Several reports emphasize the importance of age on the incidence of acute and chronic middle ear effusion. In a British study,[83] two high-incidence peaks were noted, the first in the second 6 months of life, and a second, smaller peak at 5 to 7 years of age. In a Boston study of children with middle ear infection, Feingold[84] reports that 62% of the cases occurred in children 2 years of age and younger. Other major factors in development of OME include being male, exposure to parental cigarette smoke,[85,86] race, and allergy. Day care center attendance probably increases the incidence of OME, because children in day care tend to have a higher incidence of upper respiratory infections than children in home care. The higher incidence of viral infections may contribute to the pathogenesis of OME.[87] Children who are breast-fed tend to have a lower rate of OME than bottle-fed infants.[88,89] Race appears to increase the risk of OME, with the highest incidence in Native Americans and Eskimos. Diseases of the antibody-mediated immune system, primary ciliary dyskinesia, Down's syndrome, and craniofacial abnormalities, especially cleft palate, all contribute to chronic OME. When evaluating the patient with recurrent or chronic OME, each of these conditions needs to be investigated.

Pathogenesis of OME

Multiple factors influence the pathogenesis of OME. Most studies link OME with eustachian tube (ET) dysfunction, viral and bacterial infections, abnormalities of mucociliary clearance, and allergy.

Eustachian Tube Anatomy and Physiology

The nasopharynx and middle ear are connected by the ET. The development of middle ear effusions appears to be related to functional or anatomic abnormalities of this tube. Under normal conditions, the ET has three physiologic functions: (1) ventilation of the middle ear to equilibrate pressure and replenish oxygen; (2) protection of the middle ear from nasopharyngeal sound pressure and secretions; and (3) clearance of secretions produced in the middle ear into the nasopharynx.

The ET of the infant and the young child differs markedly from that of the adult. These anatomic differences predispose infants and young children to middle ear disease. In infancy, the ET is wide, short, and more horizontal in orientation. As growth occurs, the tube narrows, elongates, and develops a more oblique course (Fig. 11-2). Usually, after 7 years of age, these physical changes lessen the frequency of middle ear inflammation.[90] In the normal state, the middle ear is free of any significant amount of fluid and is filled with air. Air is maintained in the middle ear by the action of the ET. This tube is closed at the pharyngeal end except during swallowing, when the tensor veli palatini muscle contracts and opens the ET by lifting its posterior lip (Fig. 11-3A). When the ET is opened, air passes from the nasopharynx into the middle ear, and this ventilation system equalizes air pressure on both sides of the tympanic membrane (see Fig. 11-3B).

When the ET is blocked by either functional or anatomic defects, air cannot enter the middle ear, and the remaining air is absorbed. This results in the formation of negative pressure within the middle ear and subsequent retraction of the tympanic membrane (see Fig. 11-3C). High negative pressure associated with ventilation may result in aspiration of nasopharyngeal secretions in to the middle ear, producing acute OME (see Fig. 11-3D). Prolonged negative pressure causes fluid transudation from the middle ear mucosal blood vessels (see Fig. 11-3E). With

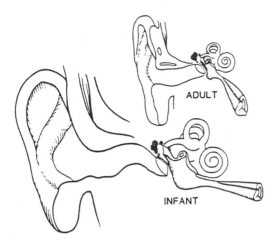

ADULT

INFANT

FIG. 11-2. Illustration showing difference in angles of eustachian tubes in infants and adults.

chronic OME, there is infiltration of lymphocytes and macrophages along with production of different inflammatory mediators. Also there is an increased density of goblet cells in the epithelium of the ET. It is thought that many children with middle ear effusions, without a demonstrable cause of ET obstruction, have a growth-related inadequate action of the tensor veli palatini muscle. Another possibility is functional obstruction from persistent collapse of the tube caused by increased tubal compliance. Nasal obstruction, either from adenoid hypertrophy or from infectious or allergic inflammation, may be involved in the pathogenesis of middle ear effusion by the "Toynbee phenomenon."[91] Studies have shown that, when the nose is obstructed, there is an increased positive nasopharyngeal pressure followed by a negative nasopharyngeal pressure on swallowing. The increased positive nasopharyngeal pressure may predispose to insufflation of secretions into the middle ear, and the secondary negative pressure in the nasopharynx may further be a factor in the inadequate opening of the ET, thereby causing obstruction.

Infection

Respiratory bacterial and viral infections are significant contributors to the pathogenesis of otitis media. The three most common bacterial isolates in AOM and OME are *Streptococcus pneumoniae*, nontypable *Haemophilus influenzae*, and *Moraxella catarrhalis*.[92] *Streptococcus pyogenes* and anaerobic cocci are isolated in less than 5% of the patients with AOM. The predominant anaerobes are gram-positive cocci, pigmented *Prevotella* and *Porphyromonas* sp, *Bacteroides* sp, and *Fusobacterium* sp. The predominant organisms isolated from chronic otitis media are *Staphylococcus aureus*, *Pseudomonas aeruginosa*, and anaerobic bacteria. In neonates, group B *Streptococci* and gram-negative organisms are common bacterial pathogens causing otitis media.[93] Most patients with chronic OME have sterile middle ear effusions. Post and associates[94] used a polymerase chain reaction to detect bacterial DNA in middle ear effusions in children undergoing myringotomy and tube placement who had failed multiple courses of antibiotics. Of the 97 specimens, 75 (77.3%) were polymerase chain reaction positive for one or more of the following bacteria: *S pneumoniae*, nontypable *Haemophilus influenzae*, and *M catarrhalis*. This suggests that active bacterial infection may be occurring in many children with chronic OME.

Viral agents are not commonly found in middle ear effusions, but are probably important in the pathogenesis of otitis media. Most studies demonstrate viral isolates in less than 5% of the aspirates from the middle ear, with the most common being respiratory syncytial virus (RSV).[95,96] Ciliary dysfunction secondary to viral infections in the upper respiratory tract can predispose to OME. Viral infections have been shown to increase bacterial adhesion in the upper respiratory tract.[97] This may allow for colonization of the upper respiratory tract with bacteria and increase the risk of otitis media. Influenza A infection has been demonstrated to contribute to the pathogenesis of experimental pneumococcal AOM.[98] Another possible mechanism for viral infections in the pathogenesis of otitis media is the production of viral-specific IgE. Welliver and coworkers[99] showed most of the 42 RSV-infected infants demonstrated anti-RSV IgE bound to exfoliated nasopharyngeal epithelial cells in the acute phase of the infection. With RSV being the most common viral agent in middle ear effusion, IgE-mediated reactions triggered by this virus may be a contributory factor to the development of OME in many patients.

Mucociliary Dysfunction

Mucociliary dysfunction from either a genetic defect or an acquired infectious or environmental condition can lead to OME. Investigations by Sadé and coworkers[100] suggest that the mucociliary transfer system is an important defense mechanism in clearing foreign particles from the middle ear and the ET. Goblet and secretory cells provide a mucous blanket to aid ciliated cells in transporting foreign particles toward the nasopharynx for phagocytosis by macrophages, or to the lymphatics and capillaries for clearance. Respiratory viral infections are associated with transient abnormalities in the structure and function of cilia.[101] Primary ciliary dyskinesia, an autosomal recessive syndrome, has been linked to over 20 different structural defects in cilia, which lead to ciliary dysfunction.[102] Both of these conditions can lead to inefficient ciliary transport, which results in mucostasis and contributes to ET obstruction and the development of middle ear effusion.

Allergy and Immunology

There is a considerable debate on whether allergic disorders play a role in the pathogenesis of OME. Many investigators believe that allergic disorders do play a prominent role, either as a cause or contributory factor, whereas others state that there is no convincing evidence that allergy leads to otitis media.[103] Allergy has been implicated as a causative factor in OME by (1) double-blind placebo-control nasal challenge studies with histamine and allergens; (2) studies on allergic children; and (3) studies on randomly selected children with OME referred to specialty clinics.[104] Kraemer and colleagues examined risk factors of OME among children with tympanostomy tubes compared with controls matched for age and showed atopy as a risk factor.[105] In another report, a series of 488 new patients referred to a pediatric allergy clinic showed that 49% had documented middle ear dysfunction.[106] In a prospective study, Bierman and Furukawa[107] demonstrated that allergic children have a high incidence of OME with conductive hearing loss. Fifty percent of their patients developed chronic effusion or AOM in a 6-month follow-up. Researchers in Japan evaluated 605 children with allergic rhinitis and found 21% with OME. They also determined that 50% of 259 children with diagnosed OME had allergic rhinitis.[108] Bernstein and Reisman[109] reviewed the clinical course of 200 randomly selected children with OME who had at least one tympanostomy with tube insertion.

Twenty-three percent were considered allergic by history, physical examination, and allergy skin testing. Other studies failed to demonstrate atopy as a risk factor for otitis media.[110,111]

The evidence that middle ear effusions are produced as a direct consequence of the mucosa of the middle ear or ET being an allergic shock organ is conflicting. Animal experiments suggest that the middle ear can serve as a shock organ. Miglets and coworkers,[112] in 1973, sensitized a squirrel monkey with human serum containing ragweed antibodies. Forty-eight hours later, this animal and a control animal were injected with Evans blue dye. Their ET orifices then were infiltrated with liquid ragweed antigen. Only the sensitized animal developed dark blue stains at the injected area. This was thought to occur secondary to an increase in capillary permeability caused by antigen–antibody interaction. Twelve of the 15 sensitized animals developed a middle ear effusion. Histologically, an early polymorphonuclear response was followed by a plasma cell infiltration. The authors conclude that the middle ear mucosa of the squirrel monkey has the capacity to act as a shock organ. Yamashita and others[113] challenged ovalbumin-sensitized guinea pigs through the nose. In this study, there was an absence of histopathologic changes in the middle ear space when only the nose was challenged. This study fails to support the theory that immediate hypersensitivity is commonly associated with middle ear effusion. Friedman and coworkers[114] studied eight patients, aged 18 to 29 years, with seasonal rhinitis but no middle ear disease. Patients underwent a blind challenged with the pollen to which the patient was sensitive or to a control. Nasal function was determined by nasal rhinomanometry and ET function by the nine-step–deflation tympanometric test. The results from this and other studies[115,116] showed that ET dysfunction can be induced by antigen and histamine challenge,[117] but no development of a middle ear effusion was demonstrated. Osur and colleagues[118] evaluated 15 children with ragweed allergy and measured ET dysfunction before, during, and after a ragweed season. A significant increase in ET dysfunction occurred during and after the ragweed season versus before the pollen season. As in the challenge studies, the ET dysfunction did not lead to OME. It appears that other variables need to be present for effusion to develop.

Much speculation on the role of allergy in contributing to the development of OME centers around the possibility of nasal obstruction from allergic rhinitis causing the Toynebee phenomenon, as previously described. This may predispose to insufflation of secretions into the middle ear.[119,120] Georgitis and associates[121] failed to show that allergen- and histamine-induced challenge leads to total nasal obstruction by the use of an anterior rhinomanometry. Bernstein[104] failed to demonstrate ET dysfunction by the nine-step ET test in 24 adults who had the test performed with nasal packing because of septoplasty for deviated septum. These studies leave in doubt that nasal obstruction from allergic rhinitis increases the likelihood of OME.

Another controversy in the pathogenesis of OME is the possible role of food allergy. Nsouli and coworkers[122] studied 104 children to assess the role food allergy in recurrent OME. These children had no history of food sensitivity and were assessed by skin prick tests, RASTs, and open food challenges. Physical examination, tympanometry, and audiometry were used to assess middle ear effusions. Seventy-eight percent of the children had food allergy by testing and went through a 16-week period of elimination of the offending foods followed by open challenge. Middle ear effusion resolved in 86% of the children when the offending food was eliminated, with 94% redeveloping OME on open food challenge. This study has been criticized because it was not controlled or blinded by the researchers.[123] The study failed to include a group of children with food allergy and OME who did not participate in an elimination diet to determine the number of children who would have had spontaneous resolution of their effusion. Bernstein and others[124] measured IgG and IgE antibodies to food substances by enzyme-linked immunosorbent assay in the serum and middle ear of otitis-prone children younger than 2 years of age and compared them with an age-related control group. There were significantly higher levels of IgG antibodies to milk, wheat, and egg white in the serum and middle ear of the otitis-prone children, but no difference in IgE levels.[124] Further research needs to be performed to clearly elicit the role of IgE hypersensitivity and IgG immune complexes to foods in the etiology of OME.

Many studies in OME involved immunoglobulin analysis of effusions.[125–127] The most prominent immunoglobulin found in effusions is secretory IgA, but IgG and IgE are elevated in some patients. In most of these investigations, patients failed to demonstrate an elevated effusion IgE level compared with the serum IgE level.[128] Although allergen-specific IgE can be found in effusions, the specificity usually is the same as that of serum. A definitive interpretation of these data is impossible, but it appears as if they, on the whole, fail to support the concept of the middle ear as a shock organ in most patients. There may be exceptions to this, because anti-ragweed[126] anti-*Alternaria*,[126] and anti-mite IgE[127] IgE have been found in effusions, but not in sera, in isolated instances. Khan and coworkers[129] compared the IgE, IgM, and IgA levels of the serum and tympanic fluid in 16 pediatric patients having OME, with the serum immunoglobulins of 32 normal children. Seven of ten patients with OME had elevated levels of IgE specific to common inhalants, compared with only 4 of 32 control patients. The elevated specific IgE found in this study may be an innocent bystander, but does provide some support for the importance of the allergic diathesis in OME.

The role of allergy in OME remains unclear. The evidence that the middle ear is rarely an allergic shock organ in OME is substantial, and most data do not support the belief that nasal obstruction causes the Toynbee phenomenon leading to OME. Available data, however, do not exclude immediate hypersensitivity as a primary etiologic factor in at least some cases. Allergy appears to be more often a contributory factor in the development of middle ear effusions. One possible mechanism is the release of chemical mediators from mast cells and basophils in allergic rhinitis, which could lead to ET inflammation and obstruction. Clearly, while the ET changes and improved muscle action of the tensor veli palatini develops in older children, the incidence of middle ear effusion dramatically decreases. The fact that the incidence of middle ear effusion declines dramatically with age, and that the incidence of allergic rhinitis rises with age, suggests that age-related factors may be more important than allergic factors in the development of middle ear effusion.

Acute and chronic suppurative otitis media are commonly part of a primary or secondary immunodeficiency syndrome. The middle ear usually is one of many locations for infection in immunodeficient patients. Of the primary immunodeficiency conditions, otitis media is more common in the humoral or B-cell disorders, such as X-linked hypogammaglobulinemia, common variable immunodeficiency, and selective IgA deficiency. A patient's incapacity to produce antibodies against pneumococcal polysaccharide antigens and a related IgG2 subclass deficiency has been associated with the development of recurrent otitis media in children.[130]

Veltri and Sprinkle[131] postulate that a type III immune complex mechanism may mediate some cases of OME. Immune complexes have been demonstrated in middle ear fluid by use of the fluorescent Raji cell assay.[132] Mravec and coworkers[133] produced an acute local inflammatory response by injecting immune complexes from rabbit and goat anti-rabbit sera into the bullae of chinchillas. Bernstein and coworkers[134] demonstrated positive immune complexes in only 2 of 41 samples of middle ear effusion using three assays: the Raji cell radioimmunoassay, direct immunofluorescence, and inhibition of anti-antibody. The literature does not support the thesis that immune complexes are fundamental in the development in middle ear effusion.

Diagnosis

Acute otitis media usually presents with fever, otalgia, vomiting, diarrhea, and irritability. In the young children, pulling at the ear may be the only manifestation of otalgia. Otorrhea, discharge from the middle ear, may occur if spontaneous perforation of the tympanic membrane occurs. AOM commonly is preceded by an upper respiratory infection. The pneumatic otoscope is an important tool for making accurate diagnosis of AOM. Classically, the tympanic membrane is erythremic and bulging without a light reflex or the ossicular landmarks visualized. Pneumatic testing fails to elicit any movement of the tympanic membrane on applying positive and negative pressure.

Most children with OME are asymptomatic. Others may complain of stopped-up or popping ears or a feeling of fullness in the ear. Older children may even observe a hearing loss. Many younger children are detected with hearing loss secondary to OME by their teachers and parents because they are noted to be inattentive, loud talkers, or slow learners. Other children may be discovered with OME in screening tests done for hearing at school. When middle ear effusions become chronic, there may be significant diminution of language development and auditory learning, with resultant poor academic achievement. On pneumatic otoscopic examination of patients with OME, the tympanic membrane may appear entirely normal. At other times, air—fluid levels and bubbles may be apparent. There often is retraction of the tympanic membrane, and the malleus may have a chalky appearance. As the disease progresses, the tympanic membrane takes on an opaque amber or bluish gray color. Alteration of the light reflex is commonly present. Mild retraction of the tympanic membrane may indicate only negative ear pressure without effusion. In more severe retraction, there is a prominent lateral process of the malleus with acute angulation of the malleus head. Tympanic membrane motility is generally poor when positive and negative pressures are applied by the pneumatic otoscopy.

Additional special tests often are performed in evaluating the patient with OME. Tympanometry is commonly used as an confirmatory test for the condition. It is a tool for indirect measuring of the compliance or mobility of the tympanic membrane by applying varying ear canal pressure from 200 to 400 mm H_2O. Patients with OME have a flat (type B) curve because of failure of the tympanic membrane to move with the changing pressure. Audiometric examination in OME often discloses a mild-to-moderate degree of conduction hearing impairment of 20 to 40 dB. The guidelines for the treatment of OME in young children from the Agency for Health Care Policy and Research[135] recommend that an otherwise healthy child with bilateral OME for 3 months should have a hearing evaluation. These guidelines fail to recommend a role for acoustic reflectometry, a test which involves a tone sweep in patient's ear, measuring reflected sound pressure to assess effusion, and tuning fork tests in the diagnosis and evaluation of OME.

The physical examination of the patient with OME should not stop at the tympanic membrane. Craniofacial anomalies may be present that predispose to OME, such as in Down's syndrome, submucous cleft palate, and bifid uvula. Stigmata of an allergic diathesis should be sought in each patient. Eye examination may illustrate injected conjunctiva seen in patients with allergic conjunctivitis. Pale, boggy turbinates with profuse serous rhinorrhea are commonly found with allergic rhinitis. When chronic middle ear effusions are associated with the signs and symptoms of allergic disease, a standard allergic evaluation is indicated. A nasal smear for eosinophils, peripheral eosinophil count, and cutaneous tests for specific allergens may be diagnostically important.

In patients with recurrent or chronic otitis media where middle ear disease is just one of many sites of infection, screening the immune system should be considered. Laboratory studies such as IgG, IgA, and IgM, naturally occurring antibodies such as isohemagglutinins, and specific antibody titers to antigens previously given in vaccines (such as tetanus), are useful in evaluating humoral immune status. Measuring specific antibody levels before and after administering a pneumococcal polyvalent vaccine is an effective means of evaluating humoral immune function. Another possible condition to consider in children with multiple sites of recurrent infection is primary ciliary dyskinesia. Examining the cilia by electron microscopic study can illustrate abnormalities of the cilia ultrastructure that can lead to ciliary dysfunction and its related chronic otitis.

Management

Management of the patient with OME requires appropriate pharmacologic and surgical intervention. The natural history of AOM and OME must be understood. Usually, the symptoms of AOM resolve in 48 to 72 hours if the organism is sensitive to the prescribed antibiotic. Two weeks into treatment, 70% of patients have a middle ear effusion; 1 month after treatment 40% continue to have effusion; but after 3 months only 10% of patients continue to have an persistent effusion.[81] Recently, the Agency of Health Care Policy and Research Guidelines published an algorithm on management of the child between the ages of 1 and 3 with OME (Fig. 11-3). This algorithm outlines a step-by-step approach to diagnosis and management of these children. In patients with OME in which allergy may be a contributing factor, the appropriate allergy treatment of avoiding particular allergens, medication, and immunotherapy may be indicated.

Pharmacology

Antimicrobial agents are the first-line therapy in AOM and may be beneficial in OME because bacterial infection is found in many cases. Amoxicillin, erythromycin-sulfisoxazole, and

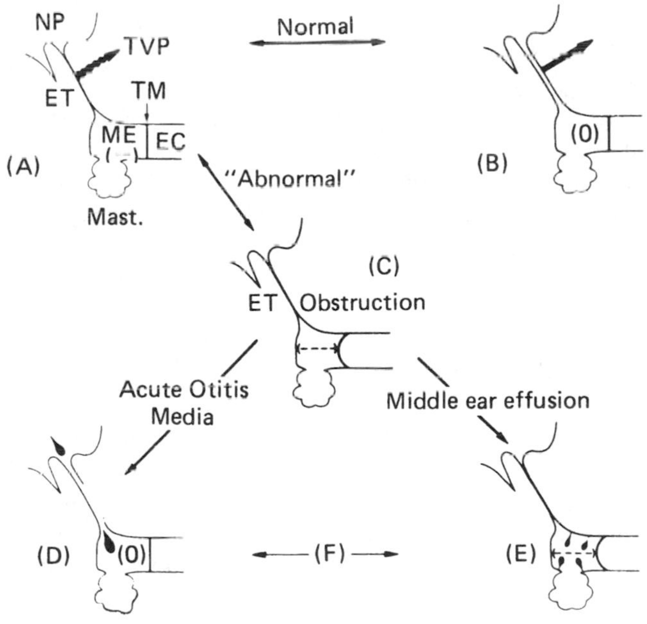

FIG. 11-3. Proposed pathogenic mechanisms of middle ear effusion. NP, nasopharynx; ET, eustachian tube; TVP, tensor veli palatini muscle; ME, middle ear; Mast., mastoid. TM, typanic membrane; EC, external canal. (Bluestone CD. Eustachian tube function and allergy in otitis media. Pediatrics 1978;61:753.)

trimethoprim-sulfamethoxazole are the antibiotics of choice in the initial treatment of these conditions. AOM usually is treated with a 7- to 10-day course of these antibiotics. Recently, reports of *S pneumoniae* resistant to penicillin, trimethoprim-sulfamethoxazole, or both raises concern of increased failure in initial treatment of AOM.[136] The Agency of Health Care Policy and Research Guidelines on OME in Young Children found by metaanalysis of the literature that there was a 14% increase in the probability that OME would resolve when antibiotic therapy was given compared with no treatment.[135] Berman[137] suggests that one of the above antibiotics be given for a 2- to 3-week course in OME. If one course of antibiotics is not effective, second and third courses may be prescribed. Another management option advocated for OME is observation of the patient for up to 4 months because of the natural history of resolution of OME in most patients. In patients with recurrent episodes of otitis media, several studies confirm that prophylactic regimens may be effective.[138–140] The suggested duration for prophylactic antibiotics is 3 to 6 months with amoxicillin, 20 mg/kg given once a day, or sulfisoxazole, 75 mg/kg given once a day.

Another therapeutic modality frequently prescribed in patients with OME is oral corticosteroids. The proper role for this agent in OME therapy is not clear. Many studies evaluate corticosteroids alone and in combination with antibiotics in clearing of middle ear effusions. Berman and others[141] performed metaanalysis comparing studies with the use of corticosteroids alone and with antibiotics and placebo. The authors found that clearance of middle ear effusion occurred in 64% with combination therapy in contrast to 39% with antibiotics only and 15% with placebo. Berman[137] recommends a 7-day trial of prednisone, 1 mg/kg/day divided into two doses, along with antibiotic therapy. The panel from the Agency of Health Care Policy and Research Guidelines on OME in Young Children[135] reviewed ten studies on the use of oral corticosteroids with and without antibiotics in OME and concluded that corticosteroid therapy is not effective in treating these children. Additional data must be obtained before a clear recommendation about the use of oral corticosteroids can be given.

Current data do not support the use of intranasal corticosteroids in the management of OME. Schwartz and associates[142] gave intranasal beclomethasone to ten children with OME and only three improved. Several studies[143,144] have shown that dexamethasone and flunisolide nasal spray in children with OME did not affect the ultimate outcome, but did facilitate rapid improvement in ET dysfunction.

Studies on the effectiveness of antihistamines and decongestants on randomly selected pediatric populations have shown no significant effect of these agents on resolution of OME.[143,145–147] Mandel and colleagues[148] compared antibiotic, antibiotic with antihistamine-decongestant, and placebo in the treatment of OME. The addition of an antihistamine-decongestant did not significantly affect the resolution of OME compared with antibiotic alone. Antihistamine-decongestant combinations are not indicated for treating OME in nonallergic patients, but studies need to be performed to determine their benefit in patients with allergic rhinitis and concomitant OME.

Environmental Control

When allergic rhinitis is associated with OME, environmental control of allergens and irritants should be advised. The most significant irritant is cigarette smoke. Parents must be urged to avoid exposing their children to cigarette smoke in the home, car, restaurant, and day-care facilities. Environmental inhalant allergens are more important to younger children because of the greater time spent in the home. Specific instructions for avoiding house dust mites, cockroaches, animal dander, and house mold spores should be given when indicated.

Surgical Treatment

Refractory cases that continue to have middle ear fluid after a 4-month trial of observation or medical management often need surgical intervention. Chronic middle ear effusion has been associated with the development of cholesteatomas, atrophy of the tympanic membrane, facial paralysis, and retention pockets. Myringotomy with the insertion of tympanostomy tubes is recommended by the Agency of Health Care Policy and Research Guidelines on OME in Young Children when children between the ages of 1 and 3 have bilateral hearing loss of at least 20 dB for 4 to 6 months. This procedure is effective in removing the effusion and restoring normal hearing in the child. Several studies[149,150–153] demonstrate the beneficial effect of tympanostomy tubes in OME. It is usually recommended that tympanostomy tubes remain in place for 6 to 18 months. The longer the tube remains in the tympanic membrane, the greater the chance of complications. These include tympanosclerosis, persistent perforation, otorrhea, and occasional cholesteatoma. Adenoidectomy has been suggested in the treatment of OME to remove blockage of the ET and improve ventilation. The Agency of Health Care Policy and Research Guidelines on OME in Young Children does not recommend adenoidectomy for children between 1 and 3 years of age with OME, although older children may benefit from the surgery. Gates and coworkers[154] demonstrated that adenoidectomy improved and reduced recurrences of OME in children older than 4 years of age. They report that the size of the adenoids did not relate to improvement of OME with adenoidectomy. Tonsillectomy is not recommended in the management of children with OME. In a study of 150 children between 2 and 9 years of age with OME, adenotonsillectomy was no more effective than adenoidectomy alone.[149]

Immunotherapy

Immunotherapy has been proved to be effective in the therapy for allergic rhinitis, when avoidance of the allergen is not possible or the symptoms are uncontrolled by medication. Many have the clinical impression that immunotherapy may be of help in OME in children with allergic rhinitis. However, there have been no controlled studies to verify this clinical impression.

In conclusion, the prognosis in OME usually is good. As the child gets older the incidence of OME tends to decrease. The medical and surgical intervention outlined for OME helps to control the condition until the child "outgrows" this disease.

REFERENCES

1. Fisher AA. Cutaneous reactions to cosmetics. In: Fisher AA, ed. Contact dermatitis. 3rd ed. Philadelphia: Lea & Febiger, 1986:77.
2. Marsh RJ, Towns S, Evans KF. Patch testing in ocular drug allergies. Trans Ophthal Soc UK 1978;98:278.
3. Mondino BJ, Salamon SM, Zaidman GW. Allergic and toxic reactions in soft contact lens wearers. Surv Ophthalmol 1982;26:337.
4. Friedlaender MH. Conjunctivitis of allergic origin: clinical presentation and differential diagnosis. Surv Ophthalmol 1993;38(Suppl):105.
5. Bonini S, Bonini S, Berruto A, et al. Conjunctival provocation test as a model for the study of allergy and inflammation in humans. Int Arch Allergy Appl Immunol 1988;998:1.
6. Proud D, Sweet J, Stein P, et al. Inflammatory mediator release on conjunctival provocation of allergic subjects with allergen. J Allergy Clin Immunol 1990;85:896. Abstract.
7. Brauninger G, Centifano Y. Immunoglobulin E in human tears. Am J Ophthalmol 1971;72:588.
8. Liotet S, Warnet VN, Arrata M. Lacrimal immunoblobulin E and allergic conjunctivitis. Opthalmologica 1983;186:31.
9. Donshik PC. Allergic conjunctivitis. Int Ophthal Clin 1988; 28:294.

10. Miller SB. Hypersensitivity diseases of the cornea and conjunctiva with a detailed discussion of phlyctenular disease. Ophthalmic Semin 1977;2:119.
11. Bonini S, Bonini S, Vecchione A, Naim D, Allansmith M, Balsano F. Inflammatory changes in conjunctival scrapings after allergen provocation in humans. J Allergy Clin Immunol 1988;82:462.
12. Bonini S, Tomassini M, Bonini S, Capron M, Balsano F. The eosinophil has a pivotal role in allergic inflammation of the eye. Int Arch Allergy Immunol 1992;99:354.
13. Bonini S, Bonini S. IgE and non-IgE mechanisms in ocular allergy. Ann Allergy 1993;71:296.
14. Bonini S, Bonini S, Berruto A, et al. Conjunctival provocation test as a model for the study of allergy and inflammation in humans. Int Arch Allergy Appl Immunol 1989;88:144.
15. Morgan SJ, Williams JH, Walls AF, Church MK, Holgate ST, McGill JI. Mast cell numbers and staining characteristics in the normal and allergic human conjunctiva. J Allergy Clin Immunol 1991;87:111. Abstract.
16. Ciprandi G, Buscaglia S, Pesce GP, Bagnasco M, Canonica GW. Ocular challenge and hyperresponsiveness to histamine in patients with allergic conjunctivitis. J Allergy Clin Immunol 1993;91:1227.
17. Woods AC. Ocular allergy. Am J Ophthalmol 1949;32:1457.
18. Friedlaender MH, Ohashi Y, Kelley J. Diagnosis of allergic conjunctivitis. Arch Ophthalmol 1984;102:1198.
19. Dechant KL, Goa KL. Levocabastine: a review of its pharmacological properties and therapeutic potential as a topical antihistamine in allergic rhinitis and conjunctivitis. Drugs 1991;41:202.
20. Stokes TC, Feinberg G. Rapid onset of action of levocabastine eye-drops in histamine-induced conjunctivitis. Clin Exp Allergy 1993;23:791.
21. Abelson MB, George MA, Schaefer K, Smith LM. Evaluation of the new ophthalmic antihistamine, 0.05% levocabastine, in the clinical allergen challenge model of allergic conjunctivitis. J Allergy Clin Immunol 1994;94:4588. Abstract.
22. Frostad AB, Olsen AK. A comparison of topical levocabastine and sodium cromoglycate in the treatment of pollen-provoked allergic conjunctivitis. Clin Exp Allergy 1993;23:406.
23. Shoel P, Freng BA, Kramer J, et al. Topical levocabastine compared with orally administered terfenadine for the prophylaxis and treatment of seasonal rhinoconjunctivitis. J Allergy Clin Immunol 1993;92:73.
24. Lanier BQ, Tremblay N, Smith JP, Defaller JM. A double-masked comparison of ocular decongestants as therapy for allergic conjunctivitis. Ann Allergy 1993;50:174.
25. Friday GA, Biglan AW, Hiles DA, et al. Treatment of ragweed conjunctivitis with cromolyn sodium 4% ophthalmic solution. Am J Ophthalmol 1993;95:169.
26. Greenbaum J, Cockcroft D, Hargreave FE, et al. Sodium cromoglycate in ragweed-allergic conjunctivitis. J Allergy Clin Immunol 1977;59:437.
27. Melamed J, Schwartz RH, Hirsch SR, Cohen SH. Evaluation of nedocromil sodium 2% ophthalmic solution for the treatment of seasonal allergic conjunctivitis. Ann Allergy 1994;73:57.
28. Juniper EF, Buyatt GH, Ferrie PJ, King DR. Sodium cromoglycate eye drops: regular versus as needed use in the treatment of seasonal allergic conjunctivitis. J Allergy Clin Immunol 1994;94:36. Abstract.
29. Montan P, Zetterström O, Eliasson E, Strömquist L-H. Topical sodium cromoglycate (Opticrom) relieves ongoing symptoms of allergic conjunctivitis within 2 minutes. Allergy 1994;49:637.
30. Ballas Z, Blumenthal M, Tinkelman DG, Kriz R, Rupp G. Clinical evaluation of ketorolac tromethamine 0.5% ophthalmic solution for the treatment of seasonal allergic conjunctivitis. Surv Ophthalmol 1993;38(Suppl):141.
31. Woodward DF, Nieves AL, Merglino G, Joseph R, Friedlaender MH. Acular: studies on its mechanism of action in reducing allergic conjunctival itching. J Allergy Clin Immunol 1995;95:360. Abstract.
32. Taudorf E, Laursen LC, Lanner A, et al. Oral immunotherapy in birch pollen hayfever. J Allergy Clin Immunol 1987;80:153.
33. Arsovski Z, Dokic D, Gavrilovski M, Dimitrovski M. The effect of immunotherapy on grass pollen allergic conjunctivitis. J Allergy Clin Immunol 1995;95:318. Abstract.
34. Abelson MB, George MA, Garofalo C. Differential diagnosis of ocular allergic disorders. Ann Allergy 1993;70:95.
35. Allansmith M, Frick OL. Antibodies to grass in vernal conjunctivitis. J Allergy 1963;34:535.
36. Allansmith MR, Baird RS, Higgenbotham EJ, Abelson MB. Am J Ophthalmol 1980;90:719.
37. Ballow M, Mendelson L. Specific immunoglobulin E antibodies in tear secretions of patients with vernal conjunctivitis. J Allergy Clin Immunol 1980;66:112.
38. Fukagawa K, Saito H, Azuma N, Tsubota K, Iikura Y, Oguchi Y. Histamine and tryptase levels in allergic conjunctivitis and vernal keratoconjunctivitis. Cornea 1994;13:345.
39. Allansmith MR, Baird RS. Mast cells, eosinophils and basophils in vernal conjunctivitis. J Allergy Clin Immunol 1978;61:154. Abstract.
40. Trocme CD, Kephart GM, Allansmith MR, Bourne WM, Gleich GJ. Conjunctival deposition of eosinophil granule major basic protein in vernal keratoconjunctivitis and contact lens associated giant papillary conjunctivitis. Am J Ophthalmol 1989;108:57.
41. Huntley CC, Fletcher WC. Current concept in therapy: vernal conjunctivitis: simple treatment. South Med J 1973;66:607.
42. Little FCS. Keeping pollen at bay. Lancet 1968;ii:512.
43. Ballow M, Donshik PC, Mendelson L, et al. IgG specific antibodies to rye, grass, and ragweed pollen antigens in the tear secretions of patients with vernal conjunctivitis. Am J Ophthalmol 1983;95:161.

44. Ballow M, Donshik PC, Mendelson L. Complement proteins and C3 anaphylatoxin in tears of patients with conjunctivitis. J Allergy Clin Immunol 1985;76:463.
45. Ballow M, Donshik PC, Rapacz P, Samartino L. Tear lactoferrin levels in patients with external inflammatory ocular disease. Invest Ophthal Vis Sci 1987;28:543.
46. Karel I, Myska V, Kvicaolva E. Ophthalmological changes in atopic dermatitis. Acta Derm Venerol (Stockh) 1965;45:381.
47. Oshinski L, Haine C. Atopic dermatitis and its ophthalmic complications. J Am Ophthalmic Assoc 1982;53:889.
48. Jay JL. Clinical features and diagnosis of adult atopic keratoconjunctivitis and the effect of treatment with sodium cromoglycate. Br J Ophthalmol 1981;65:335.
49. Reynolds RMPP. Giant papillary conjunctivitis. Trans Ophthalmol Soc N Z 1980;32:92.
50. Macivor J. Contact allergy to plastic artificial eyes. Can Med Assoc J 1950;62:164.
51. Goes F, Blockhuys S, Janssens M. Levocabastine eye drops in the treatment of vernal conjunctivitis. Doc Ophthalmol 1994;87:271.
52. Hyams SW, Bialik M, Neumann E. Clinical trial of topic disodium cromoglycate in vernal keratoconjunctivitis. J Ophthalmol 1975;12:116.
53. Collum LMT, Cassidy HP, Benedict-Smith A. Disodium cromoglycate in vernal and allergic kerato-conjunctivitis. Ir Med J 1981;74:14.
54. Foster CS, Duncan J. Randomized clinic trial of topically administered cromolyn sodium for vernal keratoconjunctivitis. Am J Ophthalmol 1980;90:175.
55. Foster CS, The Cromolyn Sodium Collaborative Study Group. Evaluation of topical cromolyn sodium in the treatment of vernal keratoconjunctivitis. Ophthalmology 1988;95:194.
56. Caldwell DR, Verin P, Hartwich-Young R, Meyer SM, Drake MM. Efficacy and safety of lodoxamide 0.1% vs. cromolyn sodium 4% in patients with vernal keratoconjunctivitis. Am J Ophthalmol 1992;113:632.
57. Abelson MC, Butrus SI, Weston J. Aspirin therapy in vernal conjunctivitis. Am J Ophthalmol 1983;95:502.
58. Meyer E, Kraus E, Zonis S. Efficacy of antiprostaglandin therapy in vernal conjunctivitis. Br J Ophthalmol 1987;71:497.
59. Trocme S, Raizman MB, Bartley GB. Medical therapy for ocular allergy. Mayo Clinic Proc 1992;67:557.
60. Allansmith MR, Lee JR, McClellan BH, et al. Evaluation of a sustained release hydrocortisone ocular insert in humans. Trans Am Acad Ophthalmol Otolaryngol 1975;79:128.
61. Foster CS, Calonge M. Atopic keratoconjunctivitis. Ophthalmology 1990;97:992.
62. Oster HB, Martin RG, Dawson CR. The use of disodium cromoglycate in the treatment of atopic disease. In: Leopold JH, Burns Rd, eds. Symposium on ocular therapy. New York: Wiley, 1977:99.
63. Amemiya T, Matsuda H, Vehara M. Ocular findings in atopic dermatitis with special reference to the clinical feature of atopic cataract. Ophthalmologica 1980;180:129.
64. Garrity JA, Liesegang TJ. Ocular complications of atopic dermatitis. Can J Ophthalmol 1984;19:21.
65. Easty D, Entwistle C, Fund A, Witcher J. Herpes simplex keratitis and keratoconums in the atopic patient: a clinical and immunological study. Trans Ophthal Soc UK 1975;95:267.
66. Meyers RL. Immunology of herpes virus infection. Int Ophthalmol Clin 1975;15:37.
67. Pavan PR, Langston D. Diagnosis and management of herpes simplex ocular infection. Int Ophthalmol Clin 1975;15:19.
68. Allansmith MI. Giant papillary conjunctivitis in contact lens wearers. Am J Ophthalmol 1977;83:697.
69. Culbertson W, Ostler BL. The floppy eyelid syndrome. Am J Ophthalmol 1981;92:568.
70. Stenson SM, ed. Contact lenses: guide to selection, fitting, and management of complications. East Norwalk, CT: Appleton & Lange, 1987:215.
71. Gudmonsson OG, Woodward DF, Fowler SA, Allansmith MR. Identification of proteins in contact lens surface deposits by immunofluorescence microscopy. Arch Ophthalmol 1985;103:196.
72. Tripathy RC, Tripathy BJ. Soft lens spoilage. Ophthalmic Forum 1984;2:80.
73. Barishak Y, Zavaro A, Samra Z, Sompolinsky D. An immunologic study of papillary conjunctivitis due to contact lenses. Current Eye Res 1984;3:1161.
74. Donshik P, Downes RT, Gotasky K, Elgebaly SA. The detection of neutrophil chemotactic factors in tear fluids of contact lens wearers with active papillary conjunctivitis. Invest Ophthalmol Vis Sci 1988;29:230.
75. Bailey CS, Buckley RJ. Nedocromil sodium in contact-lens–associated papillary conjunctivitis. Eye 1993; 7(Suppl):29.
76. Etzel R, Pattishall E, Haley N, et al. Passive smoking and middle ear effusions among children in day care. Pediatrics 1992;90:228.
77. Paparella M. Middle ear effusions: definitions and terminology. Ann Otol Rhinol Laryngol 1976;85(Suppl):8.
78. Cotton RT, Zalzal GH. Keeping otitis media and its sequelae at bay. J Respir Dis 1986;7:108.
79. Gates GA, Wachtendorf C, Hearne E, Holt G. Treatment of chronic otitis media with effusion: results of tympanosotomy tubes. Am J Otolaryngol 1985;6:249.
80. Dempster J, MacKenzie K. Tympanometry in the detection of hearing impairments associated with otitis media with effusion. Clin Otolaryngol 1991;16:157.
81. Teele O, Klein J, Rosner B, et al. Epidemiology of otitis media in children. Ann Otol Rhinol Laryngol 1980;89:5.
82. Bluestone CD, Shuring PA. Middle ear disease in children: pathogenesis, diagnosis, and management. Pediatr Clin North Am 1974;21:379.

83. Lowe JF, Baumforth JS, Pracy R. Acute otitis media: one year in general practice. Lancet 1963;31:1129.
84. Feingold M. Acute otitis media in children: bacteriological findings in middle ear fluid by needle aspiration. Am J Dis Child 1966;111:361.
85. Gulya AJ. Environmental tobacco smoke and otitis media. Otolaryngol Head Neck Surg 1994;111:6.
86. Ey J, Holberg C, Aldous M, et al. Passive smoke exposure and otitis media in the first year of life. Pediatrics 1995;95:670.
87. Thacker S, Addiss D, Goodman R, et al. Infectious diseases and injuries in child day care. JAMA 1992;268:1720.
88. Duncan B, Ey J, Holberg C, et al. Exclusive breast-feeding for at least 4 months protects against otitis media. Pediatrics 1993;91:867.
89. Aniansson G, Alm B, Andersson B, et al. A prospective cohort study on breast-feeding and otitis media in Swedish infants. Pediatr Infect Dis J 1994;13:183.
90. Strong M. The eustachian tube: basic considerations. Otol Clin North Am 1972;5:19.
91. Bluestone CD, Beery QC, Andrus S. Mechanics of the eustachian tube as it influences susceptibility to and persistence of middle ear effusions in children. Ann Otol Rhinol Laryngol 1974;83(Suppl):27.
92. Brook I. Otitis media: microbiology and management. J Otolaryngol 1994;23:269.
93. Bluestone C, Klein J. Otitis media in infants and children. Philadelphia: WB Saunders, 1988.
94. Post J, Preston R, Aul J, et al. Molecular analysis of bacterial pathogens in otitis media with effusion. JAMA 1995;273:1598.
95. Klein J, Teele D. Isolation of viruses and mycoplasmas from the middle ear effusions: a review. Ann Otol Rhinol Laryngol 1976;85(Suppl 25):140.
96. Brook I, Van de Heyning PH. Microbiology and management of otitis media. Scand J Infect Dis 1994;93(Suppl):20.
97. Fainstein V, Musager D, et al. Bacterial adherence to pharyngeal cells during viral infection. J Infect Dis 1980;142:172.
98. Giebink G, Wright P. Different virulence of influenza A virus strains and susceptibility to pneumococcal otitis media in chinchillas. Infect Immun 1983;41:913.
99. Welliver R, Kaul T, Ogra P, et al. The appearance of cell-bound IgE in respiratory tract epithelium after respiratory tract viral infection. N Engl J Med 1980;303:1198.
100. Sadé J, Halevy A, Hadas E. Clearance of middle ear effusions and middle ear pressures. Ann Otol Rhinol Laryngol 1976;85(Suppl):58.
101. Carson J, Collier A, et al. Acquired ciliary defects in nasal epithelium of children with acute viral upper respiratory infections. N Engl J Med 1985;312:463.
102. Schidlow DV. Primary ciliary dyskinesia (the immotile cilia syndrome). Ann Allergy 1994;73:457.
103. Hall L, Lukat R. Results of allergy treatment on the eustachian tube in chronic serous otitis media. Am J Otol 1981;3:116.
104. Bernstein JM. The role of IgE-mediated hypersensitivity in the development of otitis media with effusion: a review. Otolaryngol Head Neck Surg 1993;109:611.
105. Kraemer M, Richardson M, Weiss N, et al. Risk factors for persistent middle ear effusions: otitis media, catarrh, cigarette smoke exposure, and atopy. JAMA 1983;249:1022.
106. Marshall SG, Bierman CW, Shapiro GG. Otitis media with effusion in childhood. Ann Allergy 1984;53:370.
107. Bierman CW, Furukawa CT. Medical management of serous otitis in children. Pediatrics 1978;61:768.
108. Tomonaga K, Kurono Y, Mogi G, et al. The role of nasal allergy in otitis media with effusion: a clinical study. Acta Otolaryngol 1988;458(Suppl):41.
109. Bernstein J, Reisman R. The role of acute hypersensitivity in secretory otitis media. Trans Am Acad Ophthalmol Otolaryngol 1974;78:120.
110. Senturia B. Allergic manifestations and otologic disease. Laryngoscope 1960;70:285.
111. Black N. The aetiology of glue ear: a case control study. Int J Pediatr Otorhinolaryngol 1985;9:121.
112. Miglets AW, Spiegel J, Bronstein HA. Middle ear effusion in experimental hypersensitivity. Ann Otol Rhinol Laryngol 1976;85(Suppl):81.
113. Yamashita T, Okozaki N, Kumuzawa T. Relation between nasal and middle ear allergy. Ann Otol Rhinol Laryngol 1980;89(Suppl):47.
114. Friedman RA, Doyle WJ, Casselbrant ML, Bluestone C, Fireman P. Immunologic-mediated eustachian tube obstruction: a double-blind crossover study. J Allergy Clin Immunol 1983;71:442.
115. Walker SB, Shapiro GG, Bierman CW, et al. Induction of eustachian tube dysfunction with histamine nasal provocation. J Allergy Clin Immunol 1985;76:158.
116. Doyle WJ, Friedman R, Fireman P, Bluestone CD. Eustachian tube obstruction after provocative antigen challenge. Arch Otolaryngol 1984;110:508.
117. Skoner DP, Doyle WJ, Fireman P. Eustachian tube obstruction (ETO) after histamine nasal provocation: a double-blind dose-response study. J Allergy Clin Immunol 1987;79:27.
118. Osur S, Volovitz B, Dickson S, et al. Eustachian tube dysfunction in children with ragweed hayfever during natural pollen exposure. Allergy Proc 1989;10:133.
119. Cotton R. Serous otitis in children: medical and surgical aspects, diagnosis and management. Clin Rev Allergy 1984;2:329.
120. Kraemer M, Marshall S, Richardson M, et al. Etiology factors in the development of chronic middle ear effusions. Clin Rev Allergy 1984;2:319.

121. Georgitis J, Gold W, Bernstein J, et al. Eustachian tube function associated with histamine induced and ragweed induced rhinitis. Ann Allergy 1988;61:234-238.

122. Nsouli TM, Nsouli SM, Linde R, et al. Role of food allergy in serous otitis media. Ann Allergy 1994;73:215.

123. James J. Role of food allergy in serous otitis media. Ann Allergy Asthma Immunol 1995;74:277. Letter.

124. Bernstein J, Brentjens J, et al. Are immune complexes: a factor in the pathogenesis of otitis media with effusion? Am J Otolaryngol 1982;3:20.

125. Lewis DM, Schram JL, Lim DJ, Birck HG, Gleich G. Immunoglobulin E in chronic middle ear effusions: comparison of RIST, PRIST, and RIA techniques. Ann Otol Rhinol Laryngol 1978;85(Suppl):97.

126. Reisman RE, Bernstein J. Allergy and secretory otitis media: clinical and immunologic studies. Pediatr Clin North Am 1975;22:251.

127. Mogi G. Secretory IgA and antibody activities in middle ear effusions. Ann Otol Rhinol Laryngol 1976;85(Suppl):97.

128. Bernstein J, Lee J, et al. The role of IgE mediated hypersensitity in recurrent otitis media with effusion. Am J Otol 1983;5:66.

129. Khan J, Kirkwood E, Lewis L. Immunolgoical aspects of secretory otitis media in children: IgE and IgA levels in serum and glue. J Laryngol Otol 1981;95:121.

130. Umetsu D, Ambrosino D, et al. Recurrent sinopulmonary infection and impaired antibody response to bacterial capsular polysaccharide antigen in children with selective IgG-subclass deficiency. N Engl J Med 1985;313:1247.

131. Veltri RW, Sprinkle PM. Secretory otitis media: an immune complex disease. Ann Otol Rhinol Laryngol 1976;85(Suppl):135.

132. Maxim PE, Veltri RW, Sprinkle PM, Pusateri RJ. Chronic serous otitis media: an immune complex disease. Trans Am Acad Ophthalmol Otolaryngol 1977,84.234.

133. Mravec J, Lewis D, Lim D. Experimental otitis media with effusion: an immune complex mediated response. Trans Am Acad Ophthalmol Otolaryngol 1978;86:258.

134. Bernstein JM, Brentjens J, Vladutiu A. Immune complex determination in otitis media with effusion. Presented at the Midwinter Meeting of the Association of Research Otolaryngologists, St. Petersburg, FL, January 1981.

135. Stool S, Berg A, et al. Otitis media with effusion in young children. In: Clinical practice guidelines, DHHS publication no. (AHCRP) 94-0622 no. 12, 1994.

136. Leggiadro RJ. Penicillin- and cephalosporin-resistant *Streptococcus pneumoniae*: an emerging microbial threat. Pediatrics 1994;93:500.

137. Berman S. Otitis media in children. N Engl J Med 1995;332:1560.

138. Principi N, Marchisio P, Massironi E, et al. Prophylaxis of recurrent acute otitis media and middle-ear effusion. Am J Dis Child 1986;143:1414.

139. Biedel C. Modification of recurrent otitis media by short-term sulfonamide therapy. Am J Dis Child 1978;132:681.

140. Williams R, Chambers T, et al. Use of antibiotics in preventing recurrent acute otitis media and in treating otitis media with effusion: a meta-analytic attempt to resolve the brouhaha. JAMA 1993;270:1344.

141. Berman S, Roark R, et al. Theoretical cost effectiveness of management options for children with persisting middle ear effusions. Pediatrics 1994;93:353.

142. Schwartz R, Puglese J, et al. Use of a short course of prednisone for treating middle ear effusion: a double-blind crossover study. Ann Otol Rhinol Larngol 1980;89(Suppl):296.

143. Haugeto OK, Schroder KE, Mair IWS. Secretory otitis media, oral decongestant and antihistamine. J Otolaryngol 1981;10:359.

144. Shapiro GG, Bierman CW, Firilawa CT, et al. Treatment of persistent eustachian tube dysfunction in children with aerosolized nasal dexamethasone phosphate versus placebo. Ann Allergy 1982;49:81.

145. Olson AL, Klein SW, Charney E, et al. Prevention and therapy of serous otitis media by oral decongestant: a double-blind study in pediatric practice. Pediatrics 1978;61:679.

146. Cantekin E, Mandel E, Bluestone C, et al. Lack of efficacy of a decongestant–antihistamine combination for otitis media with effusion ("secretory" otitis media) in children: results of a double-blind randomized trial. N Engl J Med 1983,308.297.

147. Dusdieker L, Smith G, Booth B, et al. The long-term outcome of nonsuppurative otitis media with effusion. Clin Pediatr 1985;24:181.

148. Mandel E, Rockette H, Bluestone C, et al. Efficacy of amoxicillin with and without decongestant–antihistamine for otitis media with effusion in children: results of a double-blind, randomized trial. N Engl J Med 1987;316:4327.

149. Maw A, Herrod F. Otoscopic, impedance, and audiometric findings in glue ear treatment by adenoidectomy and tonsillectomy: a prospective randomized study. Lancet 1986;21:1399.

150. Black N, Crowther J, Freeland A. The effectiveness of adenoidectomy in the treatment of glue ear: a randomized controlled trial. Clin Otolaryngol 1986;11:149.

151. Gebhart D. Tympanostomy tubes in the otitis media prone child. Laryngoscope 1981;91:849.

152. Milner RM, Weller CR, Brenman AK. Management of the hearing impaired child with serous otitis media. Int J Pediatr Otorhinolaryngol 1985;9:233.

153. Bonding P, Tos M. Grommets versus paracentesis in secretory otitis media: a prospective, controlled study. Am J Otolaryngol 1985;6:455.

154. Gates G, Avery C, Cooper J, et al. Chronic secretory otitis media: effects of surgical management. Ann Otol Rhinol Laryngol 1989;138:2.

Allergic Diseases, 5th Edition,
edited by Roy Patterson, Leslie Carroll Grammer, and
Paul A. Greenberger. Lippincott–Raven Publishers, Philadelphia, © 1997.

12

Allergy to Stinging Insects

Robert E. Reisman

*R.E. Reisman: Departments of Medicine and Pediatrics,
State University of New York at Buffalo, Buffalo, NY 14214.*

Pearls for Practitioners
Roy Patterson

- Emergency therapy for insect sting anaphylaxis includes administration of epinephrine, 60 mg of prednisone, and hydroxyzine. The patient should then be taken to the emergency room. The same regimen should be used for anaphylaxis of other causes.

- Large local reactions to mosquito bites in northern climates may be severe in early summer and subside by later summer. Antihistamines may help. I have never seen an indication for mosquito immunotherapy.

- I have seen a case of Münchausen's anaphylaxis that was blamed on Hymenoptera stings but that was found to be self-induced by the patient with aspirin.

- Anaphylaxis from Hymenoptera stings can be frightening to patients and their parents. The availability of emergency therapy and venom immunotherapy is important for both care and reassurance.

Allergic reactions to insect stings result in about 50 recognized fatalities annually in the United States and are likely responsible for other unexplained sudden deaths. People at risk often modify their daily living patterns and life-styles. Major advances in our knowledge about the natural history of insect sting allergies have led to the appropriate diagnosis and treatment of insect sting anaphylaxis. For most affected people, this is a self-limiting disease; and for others, treatment results in a permanent cure.

THE INSECTS

The stinging insects are members of the order Hymenoptera of the class Insecta. They can be broadly divided into two families: the vespids, which include the yellow jacket, hornet, and wasp; and the apids, which include the honeybee and bumble bee. People may be allergic to one or all of the stinging insects, and identification of the insect responsible for a reaction is important in terms of the specific advice and venom immunotherapy given (see later).

    The honeybee and bumble bee are docile and tend to sting only when provoked. The bumble bee is a rare offender. Because of the common use of the honeybee for the production of honey and in plant fertilization, exposure to this insect is common. Multiple stings from honeybees can occur, particularly if their hive, which may contain thousands of insects, is in danger. The honeybee usually loses its stinging mechanism in the sting process, thereby inflicting self-evisceration and death.

The problem of multiple insect stings has been intensified by the introduction of the Africanized honeybee, the so-called killer bee, into the southwestern United States.[1] These bees are much more aggressive than the domesticated European honeybees, which are found throughout the United States. Massive sting incidents have resulted in death from venom toxicity. The Africanized honeybees entered South Texas in 1990 and are now present in Arizona and California. These bees probably will continue to spread throughout the southern United States. They are unable to survive in colder climates but may make periodic forays into the northern states during the summer months.

The yellow jacket is the most common cause of allergic insect sting reactions. These insects nest in the ground and are easily disturbed in the course of activities such as lawn mowing and gardening. They are also attracted to food and commonly are found near garbage and picnic areas. They are present in increasing numbers in late summer and fall. Hornets, which are closely related to the yellow jacket, nest in shrubs and are also easily provoked by activities such as hedge clipping. Wasps usually build honeycomb nests under eaves and rafters and are relatively few in number in these nests. In some parts of the United States, however, including Texas, wasps are the most common perpetrators of insect stings.

In contrast to stinging insects, biting insects, such as mosquitoes, rarely cause serious allergic reactions. These insects deposit salivary gland secretions that have no relation to the venom deposited by stinging insects. Anaphylaxis has occurred from bites of the deer fly, kissing bug, and bed bug. Isolated reports also have been made of mosquito bites causing anaphylaxis. Insect bites more commonly cause large local reactions, which may have an immune pathogenesis.[2]

REACTIONS TO INSECT STINGS

Normal Reactions

The usual reaction after an insect sting is mild redness and swelling at the sting site. This reaction is transient and disappears within several hours. Little treatment is needed other than analgesics and cold compresses. Insect stings, in contrast to insect bites, always cause pain at the sting site.

Large Local Reactions

Extensive swelling and erythema extending from the sting site over a large area are common reactions. The swelling usually reaches a maximum in 24 to 48 hours and may last as long as 10 days. On occasion, fatigue, nausea and malaise accompany the large local reaction. Aspirin and antihistamines are usually adequate treatment. When severe or disabling symptoms occur, steroids, such as prednisone, 40 mg/day for 2 to 3 days, may be helpful. These large local reactions have been confused with infection and cellulitis. Insect sting sites are rarely infected, and antibiotic therapy is rarely indicated.

Most people who have had large local reactions to insect stings have similar large local reactions to subsequent re-stings.[3] Generalized anaphylaxis, however, occurs in less than 5% of cases. Thus, people who have had large local reactions are not considered candidates for venom immunotherapy (discussed later) and do not require venom skin tests.

Anaphylaxis

The most serious reaction to an insect sting is anaphylaxis. Retrospective population studies suggest that the incidence of this acute allergic reaction ranges between 0.4% and 3%.[4–6] Allergic reactions can occur at any age, but most occur in people younger than 20 years of age, and twice as many occur in males as in females. These factors may reflect exposure rather than any specific age or sex predilection. Several clinical studies suggest that about one third of people who suffer systemic reactions have a personal history of atopic disease. Most allergic reactions result from stings to the head and neck, but reactions can occur from stings on any area of the body.[7–11]

In most patients, anaphylactic symptoms occur within 15 minutes after the sting, although there have been rare reports of reactions developing later. Clinical observations suggest that the sooner the symptoms occur, the more severe are the reactions. The clinical symptoms vary from patient to patient and are typical of anaphylaxis from any cause. The most common symptoms involve the skin and include generalized urticaria, flushing, and angioedema. More serious symptoms are respiratory and cardiovascular. Upper airway edema involving the pharynx, epiglottis, and trachea has been responsible for numerous fatalities. Circulatory collapse with shock and hypotension also has been responsible for mortality. Other symptoms include bowel spasm and diarrhea and uterine contractions.[9,12]

Severe anaphylaxis, including loss of consciousness, occurs in all age groups. Most deaths from sting anaphylaxis occur in adults. The reason for this increased mortality rate in adults may be the presence of cardiovascular disease or other pathologic changes associated with age. Adults may have less tolerance for the profound biochemical and physiologic changes that accompany anaphylaxis.[13–15] No clinical criteria or risk factors identify people at potential risk for insect sting anaphylaxis other than a history of a prior anaphylactic reaction.

The natural history of insect sting anaphylaxis has been well studied and is most intriguing. People who have had insect sting anaphylaxis have an approximate 60% recurrence rate of anaphylaxis after subsequent stings.[16] Viewed from a different perspective, not all people presumed to be at risk react to re-stings. The incidence of re-sting reactions is influenced by patient age and by the severity of the symptoms of the initial reaction. In general, children are less likely to have re-sting reactions than are adults. The more severe the anaphylactic symptoms, the more likely they are to recur. For example, children who have had dermal symptoms (hives, angioedema) as the only manifestation of anaphylaxis have a remarkably low re-sting reaction rate.[16,17] On the other hand, people of any age who have had severe anaphylaxis have an approximate 70% likelihood of repeat reactions.[16,18] When anaphylaxis does recur, the severity of the reaction tends to be similar to the initial reaction. No relation has been found between the occurrence and degree of anaphylaxis and the intensity of venom skin test reactions. Thus, factors other than immunoglobulin E (IgE) antibodies modulate clinical anaphylaxis.

Unusual Reactions

Serum sickness–type reactions, characterized by urticaria, joint pain, malaise, and fever, may occur about 7 days after an insect sting. On occasion, these reactions are associated with an immediate anaphylactic reaction. People who have a serum sickness–type reaction are subsequently at risk for acute anaphylaxis after repeat stings and thus are considered candidates for venom immunotherapy.[19]

Isolated reports have been made of other reactions, such as vasculitis, nephritis, neuritis, and encephalitis, occurring in a temporal relation to an insect sting. The causes of these reactions have not been established.[20]

Toxic Reactions

Toxic reactions may occur as a result of many simultaneous stings. Insect venom contains a number of potent pharmacologic agents, which can result in vascular collapse, shock, hypotension, and death.[21] The differentiation between allergic and toxic reactions sometimes can be difficult. As noted earlier, the incidence of toxic reactions in the United States probably will increase because of the Africanized honeybee. After a toxic reaction, a patient may develop IgE antibody and then be at risk for subsequent allergic sting reactions after a single sting. People who have had toxic reactions should be tested for the possibility of potential venom allergy.

IMMUNITY

Studies of immunity to insect venoms were initially carried out with beekeepers, who are stung frequently and generally have minor or no local reactions.[22] Beekeepers have high levels of serum venom-specific IgG, correlating to some extent to the amount of venom exposure (stings). These IgG antibodies are capable of blocking in vitro venom-induced histamine release from basophils of allergic people. In addition, administration of hyperimmune γ-globulin obtained from beekeepers provided temporary immunity from venom anaphylaxis in sensitive patients.[23] Successful venom immunotherapy is accompanied by the production of high titers of venom-specific IgG. These observations suggest that IgG antibodies reacting with venom have a protective function.

DIAGNOSTIC TESTS

Individual honeybee (*Apis mellifera*), yellow jacket (*Vespula* sp), yellow hornet (*Vespula arenaria*), bald-face hornet (*Vespula* maculata), and wasp (*Polistes* sp) extracts are available for the diagnosis and therapy of stinging insect allergies. Honeybee venom is obtained by electric stimulation. The vespid venoms (yellow jacket, hornet, and wasp) are obtained by dissecting and crushing the individual venom sacs. People with relevant stinging insect histories should be skin tested with the appropriate dilutions of each of the available five single Hymenoptera venom preparations. Venom dilutions must be made with a special diluent that contains human serum albumin. Testing is initiated with venom concentrations of 0.01 to 0.0001 µg/mL. The initial studies of venom skin tests concluded that an immunologically specific reaction suggesting that the patient is sensitive is a reaction of 1+ or greater at a concentration of 1 µg/mL or less, provided the 1+ reaction is greater than that of a diluent control.[24] Reactions to only 1 µg/mL must be evaluated carefully because another study of skin test reactions in an insect-nonallergic population showed that 46% reacted to this concentration of at least one venom.[25] This study suggested that 0.1 µg/mL might be a better cutoff point between immunologically specific and irritative skin test reactions. Higher concentrations of the venom tend to give nonspecific or irritative reactions and do not distinguish the normal from the allergic population.

In vitro tests have been used for the diagnosis of stinging insect allergy. IgE antibodies have been measured by the radioallergosorbent test (RAST)[26,27] and by histamine release from leukocytes.[28] About 15% to 20% of people who had positive venom skin tests do not react to the RAST. This may be a reflection of the sensitivity of the test. Conversely, the RAST results are affected by other factors, including the type and concentration of venom used for coupling and the presence of serum venom-specific IgG that could interfere by competing for the radiolabeled antisera. The RAST remains an excellent procedure for quantifying antibody titers over time. Histamine release from leukocytes is too cumbersome a laboratory procedure for routine diagnostic evaluation.

THERAPY

People who have a history of systemic reactions after insect stings and have detectable venom-specific IgE (positive skin tests or RAST) are considered at risk for subsequent reactions. Recommendations for therapy include measures to minimize exposure to insects, availability of emergency medication for medical treatment of anaphylaxis, and specific venom immunotherapy.

Avoidance

The risk of insect stings may be minimized by the use of simple precautions. People at risk should protect themselves with shoes and long pants or slacks when in grass or fields and should wear gloves when gardening. Cosmetics, perfumes, and hair sprays, which attract insects, should be avoided. Black and dark colors also attract insects; at-risk individuals should choose white or light-colored clothing. Food and odors attract insects; thus, garbage should be well wrapped and covered, and care should be taken with outdoor cooking and eating.

Medical Therapy

Acute allergic reactions from insect stings are treated in the same manner as anaphylaxis from any cause (see Chap. 20 for specific recommendations). Patients at risk are taught to self-administer epinephrine and are advised to keep epinephrine and antihistamine preparations available. Epinephrine is available in preloaded syringes (Ana-Kit, Bayer Laboratories, Spokane, WA; Epipen, Center Laboratories, Port Washington, NY) and can be administered easily. Consideration should be given to wearing an identification bracelet describing the insect allergy.

Venom Immunotherapy

Venom immunotherapy has been shown to be highly effective in preventing subsequent sting reactions.[29,30] Successful therapy is associated with the production of venom-specific IgG, which appears to be the immunologic corollary to clinical immunity. Venom immunotherapy should be administered to patients who have had sting anaphylaxis and have positive venom skin tests. As discussed earlier, studies of the natural history of the disease process in untreated patients have led to observations that may modify this recommendation. The presence of IgE antibody in a person who has had a previous systemic reaction does not neces-

TABLE 12-1. *Indications for venom immunotherapy in patients with positive venom skin tests**

Insect sting reaction	Venom immunotherapy
Normal—transient pain, swelling	No
Extensive local swelling	No
Anaphylaxis—severe	Yes
Anaphylaxis—moderate	Yes
Anaphylaxis—mild; dermal only	
Children	No
Adults	Yes†
Serum sickness	Yes
Toxic	Yes

*Venom immunotherapy is not indicated for patients with negative venom skin tests.
†Patients in this group might be managed without immunotherapy. See text.

sarily imply that a subsequent reaction will occur on reexposure. Observations relevant to the decision to use venom immunotherapy include age, interval since the sting reaction, and nature of the anaphylactic symptoms. Immunotherapy guidelines are summarized in Tables 12-1, 12-2, and 12-3.

Patient Selection

Children who have dermal manifestations as the sole sign of anaphylaxis do not require venom immunotherapy but should keep symptomatic medication available. Adults who have had mild symptoms of anaphylaxis, such as dermal reactions only, probably can be managed similarly. The documentation for the benign prognosis in adults, however, has not been as well substantiated, and this decision requires full patient concurrence. All people who have had more severe symptoms of anaphylaxis, such as respiratory distress, hypotension, or upper airway edema, should receive venom immunotherapy, regardless of the time interval since the sting reaction.

A very small number of people who have had venom anaphylaxis do not have positive venom skin tests.[31] They are not considered candidates for venom immunotherapy. The mechanism for their reactions remains unclear.

TABLE 12-2. *General venom immunotherapy dosing guidelines*

Initial dose	Administer 0.01 to 0.1 µg, depending on degree of skin test reaction.
Incremental doses	Schedules vary from "rush" therapy, administering multiple venom injections over several days, to traditional once-weekly injections.
Maintenance dose	Administer 50 to 100 µg of single venom or 300 µg of mixed vespid venom.
Maintenance interval	Every 4 weeks for the first year; every 6 weeks for the second year; every 8 weeks for the third year
Duration of therapy	Stop when skin test becomes negative, or after 3 to 5 years

TABLE 12-3. *Representative examples of venom immunotherapy dosing schedules**

	Traditional	Modified rush	Rush	
Day				
1	0.1	0.1	0.1‡	3.0
		0.3	0.3	5.0
		0.6	0.6	10
			1	20
2			35	
			50†	
			75	
3			100	
Week				
1	0.3	1		
		3		
2	1	5	100	
		10	*Repeat every 4 wks*	
3	3	20		
4	5	35		
5	10	50†		
6	20	65		
7	35	80		
8	50†	100		
9	65			
10	80	100		
11	100	*Repeat every 4 wks*		
12				
13	100			
	Repeat every 4 wks			

*Starting dose may vary depending on the patient's skin test sensitivity. Subsequent doses modified by local or systemic reactions. Doses expressed in micrograms (μg).

†50 μg may be used as maximal dose.

‡Sequential venom doses administered on same day at 20 to 30 minutes intervals.

After uneventful stings, a small percentage of people have positive skin tests, which are usually transient. In this situation, venom immunotherapy is not recommended.

Venom Selection

Since the availability of commercial venoms, the product brochure has recommended immunotherapy with each venom to which the patient is sensitive, as determined by the skin test reaction. Applying this criterion, one or multiple venoms may be administered. A mixed vespid venom preparation composed of equal parts of yellow jacket, yellow hornet, and bald face hornet venoms is available.

Controversy exists regarding whether multiple positive skin tests indicate specific individual venom allergy or reflect cross-reactivity between venoms. Extensive studies have been carried out concerning the cross-reactivity among insects. The honeybees (apids) are in a different family from the yellow jackets, hornets, and wasps (vespids). Within the vespid family, there is extensive cross-reactivity between the two hornet venoms,[32] extensive cross-reactivity between the yellow jacket and hornet venoms,[33] and limited cross-reactivity between wasp venom and other vespid venoms.[34] In my experience, most patients who have had yellow jacket sting reactions have positive skin test reactions to hornet venom and occasionally to *Polistes* venom. Thus, it is common to find multiple vespid skin test reactions in people who have reacted to one of the vespids. The product brochure recommends treatment with each of these vespid venoms. When the causative insect can be positively identified (particularly, the yellow jacket), single vespid venoms may be given with satisfactory protection.[30]

The relation between honeybee venom and yellow jacket venom is more complex.[35] RAST inhibition studies using serum from patients with coexisting titers of honeybee venom and yellow jacket venom-specific IgE have shown different patterns of reactivity ranging from no cross-reaction to fairly extensive cross-reaction. For an individual patient, this procedure is too tedious and unavailable to define the pattern. Knowledge of these results, however, may help suggest that single venom therapy would be adequate.

Dosing Schedule

The basic approach to venom immunotherapy is similar to that for other forms of allergy immunotherapy. Therapy is initiated in small doses, usually from 0.01 to 0.1 µg and incremental doses are given until a recommended dose of 100 µg is reached. Several dosing schedules have been used. The usual schedule suggests two or three injections during early visits, with doses doubled or tripled at 30-minute intervals. When higher doses are reached, a single dose is given each week. Other schedules call for more traditional dosing, with one injection per week throughout the build-up period. At the other end of the spectrum, rush desensitization has been given, with multiple doses administered to patients in a hospital setting over a period of 2 or 3 days to 1 week. The most important goal of venom therapy is to reach the recommended 100 µg dose of a single venom or 300 µg of mixed vespid venom. Maintenance doses are given every 4 weeks during the first year. Thereafter, the maintenance interval usually can be extended to 6 and even 8 weeks with no loss of clinical effectiveness or increase in immunotherapy reactions.[36,37]

In my experience, 50 µg may be used as the top venom dose. Using this maximum dose and primarily single-venom therapy, results with immunotherapy have been excellent, with an approximate 98% success rate.[30]

The more rapid schedules appear to be accompanied by a more rapid increase in venom-specific IgG production, and thus this schedule may provide protection earlier.[38] Reaction rates to venom administered by both rapid and slower schedules vary in different studies but are not significantly different.

Reactions to Therapy

As with other allergenic extracts, reactions can occur from venom immunotherapy. The usual reactions are large local reactions that last several days and immediate systemic reactions. These reactions may present more of a problem, however, because to ensure clinical protection, it is necessary to reach full maintenance doses of venom. With other allergenic extracts, such as pollen, doses are usually decreased and maintained at lower levels. Treatment of local reactions includes splitting of doses, thus limiting the amount of venom delivered to one site; cold compresses; and antihistamines.

In the large study of insect sting allergy conducted by the American Academy of Allergy, Asthma and Immunology, the incidence of venom systemic reactions was about 10%.[39] There were no identifiable factors predicting these reactions. After a systemic reaction, the next dose is reduced by about 25% to 75%, depending on the severity of the reaction, and subsequent doses are slowly increased. If patients are receiving multiple venom therapy, it may be useful to give individual venom on separate days. This may help identify the specific venom responsible for the reaction.

Another adverse reaction occasionally noted after injections of other allergenic extracts, but more frequently with venom, is the occurrence of generalized fatigue and aching often associated with large local swelling. Prevention of these reactions can usually be accomplished with aspirin, 650 mg given about 30 minutes before the venom injection and repeated every 4 hours as needed. If this therapy is ineffective, steroids may be administered at the same time as venom injection.

Most people who have had reactions to venom immunotherapy are ultimately able to reach maintenance doses. On rare occasions, systemic reactions have necessitated cessation of treatment.

No adverse reactions from long-term venom immunotherapy have been identified. Venom injections appear to be safe during pregnancy, with no adverse effect on either the pregnancy or the fetus.[40]

Cessation of Venom Immunotherapy

Definitive criteria for stopping venom injections are being developed. These include immunologic criteria and a specific time period of immunotherapy, unrelated to the persistence of a positive venom skin test.

Conversion to a Negative Skin Test

Conversion to a negative skin test is an absolute criterion for stopping immunotherapy, indicating that the IgE antibody, the immune mediator of this reaction, is no longer present. Some treated patients convert to a negative skin test after 3 to 5 years of therapy.

Fall in Serum Venom-Specific Immunoglobulin E to Insignificant Titer

Another immunologic parameter that has been applied to determine the safety of discontinuing immunotherapy is the failure to detect IgE venom antibodies in serum. Using this criterion for discontinuing therapy, re-sting reaction rates are about 10% per patient, with the average duration of venom treatment about 2 years.[41] The control for these studies was a group of patients who stopped by self-choice and received treatment for about the same period of time. In this control group, the re-sting reaction rate was about the same. These data suggest that although the fall in serum antibodies may be a reasonable criterion for stopping treatment, 2 years of treatment does reduce the risk of allergic re-sting reactions to about 10%.

Specific Time Period

Treatment for a specific period of time, 3 to 5 years, despite the presence of persistent positive skin tests also appears to be an adequate criterion for stopping therapy. Two European studies suggest that 3 years of venom therapy is sufficient.[42,43] Studies in children and adults at Johns Hopkins University concluded that 5 years of therapy is adequate.[44,45]

Specific Time Period of Treatment Related to Nature of Anaphylactic Symptoms

The nature or severity of the initial sting anaphylactic symptoms has been used as a marker to evaluate duration of treatment.[46] Data suggest that patients who have had mild to moderate venom anaphylactic symptoms can discontinue treatment after 2 to 3 years. Patients who have had more severe anaphylaxis may require longer periods of treatment. In the latter group, the re-sting reaction rate after cessation of therapy is about 15%, with most having the same or similar severe reactions. Thus, it may be prudent to treat patients who have had more severe allergic reactions, such as loss of consciousness, hypotension, and shock, and who retain positive skin tests for longer periods.

FIRE ANT AND HARVESTER ANT STINGS

Systemic reactions to the stings of the fire ant have been reported with increasing frequency.[47,48] This insect is present in growing numbers in the southeastern United States, particularly in states bordering the Gulf Coast. The fire ant attaches itself to its victim by biting with its jaws and then pivots around its head, stinging in multiple sites in a circular pattern with a stinger located on the abdomen. Within 24 hours of the sting, a sterile pustule develops that is diagnostic of the fire ant sting. Allergic symptoms occurring after stings are typical of acute anaphylaxis. Fatalities have occurred in children and adults.

Skin tests with extracts prepared from whole bodies of fire ants appear to be reliable in identifying allergic people, with few false-positive reactions in nonallergic controls. Fire ant venom, not yet commercially available, has been collected and compared with fire ant whole-body extract. The results of skin tests and in vitro tests show that the venom is a better diagnostic antigen. Whole-body extracts can be prepared, however, that apparently contain sufficient allergen and are reliable for skin test diagnosis. These results suggest that the antigens responsible for allergic reactions can be preserved in the preparation of whole-body extracts. Unfortunately, the potency of different commercial fire ant whole-body extracts has been variable. When available, fire ant venom will provide a potent, reliable extract.

Fire ant venom has been well studied and differs considerably from other Hymenoptera venoms. Studies have shown four allergenic fractions in the fire ant venom.

Immunotherapy with whole-body fire ant extract appears to be effective. Because the whole-body fire ant extract can be a good diagnostic agent, this therapeutic response can be anticipated. Control observations studying the response of subsequent stings in allergic patients not receiving venom immunotherapy have been limited. One study compared the results of fire ant re-stings in whole-body extract–treated patients and in untreated patients.[49] In the treated group, there were 47 re-stings, with 1 systemic reaction. In contrast, in the 11 untreated patients, there were 11 systemic reactions. Serologic studies defining the nature of the immunity to fire ant stings have not been conducted.

In vitro studies suggest some cross-reaction between the major allergens in fire ant venom and the winged Hymenoptera venoms. The clinical significance of this observation is still unclear; there appears to be limited clinical application. People allergic to bees and vespids do not appear to be at major risk for fire ant reactions, and similarly, fire ant allergic people are not at major risk for reactions from the winged Hymenoptera.

Anaphylaxis from the sting of the harvester ant, another nonwinged Hymenoptera present in the southwestern United States, has been described.[50] Specific IgE antibodies have been detected with direct skin tests and leukocyte histamine release using harvester ant venom.

REFERENCES

1. McKenna WR. Killer bees: what the allergist should know. Pediatr Asthma Allergy Immunol 1992;4:275.
2. Brummer-Korvenkontio H, Lappalainen P, Reunala T, Palusuo T. Detection of mosquito saliva-specific IgE and IgG$_4$ antibodies by immunoblotting. J Allergy Clin Immunol 1994;93:551.
3. Mauriello PM, Barde, SH, Georgitis JW, Reisman RE. Natural history of large local reactions (LLR) to stinging insects. J Allergy Clin Immunol 1984;74:494.
4. Golden DBK. Epidemiology of allergy to insect venoms and stings. Allergy Proc 198;10:103.
5. Chaffee FH. The prevalence of bee sting allergy in an allergic population. Acta Allergology 1970,25.292.
6. Settipane GA, Boyd GK Prevalence of bee sting allergy in 4,992 Boy Scouts. Acta Allergology 1970;25:286.
7. Brown H, Bernton HS. Allergy to the Hymenoptera. Arch Intern Med 1970;125:665.
8. Frazier CA. Allergic reactions to insect stings: a review of 180 cases. South Med J 1964:57:1028.
9. Mueller HL. Further experiences with severe allergic reactions to insect stings. N Engl J Med 1959;261:374.
10. Mueller U, Schmid WH, Rubinsztain R. Stinging insect hypersensitivity: a 20 year study of immunologic treatment. Pediatrics 1975;55:530.
11. Schwartz HJ, Kahn B. Hymenoptera sensitivity. II. The role of atopy in the development of clinical hypersensitivity J Allergy 1970;45:87.
12. Barnard JII. Nonfatal results in third degree anaphylaxis from Hymenoptera stings. J Allergy 1970;45:92.
13. Jensen OM. Sudden death due to stings from bees and wasps. Acta Pathol Microbiol Immunol Scand (A) 1962;54:9.
14. O'Connor R, Stier RA, Rosenbrook W Jr, Erickson RW. Death from "wasp" sting. Ann Allergy 1964;22:385.
15. Schenken JR, Tamisiea J, Winter FD. Hypersensitivity to bee sting. Am J Clin Pathol 1953:23:1216.
16. Reisman RE. Natural history of insect sting allergy: relationship of severity of symptoms of initial sting anaphylaxis to re-sting reactions. J Allergy Clin Immunol 1992;90:335.
17. Valentine MD, Schuberth KC, Kagey-Sobotka A, et al. The value of immunotherapy with venom in children with allergy to insect stings. N Engl J Med 1991;23:1601.
18. Lantner R, Reisman RE. Clinical and immunologic features and subsequent course of patients with severe insect sting anaphylaxis. J Allergy Clin Immunol 1989;84:900.
19. Reisman RE, Livingston A. Late onset reactions including serum sickness, following insect stings. J Allergy Clin Immunol 1989;84:331.
20. Light WC, Reisman RE, Shimizu M, Arbesman CE. Unusual reactions following insect stings. J Allergy Clin Immunol 1977;59:391.
21. Hoffman DR. Hymenoptera venoms: composition, standardization, stability. In: Levine MI, Lockey RF, ed. Monograph on insect allergy. Pittsburgh, PA: American Academy of Allergy and Immunology, 1995:27.
22. Light WC, Reisman RE, Wypych JI, Arbesman CE. Clinical and immunological studies of beekeepers. Clin Allergy 1975;5:389.
23. Lessof MH, Sobotka AK, Lichtenstein LM. Effects of passive antibody in bee venom anaphylaxis. Johns Hopkins Med J 1978;142:1.
24. Hunt KJ, Valentine MD, Sobotka AK, Lichtenstein LM. Diagnosis of allergy to stinging insects by skin testing with Hymenoptera venoms. Ann Intern Med 1976;85:56.
25. Georgitis JW, Reisman RE. Venom skin tests in insect-allergic and insect non-allergic populations. J Allergy Clin Immunol 1985;76:803.
26. Reisman RE, Wypych JI, Arbesman CE. Stinging insect allergy: detection and clinical significance of venom IgE antibodies. J Allergy Clin Immunol 1975;56:443.
27. Sobotka AK, Adkinson JF Jr, Valentine MD, Lichtenstein LM. Allergy to insect stings. V. Diagnosis by radioallergosorbent tests (RAST). J Immunol 1978;121:2477.
28. Sobotka AK, Valentine MD, Benton AW, Lichtenstein LM. Allergy to insect stings. I. Diagnosis of IgE-mediated Hymenoptera sensitivity by venom induced histamine release. J Allergy Clin Immunol 1974;53:170.
29. Valentine MD. Insect venom allergy: diagnosis and treatment. J Allergy Clin Immunol 1984:73:299.
30. Reisman RE, Livingston A. Venom immunotherapy (VIT): ten years experience with administration of single venoms and fifty micrograms maintenance doses. J Allergy Clin Immunol 1992;85:210.

31. Clayton WF, Georgitis JW, Reisman RE. Insect sting anaphylaxis in patients without detectable serum venom specific IgE. J Allergy Clin Immunol 1983;71:141.
32. Mueller U, Elliott W, Reisman RE, et al. Comparison of biochemical and immunologic properties of venoms from the four hornet species. J Allergy Clin Immunol 1981;67:290.
33. Reisman RE, Mueller U, Wypych J, et al. Comparison of the allergenicity and antigenicity of yellow jacket and hornet venoms. J Allergy Clin Immunol 1982;69:268.
34. Reisman RE, Wypych JI, Mueller UR, Grant JA. Comparison of the allergenicity and antigenicity of Polistes venom and other vespid venoms. J Allergy Clin Immunol 1982;70:281.
35. Reisman RE, Mueller UR, Wypych JI, Lazell MI. Studies of coexisting honeybee and vespid venom sensitivity. J Allergy Clin Immunol 1983;73:246.
36. Goldberg A, Reisman RE. Prolonged interval maintenance venom immunotherapy. Ann Allergy 1988:61:177.
37. Golden DBK, Kagey-Sobotka A, Valentine MD, Lichtenstein LM. Prolonged maintenance interval in Hymenoptera venom immunotherapy. J Allergy Clin Immunol 1987;67:482.
38. Golden DBK, Valentine MD, Sobotka AK, Lichtenstein LM. Regimens of Hymenoptera venom immunotherapy. Ann Intern Med 1980;92:620.
39. Lockey R, Peppe B, Barid I, Turkeltaub P. Hymenoptera venom study, safety. J Allergy Clin Immunol 1983;71:141. Abstract.
40. Schwartz HJ, Golden DBK, Lockey RF. Venom immunotherapy in the Hymenoptera allergic pregnant patient. J Allergy Clin Immunol 1990;85:709.
41. Reisman RE, Lantner R. Further observations on discontinuation of venom immunotherapy: comparisons of patients stopped because of a fall in serum venom specific IgE to insignificant levels with patients stopped "prematurely" by self-choice. J Allergy Clin Immunol 1989;83:1049.
42. M∞ller U, Berthtold E, Helbling A. Honey bee venom allergy: results of a sting challenge one year after cessation of successful venom immunotherapy in 86 patients. J Allergy Clin Immunol 1991;87:702.
43. Haugaard L, Norregaard OFH, Dahl R. In-hospital sting challenge in insect venom-allergic patients after stopping venom immunotherapy. J Allergy Clin Immunol 1991;87:699.
44. Golden DBK, Kwiterovich KD, Kagey-Sobotka A, Valentine MD, Lichtenstein LM. Discontinuing venom immunotherapy (VIT): outcome after five years. J Allergy Clin Immunol 1996;97:579.
45. Schuberth KC, Kwiterovich KA, Kagey-Sobotka A, Lichtenstein LM, Valentine MD. Starting and stopping venom immunotherapy (VIT) in children with insect sting allergy. J Allergy Clin Immunol 1988;81:200. Abstract.
46. Reisman RE. Duration of venom immunotherapy: relationship to the severity of symptoms of initial insect sting anaphylaxis. J Allergy Clin Immunol 1993;92:831.
47. Stafford CT, Hoffman DR, Rhoades RB. Allergy to imported fire ants. South Med J 1989;82:1520.
48. Stafford CT, Hutto LS, Rhoades RB, Thompson VW, Impson LK. Imported fire ant as a health hazard. South Med J 1989;82:1515.
49. Hylander RD, Ortiz AA, Freeman TM. Imported fire ant immunotherapy: effectiveness of whole body extracts. J Allergy Clin Immunol 1989;83:232.
50. Pinnas JL, Strunk RC, Wang TM, Thompson HC. Harvester ant sensitivity: in vitro and in vivo studies using whole body extracts and venom. J Allergy Clin Immunol 1977;59:10.

Allergic Diseases, 5th Edition,
edited by Roy Patterson, Leslie Carroll Grammer, and
Paul A. Greenberger. Lippincott–Raven Publishers, Philadelphia, © 1997.

13

Urticaria, Angioedema, and Hereditary Angioedema

W. James Metzger

*W.J. Metzger: Section of Allergy, Asthma, and Immunology,
East Carolina University School of Medicine, Greenville, NC 27858-4354.*

Pearls for Practitioners
Roy Patterson

- Most cases of chronic, recurrent urticaria without an obvious ingestant allergen are idiopathic, meaning they have no external cause. Patients should be encouraged to stop looking for a cause.
- Recurrent urticaria of increasing severity may be a prodrome of episodes of idiopathic anaphylaxis.
- Some cases of recurrent idiopathic urticaria are responsive to hydroxyzine, even at low doses (25 mg/d), when they are not responsive to other H1-blockers. These patients are fortunate. Recurrent idiopathic urticaria not responsive to antihistamines can be a major problem for patients and their physicians.
- Severe urticaria uncontrolled by hydroxyzine may be sufficiently problematic that an induction of remission by prednisone (as used for idiopathic anaphylaxis) becomes necessary.
- Angioedema involving the airway with possible airway obstruction is idiopathic anaphylaxis–angioedema.
- Severe angioedema involving the tongue and obstructing the airway can result from angiotensin–converting enzyme inhibitors. Often, the patient has a history of mild angioedema without angiotensin–converting enzyme inhibitors.

The earliest texts called urticaria and angioedema a "vexing problem."[1] Little has changed since that assessment. Today's clinician is still faced with a common syndrome that affects 20% of the population at some time in their lives,[2] but there is no cohesive understanding of its clinical mechanisms, presentations, or clinical management. For the clinician, this requires a broad knowledge of the many clinical forms of urticaria and an even more extensive familiarity with the creative ways that medications and treatment can be applied. Modern concepts of allergen-induced cellular inflammation, late-phase cutaneous responses, adhesion molecules, cytokines, and inflammatory autacoids may lead to a better understanding of pathogenesis and treatment. Meanwhile, clinicians should formulate a rational approach to the care of patients with these conditions.

Urticaria consists of raised, erythematous skin lesions that are markedly pruritic, tend to be evanescent in any one location, and are generally worsened by scratching. This description does not cover all forms of urticaria, but it contains the features necessary for diagnosis in most clinical situations. Angioedema is frequently associated with urticaria, but the two may occur independently. Angioedema is a reaction similar to urticaria, except that it occurs in deeper tissues and is clinically characterized by asymmetric swelling of tissue. Pruritus, however, is uncommon with angioedema, which more typically has a burning sensation. Any area of the body may be involved, although the perioral region, periorbital regions, tongue, genitalia, and extremities are involved most frequently. In this review, angioedema and urticaria are discussed jointly except where specified.

The incidence of acute urticaria is not known. Although it is said to afflict 10% to 20% of the population at some time during life, the greatest incidence occurs in young adults (15.7%).[1] Chronic urticaria occurs more frequently in middle-aged people, especially women. In a family practice office, its prevalence is 30%.[3] Of patients who have chronic urticaria for more than 6 months, 40% continue to have recurrent wheals 10 years later.[4] It is possible that the true prevalence of chronic urticaria is higher than reported owing to many acute, self-limited episodes that do not come to medical attention.

Acute urticaria is arbitrarily defined as persisting less than 6 weeks, whereas chronic urticaria refers to episodes lasting more than 6 to 8 weeks. When considering chronic urticaria, an etiologic agent or precipitating cause is established in up to 30% of patients who receive a thorough evaluation.[5] Therefore, most chronic urticaria is idiopathic. Success rates of determining an inciting agent are higher in acute forms. Because of the sometimes extreme discomfort and cosmetic problems associated with chronic urticaria, a thorough evaluation to search for etiologic factors is recommended. This evaluation must be tempered, however, by a limited laboratory evaluation, with reliance primarily on the history, physical examination, and response to therapy (Fig. 13-1).

PATHOGENESIS

No unifying concept has been determined to account for all forms of urticaria. Histamine plays a major role in many forms, based first on the observations by Lewis[6] of a cutaneous triple response characterized by erythema, edema, and flare due to an axon reflex that is mediated, perhaps, by substance P. Erythema and edema are mimicked by intracutaneous injection of histamine, causing localized pruritus, a major characteristic of urticaria. The hypothesis that histamine is the central mediator of urticaria is bolstered by (1) the cutaneous response to injected histamine, (2) the frequent clinical response to various forms of urticaria and to therapeutic antihistamines, (3) the documented elevation of plasma histamine or local histamine release from urticating tissue in some forms of the condition, and (4) the apparent degranulation of skin mast cells. An association with histamine release has not been made in many forms of urticaria.

Various forms of chronic urticaria have been associated with eosinophil granule proteins[7] presumed to be capable of prolonged inflammation of the skin. Cytokines, such as interleukin-5, may be responsible for the attraction to and maintenance of activated eosinophils at the skin site.[7,8] Platelet-activating factor[9,10] may also be integral to certain urticarias because of its potent eosinophilic and chemotactic properties[11] and because effective medications such as doxepin have platelet-activating factor antagonist activity, among other inhibitory effects.[12]

If any central hypothesis for pathogenesis can be formulated, histamine and the skin mast cell certainly play a crucial role in several forms of urticaria.[8,13,14] Whether certain subtypes of skin mast cells are characterized by their content of tryptase or chymase[8,15] requires further investigation. Although helper T cells are increased,[16] activation of T cells is not demonstrable. Dysregulation of E-selectin, ICAM-1, and VCAM-1 adhesion molecules may account for the former and may be precipitated by mast cell–released cytokines.[3,16,17] Autoactivation by discharged substance P may perpetuate the urticaria.[9]

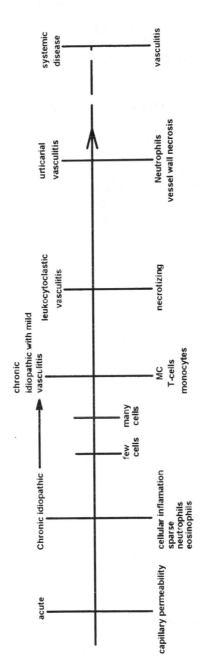

CONTINUUM OF ACUTE URTICARIA TO URTICARIAL VASCULITIS

FIG. 13-1. A hypothetical model for describing the range of histology of chronic idiopathic urticaria. MC, mast cells.

Several potential mechanisms for mast cell activation in the skin are summarized in Table 13-1 and include: (1) immunoglobulin E (IgE) immediate hypersensitivity, (2) activation of the classic or (3) alternative complement cascades, and (4) direct mast cell membrane activation. The presence of major basic protein in biopsy specimens of chronic urticaria[7] makes the eosinophil suspect as an effector cell. Greaves[17] identified autoimmune chronic urticaria, mediated by anti-FcεRIα, anti-IgE antibodies of the IgG class, or both, which crosslink adjacent mast cell receptors or IgE molecules up to 48% of the time in chronic idiopathic urticaria. This entity can be identified by cutaneous injections of autologous serum. Thyroid autoimmunity has been reported in 14% of chronic idiopathic urticaria, with nearly half of patients having clinical disease.[18] Prolonged response to histamine, but not leukotrienes, in the skin of patients with chronic urticaria suggests abnormal clearance of mediators locally.[19]

Nonspecific factors that may aggravate urticaria include fever, heat, alcohol ingestion, exercise, emotional stress, premenstrual or postmenopausal status, and hyperthyroidism. Chronic anaphylaxis with urticaria due to progesterone has been described,[20] and progesterone has also been used to treat chronic cyclic urticaria and eosinophilia.[21] Certain food preservatives may also aggravate chronic urticaria.[8,22] Some experts believe that progesterone is not a cause or a treatment and that food preservatives do not aggravate chronic urticaria.

The kinin-generating system may be important in hereditary angioedema (HAE)[23] or in angioedema resulting from angiotensin-converting enzyme inhibitors.[8]

TABLE 13-1. *Potential mechanisms of mast cell activation in urticaria or angioedema*

Type	Cause	Mediators
IgE immediate hypersensitivity	Allergens[80] Modified IgE IgG$_4$ Autoimmune anti-IgE or FcεRIα FcεRII (CD23) on platelets, lymphocytes, or eosinophils	Histamine leukotrienes, prostaglandin D$_2$,[39] platelet-activating factor,[9] eosinophil chemotactic factor of anaphylaxis,[81] and histamine-releasing factor[82]
Activation of classic pathway of complement	Antigen–antibody complexes (IgM, IgG$_1$, IgG$_2$, or IgG$_3$)	C3a, C4a, C5a (anaphylatoxins) cause release of mast cell mediators
Activation of alternative pathway of complement	IgA–antigen complexes Complex polysaccharides Lipopolysaccharides	C3a, C4a, C5a (anaphylatoxins) cause release of mast cell mediators
Direct activation of mast cell membrane	Morphine, codeine, D-turbocuarine polymyxin antibiotics, thiamine, certain foods containing histamine-releasing factors	Opiates act through specific receptors to release histamine Others nonspecifically activate cell membrane to release or generate mast cell mediators
Plasma–kinin generating system	Activation of plasma or tissue kallikrein or coagulation pathway, negatively charged surfaces, collagen vascular basement membrane, or endotoxin	Bradykinin and thrombin activation, especially for hereditary angioedema[8,23]

BIOPSY

Biopsy of urticarial lesions has accomplished less than expected to improve our understanding of the pathogenesis of urticaria. Three major patterns are recognized (Table 13-2). Further longitudinal and pathogenetic studies may determine whether these several pathologic forms of urticaria represent a continuum of disease (see Fig. 13-1) or separate pathophysiologic entities.

CLASSIFICATION

Classification in terms of known causes is helpful in evaluating patients with urticaria. Table 13-3 presents one classification that may be clinically useful. Additional knowledge of precipitating events or mechanisms may simplify this classification.[24]

Nonimmunologic Urticaria

Dermographism

Dermographism literally means "write on skin." This phenomenon may be detected unexpectedly on routine examination, or patients may complain of pruritus and rash, frequently characterized by linear wheals. When questioned carefully, they may admit that itching precedes the rash, causing them to scratch and worsen the condition. The cause of this lesion is unknown, but because it appears in about 5% of people, it may be a normal variant. Its onset has been described after severe drug reactions and may be confused with vaginitis in evaluating genital pruritus.[25] A delayed form has been recognized, with onset of lesions 3 to 8 hours after stimulus to the skin, which may be related to delayed pressure urticaria. It may accompany other forms of urticaria. The lesion is readily demonstrated by lightly stroking the skin of an affected patient with a pointed instrument. A dermatographometer (Hook & Tucker Ltd, Croydon, England) can be used to quantify this response. This produces erythema, pruritus, and linear streaks of edema or wheal formation. No antigen, however, has been shown to initiate the response, but dermographism has been passively transferred. Antihistamines usually ameliorate symptoms. Cutaneous mastocytosis may be considered under the heading of dermographism because stroking the skin results in significant wheal formation (Darier's sign). This disease is characterized by a diffuse increase in cutaneous mast cells. The skin may appear normal but is usually marked by thickening and accentuated skin folds.

TABLE 13-2. *Biopsy patterns of urticaria and angioedema lesions*

Type	Description
Acute urticaria or angioedema	Dilation of small venules and capillaries in superficial dermis (urticaria) or subcutaneous tissue (angioedema); Flattening of rete pegs; swollen collagen fibrils[8]
Chronic idiopathic urticaria	Mild cellular inflammation, including activated T lymphocytes, monocytes, and mast cells; delayed-onset urticaria may be mediated by cytokines (e.g., IL-1, IL-3, IL-5, or histamine-releasing factor[82])
Urticarial vasculitis	Neutrophil infiltration with vessel wall necrosis; occasional deposition of immunoglobulin and complement[8,83]

TABLE 13-3. *Classification of urticaria*

Nonimmunologic

Dermographism	*Hereditary urticaria*	*Miscellaneous*
Idiopathic	Hereditary angioedema	Infections
Cutaneous mastocytosis	Hereditary vibratory angioedema	Vasculitis
Adrenergic		Neoplasm
Physical urticaria	Urticaria, deafness, amyloidosis syndrome	Anaphylaxis
Pressure	Familial localized heat urticaria	Recurrent idiopathic
Vibratory		Exercise induced
Solar	C3b-inactivator deficiency	
Cholinergic	Porphyria	
Local heat	Papular urticaria	
Cold	Urticaria pigmentosa	

Immunologic

Food	Transfusion reactions
Drugs	Schnitzler's syndrome[84]
Autoimmune anti-IgE or anti-FcεRI	Atopy
Insect stings	Acquired C1-inhibitor deficiency

Identifiable agents (uncertain mechanisms)

Aspirin	Metabisulfites
Opiates	Tartrazine

Physical Urticaria

The physical urticarias are a unique group that constitute up to 17% of chronic urticarias.[13,26,27] They are frequently missed as a cause of chronic urticaria, and more than one type may occur together in the same patient. Most forms (except delayed pressure urticaria) occur as simple hives without inflammation, and individual lesions resolve within 24 hours. As a group, they can be reproduced by various physical stimuli, which have been standardized in some cases (Table 13-4). A new form of autonomic urticaria, called *adrenergic urticaria*, has been described and can be reproduced by intracutaneous injection of noradrenaline, 0.5×10^{-6} M.[28] This unique form of urticaria is characterized by a halo of white skin surrounding a small papule. It may have been previously misdiagnosed as cholinergic urticaria because of its small lesions, and it is caused by stress. In this case, however, relief can be found with β-blockers.

Delayed pressure urticaria, with or without angioedema, is clinically characterized by the gradual onset of wheals or edema in areas where pressure has been applied to the skin. Onset is usually 4 to 6 hours after exposure, but wide variations may be noted. An immediate form of pressure urticaria has been observed. The lesion of delayed pressure urticaria can be reproduced by applying pressure with motion for 20 minutes.[29] Delayed pressure urticaria may be associated with malaise, fevers, chills, arthralgia, and leukocytosis. When chronic urticaria is also present, foods occasionally have been recognized to precipitate episodes. The mechanism of these reactions is unknown, but biopsy specimens of lesions closely resemble aspects of the late cutaneous response.[30] Treatment is based on avoidance of situations that precipi-

TABLE 13-4. *Test procedures for physical and chronic idiopathic urticaria*

Test	Procedure
Dermographism	Firmly stroke interscapular skin with tongue blade or dermatographometer.
Delayed pressure urticaria	Hang 15-lb weight across shoulder while walking for 20 minutes.
Solar urticaria	Expose skin to defined wavelengths of light.
Cholinergic urticaria	1. Use methacholine skin test.
	2. Immerse in hot bath (42°C) to raise body temperature 0.7°C.
Local heat urticaria	Apply warm compress to forearm.
Cold urticaria	1. Apply ice cube to forearm for 4 minutes; observe rewarming for 10 minutes.
	2. Exercise in cold and observe for cholinergic-like urticaria (cold-induced cholinergic urticaria)
Aquagenic	Apply water compresses (35°C) for 30 minutes.
Vibratory	Apply laboratory vortex gently to mid-forearm for 4 minutes.
Autoimmune	Give intradermal injection of autologous serum.

tate the lesions. Antihistamines are generally ineffective, and a low-dose, alternate-day corticosteroid is usually necessary for the more severe cases. Nonsteroidal antiinflammatory drugs[31] with the addition of a histamine-2 (H_2) blocker may be helpful.

Solar urticaria is clinically characterized by development of pruritus, erythema, and edema within minutes of exposure to light. The lesions are typically present only in exposed areas and have been classified into six types according to the wavelength of light that elicits the lesions: I, 2800 to 3200 nm; II, 3200 to 4000 nm; III, 4000 to 5000 nm; IV, 4000 to 5000 nm; V, 2800 to 5000 nm; and VI, 4000 nm. The mechanism of these lesions is not known. Types I and IV can be passively transferred. Type VI is a metabolic abnormality recognized as erythropoietic protoporphyria. Diagnosis can be established using broad-spectrum light with various filters or a spectrodermograph to document the eliciting wavelength. Treatment includes avoidance of sunlight, wearing protective clothing, and applying various sunscreens or blockers, depending on the wavelength eliciting the lesion. An antihistamine taken 1 hour before exposure may be helpful in some forms, and induction of tolerance is possible.

Cholinergic urticaria (generalized heat) is a common form of urticaria (5% to 7%), especially in teenagers and young adults (11.2%). Clinically, it is characterized by small, punctate hives surrounded by an erythematous flare. These lesions may be clustered initially but can coalesce and usually become generalized in distribution, primarily over the upper trunk and arms. Pruritus is generally severe. The onset of the rash is frequently associated with hot showers, sudden temperature change, exercise, sweating, or anxiety. A separate entity with similar characteristic lesions induced by cold has been described.[32] Rarely, systemic symptoms may occur. The mechanism of this reaction is not certain, but cholinergically mediated thermodysregulation resulting in a neurogenic reflex has been postulated because it can be reproduced by increasing core body temperature 0.7° to 1°C.[33] Histamine and other mast cell mediators have been documented in some patients,[34] and increased muscarinic receptors have been reported in lesion sites of a patient with cholinergic urticaria.[35] The appearance and description of the rash are highly characteristic and are reproduced by an intradermal methacholine skin test, but only in one third of patients. Exercise in an occlusive suit or submersion in a warm bath is a more sensitive method of reproducing the urticaria. Passive heat can be used to differentiate this syndrome from exercise anaphylaxis. Hydroxyzine is considered the treatment of choice, but if it is ineffective, other antihistamines or combinations may be tried.

Local heat urticaria, a rare form of heat urticaria,[36] can be demonstrated by applying localized heat to the skin. A familial localized heat urticaria has also been reported[37] and is manifested by the delayed onset (4 to 6 hours) of urticarial lesions after local heat exposure.

Cold urticaria is clinically characterized by the rapid onset of urticaria or angioedema after cold exposure. Lesions are generally localized to exposed areas, but sudden total body exposure, as in swimming, may cause hypotension and result in fatalities.[38] Although usually idiopathic, cold urticaria has been associated with cryoglobulinemia, cryofibrinogenemia, cold agglutinin disease, and paroxysmal cold hemoglobinuria. The mechanism of cold urticaria is not known. Release of histamine and several other mediators has been demonstrated in selected patients after cold exposure.[39] In patients with abnormal proteins, passive transfer of the cold sensitivity has been accomplished.[40,41] Some cryoprecipitates can fix complement and thus may induce anaphylatoxin production. Diagnosis of cold urticaria frequently can be confirmed by placing an ice cube on the forearm for 4 minutes (see Table 13-4). Several coexisting cold-induced urticarias do not respond to an ice-cube test.[42] Treatment should consist of limited cold exposure (e.g., the patient should enter swimming pools cautiously), proper clothing, and oral cyproheptadine,[43] although other antihistamines, such as doxepin, may be useful.[44] In cases in which an abnormal protein is present, treatment of an underlying disease may be indicated. Delayed-onset hypersensitivity to cold has also been reported.[45]

Hereditary Urticaria

Hereditary angioedema is clinically characterized by recurrent episodes of angioedema involving any part of the body. Urticaria is not a feature of this disease. Laryngeal edema is common and is the major cause of death. Angioedema of the gastrointestinal tract may frequently cause abdominal discomfort and can mimic an acute abdomen. Type I HAE (Table 13-5) is inherited as an autosomal codominant trait, manifested by the absence of C1 inhibitor. Type II HAE is

TABLE 13-5. *Forms of hereditary and acquired angioedema*

Disease	Mechanism	Diagnosis
Type I hereditary angioedema	Autosomal codominant Deficiency of C1-inhibitor	Low C4,[85] undetectable during an attack
	Bradykinin[23] and possible C2b-derived kinin[33]	Low or absent C2[86], when symptomatic
Type II hereditary angioedema	Anaphylatoxin-generated histamine	Normal C1 level
	Functionally inactive C1-inhibitor	Low C4
	20% of cases of hereditary angioedema	Present but inactive C1-inhibitor (functional assay necessary)
Acquired angioedema[49,50]	Reduced C1q levels by excessive activation of C1 (e.g., lymphoma) through autoimmune immunoglobulin	Low C1q levels; low C1-inhibitor
Autoimmune acquired angioedema[5]	Autoantibody (IgG) against C1-inhibitor	Normal C1 level; low C4, C1-inhibitor; absent family history

characterized by the functional absence of this inhibitor, which allows activation of the complement cascade and results in the clinical features noted in Table 13-5. The diagnosis usually is established by a history of angioedema, a family history of similar disease or early death because of laryngeal obstruction, and appropriate complement studies. The usual forms of treatment for angioedema, including epinephrine, are generally ineffective for HAE. Tracheostomy may be necessary in urgent situations when laryngeal edema has occurred. Supportive therapy, such as intravenous fluids or analgesics, may be required for other manifestations of the disease.

Danazol[46] and stanozolol[47] have been used successfully on a chronic basis to treat HAE. Each of these attenuated androgens appears to reduce the number and severity of acute exacerbations and to raise C4 levels. Often, sufficient clinical improvement may be obtained with minimal doses so that the C4 level is normalized, but the C1 inhibitor level is not significantly increased. Long-term minimal-dose (2 mg/day or less) stanozolol or danazol for hereditary HAE is remarkably safe. Even when given during the last 8 weeks of pregnancy, a mother suffered no ill effects, and virilization of the infant was transient.[48]

Acquired forms of HAE[49,50] may require larger doses of medication, and autoimmune acquired angioedema with autoantibody against C1 inhibitor may require plasmapheresis or immunosuppressive agents.[51] For intermittent attacks, prophylaxis for surgery, children, and pregnant women, purified C1 inhibitor should become the ideal form of replacement therapy and already has met with success in limited trials.[52,53]

Hereditary vibratory angioedema is clinically characterized by localized pruritus and swelling in areas exposed to vibratory stimuli.[54] It appears to be inherited as an autosomal dominant trait and generally is first noted in childhood. The mechanism is not certain, but histamine release has been documented during experimental induction of a lesion.[55] Treatment consists of avoidance of vibratory stimuli and use of antihistamines in an attempt to reduce symptoms.

A nonhereditary (acquired) form of vibratory angioedema has been described separately in two Mexican-American males. This form resulted intermittently in median nerve compression in one patient,[56] and it responded to desensitization by regular stimulation in the other.[57] Histamine was implicated as a potential inflammatory mediator in each situation, as it was for hereditary vibratory angioedema.

Papular urticaria is clinically characterized by slightly erythematous, highly pruritic papular lesions of various sizes. Each lesion tends to be persistent, in contrast to most urticarial conditions. The lower extremities are involved most often, although the trunk may also may be affected, especially in young children. The mechanism is unknown, but the rash is thought to be caused by insect bites. In my experience, it is frequently associated with unrecognized dermatographism. Treatment is supportive: antihistamines are given, often prophylactically, in an attempt to reduce pruritus. Good skin care is essential to prevent infection caused by scratching. Examination of the patient's sleeping quarters and especially of children's play areas for insects may provide a clue to the cause.

Pruritic urticaria papules and plaques of pregnancy is a bothersome condition of typically primigravida women. It is intensely pruritic and should be differentiated from herpes gestationis by biopsy.[8]

Urticaria pigmentosa is characterized by persistent, pigmented, maculopapular lesions that urticate when stroked (Darier's sign). These lesions generally have their onset in childhood. Rare familial forms have been described. On biopsy examination, there appear to be small clusters of mast cells. The diagnosis may be established by their typical appearance, Darier's sign, and skin biopsy. Occasionally, it complicates other forms of anaphylaxis, such as Hymenoptera venom sensitivity, causing severe reactions with sudden vascular collapse. These cutaneous lesions may be seen in systemic mastocytosis, which is a generalized form of mast cell infiltration into bone, liver, lymph nodes, and spleen.

Other Forms of Urticaria, Including Immunologic Forms

The remaining forms of urticaria are associated with many diverse causes (see Table 13-3). Diagnosis is established by history and physical examination based on knowledge of the possible causes. Laboratory evaluation is occasionally helpful in establishing a diagnosis and identifying the underlying disease. Treatment is based on the underlying problem, and may include avoidance, antihistamines, and corticosteroid therapy or other forms of antiinflammatory drugs.

CLINICAL APPROACH

History

The clinical history is the single most important aspect of evaluating patients with urticaria. The history generally provides important clues to the cause; therefore, an organized approach is essential.

If the patient has no rash at the time of evaluation, urticaria or angioedema usually can be established historically with a history of hives, welts, or wheps resembling mosquito bites; raised, erythematous, pruritic lesions; evanescent symptoms; potentiation of lesions by scratching; and lesions that coalesce. By contrast, angioedema is asymmetric, often involves nondependent areas, recurs in different sites, is transient, and is associated with little pruritus. Urticaria and angioedema may occur together. Cholinergic or adrenergic urticaria, papular urticaria, dermographism, urticaria pigmentosa, jaundice with urticaria, and familial cold urticaria, however, do not fit the typical pattern.

Both papular urticaria and urticaria pigmentosa most often arise in childhood. HAE and hereditary vibratory angioedema may also occur during childhood but are readily recognized by the absence of urticaria in both diseases. Other etiologic factors in childhood urticaria have been reviewed.[58,59]

Once the diagnosis of urticaria is established on the basis of history, etiologic mechanisms should be considered. The patient with dermographism usually has a history of rash after scratching. Frequently, the patient notices itching first, scratches the offending site, and then develops linear wheals. Stroking the skin with a pointed instrument without tearing the skin confirms the diagnosis. In most patients, the physical urticarias may be eliminated quickly as a possible diagnosis by asking about the association with light, heat, cold, pressure, or vibration, or by using established clinical tests (see Table 13-4). Cholinergic urticaria is usually recognized by its characteristic lesions and relation to rising body temperature or stress. Hereditary forms of urticaria are rare. Familial localized heat urticaria is recognized by its relation to the local application of heat, and familial cold urticaria is diagnosed by the unusual papular skin lesions and by the predominance of a burning sensation instead of pruritus. Porphyria is a light-sensitive reaction. C3b-inactivator deficiency is rare and can be recognized only by special complement studies. Patients with idiopathic anaphylaxis may have histaminuria, and those with systemic mastocytosis may have elevated tryptase levels. Thus, after a few moments of discussion with the patient, a physical urticaria or hereditary form usually can be suspected or established.

Relatively few patients have immunologic causes of urticaria, but more patients have this form than the hereditary forms or physical urticarias. A cause of acute urticaria is found more often than is a cause of chronic urticaria. Each of the items in Table 13-3 may be involved.

Food may be identified as a cause of acute urticaria. Great patience and effort are necessary, along with repeated queries, to detect drug use. Over-the-counter preparations are not regarded as drugs by many patients and must be specified when questioning the patient. Penicillin still heads the list, but aspirin or nonsteroidal antiinflammatory drugs are frequently recognized as a cause or aggravator of urticaria. Drug-induced episodes of urticaria are usually acute. Angiotensin-converting enzyme inhibitor drugs, which are used primarily for hypertension, can also cause urticaria. Infections that can cause urticaria include infectious mononucleosis, viral hepatitis B and C, and parasitic invasions. Chronic infection rarely causes chronic urticaria, but chronic hepatitis has been called into question.[60] If the history does not reveal significant clues, the patient's urticaria generally is labeled *chronic idiopathic urticaria*; this category includes most patients with chronic urticaria.

Physical Examination

A complete physical examination should be carried out in all patients with urticaria. The purposes of the examination are to identify typical urticarial lesions, if present; to establish the presence or absence of dermographism; to identify the characteristic lesions of cholinergic and papular urticaria; to characterize atypical lesions; to determine the presence of jaundice, urticaria pigmentosa (Darier's sign), or familial cold urticaria; to exclude other cutaneous diseases; to exclude evidence of systemic disease; and to establish the presence of coexisting diseases.

It is difficult to outline an acceptable diagnostic program for all patients with urticaria. Each diagnostic work-up must be individualized, depending on the results of the history and physical examination. An algorithm may become a useful adjunct in this often unrewarding diagnostic endeavor (Fig. 13-2).

Diagnostic Studies

Foods

Four diagnostic procedures may be considered when food is thought to be a cause of urticaria (Table 13-6). These include: (1) avoidance, (2) restricted diet, (3) diet diary, and (4) skin testing with food extracts or fresh foods.

Routine food skin tests used in evaluating urticaria are at best of unproven value. Because the cause of chronic urticaria is established in only an additional 5% of patients,[33] and only some of these cases are related to food, the diagnostic yield from skin testing is low. In addition, both false-positive and false-negative skin tests are common. Important studies of food-induced atopic dermatitis[61] have revealed a few selected foods that are most commonly associated with symptoms; these are egg, peanut, fish, soy, pork, milk, wheat, beef, and chicken. If no food skin tests are positive, then foods are probably not a cause. If all food skin tests are positive, dermatographism is probably present. Whether these data can be applied directly to food allergies has not been tested, but they help temper our thinking about food sensitivity causing chronic urticaria. For patients in whom a mixed food (combination of ingredients) is thought to be the problem, food tests may isolate the particular item (e.g., soybeans). An extensive battery of food tests cannot be recommended on a routine basis and must be used with clinical discretion. For oral allergy syndrome, skin tests using ripe fruit into which the

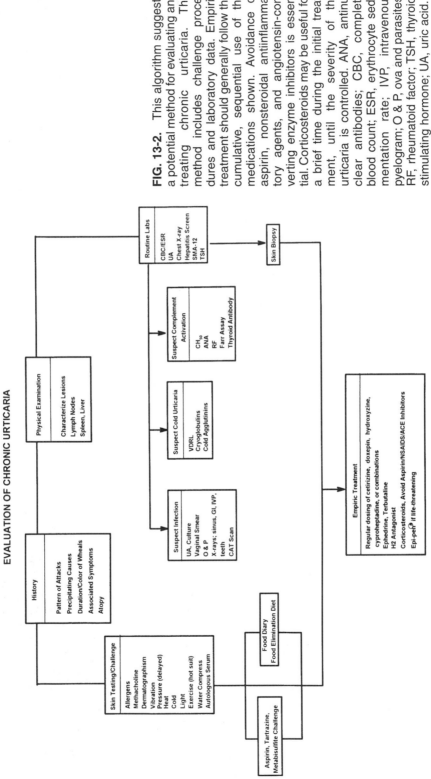

EVALUATION OF CHRONIC URTICARIA

History
Pattern of Attacks
Precipitating Causes
Duration/Color of Wheals
Associated Symptoms
Atopy

Physical Examination
Characterize Lesions
Lymph Nodes
Spleen, Liver

Skin Testing/Challenge
Allergens
Methacholine
Dermatographism
Vibration
Pressure (delayed)
Heat
Cold
Light
Exercise (hot suit)
Water Compress
Autologous Serum

Aspirin, Tartrazine,
Metabisulfite Challenge

Food Diary
Food Elimination Diet

Suspect Infection
UA, Culture
Vaginal Smear
O & P
X-rays; sinus, GI, IVP,
teeth
CAT Scan

Suspect Cold Urticaria
VDRL
Cryoglobulins
Cold Agglutinins

Suspect Complement Activation
CH$_{50}$
ANA
RF
Farr Assay
Thyroid Antibody

Routine Labs
CBC/ESR
UA
Chest X-ray
Hepatitis Screen
SMA-12
TSH

Skin Biopsy

Empiric Treatment
Regular dosing of cetirizine, doxepin, hydroxyzine,
cyproheptadine, or combinations
Ephedrine, Terbutaline
H2 Antagonist
Corticosteroids, Avoid Aspirin/NSAIDS/ACE Inhibitors
Epi-pen® if life-threatening

FIG. 13-2. This algorithm suggests a potential method for evaluating and treating chronic urticaria. The method includes challenge procedures and laboratory data. Empiric treatment should generally follow the cumulative, sequential use of the medications shown. Avoidance of aspirin, nonsteroidal antiinflammatory agents, and angiotensin-converting enzyme inhibitors is essential. Corticosteroids may be useful for a brief time during the initial treatment, until the severity of the urticaria is controlled. ANA, antinuclear antibodies; CBC, complete blood count; ESR, erythrocyte sedimentation rate; IVP, intravenous pyelogram; O & P, ova and parasites; RF, rheumatoid factor; TSH, thyroid-stimulating hormone; UA, uric acid.

TABLE 13-6. *Diagnostic studies of food-induced urticaria*

Study or Test	Treatment
Avoidance (acute): use patient's history.	Eliminate 1 or 2 foods; urticaria should clear.
Restricted diet (chronic relapsing): use standardized rice and lamb or other restrictive diets; elemental diet may be useful.	Reinstitute one food every 3–5 days; duplicate, if successful.
Diet diary: (intermittent episodes for extended period): list all foods and events for 24 hours before episode on several occasions.	Eliminate suspected food; duplicate, if successful.
Skin tests (chronic, unknown cause): use a brief battery of food skin tests based on patient's history. Certain inhalant or latex allergens may suggest cross-reacting foods. Use fresh foods as allergen source for oral allergy syndrome.	Eliminate suspected test-positive foods. A battery of negative skin tests suggests no food hypersensitivity.

prick testing needle is inserted are most helpful.[62] Additionally, certain foods have been shown to cross-react with pollen allergens[63] or latex allergens,[64] to which a patient may be exquisitely sensitive.

Drugs

With the exception of penicillin, foreign sera, and insulin, there are no reliable diagnostic tests for predicting or establishing clinical sensitivity (as hives) to a drug. In patients with urticaria, drugs must always be considered as etiologic agents. The only evaluation of value is avoidance of the drug. This can be accomplished safely and effectively in most patients, even when multiple drugs are involved and coexisting diseases are present. Substitute drugs with different chemical structures are frequently available and may be used. Not all drugs need to be stopped simultaneously unless the allergic reaction is severe.

Infections

As noted previously, viral infections and parasites may cause urticaria. Patients with infectious mononucleosis or hepatitis generally have other symptoms, and appropriate laboratory studies confirm the diagnosis. Many of the parasitic infections demonstrate peripheral blood eosinophilia, high serum IgE levels, or positive stool specimens. An extensive search for occult infection is of no value. If history or examination suggests undiagnosed infection, appropriate laboratory studies can be undertaken (see Fig. 13-2).

Penetrants

The medical literature is filled with numerous case reports of urticaria after contact. The only tests that should be performed involve actual contact with the agent and demonstration of a localized skin eruption in the area of contact. Usually, these cases of urticaria result from penetration of the skin by antigen or a mediator releasing substance from animal hairs or stingers. Examples of agents causing such urticaria include drugs and occupationally employed chemicals.[65]

Insect Stings

Urticaria may present as a result of insect stings, and this history generally is obtained easily. Appropriate skin tests with Hymenoptera venoms may be indicated in cases of generalized urticaria and anaphylaxis to demonstrate immediate hypersensitivity. One should consider fire ant stings owing to their continued migration into more northern latitudes. Whole-body extract skin testing or a radioallergosorbent test for venom may be helpful diagnostically.

Neoplasm

If neoplasm is suspected by history or examination, standard evaluation should be undertaken and perhaps repeated on several occasions.

Vasculitis

In a patient with vasculitis, complete blood count, sedimentation rate, urinalysis, and tissue biopsy are indicated. Tests for antinuclear antibody and rheumatoid factor, complement studies, and screening for hepatitis and mononucleosis are generally indicated. A highly sensitive thyroid-stimulating hormone test should also be performed because of the association with autoimmune thyroiditis.[66,67] Urticarial vasculitis must be differentiated from chronic idiopathic urticaria.[8]

Serum Sickness

The clinical picture with serum sickness is usually clear. Complete blood count, urinalysis, and sedimentation rate are indicated.

The more difficult and more common problem regarding diagnostic tests relates to patients who appear to have idiopathic disease. Laboratory studies are probably unnecessary in the absence of abnormal features in the history or physical examination. Most of these episodes are self-limited and resolve spontaneously.

In patients with chronic idiopathic urticaria, the discomfort, inconvenience, and disfigurement of the disease generally warrant further evaluation. The following tests should be considered but not necessarily carried out in all patients: complete blood count with differential, urinalysis, chest radiograph, sedimentation rate, complement studies, examination of stool for ova and parasites, antinuclear antibody, VDRL, hepatitis screen, and skin biopsy. Because thyroid disease (particularly Hashimoto's thyroiditis) is more common in chronic urticaria, thyroid function tests (T_3, T_4, ultrasensitive thyroid stimulating hormone, antibodies for thyroglobulin, and microsomes) may be considered in anyone with a palpable goiter, family history of thyroid disease, or evidence for thyroid dysfunction.[18]

Urinalysis (cells or protein), complete blood count (anemia, leukocytosis, or eosinophilia), and chest radiograph are most likely to demonstrate significant abnormalities. The sedimentation rate may be elevated in active vasculitis. Circulating hepatitis-related antibodies may indicate acute or chronic disease. Complement abnormalities are common in reports of chronic idiopathic urticaria, although the underlying mechanisms are unclear, and their relevance is uncertain.

Skin biopsy is suggested for chronic idiopathic urticaria that is difficult to manage, and it is probably indicated in patients with connective tissue disease or a complement abnormality. Acute urticaria should not undergo biopsy, and chronic urticaria should not undergo biopsy when laboratory studies are normal.

THERAPY

Drug therapy is the main form of treatment for urticaria and angioedema (Table 13-7). As in other forms of allergic disease, however, if an allergen has been identified, avoidance is the most effective treatment. Avoidance techniques for specific forms of urticaria have been reviewed previously.[8] For most urticaria patients, three types of drugs are adequate to obtain symptomatic control: sympathomimetic agents, antihistamines, and corticosteroids.

The sympathomimetic agents, notably epinephrine and ephedrine, have α-agonist properties that cause vasoconstriction in superficial cutaneous and mucosal surfaces, which directly opposes the effect of histamine on these end organs. Normally, they are used for acute urticaria or in conjunction with antihistamines.

Antihistamines (H_1-blockers) are useful in most cases of urticaria. They are competitive inhibitors of histamine, reducing the end-organ effect of histamine even if histamine release continues. Although documentation of histamine release is not available for all forms of urticaria, antihistamines are the mainstay of symptomatic improvement or control of urticaria. Notably, low-dose antidepressants, especially doxepin, are unique in their potent H_1- and H_2-antagonist effects and inhibit other mediators, such as platelet-activating factor. Their main side effect is sedation, but when administered in small doses (10 to 25 mg) at bedtime, this is usually avoided. A trial of therapy with representative agents from the different classes of antihistamines may be required to select the proper drug.

The newer nonsedating antihistamines offer some valuable options.[68,69] Astemizole is approved for urticaria, but it causes weight gain in about 10% of patients. Terfenadine is probably as effective in most situations. Both drugs in rare cases can cause torsade de pointe arrhythmia if doses become toxic. Loratadine has not been implicated in this mechanism of potential toxicity. Ketotifen[70] and cetirizine[71–73] offer effective alternatives with little sedation for chronic idiopathic urticaria, especially physical urticaria.[14] Only cetirizine, however, an active metabolite of hydroxyzine, is available in the United States. Acrivastine, a side-chain reduced metabolite of triprolidine, is another nonsedating alternative.[68]

Hydroxyzine has clinical antihistaminic effects as well as experimental anticholinergic and antiserotonin effects. This agent is considered the drug of choice for cholinergic urticaria and is also effective in many other forms of chronic urticaria. Often, the initially effective dose

TABLE 13-7. *Treatment of chronic idiopathic urticaria*

Avoid triggers.
Keep diary of flares.
Use of antihistamines regularly for 3–6 months.
Add ephedrine or β-agonists.
Add H_2-blockers.
β-Blockers (adrenergic urticaria only).
Use corticosteroids cautiously.

TABLE 13-8. *Treatment of chronic idiopathic urticaria: use of secondary options*

Cautiously use corticosteroids (low dose or every other morning).

Add stanozolol to corticosteroid.

Add sulfasalazine.

Add nifedipine.

Use antiinflammatory drugs.

can be reduced or used only at night for chronic therapy. Because sedation from this drug is frequently not as severe as from the other antihistamines, it is a good choice for initial therapy of acute or chronic urticaria. Normally, less than 100 mg/day is needed.

Cyproheptadine is a serotonin and histamine antagonist and also has anticholinergic effects. Its mechanism of action in urticaria is uncertain, but it appears to be effective in some cases. It is most commonly employed to treat cold urticaria,[43] but it may be useful in other forms of urticaria, especially in combination with other drugs.

Corticosteroids, such as oral prednisone, may be necessary in the management of urticaria. Because of their potential for significant long-term side effects, these drugs should be used chronically only after a demonstrated failure of both high-dose antihistamines and sympathomimetic agents to control urticaria. Based on clinical experience, moderate-dose steroid therapy (30 to 40 mg prednisone) may be required initially to control the urticaria. Thereafter, alternate-day therapy generally provides control on a long-term basis, often with decreasing doses. As in all forms of therapy, the risk/benefit ratio must be assessed when using steroid therapy for long-term treatment. Short-term prednisone has limited side effects and is often useful for control of acute urticaria not responding to antihistamines and ephedrine. Delayed pressure urticaria frequently requires the use of low-dose or every-other-day corticosteroids to maintain the patient's activity, and a cautious trial of a nonsteroidal antiinflammatory drug may be helpful.

The choice of agents and the route of administration of drugs depend on the clinical situation. The adult patient who presents in an emergency room or physician's office within hours of the onset of significant urticaria can be treated with epinephrine, 0.3 mL (1:1000) subcutaneously, and hydroxyzine, 25 to 50 mg orally. This approach gives prompt relief from symptoms in many patients. After evaluation for a precipitating agent (e.g., drug or food), the patient may be given a long-acting epinephrine preparation, such as Sus-Phrine, and released with instructions to take oral ephedrine and hydroxyzine for 24 to 48 hours. A brief burst of corticosteroids may be judicious and is essential if there have been associated signs of anaphylaxis. Ambulatory medical follow-up is required.

The patient who presents with urticaria of several days' duration may be treated with regular doses of antihistamines, such as 10 to 30 mg of doxepin at bedtime. A small weight gain may cause some patients to be unhappy, however. Ephedrine, terbutaline, or H_2-antagonists may be prescribed with the initial antihistamine, or an additional antihistamine may be prescribed. Failure to respond in a few days to this therapy may indicate a short course of prednisone. Many patients respond to this therapy, but the antihistamines should be continued for a period after the prednisone is stopped.

The patient with a history of chronic urticaria presents a more complicated therapeutic problem (Table 13-8). After evaluation for a cause, therapy is usually initiated with regular dosing of a potent antihistamine (often hydroxyzine, cetirizine, or doxepin) and possibly an H_2-antagonist. Failure to respond suggests that moderate-dose prednisone should be initiated if the symptoms are severe. Every effort to use alternate-day therapy should be made, but this is often initially inadequate. When control is achieved, the steroids are slowly withdrawn to determine whether chronic steroid therapy is required.

Other antiinflammatory medications have been reported useful in refractory patients. Stanozolol,[74] nifedipine,[75] and other antiinflammatory drugs, including cyclosporine[76] and methotrexate,[77] have been used experimentally for inflammatory urticaria and have been reviewed.[14] Sulfasalazine[78,79] has been effective in case studies of delayed pressure urticaria and angioedema.

Patients with urticaria are uncomfortable, have difficulty sleeping, and complain of cosmetic problems. Aggressive and consistent therapy for at least several months provides relief in many cases.

In summary, chronic idiopathic urticaria may be unpleasant, annoying, and frightening to patients. Often, these patients seek help from various physicians for an allergen that does not exist. At times, they receive expensive, inappropriate tests and treatments that are of no value and perhaps dangerous. These patients need reassurance. Treatment with prednisone in doses that induce remission, followed by 3 to 6 months of a nightly dose of a potent antihistamine (e.g., doxepin), often results in a good outcome.

REFERENCES

1. Sheldon JM, Mathews KP, Lovell RG. The vexing urticaria problem: present concepts of etiology and management. J Allergy 1954;25:525.
2. Mathews KP. Urticaria and angioedema. J Allergy Clin Immunol 1983;72:11.
3. Cooper KD. Urticaria and angioedema: diagnosis and evaluation. J Am Acad Dermatol 1991;25:166.
4. Champion RH, Roberts SOB, Carpenter RG, Roger JH. Urticaria and angioedema: a review of 554 patients. Br J Dermatol 1969;81:588.
5. Green GR, Koelsche GA, Kierland RR. Etiology and pathogenesis of chronic urticaria. Ann Allergy 1965;23:30.
6. Lewis T. The blood vessels of the human skin and their responses. London: Shaw & Sons, 1927.
7. Peters MS, Schroeter AL, Kaphart GM, Gleich GJ. Localization of eosinophilic granule major basic protein in chronic urticaria. J Invest Dermatol 1983;81:39.
8. Charlesworth EN. The spectrum of urticaria. Immunol Allergy Clin North Am 1995;15:641.
9. Bressler RB. Pathophysiology of chronic urticaria. Immunol Allergy Clin North Am 1995;15:659.
10. Grandel KE, Farr RS, Wanderer AA, Eisenstadt JC, Wasserman SI. Association of platelet activation factor with primary, acquired cold urticaria. N Engl J Med 1985;313.405.
11. Juhlin L. Late phase cutaneous reactions to platelet activating factor and kallikrein in urticaria. Clin Exp Allergy 1990;90:9.
12. Goldsobel AB, Rohr AS, Siegel SC, et al. Effect of doxepin in the treatment of chronic idiopathic urticaria. J Allergy Clin Immunol 1986;78:867.
13. Greaves MW. The physical urticarias. Clin Exp Allergy 1991;21:1.
14. Fox RW. Update on urticaria and angioedema (hives). Allergy Proc 1995;16.289.
15. Smith CH, Kepley C, Schwartz LB, Lee TK. Mast cell membrane and phenotype in chronic urticaria. Allergy Clin Immunol 1995;96:360.
16. Barlow RJ, Ross EL, MacDonald DM, Black AK, Greaves MW. Mast cells and T lymphocytes in chronic urticaria. Clin Exp Allergy 1994;25:317.
17. Greaves MW. Chronic urticaria: current concepts. N Engl J Med 1995;332:1767.
18. Leznoff A, Sussman GL. Syndrome of idiopathic chronic urticaria and angioedema with thyroid autoimmunity: a study of 90 patients. J Allergy Clin Immunol 1989;84:66.
19. Maxwell DL, Atkinson BA, Spur BW, Lessof MH, Lee TH. Skin responses to intradermal histamine and leukotrienes C4, D4 and E4 in patients with chronic idiopathic urticaria and in normal subjects. J Allergy Clin Immunol 1990;86:759.
20. Meggs WJ, Pescovitz OR, Metcalfe DD, Loriaux DL, Cutler G, Kaliner MA. Progesterone sensitivity as a cause of recurrent anaphylaxis. N Engl J Med 1984;311:1236.
21. Mittman RJ, Berstein DI, Steinberg DR, Enrione M, Bernstein IL. Progesterone-responsive urticaria and eosinophilia. J Allergy Clin Immunol 1989;84:304.
22. Goodman DL, McDonnell JT, Nelson HS, Vaughan TR, Weber RW. Chronic urticaria exacerbated by the antioxidant food preservatives, butylated hydroxyanisole (BHA) and butylated hydroxytoluene (BHT). J Allergy Clin Immunol 1990;86:570.

23. Fields T, Ghebrehiwet B, Kaplan AP. Kinin formation in hereditary angioedema plasma: evidence against kinin derivation from C2 and in support of "spontaneous" formation of bradykinin. J Allergy Clin Immunol 1983;72:54.

24. Vaughn MP, DeWalt AC, Diaz JD. Urticaria associated with systemic disease and psychological factors. Immunol Allergy Clin North Am 1995;15:725.

25. Sherertz EF. Clinical pearl: symptomatic dermatographism as a cause of genital pruritus. J Am Acad Dermatol 1994;31:1040.

26. Casale TB, Sampson HA, Honifan J, et al. Guide to physical urticarias. J Allergy Clin Immunol 1988;82:758.

27. Schafer CM. Physical urticaria. Immunol Allergy Clin North Am 1995;15:679.

28. Shelley WB, Shelley EO. Adrenergic urticaria: a new form of stress induced hives. Lancet 1985;2:1031.

29. Ryan TJ, Shim-Young N, Turk JL. Delayed pressure urticaria. Br J Dermatol 1968;80:485.

30. Mekori YA, Dobozin BS, Schocket AL, et al. Delayed pressure urticaria histologically resembles cutaneous late phase reactions. Arch Dermatol 1988;124:230.

31. Sussman GL, Harvey RP, Schocket AL. Delayed pressure urticaria. J Allergy Clin Immunol 1982;70:337.

32. Kaplan AP, Garofalo J. Identification of a new physically induced urticaria: cold-induced cholinergic urticaria. J Allergy Clin Immunol 1981;68:438.

33. Kaplan AP. Urticaria and angioedema. In: Middleton E Jr, et al, eds. Allergy: principles and practice. 4th ed. St Louis: CV Mosby, 1993:1553.

34. Kaplan AP, Gray L, Shaff RE. *In vivo* studies of mediator release in cold urticaria and cholinergic urticaria. J Allergy Clin Immunol 1975;55:394.

35. Shelley WB, Shelley EO, Ho AKS. Cholinergic urticaria: acetylcholine-receptor-dependent immediate-type hypersensitivity reaction to copper. Lancet 1983;i:843.

36. Greaves MW, Kaplan AP. Urticaria and angioedema. In: Samter M, et al, eds. Immunological diseases. 4th ed. Boston: Little, Brown, 1988:1187.

37. Michaelson G, Ros A. Familial localized heat urticaria of delayed type. Acta Derm Venereol (Stockh) 1971;51:279.

38. Horton BT, Brown GE, Roth GM. Hypersensitivities to cold with local and systemic manifestations of a histamine-like character: its amenability to treatment. JAMA 1936;107:1263.

39. Ormerod AD, Black AK, Dawes J, et al. Prostaglandin D2 and histamine release in cold urticaria unaccompanied by evidence of platelet activation. J Allergy Clin Immunol 1988;82:586.

40. Costanzi JJ, Cottman JC Jr, Donaldson VH. Activation of complement by a monoclonal cryoglobulin associated with cold urticaria. J Lab Clin Med 1969;74:902.

41. Costanzi JJ, Cottman JC Jr. Kappa chain precipitable immunoglobulin G (IgG) associated with cold urticaria. I. Clinical observations. Clin Exp Immunol 1967;2:167.

42. Kaplan AP. Urticaria and angioedema. In: Kaplan AP, ed. Allergy. New York: Churchill Livingstone, 1985:439.

43. Sigler RW, Evans R, Hoarkova Z, et al. The role of cyproheptadine in the treatment of cold urticaria. J Allergy Clin Immunol 1980;65:309.

44. Bentley B II. Cold-induced urticaria and angioedema: diagnosis and management. Am J Emerg Med 1993;11:43.

45. Sarkany I, Turk JL. Delayed type hypersensitivity to cold. Proc R Soc Med 1965;58:622.

46. Gelfand JA, Sherms RJ, Allevy DW, et al. Treatment of hereditary angioedema with danazol: reversal of clinical and biochemical abnormalities. N Engl J Med 1976;295:1444.

47. Sheffer AL, Feron DT, Austen KF. Clinical and biochemical effects of stanozolol therapy for hereditary angioedema. J Allergy Clin Immunol 1981;68:181.

48. Cicardi M, Bergamaschini L, Cugno M, Hack E, Agostoni G, Agostoni A. Long-term treatment of hereditary angioedema with attenuated androgens: a survey of a 13-year experience. J Allergy Clin Immunol 1991;87:768.

49. Gelfand JA, Boss GR, Conley CL, et al. Acquired C1 esterase inhibitor deficiency and angioedema: a review. Medicine 1979;58:321.

50. Frigas E. Angioedema with acquired deficiency of the C1 inhibitor: a constellation of syndromes. Mayo Clin Proc 1989;64:1269.

51. Donaldson VH, Wagner CJ, David AE III. An autoantibody to C-1 inhibitor recognizes the reactive center of the inhibitors. J Lab Clin Med 1996;127:229.

52. Bork K, Witzke G. Long-term prophylaxis with C1-inhibitor (C1 INH) concentrate in patients with recurrent angioedema caused by hereditary and acquired C1-inhibitor deficiency. J Allergy Clin Immunol 1989;83:677.

53. Gadek JE, Hosea SW, Gelfand JA, et al. Replacement therapy in hereditary angioedema: successful treatment of acute episodes with partially purified C1 inhibitor. N Engl J Med 1976;295:1444.

54. Patterson R, Mellies CJ, Blankenship ML, et al. Vibratory angioedema: a hereditary type of physical hypersensitivity. J Allergy Clin Immunol 1972;50:174.

55. Metzger WJ, Kaplan AP, Beaven MA, et al. Hereditary vibratory angioedema: confirmation of histamine release in a type of physical hypersensitivity. J Allergy Clin Immunol 1976;57:605.

56. Wener MH, Metzger WJ, Simon RA. Occupationally acquired vibratory angioedema with secondary carpal tunnel syndrome. Ann Intern Med 1983;98:44.

57. Ting S, Reimann BEF, Rauls DO, Mansfield LE. Non-familial, vibration-induced angioedema. J Allergy Clin Immunol 1983;71:546.

58. Ghosh Schabani, Kanwar AJ, Kaur S. Urticaria in children. Pediatr Dermatol 1993;10:107.

59. Volonakis M, Katsarou-Katsari A, Stratigos J. Etiologic factors in childhood chronic urticaria. Ann Allergy 1992;69:61.
60. Vaida, GA, Goldman MA, Blockk KJ. Testing for hepatitis B in patients with chronic urticaria and angioedema. J Allergy Clin Immunol 1983;72:193.
61. Sampson HA. The role of food allergy and mediation release in atopic dermatitis. J Allergy Clin Immunol 1988;81:635.
62. Telez-Diaz G, Ellis MH, Morales-Russo R, Heiner DC. Prevalence of avocado allergy among atopic patients. Allergy 1995;16:241.
63. Bush RK, Hefle SL. Lessons and myths regarding cross-reacting foods. Allergy Proc 1995;16:245.
64. Dompmartin A, Szczurko C, Michel M, et al. 2 Cases of urticaria following fruit ingestion, with cross-sensitivity to latex. Contact Dermatitis 1994;30:250.
65. Vonkrog HG, Maiback HI. Contact urticaria. In: Adams RM. ed. Occupational skin disease. New York: Grune & Stratton, 1983:69.
66. Altus P, Blandon R, Wallach PM, Flannery MT. Case report: the spectrum of autoimmune thyroid disease with urticaria. Am J Med Sci 1993;306:379.
67. Rumbyrt JS, Katz JL, Schocket AL. Resolution of chronic urticaria in patients with thyroid autoimmunity. J Allergy Clin Immunol 1995;96:901.
68. Ormerod AD. Urticaria: recognition, causes and treatment. Drugs 1994;48:5.
69. Soter NA. Treatment of urticaria and angioedema: low-sedating H1-type antihistamines. J Am Acad Dermatol 1991;24:1084.
70. Grant SM, Goa KL, Fitton A, Sorkin EM. Ketotifen: a review of its pharmacodynamic and pharmacokinetics properties, and therapeutic use in asthma and allergic disorders. Drugs 1990;40:412.
71. Campoli-Richards DM, Buckley MM-T, Fitton A. Cetirizine: a review of its pharmacological properties and clinical potential in allergic rhinitis, pollen-induced asthma, and chronic urticaria. Drugs 1990;40:762.
72. Breneman D, Bronsky EA, Bruce S, et al. Cetirizine and astemizole therapy for chronic idiopathic urticaria: a double-blind, placebo-controlled, comparative trial. J Am Acad Dermatol 1995;33:192.
73. Townley RG. Cetirizine: a new H1 antagonist with antieosinophilic activity in chronic urticaria. J Am Acad Dermatol 1991;25:668.
74. Brestel EP, Thrush LB. The treatment of glucocorticosteroid-dependent chronic urticaria with stanozolol. J Allergy Clin Immunol 1988;82:265.
75. Bressler RB, Sowell K, Huston DP. Therapy of chronic idiopathic urticaria with nifedipine: demonstration of beneficial effect in a double-blinded, placebo-controlled, crossover trial. J Allergy Clin Immunol 1989;83:756.
76. Fradin MS, Ellis CN, Goldfarb MT, Voorhees JJ. Oral cyclosporine for severe chronic idiopathic urticaria and angioedema. J Am Acad Dermatol 1991;25.1065.
77. Weiner MJ. Methotrexate in corticosteroid-resistant urticaria. Ann Intern Med 1989;110:848.
78. Engler RJM, Squire E, Benson P. Chronic sulfasalazine therapy in the treatment of delayed pressure urticaria and angioedema. Ann Allergy Asthma Immunol 1995;74:1557.
79. Jaffer AM. Sulfasalazine in the treatment of corticosteroid-dependent chronic idiopathic urticaria. J Allergy Clin Immunol 1991;88:964.
80. Zavadak D, Tharp Md. Chronic urticaria as a manifestation of the late phase reaction. Immunol Allergy Clin North Am 1995;15:745.
81. Wasserman SI, Austen F, Soter NA. The functional and physicochemical characterization of three eosinophilotactic activities released into the circulation by cold challenge of patient with cold urticaria. Clin Exp Immunol 1982;47:570.
82. Lichtenstein LM. Histamine releasing factors and IgE heterogeneity. J Allergy Clin Immunol 1988;81:814.
83. Dohl MV. Clinical pearl: diascopy helps diagnose urticarial vasculitis. J Am Acad Dermatol 1994;30:481.
84. Berdy SS, Bloch KJ. Schnitzler's syndrome: a broader clinical spectrum. J Allergy Clin Immunol 1991;87:849.
85. Sism TC, Grant JA. Hereditary angioedema: its diagnosis and management perspective. Am J Med 1990;88:656.
86. Austen KF, Sheffer AL. Detection of hereditary angioneurotic edema by demonstration of a reduction in the second component of human complement. N Engl J Med 1965;272:649.

Allergic Diseases, 5th Edition,
edited by Roy Patterson, Leslie Carroll Grammer, and
Paul A. Greenberger. Lippincott–Raven Publishers, Philadelphia, © 1997.

14

Food Allergy

Anne M. Ditto and Leslie C. Grammer

*A.M. Ditto and L.C. Grammer: Division of Allergy-Immunology,
Northwestern University Medical School, Chicago, IL 60611.*

Pearls for Practitioners
Roy Patterson

- True IgE-mediated food allergy results in immediate symptoms of urticaria, angioedema, asthma, or anaphylaxis. Symptoms occurring several hours later are unlikely to be due to IgE-mediated allergy. Symptoms occurring days later are not due to IgE-mediated allergy.
- As in other allergic diseases, the term *allergy* related to foods requires that there is an immunologic basis for the reaction.
- IgE-mediated food allergy is extremely important because fatal anaphylaxis may occur.
- Nuts, shellfish, and fish are important foods in causing anaphylaxis, and reactions can persist throughout life in some patients.
- Milk, eggs, and soy allergies are important in children and frequently disappear by 2 to 3 years of age.
- The emergency program of (1) epinephrine (Epipen), (2) prednisone, (3) hydroxyzine, and (4) emergency room treatment, developed for idiopathic anaphylaxis (See Chap. 21), is appropriate for patients with severe food anaphylaxis.
- Be careful with skin tests in a patient with a history of food anaphylaxis.
- Positive skin tests to foods may not correlate with symptoms but may only demonstrate the presence of IgE antibody.
- Many patients believe they have "food allergies" when there is no immunologically mediated problem.
- Food is so important nutritionally, psychologically, and as a cause of morbidity (as an ingestant or by avoidance) that the syndromes reviewed in this chapter deserve careful study.

The term *adverse food reaction* includes a variety of reactions to food, only some of which are the result of a true food allergy. The American Academy of Allergy and Immunology and the National Institutes of Health have defined food reactions in an attempt to standardize the nomenclature used in scientific literature.[1] An adverse food reaction is any untoward reaction to food or food additive ingestion. These reactions can be further subdivided into food allergy and food intolerance. A *food allergy* is any adverse food reaction due to an immunologic mechanism. *Food intolerance* is any adverse reaction due to a physiologic or nonimmunologic mechanism. This may be the result of pharmacologic properties of the food (e.g., caffeine in irritable bowel, tyramine-induced nausea, emesis and headache), toxins in the food, usually from improper food handling (e.g., histamine in scombroid fish poisoning, *Staphylococcus* sp food poisoning), or metabolic disorders (e.g., lactase deficiency, phenylketonuria).

PREVALENCE

The true prevalence of food allergy is not known, but the public perception exceeds the prevalence noted in several clinical studies. According to one prospective survey, at least one in four atopic adults report an adverse reaction to food they have ingested or handled.[2] Similarly, 28% of mothers in one study perceived their children to have had at least one adverse reaction to food.[3] Only 8% of these children had reactions confirmed by double-blind placebo-controlled food challenge (DBPCFC)[3]—one third of the patients whose history was suggestive of food allergy. A study of an unselected population of more than 1700 Danish children reported that 6.7% had symptoms suggestive of cow's milk allergy in the first year of life, with 2.2% confirmed by open challenge.[4] Buckley reports that in the general population, food allergy prevalence is estimated to be between 0.3% to 7.5% and that it is less in adults.[5] Studies like these have not been done in adults, but some surveys suggest the prevalence of food allergy in adults to be 1% to 2%.

FATAL FOOD ANAPHYLAXIS

The most easily recognized food hypersensitivity reactions and the best characterized are the immunoglobulin E (IgE) mediated type I reactions in the Gel and Coombs rubric.[6] These account for most food allergies. They are notable for their immediate onset; most manifest within 1 hour, but frequently within minutes. As with other IgE-mediated reactions, food hypersensitivity reactions can also manifest an additional late phase response 4 to 6 hours later. Protracted anaphylaxis relatively resistant to epinephrine has been noted with food hypersensitivity and has also been described with bee sting anaphylaxis.[7] Reactions can be severe, even fatal. Historically, the incidence of fatal and near-fatal food-induced anaphylaxis has been difficult to ascertain, primarily owing to a lack of coding in the International Classification of Disease. Sampson and associates[8] reported a series of 13 cases of fatal and near-fatal reactions to foods in children and adolescents. Peanuts, tree nuts, fish, and shellfish were the foods responsible for the most severe, life-threatening anaphylactic reactions. Factors that appeared to contribute to a fatal outcome were a concomitant diagnosis of asthma and a delay in the administration of epinephrine. The latter was also described in a study by Yunginger and associates[9] of seven adult patients, whose risk of death was also correlated with denial of symptoms and treatment with antihistamines alone.

PATHOPHYSIOLOGY

The gastrointestinal tract is exposed to many foreign proteins, including bacteria, parasites, and viruses as well as food. Its function is to digest food into forms more easily absorbed and available for energy and cell growth. In this process, it must provide a defensive barrier against any pathogens entering by this route, yet simultaneously tolerate the many foreign proteins in foods to which it is exposed. The fact that the gastrointestinal tract is exposed to a multitude of potentially allergenic proteins daily, yet food hypersensitivity is rare, attests to the efficiency with which this process is carried out.

Multiple nonimmunologic and immunologic barriers within the gastrointestinal tract operate to reduce systemic exposure to foreign antigens. Nonimmunologic or mechanical barriers include gastric acid secretions and proteolytic enzymes. These digest proteins into molecules that are less antigenic, either by reducing the size[10] or by altering the structure[4,10] (see later). Other physical barriers include mucus production and secretion and peristalsis. These decrease contact of potential allergens with the gastrointestinal mucosa.[10] The gut epithelium provides a barrier against significant macromolecular absorption.[11] Physical factors that increase the rate of absorption are alcohol ingestion and decreased gastric acid secretion. Increased acid production and food ingestion both decrease the rate of absorption.[12]

In addition to the physical barriers are immunologic barriers. The gastrointestinal tract is supplied with a local immune system referred to as the *gut-associated lymphoid tissue* or GALT.[13] The gut-associated lymphoid tissue is composed of the following: (1) discrete aggregates of lymphoid follicles distributed throughout the intestinal mucosa, including Peyer's patches and the appendix; (2) intraepithelial lymphocytes; (3) lymphocytes, plasma cells, and mast cells throughout the lamina propria; and (4) mesenteric lymph nodes.[13] Increased production and release of antibodies can occur within the gut after food ingestion, but the predominant response is increase in IgA production,[14] with suppression of IgG, IgM, and IgE.[10,15,16] This is largely in the form of dimeric secretory IgA and serves to bind proteins, forming complexes and thereby decreasing the rate of absorption.[17] IgA is found in high quantities in the mucus, adding to barrier protection. The functional significance of other antibodies is not known. For the approximately 2% of macromolecules that are absorbed as intact antigens,[15] oral tolerance develops. Tolerance is an immunologic unresponsiveness to a specific antigen,[18] in this case food proteins.

Both the local and systemic immune systems appear to play a significant role in the development of oral tolerance,[18] although the exact mechanisms are not well understood. The processing of antigens by the gut into a nonallergenic or "tolerogenic" form is important.[19] This form has a slightly different structure and appears to cause a decreased immune response in cell-mediated immunity through stimulation of CD8+ T cells.[20] This has been shown in studies of mice fed ovalbumin, which is shown to be immunogenic when administered parenterally. Within 1 hour after ingestion, a form similar in molecular weight to native ovalbumin was recovered from the serum. This tolerogenic form of ovalbumin induced suppression of cell-mediated responses but not antibody responses to native ovalbumin in recipient mice.[19] This intestinally processed ovalbumin is distinct from systemic antigen processing.[19] Lymphoid cells appear to be necessary for this process. Mice that were first irradiated were unable to process the ovalbumin into a tolerogenic form. With infusion of spleen cells, however, they regained this ability.[20] Antigen-presenting cells also appear to play an important role. With an increase in antigen presentation, there are decreases in CD8+ T cells and in tolerance.[21] Depletion of CD8+ T cells with cyclophosphamide prevents the development of oral tolerance,[22] with resultant cell-mediated immune responses, further supporting a role for CD8+ T cells in the development of tolerance.

Food hypersensitivity is the result of a loss or lack of tolerance, the cause of which is likely multifactorial. An increased incidence is noted in infants and children, and this may be due to immaturity of both the immune system and the physiologic functions of the gastrointestinal tract. Until recently, some of this immaturity was thought to lead to increased absorption of macromolecules from the infant gut, but studies now indicate that this is not likely.[23,24] There is, however, a decrease in IgA in the immature gut,[25] and perhaps this, combined with a relative decrease in CD8+ T cells or suppressor macrophage activity in youth,[26–28] may, in genetically prone individuals, contribute to the increased incidence of food allergy noted in children.[29] The importance of local IgA is further supported by the finding of an increase in incidence of food allergy associated with IgA deficiency.[29] Also, compared with adults, infants have decreased acid secretion[30]; less effective mucus secretion, with differences in both chemical and physical properties of the glycoproteins[31]; and decreased enzymatic activity.[32] These factors, combined with immunologic immaturity, may increase the risk of development of allergies. Interruption of the physical barrier of the gastrointestinal tract could lead to increased absorption.

An increase in systemic antibody production, generally food-specific IgM and IgG, occurs in patients with inflammatory bowel disease and celiac disease.[29] The significance of these antibodies is not known, however, because patients often tolerate these foods well.[33,34] Food-specific antibodies are also found in normal individuals, although usually of less quantity.[33] They may reflect dietary intake and not specific allergens.

The handling of food by the gastrointestinal tract is complex, and the development of food hypersensitivity is likely multifactorial. For sensitization to occur, an antigen must come in contact with lymphocytes either in the lamina propria, Peyer's patches, lymph nodes, spleen, or circulation.[35] Any disruption of the immunologic or nonimmunologic barriers could alter the handling of antigen and lead to an increased production of systemic antibodies. In patients with genetic predisposition to atopy, this could lead to IgE production and resultant food hypersensitivity reactions on reexposure.[36] Many more human studies need to be done before mechanisms are elucidated.

ALLERGENS

Food antigens are composed of proteins, carbohydrates, and fats. The glycoprotein in food is the component most implicated in food allergies. Glycoproteins that are allergenic have molecular weights of 10,000 to 67,000 daltons. They are water soluble, predominantly heat stable, and resistant to acid and proteolytic digestion.[37] Although many foods are potentially antigenic, most food allergies involve only a few foods.[38]

The combined results of double-blind placebo-controlled food challenges performed in the United States primarily in children showed that eight foods were responsible for 93% of reactions.[38] These foods, listed in order of frequency, are egg, peanut, milk, soy, tree nuts, fish, crustaceans, and wheat.[38] Allergy to chocolate, previously thought to be responsible for food reactions, was not found in any of the 710 patients tested.[38] In adults and older children, peanuts, crustaceans, tree nuts, and fish (in order of frequency) were reported to be responsible for most fatal anaphylactic reactions.[9] There have not been any well-studied DBPCFCs in this age group.

Allergens found commonly in children but not in adults (egg, soy, milk, and wheat) are usually outgrown with strict elimination for 1 or more years,[39] although evidence of IgE antibodies may persist.[40] Those with histories of severe reactions may take longer to develop clinical tolerance, up to several years.[39,41] The others (peanut,[42] tree nut, crustaceans,[43] and fish[44]) tend to be lifelong and thus are common to both populations.

Food processing can alter antigenicity in certain foods. Some whey proteins found in milk are denatured by heating and routine processing, while others are rendered more allergenic.[45] Fish allergens may be changed with the canning process, and patients who cannot tolerate fresh fish may tolerate canned tuna and other fish.[46] Lyophilization can also change fish allergens. This process is often used in food preparation for DBPCFCs, so great caution should be taken in interpreting a negative result of a DBPCFC to fish.[47] A different preparation may be needed. Peanut allergen is remarkably resistant to any kind of processing, retaining its allergenicity.[46] Peanut oil has been shown to be tolerated by 10 peanut-allergic patients,[48] but there have not been adequate studies ensuring its safety.

Allergen cross-reactivity is readily demonstrated by skin test, radioallergosorbent technique (RAST), RAST inhibition, and immunoblotting techniques and varies with the different food groups.[1,49–51] It does not, however, always reflect clinical cross-reactivity. For example, immunologic cross-reactivity between peanuts and other legumes is common,[50] but clinical allergic reactions (as demonstrated by DBPCFC) to more than one legume is rare.[49]

In a study of fish-allergic patients, of 11 patients with multiple positive prick skin tests, 7 patients reacted to only one fish when challenged with DBPCFC.[51] Extensive cross-reactivity among cereal grains (wheat, rye, oat, barley, rice, and corn) was noted, with less than 25% of cases confirmed by DBPCFC in one study.[52] Crustaceans also show considerable cross-reactivity,[53] but the clinical significance remains unknown due to a lack of controlled food challenges. Many children with allergy to cow's milk protein also react to milk from goats,[54] and in vitro studies have shown cross-reactivity between eggs from different animals.[55]

IgE-MEDIATED REACTIONS

Food hypersensitivity IgE-mediated reactions are the result of mast cell and basophil mediator release. Food-specific IgE bound to mast cells or basophils by the high-affinity FcɛRI is crosslinked by the food allergen, resulting in the release of preformed mediators such as histamine and newly formed mediators such as leukotrienes and prostaglandins. These result in smooth muscle contraction, vasodilation, microvascular leakage, and mucus secretion. Cytokines are also generated over several hours and thought to play a significant role in the late-phase response. Eosinophils, monocytes, and lymphocytes are recruited to the area affected in the late-phase response and release a variety of cytokines and inflammatory mediators. Clinical manifestations of IgE-mediated food allergy depend on the organ systems involved. Reactions can occur in isolation, in combination, or as part of a generalized anaphylactic reaction.

Cutaneous Manifestations

Cutaneous manifestations are the most common reaction. These range from acute urticaria or angioedema or both to a morbilliform pruritic rash. Chronic urticaria is rarely caused by food allergy.[56] Food allergies have been confirmed by DBPCFC in about one third of children with atopic dermatitis.[57] In one study, in which 210 children were evaluated and followed to determine a relation between food allergy and exacerbations of their atopic dermatitis, 62% of children had a reaction to at least one food. Of all reactions that occurred within 2 hours of a DBPCFC, 75% were cutaneous.[58] Urticaria was rare, and cutaneous manifestations were predominantly erythema and pruritus, leading to scratching and exacerbation of the atopic dermatitis.

Sampson and Broadbent reported[59] an increase in histamine releasability in basophils in patients with atopic dermatitis who repeatedly ingest a food allergen. This is due to the stimulation of mononuclear cells to secrete histamine-releasing factors, some of which interact with IgE molecules bound to the surface of basophils. Increased histamine-releasing factor production has been associated with an increase in symptoms as well as increased lung and skin hyperreactivity.

Gastrointestinal Manifestations

Gastrointestinal symptoms are the second most frequently noted manifestation of food allergy. Clinical presentations include nausea, vomiting, diarrhea, and abdominal pain and cramping. These symptoms may occur alone or in combination with other organ system symptoms. Studies in humans have elucidated some possible mechanisms, but much remains unknown. Radiologic data have shown alteration in gastrointestinal motility in allergic individuals in response to specific foods[60] as well as hypotonia and retention of the allergen test meal and prominent pylorospasm.[61] Direct visualization of the gastric mucosa during food allergen challenge revealed hyperemia, edema, petechiae, increased mucus, and decreased peristalsis.[62] Studies of passive sensitization of rectal mucosa, ileostomies, and colostomies in nonatopic patients revealed local erythema, edema, and increased mucus secretion within minutes of allergen ingestion.[63,64]

The *oral allergy syndrome* is considered to be a form of contact urticaria with symptoms resulting from contact of the food allergen with the oral mucosa. Symptoms include pruritus with or without angioedema of the lips, tongue, palate, and posterior oropharynx. It is associated with the ingestion of fresh fruits and vegetables and is the result of cross-allergenicity between the fruit or vegetable and some pollen. Shared allergen sensitivities have been reported between ragweed and the gourd family (watermelon, cantaloupe, honey-dew melon, zucchini, and cucumbers) and banana.[65] Oral allergy syndrome has been described with ingestion of apples[66], carrots, parsnips, celery, hazelnuts, potatoes,[67,68] and kiwi[69] in patients sensitive to birch pollen, and with ingestion of apples, tree nuts, peaches, oranges, pears, cherries, fennel, tomatoes, and carrots in patients allergic to tree and grass pollens.[70] Oral allergy symptoms resolve rapidly and rarely involve any other target organs. Pruritus of the mouth and lips, however, can be the initial symptoms of more severe food allergy, especially in those foods most commonly implicated in food anaphylaxis.

Allergic eosinophilic gastroenteropathy is manifested by eosinophilic infiltration of the gastrointestinal tract. Symptoms depend on the layer of gastrointestinal tract involved and are intermittent. Often, this is associated with peripheral eosinophilia and rarely involves other organs. Patients with other organ involvement do not meet criteria for hypereosinophilic syndrome.[71] Eosinophilic infiltration of the mucosal layer is most common and can be seen in any part of the gastrointestinal tract. Clinical symptoms include abdominal pain, postprandial nausea, vomiting, diarrhea, weight loss, failure to thrive, occult or gross blood loss in the stool, anemia, hypoalbuminemia, and peripheral edema.[71,72] Involvement of the submucosal and muscular regions is more common in the prepyloric region of the gastric antrum and the distal small intestine.[73] These patients may also have symptoms of gastric outlet obstruction, a mass lesion with epigastric tenderness, and even perforation of the intestinal wall.[71,74] Rarely, eosinophilic infiltration involves the serosal surface presenting with prominent ascites.[71–73] Patients in whom eosinophilic gastroenteropathy is thought to be IgE mediated (about half of adult cases) tend to have a history of atopy, including asthma and allergic rhinitis, and elevated IgE levels. These patients tend to have multiple food intolerances and positive skin tests to multiple foods.[75] Repeated degranulation of mast cells resulting from multiple food allergies is thought to be the cause of this disease in these atopic patients. Food-induced symptoms are thought to be more common in children, although the prevalence is not known.[76]

Infantile colic is a syndrome that occurs in infants younger than 3 months of age and is characterized by recurrent attacks of fussiness, inconsolable crying, drawing up of the legs, abdominal distension, and excess gas. Often, symptoms appear to be relieved with the passage of feces and flatus.[77] Symptoms commonly occur in the late afternoon or evening after feeding and last for several hours. Several double-blind crossover trials have supported IgE-mediated food hypersensitivity as a mechanism in a minority of cases,[78–80] in both breastfed and formula-fed babies. The syndrome, however, is poorly defined and is likely multifactorial with no treatment that consistently relieves symptoms. Social factors, emotional factors, environment, feeding techniques, overfeeding, and underfeeding have all been implicated. True food allergy is thought to be responsible for only 10% to 15% of cases.[81]

Respiratory Manifestations

Respiratory manifestations of food allergy usually present as part of a generalized anaphylactic reaction. Symptoms include sneezing; rhinorrhea; ocular, otic, and palatal pruritus; bronchospasm; and laryngeal edema. Isolated airway symptoms are rarely manifestations of food allergy.[82]

NON–IgE-MEDIATED REACTIONS

Food-Induced Enterocolitis

Food-induced enterocolitis syndrome presents as protracted vomiting and diarrhea in children 2 days to 3 months of age. Symptoms occur 1 to 8 hours after ingestion of the allergen, leading to a clinical picture of chronic diarrhea, eosinophilia, and malabsorption. Severe symptoms can lead to dehydration.[83] Allergy to cow's milk protein is the most common cause, although soy allergy is frequently implicated. Occasionally, this condition is seen in breastfed infants due to the antigens passed on through the mother's milk. Children who develop cow's milk–induced enterocolitis can subsequently develop soy-induced enterocolitis with a change in formula.[83,84] Stools contain erythrocytes, neutrophils, eosinophils, and not infrequently, reducing substances.[83] Jejunal biopsy reveals partial villous atrophy, lymphocytosis,[85] and plasma cells containing IgM and IgA.[85,86] Skin prick tests are characteristically negative, supporting the idea that the immunologic mechanism is not IgE-mediated. However, some investigators propose a localized IgE mechanism with resultant mast cell degranulation.[87,88] Some children also have a component of IgE sensitivity to milk or soy, and there is increased atopy among family members. Symptoms resolve within 72 hours after elimination of the allergen; diarrhea may persist longer owing to the secondary development of disaccharidase deficiency. Rechallenge is hallmarked by a recurrence of symptoms within 1 to 8 hours, fecal leukocytes and erythrocytes, and an increase in peripheral blood leukocytes by 3500 cells/m³.[83]

Food-Induced Colitis

Food-induced colitis is similar to enterocolitis with the same allergens responsible (milk and soy)[89–91] but with involvement limited to the colon.[90,92] It is also seen in infants exclusively breastfed for reasons described earlier.[93] It appears in the same age group, but there is no diarrhea and marked dehydration, and the symptoms are less severe.[90,91] Clinical findings are hematochezia or occult blood in the stool.[92,91,94] Sigmoidoscopy findings depend on the extent of involvement, ranging from areas of patchy mucosal injection to severe friability with bleeding and aphthous ulcers.[92,93] Colonic biopsies characteristically reveal eosinophilic infiltrate in the crypt epithelium and lamina propria, with destruction of crypts and neutrophils demonstrated in severe lesions.[91,93] Blood loss usually resolves within 72 hours of discontinuing the allergen, but resolution of mucosal lesions may take as long as 1 month.

Malabsorption Syndromes

Food hypersensitivity has been associated with malabsorption; cow's milk, soy, egg, and wheat are the most common offenders.[95] Symptoms usually present in the first few months of life, and are the same regardless of etiology. Symptoms range from steatorrhea to protracted diarrhea, poor weight gain, and failure to thrive.[95] Stools have increased fecal fat and reducing substances. Small intestinal findings frequently reveal areas of villous atrophy interspersed with areas of normal mucosa, referred to as a *patchy enteropathy*.[95,96] Severe, confluent, subtotal villous atrophy as seen in gluten-sensitive enteropathy is uncommon. The epithelium is hypercellular, with a predominant mononuclear round cell infiltrate and few eosinophils. Challenge with the allergen does not produce immediate symptoms; symptoms may appear days or weeks later.[95] Likewise, resolution of symptoms after antigen elimination is slow; resolution of lesions may take 6 to 18 months.[95]

Celiac Disease

Celiac disease, also known as *gluten-sensitive enteropathy* and *celiac sprue,* is characterized by malabsorption secondary to gluten ingestion.[97,98] The allergen known to be the cause is gliadin, the alcohol-soluble portion of gluten found in wheat, oats, rye, and barley. The small intestine is involved with characteristic lesions[99] that resolve totally with elimination of gluten. The disease often presents in children between 6 months and 2 years of age. Less severe disease may go unrecognized, not presenting until adulthood.[100] The small intestine is involved to varying degrees; the proximal portion is most often involved.[101] Clinical symptoms are those of malabsorption and are indistinguishable from other causes of malabsorption. The severity of symptoms correlates directly with the amount of intestine involved. Symptoms may be mild, such as ill-defined, vague symptoms of not feeling well; or patients may present with anemia secondary to vitamin B_{12} or folate malabsorption or both. Patients may have more classic symptoms of malabsorption, such as an increase in stool frequency or volume; foul-smelling or rancid, frothy stools; weight loss; and weakness.[102] In the most severe cases, the total small intestine is involved resulting in severe, life-threatening malnutrition, anemia, vitamin deficiencies, electrolyte imbalances, acidosis, and in children, dehydration, and failure to thrive.[102] Extraintestinal manifestations, such as cheilosis, glossitis, and osteopenia, may be present reflecting severe malabsorption.[102]

Lesions of the small intestine are contiguous and not patchy and most often involve the mucosa only, sparing the submucosa, muscularis, and serosa.[100] Shortening of the microvilli and flattening of the villi frequently give them a fused appearance.[103] The crypts are hyperplastic with cytologically abnormal surface cells.[103] The lamina propria is hypercellular with a predominance of lymphocytes and plasma cells.[100,103] These plasma cells are increased two-fold to six-fold and produce IgA, IgM, and IgG, with a predominance of IgA-producing cells as is found normally.[104] Basophils, eosinophils, and mast cells are also present.[105]

In addition to the classic intestinal lesions, serologic markers are often present in this disease. IgA antibodies to reticulin and smooth muscle endomysium[106] and circulating IgG and IgA antibodies to gliadin are found in most patients.[107] Antigliadin antibodies are shown to be synthesized in vitro in cultured biopsy specimens taken from the mucosa of patients with untreated celiac disease.[108] Total IgA levels are frequently elevated and total IgM levels decreased in many untreated patients. Titers to IgA antigliadin, IgA antireticulin, and IgA antiendomysial antibodies decrease or disappear after gluten elimination and therefore can be used to follow response to treatment or to monitor compliance.[109,110]

The clinical and pathophysiologic findings are consistent with an immunologic process in response to gluten ingestion: increased plasma cells and lymphocytes in the small intestine, destruction of the normal structure of the intestinal mucosa, specific antibodies to gliadin in the mucosa and serum, and the reversal of mucosal lesions and serologic markers with the elimination of gluten, with recurrence on rechallenge. The exact mechanism, however, is unknown. First thought to be immune complex–mediated with the finding of specific antibodies, there is now evidence for T-cell–mediated mechanisms as well.[111–113]

Dermatitis Herpetiformis

Dermatitis herpetiformis is a food hypersensitivity manifested by a pruritic rash in association with gluten-sensitive enteropathy.[114] It occurs most commonly in children ages 2 to 7 years. The rash is described as an erythematous, pleomorphic eruption involving predominantly the knees, elbows, shoulders, buttocks, and scalp. Lesions can be urticarial, papular, vesicular, or bullous.[115] They may be hemorrhagic on the palms and soles, but mucous membranes are spared. Gluten-sensitive enteropathy is reported in 75% to 90% of cases. The remainder of patients usually have subclinical symptoms of celiac disease, which is unmasked with aggressive gluten challenge.

The immunologic mechanism is unknown; but in addition to its association with gluten sensitivity, there is other evidence for an immune-mediated process. IgA deposition in either a granular (85% to 90%) or linear (10% to 15%) pattern and C3 cells are found on immunofluorescent staining of dermal papillary tips in both normal and affected skin.[114] Immune complexes are frequently found in the sera, although what role they play is uncertain.[115] IgA antibodies against smooth muscle endomysium are found in about 70% of patients, and titers correlate with the severity of the intestinal disease. There is also an association with HLA-B8 (80% to 90%),[115,116] and about 75% of patients are positive for HLA-DW3.[116] Both the cutaneous lesions and the enteropathy respond to gluten elimination. The cutaneous lesions, however, may respond more slowly to treatment and may also appear more slowly with rechallenge. Sulfones are the mainstay of therapy for the cutaneous lesions and may relieve pruritic symptoms within 24 hours.[115]

Heiner's Syndrome

Heiner's syndrome is a form of primary pulmonary hemosiderosis associated with cow's milk sensitivity. It is rare, occurs in infants and young children, and is characterized by wheezing, chronic cough, recurrent pulmonary infiltrates, hypochromic microcytic anemia, and failure to thrive.[117] Patients may also have rhinitis, hypertrophied nasopharyngeal tissue with resultant cor pulmonale,[118] recurrent otitis media, variable gastrointestinal symptoms, and growth retardation.[119] Consistent with hemosiderosis, hemosiderin-laden macrophages may be seen in biopsy specimens of the lung or in stomach aspirates.[117] Patients have positive skin tests to cow's milk proteins and may have unusually high titers of precipitins to many cow's milk proteins as well as eosinophilia. The titers, however, do not correlate with disease severity, and their significance is unknown.[118] Symptoms improve when milk is eliminated from the diet and recur with rechallenge. With severe disease and acute gastrointestinal symptoms, corticosteroids may be needed.

Some patients with positive precipitins do not respond to milk elimination, while some with no titers do respond.[120] In general, patients who have high titers of precipitins to cow's milk constituents respond to treatment and have a better prognosis than patients with other forms of pulmonary hemosiderosis.[120] Although pulmonary hemosiderosis may have other causes, the presence of severe anemia should raise the suspicion of cow's milk sensitivity.

IgE-MEDIATED ASTHMA FROM FOOD ALLERGEN INHALATION

IgE-mediated food reactions can result from inhalation of aerosolized antigens, usually in an occupational setting. The resultant symptoms are the same as respiratory symptoms seen with aeroallergens (rhinoconjunctivitis, asthma), but the asthma is a more prominent symptom. Patients typically have IgE antibody to the food as demonstrated by skin tests or RAST. Baker's asthma, the first described occupational food allergy, was noted in 1705 by Bernadino Ramazzini in his treatise, "De Moribus Artifucum Diatriba" (Disease of Workers).[121] This is the most common food-related lung disease and affects workers who are regularly exposed to flour. Wheat is the most common allergen, and IgE antibody to wheat flour has been demonstrated in patients with Baker's asthma.[122-124] Bronchial provocation has shown sensitivity to flour and also to contaminants such as insects or molds.[125-127] A study with crab processors showed that the IgE sensitization is through exposure to aerosolized proteins, in this case, in the steam of cooking water, thus explaining the resultant respiratory symptoms.[128] This may also explain some adverse reactions that food-sensitive patients have experienced when smelling the food or when in close vicinity while it is cooked. Of interest, 12 of 54 snow crab workers, who were sensitized by inhalation and developed asthma, experienced the same reaction with ingestion of the snow crab.[128] This has been described in a garlic worker as well.[129] This, however, is not common because most patients with Baker's asthma do not experience symptoms with wheat ingestion.[123] Of note, there have been isolated reports of anaphylaxis from ingestion of food contaminated with an aeroallergen.[130,131] Table 14-1 lists allergens implicated in food-related occupational lung disease.

FOOD-RELATED EXERCISE-INDUCED ANAPHYLAXIS

Exercise-induced anaphylaxis is a unique syndrome characterized by generalized body warmth, erythema, and pruritus that, with continued exertion, progresses to fulminant anaphylaxis with confluent urticaria, laryngeal edema, bronchospasm, gastrointestinal symptoms, and even vascular collapse.[132] A subset of patients have these symptoms only if exercise is within 2 hours of food ingestion.[133] With food alone or exercise alone, there is no anaphylaxis.[133,134] For some patients, this postprandial exercise-induced anaphylaxis may occur with any food ingestion followed by exercise.[133,134] Others have exercise-induced anaphylaxis only associated with the

TABLE 14-1. *Foods associated with upper respiratory diseases*

Food	Associated occupation
Buckwheat flour	Food processors
Castor bean	Longshoremen, fertilizer workers, oil industry workers
Coffee bean	Longshoremen, food processors
Egg	Egg-processing workers
Garlic	Spice factory workers
Grain dust	Granary workers, farmers, millers, bakers
Guar gum	Carpet manufacturers
Gum acacia	Printers
Mushroom	Mushroom growers
Papain	Food processors

ingestion of specific foods, that is, celery[133] and shellfish.[135] These patients are skin test positive to the foods, yet they have no allergic reactions unless ingestion is followed by or proceeded by rigorous exercise.[133,135] Symptoms may be intermittent. For all food-related exercise-induced anaphylaxis, episodes are prevented with avoidance of food ingestion 4 hours before or after exercise.[134] Treatment also includes carrying self-injectable epinephrine and exercising with a companion. The mechanism of this type of anaphylaxis is not well understood, but it is thought to be mediated by mast cell degranulation.[132]

FOOD-RELATED REACTIONS OF UNCERTAIN CAUSE

Food Additives

Allergic reactions to food additives are rare yet overestimated. Many symptoms are suggestive of food intolerance, such as mood changes and behavioral changes, and are not substantiated by DBPCFC. In one study, 132 patients who responded to a survey stating they had an adverse reaction to food additives underwent different oral challenges with additives mixed in combination and with placebo capsules. Of these, only 3 patients had consistent reactions—2 to the natural yellow-orange annatto and 1 to the azo dye and the antioxidants.[136]

Metabisulfite reactions in asthmatic patients are both rare and variable.[137] Oral challenge of metabisulfite in 12 patients with idiopathic anaphylaxis and in 1 patient with chronic urticaria who had reactions temporally related to restaurant meals showed no reaction in any of the patients.[138] Two multicenter trials were conducted to evaluate claims of hypersensitivity to aspartame. These were double-blind, placebo-controlled crossover trials; one involved 40 patients presenting with headache after aspartame injection, and the other involved 21 patients with urticaria or angioedema or both associated with aspartame ingestion. Both studies showed that aspartame was no more likely than placebo to cause the adverse reactions.[139,140]

Other

Other diseases that appear to be exacerbated by certain foods have been reported in the literature. Some have been reported to be documented by DBPCFC, such as 1 case of arthritis[141] and 16 pediatric patients with migraine and epilepsy, 15 of whom had symptoms with exposure to several foods, 8 of whom had seizures.[142] Although these DBPCFCs show an association, they do not necessarily suggest an immunologic cause. Other symptoms, such as fatigue, hyperreactivity, enuresis, and mood changes, have not been substantiated by DBPCFC.

DIAGNOSIS

Diagnosis of food allergy requires a thorough history to differentiate between food intolerance and a true hypersensitivity reaction. Table 14-2 lists important data to obtain.

Multiple food allergies are rare. Complaints of these, unusual clinical manifestations, and excessive weight loss with elimination diets may all be manifestations of food aversion, possibly of a psychological nature. Histories may more reliably implicate the offending agent in immediate-type reactions and may not be helpful in chronic diseases such as atopic dermatitis.[143] The physical examination may be helpful if a reaction is occurring and should also be used to rule out other disease processes.

TABLE 14-2. *Data important in the evaluation of food allergy*

Implicated foods

Amount of food required to elicit a reaction

History of a reaction with each exposure

Amount of time between the exposure and the reaction (especially useful for an IgE-mediated reaction, which is usually immediate in onset but may occur up to 2 hours after ingestion)

Clinical manifestations consistent with food allergy

Resolution of symptoms with elimination of the food

Duration of symptoms

Medications, if any, needed to treat reactions

A variety of in vivo and in vitro tests can help confirm a suspected food allergy. In vivo tests include prick skin testing and elimination diets. Skin testing is recommended for histories suggestive of IgE-mediated food hypersensitivity. They are highly reliable[144,145] and give useful information in a short period of time.[145,146] A drop of glycerinated food allergen extract (1:20 to 1:10 w/v dilution) is placed on the skin and the prick or puncture technique applied.[146] Histamine and saline are used as positive and negative controls, respectively. Fruit and vegetable extracts are labile, and therefore fresh fruits and vegetables are recommended.[70] The food can be rubbed on the skin, which is then pricked, or the needle can first be introduced into the food with subsequent pricking of the skin. A wheal 3 mm greater than the negative control is considered positive.[146] With reliable extracts, the incidence of false-negative results is low, rendering the negative predictive value higher than 95%.[147] The positive predictive value, however, is significantly lower—about 60% in patients in whom the prevalence of food allergies is fairly high,[147] and as low as 3% in patients in whom the prevalence is low and in whom there is no suggestive history.[147] In this same population, however, the negative predictive value of the prick test for foods approaches 100%.[147,148] Intradermal food skin testing has a higher chance of inducing systemic symptoms and a greater false-positive rate then prick skin testing when compared with DBPCFC.[146,148]

Elimination diets are 7- to 14-day diets in which all foods suspected of causing an allergic reaction are eliminated. If multiple foods are suspected, the elimination diet may have to be repeated, with only several foods eliminated each time. This may be helpful in chronic conditions, such as atopic dermatitis, or in children in whom specific foods may be difficult to implicate. If there is no resolution in symptoms, the foods are thought not to be responsible. Foods that are implicated may be reintroduced one at a time at 24- to 48-hour intervals to determine which foods are responsible. Elimination diets rarely diagnose food allergies and can be tedious and time-consuming. Foods thought to be implicated should generally be confirmed by skin testing and possibly DBPCFC because persistent elimination of foods can lead to nutritional inadequacies, especially in children.[149] Diet diaries are occasionally useful when the cause-and-effect relation is not initially perceived. Data of all foods ingested and any associated symptoms are recorded prospectively. Although there is no risk of nutritional inadequacies, these tend to yield little reward for the effort involved.

Occupational food-induced respiratory allergies (allergic rhinoconjunctivitis or asthma) may also require spirometry to document asthma. Many patients have symptoms only in the workplace initially and may benefit from serial peak flow monitoring or even spirometry at the workplace.[150] Bronchial allergen challenges may be used, but patients can have severe life-threatening bronchospasm, so this should be done in a medical setting and only if necessary.

In vitro tests consist of RAST measurement of specific serum IgE. This is less specific[147] than prick skin tests, considerably more expensive, and yields less immediate results. It may be considered, however, in cases of severe atopic dermatitis or dermatographism, in which skin testing is more difficult.

DBPCFC is considered the gold standard for the definitive diagnosis of food allergies.[38] With foods that are not likely to cause an allergy or with negative skin tests or RAST tests, open or simple-blinded oral challenges may be used in the office setting and are much more practical. In the case of multiple positive results, however, DBPCFC may be used to confirm results, especially in children, in whom elimination of multiple foods may lead to nutritional deficiencies.[149] The choice of foods selected for the DBPCFC should be determined by the history, skin test, or RAST test or by results of an elimination diet. Foods should be eliminated for 7 to 14 days, and all medication that may interfere with interpretation of symptoms (i.e., antihistamines, corticosteroids) should be discontinued. A standard scoring system[38] should be used, and there must be access to emergency medical treatment in case anaphylaxis occurs. Patients with a history consistent with an immediate reaction to food (especially those with a life-threatening reaction) and a positive skin test (or RAST test) should not be challenged.

The DBPCFC is administered in the fasting state. Lyophilized food is often used, and it is blinded to the patient and medical personnel as either a capsule or liquid. The starting dose is usually 125 to 500 mg of lyophilized food, which is then doubled every 15 to 60 minutes. Symptoms are recorded using a standard scoring system, usually categorized by organs involved.[38] A study is considered negative if 10 g of the substance has been tolerated. All blinded negative challenges must be confirmed by an open feeding under observation to rule out a false-negative reaction. This is rare, however, and may be secondary to the food processing (i.e., lyophilization with fish). In summary, the DBPCFC may be especially useful in determining suspected food allergies that are not apparent by history supplemented by skin

TABLE 14-3. *Diagnosis of non-IgE–mediated food allergy*

Manifestation	Diagnostic criteria
Food-induced enterocolitis	Resolution of symptoms within 72 hours after elimination of the allergen (usually milk or soy); symptoms may persist if a secondary dissacharidase deficiency develops.
	Open oral challenge, if elimination is inconclusive, consisting of 0.6 mg/kg protein with simultaneous monitoring of the white blood count (WBC) and stools; symptoms of vomiting and diarrhea appear in 1–6 h and can be *severe;* peripheral WBC increases by 3500 cells/m³, and polymorphonuclear cells and eosinophils can be found in the stool.
Food-induced colitis	Same as above, but symptoms may take hours or days to appear and are not as severe. Biopsy
Malabsorption syndromes	Same as above, including biopsy
Celiac disease	Biopsy required for diagnosis with resolution of characteristic villous atrophy after 6–12 wk of a gluten-free diet IgA levels useful for screening and monitoring the disease (i.e., compliance)
Allergic eosinophilic gastroentritis	Biopsy-proven eosinophilic infiltration of the gastrointestinal wall; multiple biopsies (as many as 10) may be needed because lesions are sporadic. Some patients have IgE to specific foods with improvement of symptoms and intestinal lesions after 6–12 wk of elimination.

testing, RAST testing, or an elimination diet. It may also be helpful in interpreting positive skin tests that do no correlate with the patient's history.

Non-IgE–mediated food allergies involving the gastrointestinal tract are diagnosed predominantly by response to elimination of the allergen from the diet, although some diseases require biopsies as well (Table 14-3). Food-induced enterocolitis and colitis resolve within 72 hours after elimination of the suspected antigen from the diet, although symptoms may persist if a secondary disaccharide deficiency has developed. Malabsorption syndromes may take days or weeks for symptoms to resolve. An oral food challenge can be used to confirm the diagnosis of enterocolitis. This consists of administering 0.6 g allergen/Kg, with simultaneous monitoring of the peripheral white blood cell count. Vomiting and diarrhea occur within 1 to 6 hours, and the absolute leukocyte count increases by 3500 cells/m^3 if the challenge is positive. Polymorphonuclear leukocytes and eosinophils can be found in the stool as well. Reactions to an oral challenge can be severe, leading to dehydration and hypotension; therefore, such challenges need to be done in a medical setting and should only be performed if the diagnosis is still in question after elimination of the allergen. In the case of food-induced colitis, symptoms may take hours to days to reappear with this oral challenge and are not as severe as those seen with enterocolitis. Both colitis and malabsorption syndromes can be confirmed by biopsy.

Celiac disease requires biopsy showing characteristic villous atrophy with resolution after 6 to 12 weeks of a gluten-free diet. IgA levels can be used for screening and following a patient's progress, but celiac disease can only be diagnosed by biopsy.

Allergic eosinophilic gastroenteritis is diagnosed with biopsy-proven eosinophilic infiltration of the gastrointestinal wall. Multiple biopsies, in some cases as many as 10, may be needed because the eosinophilic infiltrate is often sporadic and may be missed on a single biopsy. Some patients may also have positive skin tests or RAST tests to specific foods, with improvement in symptoms and normalization of intestinal lesions after 6 to 12 weeks of elimination of the food.

Other tests that have been reported in the evaluation of food allergies are basophil histamine release, IgG$_2$ and IgG$_4$ antibodies, antigen–antibody complexes, plasma histamine level, neutrophil chemotaxis, lymphocyte stimulation studies, and special intestinal biopsies. These tests are predominantly research tools, are not widely available, and although appropriate for investigational purposes, are not sufficiently reliable to be used in clinical practice.[151] Several tests, including subcutaneous or sublingual provocation, the leukocytotoxicity assay, and intracutaneous or low-level modified RAST titration, are widely promoted by some practitioners and laboratories for the diagnosis and treatment of food allergy. No generally accepted body of literature, however, has documented any diagnostic or treatment value using these methods.[151,152]

TREATMENT

Once food hypersensitivity is diagnosed, the offending allergen must be strictly eliminated from the diet. This is the only proven treatment for food allergy. Patients and their families need to be properly educated in food avoidance, including hidden food sources. Patients with IgE-mediated reactions should be given injectable epinephrine (e.g., Epipen®) to be carried at all times, and its use should be demonstrated in the office. They should be instructed to use the epinephrine in case of accidental exposure. Because reactions can progress and late-phase reactions can occur, patients should go immediately to an emergency room for further evaluation. Patients should be observed there four additional hours after a reaction. School children should have their injectable epinephrine at school. The school administrators, nurse, and the patient's teachers should be made aware of the allergy and what symptoms to look for in case of exposure. They should also be instructed in emergency treatment. These recommendations are extremely important because studies show that food anaphylaxis usually results from accidental exposure to a known allergen, and the risk for a fatal outcome is increased with a delay in treatment.[8,9]

As previously mentioned, many food allergies diagnosed in childhood are not lifelong (with the exception of peanuts, shellfish, nuts, and fish), and reevaluation with skin test, RAST test, or oral challenges should be considered every 1 to 3 years. This is not true for celiac disease, dermatitis herpetiformis, Heiner's syndrome, and allergic eosinophilic gastroenteritis, for which the allergens must always be avoided. Pharmacologic agents are used to treat symptoms of anaphylaxis, but none has been shown reliably effective in preventing anaphylaxis.[153] These include H_1 and H_2 antihistamines, oral cromolyn glycate, ketotifen, and antiprostaglandins. Immunotherapy was reported in one double-blind placebo-controlled study to be efficacious in three peanut-allergic patients.[154] The rate of adverse systemic reactions, however, was three times that of aeroallergen rush immunotherapy. This study was discontinued, and the long-term effect of immunotherapy was not evaluated.

PREVENTION

The role of dietary manipulation in the prevention of atopic disease in infants of allergic parents has been under debate since 1936, when Grulee and Sanford[155] noted a decreased incidence of atopy and food allergy among infants who were exclusively breastfed. In 1989, Zeiger and associates[156] prospectively studied dietary manipulation in infants of atopic parents. With both maternal and infant avoidance of foods, the number of food-related symptoms (particularly atopic dermatitis, urticaria, and gastrointestinal disease) were significantly reduced in the first 12 months of life and less so at 2 years.[156] These, however, became similar at 3 and 4 years of age[157] and again at a 7-year follow-up.[158] There was no difference in the incidence of asthma or rhinitis in the two groups at any time.[156–158]

NATURAL HISTORY

Since the 1980s, much has been learned about the natural history of food allergy. Children tend to lose their clinical reactivity to milk, soy, egg, and wheat as they get older. In a prospective study of 501 children, only 2 of 15 patients with allergy proven by DBPCFC during the first year of life remained reactive at 13 to 24 months of age.[39] After 24 months of age, none retained reactivity. In another study of patients who had severe reactions to egg and milk, clinical reactivity lasted for years, but tolerance was eventually achieved.[41] Despite clinical tolerance, often the presence of IgE as detected by skin test or RAST still exists.[39,41] Unlike with milk, soy, egg, and wheat, hypersensitivity to peanut, fish, tree nuts, and shellfish tends to remain. One long-term follow-up study of peanut-allergic patients reported that clinical reactions persist for a minimum of 14 years.[42] Similar results were obtained from studies of patients with life-threatening anaphylaxis from fish,[44] tree nuts, and crustaceans.[43] These food allergies are considered lifelong and patients must always carry emergency medicine.

REFERENCES

1. Anderson JA, Sogn DD, eds. Adverse reactions to foods. American Academy of Allergy and Immunology NIAID. NIH Publication 1984;84:2442
2. Eriksson NE. Food sensitivity reported by patients with asthma and hay fever. Allergy 1978;33:189.

3. Bock SA. Prospective appraisal of complaints of adverse reactions to foods in children during the first 3 years of life. Pediatrics 1987;79:683.
4. Høst A, Halken S. A prospective study of cow milk allergy in Danish infants during the first 3 years of life. Allergy 1990;45:587.
5. Buckley RH, Metcalfe DD. Food allergy. JAMA 1982;248:2627.
6. Hypersensitivity: type I. In: Roitt I, Brostoff J, Male D, eds. Immunology. 4th ed. Chicago: Mosby, 1996:22.
7. Smith PL, Kagey-Sobotka A, Bleeker ER, et al. Physiologic manifestations of human anaphylaxis. J Clin Invest 1980;66:1072.
8. Sampson HA, Mendelson L, Rosen JP. Fatal and near-fatal anaphylactic reactions to food in children and adolescents. N Engl J Med 1992;327:380.
9. Yunginger JW, Sweeney KG, Sturner WQ, et al. Fatal food-induced anaphylaxis. JAMA 1988;260:1450.
10. Walker WA. Pathophysiology of intestinal uptake and absorption of antigens in food allergy. Ann Allergy 1987;59:7.
11. Walker WA. Antigen handling by the small intestine. Clin Gastroenterol 1986;15:1.
12. Walzer M. Allergy of the abdominal organs. J Lab Clin Med 1941;26:1867.
13. The lymphoid system. In: Roitt I, Brostoff J, Male D, eds. Immunology. 4th ed. Chicago: Mosby, 1996:3.2.
14. Gearhart PJ, Cebra JJ. Differentiated B-lymphocytes: potential to express particular antibody variable and constant regions depends on site of lymphoid tissue and antigen load. J Exp Med 1979;149:216.
15. Mowat AM. The regulation of immune responses to dietary protein antigens. Immunol Today 1987;8:93.
16. Mowat AM, Strobel S, Drummond HE, Ferguson A. Immunological responses to fed protein antigens in mice. I. Reversal of oral tolerance to ovalbumin by cyclophosphamide. Immunology 1982;45:105.
17. Kleinman RE, Walker WA. The enteromammary immune system: an important new concept in breast milk host defense. Digest Dis Sci 1979;24:876.
18. Asherson GL, Zembala M, Perera MA, et al. Production of immunity and unresponsiveness in the mouse by feeding contact sensitizing agents and the role of suppressor cells in the Peyer's patches, mesenteric lymph nodes, and other tissues. Cell Immunol 1977;33:145.
19. Bruce MG, Ferguson A. Oral tolerance to ovalbumin in mice: studies of chemically modified and `biologically filtered' antigen. Immunology 1986;57:627.
20. Bruce MG, Strobel S, Hanson DG, Ferguson A. Irradiated mice lose the capacity to `process' fed antigen for systemic tolerance of delayed-type hypersensitivity. Clin Exp Immunol 1987;70:611.
21. Stobel S, Mowat AM, Ferguson A. Prevention of oral tolerance induction to ovalbumin and enhanced antigen presentation during a graft-versus-host reaction in mice. Immunology 1985;56:57.
22. Mowat AM, Ferguson A. Migration inhibition of lymph node lymphocytes as an assay for regional cell-mediated immunity in the intestinal lymph nodes of mice immunized orally with ovalbumin. Immunology 1982;47:365.
23. Heyman M, Grasset E, Ducroc R, Desjeux J-F. Antigen absorption by the jejunal epithelium of children with cow's milk allergy. Pediatr Res 1988;24:197.
24. Powell GK, McDonald PJ, Van Sickle GJ, Goldblum RM. Absorption of food protein antigen in infants with food protein-induced enterocolitis. Digest Dis Sci 1989;34:781.
25. Selner JC, Merrill DA, Claman HN. Salivary immunoglobulin and albumin: development during the newborn period. J Pediatr 1968;72:685.
26. Kerner JA Jr. Formula allergy and intolerance. Gastroenterol Clin North Am 1995;24:1.
27. Ohsugi Y, Gershwin ME. The IgE response of New Zealand black mice to ovalbumin: an age-acquired increase in suppressor activity. Clin Immunol Immunopathol 1981;20:296.
28. Strobel S, Ferguson A. Immune responses to fed protein antigens in mice. 3. Systematic tolerance or priming is related to age at which antigen is first encountered. Pediatr Res 1984;18:588.
29. Businco L, Benincori N, Cantani A. Epidemiology, incidence and clinical aspects of food allergy. Ann Allergy 1984;53:615.
30. Hyman EPE, Clarke DD, Everett SL, et al. Gastric acid secretory function in pre-term infants. J Pediatr 1985;106:467.
31. Shub MD, Pang KY, Swann DA, Walker WA. Age-related changes in chemical composition and physical properties of mucous glycoproteins from rat small intestine. Biochem J 1983;215:405.
32. Lebenthal E, Lee PC. Development of functional response in human exocrine pancreas. Pediatrics 1980;66:556.
33. Johansson SGO, Dannaeus A, Lilja G. The relevance of anti-food antibodies for the diagnosis of food allergy. Ann Allergy 1984;53:665.
34. May CD, Remigio L, Feldman J, Bock SA, Carr RI. A study of serum antibodies to isolated milk proteins and ovalbumin in infants and children. Clin Allergy 1977;7:583.
35. Parrott DMV. The gut as a lymphoidal organ. Clin Gastroenterol 1976;5:211.
36. Marsh DG, Meyers DA, Bias WB. The epidemiology and genetics of atopic allergy. N Engl J Med 1981;305:1551.
37. Lemanske RF Jr, Taylor SL. Standardized extracts, foods. Clin Rev Allergy 1987;5:23.
38. Bock SA, Sampson HA, Atkins FM, et al. Double-blind, placebo-controlled food challenge (DBPCFC) as an office procedure: a manual. J Allergy Clin Immunol 1988;82:986.
39. Bock SA. The natural history of adverse reaction to foods. N Engl Reg Allergy Proc 1986;7:504.
40. Foucard T. Developmental aspects of food sensitivity in childhood. Nutr Rev 1984;42:98.

41. Bock SA. Natural history of severe reactions to foods in young children. J Pediatr 1985;107:676.
42. Bock SA, Atkins F. The natural history of peanut allergy. J Allergy Clin Immunol 1989:83:900.
43. Atkins FM, Steinberg SS, Metcalfe DD. Evaluation of immediate adverse reactions to foods in adult patients. II. A detailed analysis of reaction patterns during oral food challenge. J Allergy Clin Immunol 1985;75:356.
44. Dannaeus A, Inganäs M. A follow-up study of children with food allergy: clinical course in relation to serum IgE- and IgG-antibody levels to milk, egg and fish. Clin Allergy 1981;11;533.
45. Bleumink E, Young E. Identification of the atopic allergen in cow's milk. Int Arch Allergy 1968;34:521.
46. Nordlee JA, Taylor SL, Jones RT, Yunginger JW. Allergenicity of various peanut products as determined by RAST inhibition. J Allergy Clin Immunol 1981;68:376.
47. Bernhisel-Broadbent J, Strause D, Sampson HA. Fish hypersensitivity. II. Clinical relevance of altered fish allergenicity caused by various preparation methods. J Allergy Clin Immunol 1992;90:622.
48. Taylor SL, Busse WW, Sachs MI, Parker JL, Yunginger JW. Peanut oil is not allergenic to peanut-sensitive individuals. J Allergy Clin Immunol 1981;68:372.
49. Bernhisel-Broadbent J, Sampson HA. Cross-allergenicity in the legume botanical family in children with food hypersensitivity. J Allergy Clin Immunol 1989;83:435.
50. Bernhisel-Broadbent J, Taylor S, Sampson HA. Cross-allergenicity in the legume botanical family in children with food hypersensitivity. II. Laboratory correlates. J Allergy Clin Immunol 1989;84:701.
51. Bernhisel-Broadbent J, Scanlon SM, Sampson HA. Fish hypersensitivity. I. In vitro and oral challenge results in fish-allergic patients. J Allergy Clin Immunol 1992;89:730.
52. Jones SM, Magnolfi CF, Cooke SK, Sampson HA. Immunologic cross-reactivity among cereal grains and grasses in children with food hypersensitivity. J Allergy Clin Immunol 1995;96:341.
53. Waring NP, Daul CB, deShazo RD, McCants ML, Lehrer SB. Hypersensitivity reactions to ingested crustacea: clinical evaluation and diagnostic studies in shrimp-sensitive individuals. J Allergy Clin Immunol 1985;76:440.
54. Clein NW. Cow's milk allergy in infants and children. Int Arch Allergy 1958;13:245
55. Langeland T. A clinical and immunological study of allergy to hen's egg white. VI. Occurrence of proteins crossreacting with allergens in hen's egg white as studied in egg white from turkey, duck, goose, seagull, and in hen egg yolk, and hen and chicken sera and flesh. Allergy 1983;38:399.
56. Champion RH, Roberts SOB, Carpenter RG, Roger JH. Urticaria and angio-oedema: a review of 554 patients. Br J Dermatol 1969;81:588.
57. Burks AW, Mallory SB, Williams LW, Shirrell MA. Atopic dermatitis: clinical relevance of food hypersensitivity reactions. J Pediatr 1988;113:447.
58. Sampson HA. Food hypersensitivity and atopic dermatitis. Allergy Proc 1991;12:327.
59. Sampson HA, Broadbent K. "Spontaneous" basophil histamine release (SBHR) and histamine releasing factor (HRF) in patients with atopic dermatitis (AD) and food hypersensitivity (FH). J Allergy Clin Immunol 1987;79:497. Abstract.
60. Liu H-Y, Whitehouse WM, Giday Z. Proximal small bowel transit pattern in patients with malabsorption induced by bovine milk protein ingestion. Radiology 1975;115:415.
61. Fries JH, Zizmor J. Roentgen studies of children with alimentary disturbances due to food allergy. Am J Dis Child 1937;54:1239.
62. Pollard HM, Stuart GJ. Experimental reproduction of gastric allergy in human beings with controlled observations on the mucosa. J Allergy 1942;13:467.
63. Gray I, Walzer M. Studies in mucous membrane hypersensitiveness. III. The allergic reaction of the passively sensitized rectal mucous membrane. Am J Diff Dis 1938;4:707.
64. Gray I, Harten M, Walzer M. Studies in mucous membrane hypersensitiveness. IV. The allergic reaction in the passively sensitized mucous membranes of the ileum and colon in humans. Ann Intern Med 1940;13:2050.
65. Enberg RN, Leickly FE, McCullough J, Bailey J, Ownby DR. Watermelon and ragweed share allergens. J Allergy Clin Immunol 1987;79:867.
66. Lahti A, Björkstén F, Hannuksela M. Allergy to birch pollen and apple, and cross-reactivity of allergens studied with the RAST. Allergy 1980;35:297.
67. Anderson KE, Lowenstein H. An investigation of the possible immunological relationship between allergen extracts from birch pollen, hazelnut, potato and apple. Contact Derm 1978;4:73.
68. Halmepuro L, Lowenstein H. Immunological investigation of possible structural similarities between pollen antigens and antigens in apple, carrot, and celery tuber. Allergy 1985;40:264.
69. Gall H, Kalveram K-J, Forck G, Sterry W. Kiwi fruit allergy: a new birch pollen–associated food allergy. J Allergy Clin Immunol 1994;94:70.
70. Ortolani C, Ispano M, Pastorello EA, Ansaloni R, Magri GC. Comparison of results of skin prick tests (with fresh foods and commercial food extracts) and RAST in 100 patients with oral allergy syndrome J Allergy Clin Immunol 1989;83:683.
71. Steffen RM, Wyllie R, Petras RE, et al. The spectrum of eosinophilic gastroenteritis. Clin Pediatr 1991;30:404.
72. Talley NJ, Shorter RG, Phillips SF, Zinsmeister AR. Eosinophilic gastroenteritis: a clinicopathological study of patients with disease of the mucosa, muscle layer and subserosal tissue. Gut 1990;31:54.
73. Pathology of the gastrointestinal tract. In: Goldman H, Ming S-C, eds. Philadelphia: WB Saunders, 1992:171.
74. Snyder JD, Rosenblum N, Wershil B, Goldman H, Winter HS. Pyloric stenosis and eosinophilic gastroenteritis in infants. J Pediatr Gastroenterol Nutr 1987;6:543.
75. Kettlehut BV, Metcalfe DD. Adverse reactions to foods. In: Middleton E, Reed CE, Ellis EF, Adkinson NF, Yunginger JW, eds. Allergy: principles and practice. 3rd ed. St Louis: CV Mosby, 1988:1481.

76. James JM, Sampson HA. An overview of food hypersensitivity. Pediatr Allergy Immunol 1991;3:67.
77. First year feeding problems. In: Nelson WE, Behrman RE, Kliegman RM, Arvin AM, eds. Textbook of pediatrics. 15th ed. Philadelphia: WB Saunders, 1996:165.
78. Forsyth BWC. Colic and the effect of changing formulas: a double-blind multiple-crossover study. J Pediatr 1989;115:521.
79. Lothe L, Lindberg T. Cow's milk whey protein elicits symptoms of infantile colic in colicky formula-fed infants: a double-blind crossover study. Pediatr 1989;83:262.
80. Jakobsson I, Lindberg T. Cow's milk proteins cause infantile colic in breast-fed infants: a double-blind crossover study. Pediatrics 1983;71:268.
81. Sampson HA. Infantile colic and food allergy: fact or fiction? J Pediatr 1989;115:583.
82. Bock SA, Atkins FM. Patterns of food hypersensitivity during sixteen years of double-bind, placebo-controlled food challenges. J Pediatr 1990;117:561.
83. Powell GK. Milk- and soy-induced enterocolitis of infancy: clinical features and standardization of challenge. J Pediatr 1978;93:553.
84. Jakobsson I, Lindberg T. A prospective study of cow's milk protein intolerance in Swedish infants. Acta Pediatr Scand 1979;68:853.
85. Perkkio M, Savilahti E, Kuitunen P. Morphometric and immunohistochemical study of jejunal biopsies from children with intestinal soy allergy. Eur J Pediatr 1981;137:63.
86. Pearson JR, Kingston D, Shiner M. Antibody production to milk proteins in the jejunal mucosa of children with cow's milk protein intolerance. Pediatr Res 1983;17:406.
87. Selbekk BH. A comparison between in vitro jejunal mast cell degranulation and intragastric challenge in patients with suspected food intolerance. Scand J Gastroenterol 1985;20:299.
88. Nolte H, Schiotz PO, Kruse A, Skovp. Comparison of intestinal mast cell and basophil histamine release in children with food allergic reactions. Allergy 1989;44:554.
89. Jenkins HR, Pincott JR, Soothill JF, Milla PJ, Harries JT. Food allergy: the major cause of infantile colitis. Arch Dis Child 1984;59:326.
90. Berezin S, Schwarz SM, Glassman M, Davidian M, Newman LJ. Gastrointestinal milk intolerance of infancy. Am J Dis Child 1989;143:361.
91. Goldman H, Proujansky R. Allergic proctitis and gastroenteritis in children: clinical and mucosal features in 53 cases. Am J Surg Pathol 1986;10:75.
92. Gryboski JD. Gastrointestinal milk allergy in infants. Pediatr 1967;40:354.
93. Lake AM, Whitington PF, Hamilton SR. Dietary protein-induced colitis in breast-fed infants. J Pediatr 1982;101:906.
94. Silber GH, Klish WJ. Hematochezia in infants less than 6 months of age. Am J Dis Child 1986;140:1097.
95. Kuitunen P, Visakorpi JK, Savilahti E, Pelkonen P. Malabsorption syndrome with cow's milk intolerance: clinical findings and course in 54 cases. Arch Dis Child 1975;50:351.
96. Manuel PD, Walker-Smith JA, France NE. Patchy enteropathy in childhood. Gut 1979;20:211.
97. Van de Kamer JH, Weyers HA, Dicke KW. Coeliac disease. IV. An investigation into injurious constituents of wheat in connection with their action on patients with coeliac disease. Acta Pediatr 1953;42:223.
98. Anderson CM, Frazer AC, French JM, Gerrard JW, Sammons HG, Smellie JM. Coeliac disease: gastrointestinal studies and the effects of dietary wheat flour. Lancet 1952;1:836.
99. Paulley LW. Observations on the aetiology of idiopathic steatorrhea. Br Med J 1954;2:1328.
100. Rubin CE, Brandborg LL, Phelps PC, Taylor HC Jr. Studies of celiac disease. I. The apparent identical and specific nature of the duodenal and proximal jejunal lesion in celiac disease and idiopathic sprue. Gastroenterology 1960;38:28.
101. MacDonald WC, Brandborg LL, Flick AL, Trier JS, Rubin CE. Studies of celiac sprue. IV. The response of the whole length of the small bowl to a gluten-free diet. Gastroenterology 1964;47:573.
102. Trier JS. Celiac sprue. In: Sleisenger MH, Fordtran JS, eds. Gastrointestinal disease: pathophysiology, diagnosis, management. 5th ed. Philadelphia: WB Saunders, 1993:1078.
103. Yardley JH, Bayless TM, Norton JH, Hendrix TR. A study of the jejunal epithelium before and after a gluten-free diet. N Engl J Med 1962;267:1173.
104. Baklien K, Brandtzaeg P, Fausa O. Immunoglobulins in jejunal mucosa and serum from patients with adult coeliac disease. Scand J Gastroenterol 1977;12:149.
105. Marsh MN, Hinde J. Inflammatory component of celiac sprue mucosa. I. Mast cells, basophils and eosinophils. Gastroenterology 1985;89:92.
106. Kumar V, Lerner A, Valeski JE, Beutner EH, Chorzelski TP, Rossi T. Endomysial antibodies in the diagnosis of celiac disease and the effect of gluten on antibody titers. Immunol Invest 1989;18:533.
107. Levenson SD, Austin RK, Dietler MD, Kasarda DD, Kagnoff MF. Specificity of antigliadin antibody in celiac disease. Gastroenterol 1985;89:1.
108. Ciclitira PJ, Ellis HJ, Wood GM, Howdle PD, Losowsky MS. Secretion of gliadin antibody by coeliac jejunal mucosal biopsies cultured in vitro. Clin Exp Immunol 1986;64:119.
109. O'Farrelly C, Feighery C, O'Briain DS, et al. Humoral response to wheat protein in patients with coeliac disease and enteropathy associated T cell lymphoma. Br Med J 1986;293:908.
110. Walker-Smith JA, Guandalini S, Schmitz J, Shmerling DH, Visakorpi JK. Revised criteria for diagnosis of coeliac disease. Arch Dis Child 1990;65:909.

111. Howdle PD, Bullen AW, Losowsky MS. Cell mediated immunity to gluten within the small intestinal mucosa in coeliac disease. Gut 1982;23:115.
112. MacDonald TT, Spencer J. Evidence that activated mucosal T cells play a role in the pathogenesis of enteropathy in human small intestine. J Exp Med 1988;167:1341.
113. Marsh MN. The immunopathology of the small intestinal reaction in gluten-sensitivity. Immunol Invest 1989;18:509.
114. Hall RP. The pathogenesis of dermatitis herpetiformis: recent advances. J Am Acad Dermatol 1987;16:1129.
115. Katz SI, Hall RP III, Lawley TJ, Strober W. Dermatitis herpetiformis: the skin and the gut. Ann Intern Med 1980;93:857.
116. Solheim BG, Ek J, Thune PO, Baklien K, et al. HLA antigens in dermatitis herpetiformis and coeliac disease. Tissue Antigens 1976;7:57.
117. Heiner DC, Sears JW. Chronic respiratory disease associated with multiple circulating precipitins to cow's milk. Am J Dis Child 1960;100:500.
118. Boat TF, Polmar SH, Whitman V, Kleinerman JI, Stern RC, Doershuk CF. Hyperreactivity to cow milk in young children with pulmonary hemosiderosis and cor pulmonale secondary to nasopharyngeal obstruction. J Pediatr 1975;87:23.
119. Heiner DC, Sears JW, Kniker WT. Multiple precipitins to cow's milk in chronic respiratory disease: a syndrome including poor growth, gastrointestinal symptoms, evidence of allergy, iron deficiency anemia and pulmonary hemosiderosis. Am J Dis Child 1962;103:634.
120. Lee SK, Kniker WT, Cook CD, Heiner DC. Cow's milk-induced pulmonary disease in children. Adv Pediatr 1978;25:39.
121. Cohen SG. Landmark commentary: Ramazzini on occupational disease. Allergy Proc 1990;11:49.
122. Blands J, Diamant B, Kallos P, et al. Flour allergy in bakers. Int Arch Allergy Appl Immunol 1976;52:392.
123. Hendrick DJ, Davies RJ, Pepys J. Baker's asthma. Clin Allergy 1976;6:241.
124. Walker CL, Grammer LC, Shaughnessy MA, Patterson R. Baker's asthma: report of an unusual case. J Occup Med 1989;31:439.
125. Frankland AW, Lunn JA. Asthma caused by the grain weevil. Br J Ind Med 1965;22.157.
126. Weiner A. Occupational bronchial asthma in a baker due to Aspergillus. Ann Allergy 1960;18:1004.
127. Stressman E. Results of bronchial testing in bakers. Acta Allergol 1967;22(Suppl 8).99.
128. Cartier A, Malo J-L, Ghezzo H, McCants M, Lehrer S. IgE sensitization in snow crab processing worker. J Allergy Clin Immunol 1986;78:344.
129. Lybargar JA, Gallagher JS, Pulver DW, Litwin A, Brooks S, Bernstein IL. Occupational asthma induced by inhalation and ingestion of garlic. J Allergy Clin Immunol 1982;69:448.
130. Erben AM, Rodriguez JL, McCullough J, Ownby DR. Anaphylaxis after ingestion of beignets contaminated with Dermatophagoides farinae. J Allergy Clin Immunol 1993;92:846.
131. Matsumoto T, Hisano T, Hamaguchi M, Miike T. Systematic anaphylaxis after eating storage-mite-contaminated food. Arch Allergy Immunol 1996;109:197.
132. Sheffer AL, Tong AK, Murphy GF, Lewis RA, McFadden ER Jr, Austen KF. Exercise-induced anaphylaxis: a serious form of physical allergy associated with mast cell degranulation. J Allergy Clin Immunol 1985;75:479.
133. Kidd JM 3d, Cohen SH, Sosman AJ, Fink JN. Food-dependent exercise-induced anaphylaxis. J Allergy Clin Immunol 1983;71:407.
134. Novey HS, Fairshter RD, Salness K, Simon RA, Curd JG. Postprandial exercise-induced anaphylaxis. J Allergy Clin Immunol 1983;71:498.
135. Maulitz RM, Pratt DS, Schocket AL. Exercise-induced anaphylactic reaction to shellfish. J Allergy Clin Immunol 1979,63:433.
136. Young E, Patel S, Stoneham M, Rona R, Wilkinson JD. The prevalence of reaction to food additives in a survey population. J R Coll Physicians London 1987;21:241.
137. Taylor SL, Bush RK, Selner JC, et al. Sensitivity to sulfited foods among sulfite-sensitive subjects with asthma. J Allergy Clin Immunol 1988;81·1159.
138. Sonin L, Patterson R. Metabisulfite challenge in patients with idiopathic anaphylaxis. J Allergy Clin Immunol 1985;75;67.
139. Schiffman SS, Buckley CE III, Sampson HA, et al. Aspartame and susceptibility to headache. N Engl J Med 1987;317:1181.
140. Geha R, Buckley CE, Greenberger P, et al. Aspartame is no more likely than placebo to cause urticaria/angioedema: results of a multicenter, randomized, double-blind, placebo-controlled, crossover study. J Allergy Clin Immunol 1995;95:639.
141. Panush RS, Stroud RM, Webster EM. Food-induced (allergic) arthritis. Inflammatory arthritis exacerbated by milk. Arthritis Rheum 1986;29:220.
142. Egger J, Carter CM, Soothill JF, Wilson J. Oligoantigenic diet treatment of children with epilepsy and migraine. J Pediatr 1989;114:51.
143. Sampson HA. Role of immediate food hypersensitivity in the pathogenesis of atopic dermatitis. J Allergy Clin Immunol 1983;71:473.
144. Taudorf E, Malling H-J, Laursen LC, Lanner A, Weeke B. Reproducibility of histamine skin prick test: inter- and intravariation using histamine dihydrochloride 1, 5, and 10 mg/ml. Allergy 1985;40:344.

145. Bock SA, Lee W-Y, Remigio L, Holst A, May CD. Appraisal of skin tests with food extracts for diagnosis of food hypersensitivity. Clin Allergy 1978;8:559.
146. Bock SA, Buckley J, Holst A, May CD. Proper use of skin tests with food extracts in diagnosis of hypersensitivity to food in children. Clin Allergy 1977;7:375.
147. Sampson HA, Albergo R. Comparison of results of skin tests, RAST, and double-blind placebo-controlled food challenges in children with atopic dermatitis. J Allergy Clin Immunol 1984;74:26.
148. May CD. Objective clinical and laboratory studies of immediate hypersensitivity reactions to foods in asthmatic children. J Allergy Clin Immunol 1976;58:500.
149. Roesler TA, Barry PC, Bock SA. Factitious food allergy and failure to thrive. Arch Pediatr Adolesc Med 1994;148:1150.
150. Ditto AM, Grammer LC. Immunologic evaluation of environmental lung disease. Clin Pulm Med 1995:2;276.
151. Bahna SL. Diagnostic tests for food allergy. Clin Rev Allergy 1988;6:259.
152. Grieco MH. Controversial practices in allergy. JAMA 1982:247:3106.
153. Sogn DD. Medications and their use in the treatment of adverse reactions to foods. J Allergy Clin Immunol 1986;78:238.
154. Oppenheimer JJ, Nelson HS, Bock SA, Christensen F, Leung DY. Treatment of peanut allergy with rush immunotherapy. J Allergy Clin Immunol 1992;90:256.
155. Grulee EG, Sanford HN. The influence of breast and artificial feeding on infantile eczema. J Pediatr 1936;9:223.
156. Zeiger RS, Heller S, Mellon MH, et al. Effect of combined maternal and infant food-allergen avoidance on development of atopy in early infancy: a randomized study. J Allergy Clin Immunol 1989;84:72.
157. Zeiger RS, Heller S, Sampson HA. Genetic and environmental factors affecting the development of atopy from birth through age 4 in a prospective randomized controlled study of dietary avoidance. J Allergy Clin Immunol 1992;89:192. Abstract.
158. Zeiger RS, Heller S. The development and prediction of atopy in high-risk children: follow-up at age seven years in a prospective randomized study of combined maternal and infant food allergen avoidance. J Allergy Clin Immunol 1995;95:1179.

Allergic Diseases, 5th Edition,
edited by Roy Patterson, Leslie Carroll Grammer, and
Paul A. Greenberger. Lippincott–Raven Publishers, Philadelphia, © 1997.

15

Atopic Dermatitis

Leslie C. Grammer

*L.C. Grammer: Division of Allergy-Immunology, Northwestern University,
Chicago, IL 60611.*

Pearls for Practitioners
Roy Patterson

- Spontaneous remission often occurs in patients with atopic dermatitis between the ages of 2 and 3 years.
- Persistence of atopic dermatitis into adulthood is often a lifelong, unpleasant condition.
- Food allergy in young children may exacerbate atopic dermatitis in some cases. This occurs rarely in adults, and dietary management of food allergy is seldom helpful.
- Inhalant allergens may contribute to the cutaneous problem by contact of allergens with open skin lesions.
- Exacerbation of atopic dermatitis is often associated with infection, and both infection and inflammation must be treated.
- Atopic dermatitis should be treated without use of chronic systemic corticosteroids.
- Rarely, atopic dermatitis is so severe in terms of discomfort, disfigurement, and risk of infection that chronic alternate day prednisone is warranted at the lowest possible maintenance dose.
- If an acute exacerbation of atopic dermatitis does not respond to oral steroids, then the diagnosis is wrong, the dose is too low, or the patient is not taking the prednisone.

Atopic dermatitis, also called *atopic eczema* or *allergic eczema,* is a chronic or recurrent, pruritic, eczematous eruption that generally begins in the first few years of life and usually resolves before the fourth decade. In 1892, Besnier[1] described the association of this disease with asthma, allergic rhinitis, and familial predisposition. The term *atopy* was introduced by Coca and Cooke in 1923[2] to describe the clinical manifestations of the recognized hypersensitivity of asthma and allergic rhinitis. The term *atopic dermatitis* was probably first used by Wise and Sulzberger in 1933[3] and is currently the most common appellation.

EPIDEMIOLOGY

The incidence of atopic dermatitis in the United States is estimated to be between 0.7% and 2.4%.[4] The incidence is higher in children and may approach 3% to 5%.[5] Atopic dermatitis typically begins in childhood; it develops in 60% of patients in the first year of life and in 30% between the ages of 1 and 5 years.[6] About half of patients with atopic dermatitis develop or have asthma or allergic rhinitis.[6] Most patients have a personal or family history of atopy. Although the mode of genetic inheritance remains unclear, twin studies have provided strong support for the heritability of atopic dermatitis. There is 86% concordance in monozygotic pairs, and no greater concordance in dizygotic twin pairs than in controls.[7] There have been no reports of statistically significant associations between HLA antigens and atopic dermatitis.[8,9] The course of atopic dermatitis is unpredictable, but about half of patients no longer have manifestations by the age of 15 years.[10] Factors that appear to be associated with more persistent disease include late onset of disease, increased immunoglobulin E (IgE) level, concurrent asthma or allergic rhinitis, and family history of atopic dermatitis.[11]

PATHOGENESIS

The primary defect in atopic dermatitis remains unknown. Many of the observations that have been made about patients with atopic dermatitis may be epiphenomena rather than causal or pathogenic defects. Alterations are seen in nerve fibers and neurokinins, such as calcitonin gene–related peptide and substance P.[12] The skin of patients with atopic dermatitis is dry, with increased transepidermal water loss.[13] When the skin of patients with atopic dermatitis is stroked, a white line appears rather than the normal red triple response of Lewis. This is called *white dermatographism* and is almost certainly secondary to cutaneous inflammation and not a primary pharmacologic abnormality.[5]

More than half of patients with atopic dermatitis have elevated IgE levels.[14] The discovery that Langerhans cells possess both high-affinity and low-affinity IgE receptors (FcεRI and FcεRII) suggests that allergen presentation by epidermal Langerhans cells is IgE mediated.[15] In atopic dermatitis lesions, activated CD4+ cells of the TH$_2$ phenotype predominate.[16] These TH$_2$ cells likely contribute to the known B-cell IgE overproduction. About three quarters of patients with atopic dermatitis described by Rajka[17] had positive immediate cutaneous reactions to common aeroallergens or foods. Atopic dermatitis obviously bears little resemblance to an immediate-type, IgE-mediated reaction. However, as Sampson[18] indicates, perhaps delayed or late-phase IgE-mediated reactions are important in some patients with atopic dermatitis. However, there are important histologic differences between atopic dermatitis and IgE-mediated cutaneous late-phase reactions. Some controversy has related to the relative prevalence of food allergy as a cause of, or major contributing factor in, patients with atopic dermatitis. In 1965, Holt[19] reported that food allergy was not a cause of atopic dermatitis in most patients. In 1977, Bock and colleagues[20] reported that four of seven children with atopic dermatitis had exacerbations with food challenge. Sampson and McCaskill[21] reported that more than half of children they evaluated for atopic dermatitis had positive food challenges. In general, only one to four foods resulted in positive challenges; six foods accounted for 90% of positive food challenges: soy, milk, wheat, egg, peanut, and fish. Positive skin test results or in vitro tests were not always highly predictive of positive food challenges,[18] and thus food challenges may be indicated even with negative cutaneous tests.

The possible role of inhalant allergens, such as mite or animal dander, has been suggested.[22] It is possible that exacerbation of pruritus occurs in patients with atopic dermatitis whose abraded skin is exposed to common aeroallergens, such as animal dander or house dust mite. About half of patients with atopic dermatitis have IgE against staphylococcal proteins, such as the enterotoxin, which is also a superantigen.[23] More than 90% of patients with atopic dermatitis are colonized with *Staphylococcus aureus*.[24] Thus, immunologic mechanisms involving IgE, superantigens, or both could be operative in atopic dermatitis.

Patients with atopic dermatitis clearly have cutaneous abnormalities in cell-mediated immunity. In peripheral blood, they are known to have reduced numbers of CD3+ and CD8+

lymphocytes and natural killer cells.[25] Clinically, this may present as diffuse, cutaneous infection with herpes simplex; increased likelihood of contracting other viral-type cutaneous infections, such as warts; and decreased likelihood of contact dermatitis and delayed-type cutaneous sensitivity to antigens such as *Candida* sp and streptococci. Interestingly, patients with atopic dermatitis do not appear to be predisposed to systemic fungal infection or other stigmata of depressed systemic cellular immunity.

HISTOPATHOLOGY AND IMMUNOLOGIC TESTS

No single confirmatory immunologic test nor battery of tests are useful in the diagnosis of atopic dermatitis.[11] Similarly, the histopathology is not pathognomonic. With light microscopy, acute lesions feature epidermal spongiosis and dermal perivascular inflammatory cell infiltration, while chronic lesions feature thickened epidermis and elongated fibrotic rete ridges.[11,18,19] Using immunohistologic techniques, it has been determined that most of the lymphocytes present are activated TH_2.[25] Major basic protein, eosinophil cationic protein, and eosinophil-derived neurotoxin, with few intact eosinophils, are found.[19]

Most patients with atopic dermatitis have elevated levels of serum IgE (more than 200 IU/mL).[14] Many have an increase in peripheral blood eosinophils; however, increased tissue eosinophils are not seen in patients with atopic dermatitis.[19] Patients with atopic dermatitis have decreased delayed hypersensitivity to dinitrochlorobenzene and many bacterial and fungal antigens.[11] Increased levels of histamine-releasing factor have also been reported in patients with atopic dermatitis.[18] A synopsis of immunologic findings in atopic dermatitis is presented in Table 15-1. Generally, neither biopsy nor immunologic tests are necessary for the diagnosis, evaluation, or management of patients with atopic dermatitis.

CLINICAL MANIFESTATIONS AND DIAGNOSIS

No specific or pathognomonic lesion characterizes atopic dermatitis; papules, scaling, minute epidermal vesicles, erythematous patches, crusting, and lichenification may all occur. Intense pruritus is a characteristic feature and that generally leads to a scratch-itch cycle. It is quoted that atopic dermatitis is the itchiness that erupts, not the eruption that itches; that is the itch-scratch cycle. The patient's reaction to the pruritus, in terms of how much scratching and abrasion occur, is a significant determinant of the severity of disease. The clinical manifestations, especially distribution, of atopic dermatitis vary with the age of the patient.

TABLE 15-1. *Immunologic features of patients with atopic dermatitis*

Elevated serum IgE
Decreased blood lymphocytes bearing CD_3 and CD_8 cells
Activated CD4+ lymphocytes of TH_2 phenotype in skin lesions
Major basic protein, eosinophil cationic protein, and eosinophil-derived neurotoxin in skin lesions
Decreased cutaneous delayed hypersensitivity
Decreased blood natural killer cells
Increased blood but not tissue eosinophilia
Increased histamine-releasing factors

TABLE 15-2. *Diagnostic characteristics of atopic dermatitis*

Major criteria (must have four):

   Pruritus

   Age-appropriate distribution and morphology

      Infants, children: extensor and facial involvement

      Adolescents, adults: flexural involvement with lichenification

   Chronic or recurrent dermatitis

   Early age onset

   Personal or family history of atopy

Hanifin JM, Rajka G. Diagnostic features of atopic dermatitis. Acta Derm Venereol 1980;92(Suppl):44.

The criteria that are often cited as the most useful for diagnosing atopic dermatitis are those proposed by Hanifin and Rajka[26] (Table 15-2). In these criteria, the minimum duration of cutaneous lesions is 6 weeks, and patients must have four of five major features. In the absence of four major criteria, a variety of minor, less specific features may be involved.

The differential diagnosis of atopic dermatitis is potentially broad. In infants, a number of rare immunodeficiency diseases are associated with cutaneous eruptions. These eruptions generally do not resemble atopic dermatitis but are often listed in the differential diagnosis because they may present diagnostic difficulties.[5,27] Examples of such diseases are ataxia-telangiectasia, Wiskott-Aldrich syndrome, histiocytosis X, Swiss-type agammaglobulinemia, hyperimmunoglobulin E syndrome, and chronic granulomatous disease.[28] Besides atopic dermatitis, the other common chronic dermatitis in infants is seborrheic dermatitis. Important distinguishing features include lack of pruritus and prominent involvement of diaper area and scalp.

In any age group, contact dermatitis may be a differential problem. Generally, the distribution of the lesions of contact dermatitis would be expected to be different than that of atopic dermatitis. Other cutaneous diseases, including psoriasis, scabies, and dermatitis herpetiformis, may also occasionally mimic atopic dermatitis.[5,11] Certain nutritional deficiencies, including fatty acid and zinc deficiencies, may present with lesions similar to those of atopic dermatitis.[11]

COMPLICATIONS

The most common complication of atopic dermatitis is that of secondary infection. The most usual secondary infections are bacterial, with staphylococci and streptococci heading the list and being causally related to some clinical flares of disease. Bacteremia may develop and requires emergent hospitalization for parenteral antibiotics.

Viral infections are also more common, probably due to depressed cellular immunity. Some viruses, such as warts and molluscum contagiosum, tend to be similar in intensity and treatment to those seen normally. Rare patients, however, develop severe disseminated infections, such as herpes simplex virus, which can result in permanent neurologic sequelae or even death.

Although contact dermatitis is relatively rare in patients with atopic dermatitis, probably owing to depressed cutaneous cellular immunity, the abraded epidermis can be a problem. Several medications, including topical antibiotics and topical anesthetics, can be especially troublesome.[5] They should be avoided if possible. When clinical flares occur in patients taking topical medications, consideration should be given to the possibility that the medication is causing the contact dermatitis.

TABLE 15-3. *Factors reported to exacerbate atopic dermatitis*

Infection

Irritants (scratchy clothing, acids, alkali, solvents)

Sweating or extreme dryness

Scratching or vigorous scrubbing

Occlusive clothing

Hot water

Frequent handwashing

Foods, in a minority of patients

TREATMENT

As is the case with other allergic diseases, there are two general phases of management of atopic dermatitis: acute management of flares in disease and chronic management to maintain control of the disease.

The following approaches to chronic management are useful in most patients.[11,17,28] First, it is imperative that the patient or parent recognize that atopic dermatitis is a chronic condition requiring chronic interventions that are specifically aimed at breaking the itch–scratch cycle. Patients should avoid such irritants as harsh soaps, scratchy clothing like wool, and extremes of temperatures and humidity that are likely to induce significant sweating or alternatively dryness (Table 15-3). Fingernails should be trimmed short to minimize the ability to scratch; showers or baths with tepid water and mild soaps such as Dove or Basis should be followed by a bland emollient such as Eucerin or Aquaphor. A topical corticosteroid in an ointment or cream base should be applied to affected areas. The lowest potency corticosteroid and the lowest dose that will control the dermatitis should be used. If possible, nonfluorinated preparations, such as hydrocortisone cream, should be used. If that is not sufficient, fluorinated steroids should be applied only to problem areas, as infrequently as possible, and never on the face, owing to problems with cutaneous atrophy and cosmetic disfigurement. Rarely, in severe cases, a regimen of low-dose alternate-day oral corticosteroids may be useful. For additional control of pruritus, antihistamines, such as diphenhydramine or hydroxyzine, are often useful, especially at night. If foods such as soy or milk have been identified as important aggravating factors, they should be avoided. There is no evidence for efficacy of allergen immunotherapy in the treatment of atopic dermatitis (Table 15-4).

TABLE 15-4. *Chronic management of atopic dermatitis*

Short fingernails

Tepid water

Mild soap

Bland emollient

Antihistamines for pruritus control

Lowest-potency topical corticosteroid in lowest possible dose

On face, nonfluorinated corticosteroids

Avoid exacerbating factors

Despite careful chronic management, flares of atopic dermatitis, including pruritus, erythema, and exudative lesions, may occur. The following general approaches usually result in prompt, dramatic relief.[5,11,28] Wet dressing of aluminum acetate solution, such as Domeboro powder, and water should be applied to exudative lesions several times a day. Between dressings, a fluorinated steroid should be applied to affected areas but not on the face. In severe cases, systemic corticosteroids may be required. Systemic antibiotics should be administered for any significant secondary bacterial infection.

Other therapies useful in some situations include tar application, Retin-A, psoralens and ultraviolet light (PUVA), the Goederman treatment (tar and ultraviolet light), antimetabolites such as azathioprine, thymopoietin, phototherapy, γ-interferon, and cyclosporine.[5,11,29]

REFERENCES

1. Besnier E. Premiere note et observations preliminairies pour servir d'introduction a' l'etude diathesique. Ann Dermatol Syphiligr (Paris) 1892;4:634.
2. Coca RF, Cooke RA. On the classification of the phenomena of hypersensitiveness. J Immunol 1922;8:163.
3. Wise F, Sulzberger MB. Editorial remarks. In: Yearbook of Dermatology and Syphilology. Chicago: Year Book Medical Publishers, 1933:59.
4. Johnson ML. Prevalence of dermatologic disease among persons 1–74 years of age: United States. Advance data from vital and health statistics of the National Center for Health Statistics. 1977:4.
5. Oakes RC, Cox AD, Burgdorf WHC. Atopic dermatitis: a review of diagnosis, pathogenesis, and management. Clin Pediatr 1983;22:467.
6. Rajka G. Atopic dermatitis. In: Rook A, ed. Major problems in dermatology. London: WB Saunders, 1975:2.
7. Schultz-Larsen F. Atopic dermatitis: a genetic-epidemiologic study in a population-based twin sample. J Am Acad Dermatol 1993;28:719.
8. Blumenthal MN, Mendell N, Unis E. Immunogenetics of atopic diseases. J Allergy Clin Immunol 1980;65:403.
9. Saeki H, Kuwata S, Nakagawa H, et al. HLA and atopic dermatitis with high serum IgE levels. J Allergy Clin Immunol 1994;94:575.
10. Musgrove K, Morgan JK. Infantile eczema: a long-term follow-up study. Br J Dermatol 1976;95:365.
11. Leung DYM, Rhodes AR, Geha RS. Atopic dermatitis. In: Fitzpatrick TB, Eisen A, Wolff K, Freedberg IM, Austen KF, eds. Dermatology in general medicine. 3rd ed. New York: McGraw Hill, 1987:1385.
12. Tobin D, Nabarra G, Baart de la Faille H, Jan Vloten W, van der Putte SC, Schuurman HJ. Increased number of immuno-reactive nerve fibers in atopic dermatitis. J Allergy Clin Immunol 1992;90:613.
13. Blaylock WK. Atopic dermatitis: diagnosis and pathobiology. J Allergy Clin Immunol 1976;57:62.
14. Wittig HJ, Belloit J, DeFillippi I, Royal G. Age-related serum immunoglobulin E levels in healthy subjects and in patients with allergic disease. J Allergy Clin Immunol 1980;66:305.
15. Mudde GC, Van Reijsen FC, Boland GJ. Allergen presentation by epidermal Langerhans' cells from patients with atopic dermatitis is mediated by IgE. Immunology 1990;69:335.
16. Furue M. Atopic dermatitisÄimmunologic abnormality and its background. J Derm Sci 1994;7:159.
17. Rajka G. Prurigo Besnier (atopic dermatitis) with special reference to the role of allergic factors. II. The evaluation of the results of skin reactions. Acta Derm Venereol (Stockholm) 1961;41:1.
18. Sampson HA. Late-phase response to food in atopic dermatitis. Hosp Pract 1987;22:111.
19. Holt LE. Conference on infantile eczema. J Pediatr 1965;66:153.
20. Bock SA, Buckley J, Holst A, May CD. Proper use of skin tests with food extracts in diagnosis of hypersensitivity to food in children. Clin Allergy 1977;7:375.
21. Sampson HA, McCaskill CC. Food hypersensitivity and atopic dermatitis: evaluation of 113 patients. J Pediatr 1985;107:669.
22. Mitchell EB, Chapman MD, Pope FM, Crow J, Jouhal SS, Platts-Mills TAE. Basophils in allergen-induced patch skin test sites in atopic dermatitis. Lancet 1982;1:127.
23. Leung DYM, Harbeck R, Bina P, et al. Presence of IgE antibodies to staphylococcal exotoxins on the skin of patients with atopic dermatitis: evidence for a new group of allergens. J Clin Invest 1993;92:1374.
24. Aly R, Maibach HI, Shinefield HR. Microbial flora of atopic dermatitis. Arch Dermatol 1977;133:780.
25. Leung DYM. Immunopathology of atopic dermatitis. Springer Semin Immunopathol 1992;13:427.
26. Hanifin JM, Rajka G. Diagnostic features of atopic dermatitis. Acta Derm Venereol 1980;92(Suppl):44.
27. Rostenberg A Jr, Solomon LM. Infantile eczema and systemic disease. Arch Dermatol 1968;98:41.
28. Sparks DB. Atopic dermatitis. In: Patterson R, ed. Allergic diseases: diagnosis and management. 3rd ed. Philadelphia: JB Lippincott, 1985:491.
29. Cooper KD. Atopic dermatitis: recent trends in pathogenesis and therapy. J Invest Dermatol 1994;102:128.

Allergic Diseases, 5th Edition,
edited by Roy Patterson, Leslie Carroll Grammer, and
Paul A. Greenberger. Lippincott–Raven Publishers, Philadelphia, © 1997.

16

Stevens-Johnson Syndrome and Erythema Multiforme

Roy Patterson and Sarah Cheriyan

*R. Patterson: Division of Allergy-Immunology,
Northwestern University Medical School, Chicago, IL 60611.
S. Cheriyan: Allergy & Asthma Clinic, Lufkin, TX 75901.*

Pearls for Practitioners
Roy Patterson

- For Stevens-Johnson syndrome due to a drug reaction: Stop the drug! Start corticosteroids at a minimum of 60 mg/d for mild cases or four to six times that dose intravenously for severe cases! Hospitalize the patient.
- For Stevens-Johnson syndrome with ocular involvement, get an ophthalmology consult for care of the eyes.

Stevens-Johnson syndrome (SJS) and erythema multiforme (EM) are often caused by an allergic drug reaction and are best managed as such. In some cases, the cause is viral, but management is the same, with the addition of an antiviral agent. To date, 60 cases of SJS have been managed by the Northwestern University Allergy Service, with no fatalities and with sufficient documentation to emphasize that the programs described in this chapter are the appropriate standards of care.

Our interest in SJS and EM began about two decades ago when we observed the severity of SJS in some cases, the obvious correlation with drug allergy in many cases, and the rapid improvement that occurred when adequate doses of corticosteroids were used for therapy early and when the offending drug was stopped immediately. Simultaneously, we noted the controversy about the use of corticosteroids in the treatment of SJS. This was apparent in the medical literature and at the bedside when dermatologic consultants advised against the use of corticosteroids, even when the patient with SJS had already demonstrated improvement with this therapy.

DEFINITIONS

The terminology in the medical literature relative to EM and SJS is confusing, so we define *erythema multiforme* as an erythematous, maculopapular, cutaneous eruption of various forms.[1] Classically, there is a target lesion with a predilection for the extremities. EM may occur as a mild, self-limiting, cutaneous manifestation, or it may progress to more serious vesicular and bullous lesions. Mucosal lesions involve selected or all mucosal surfaces. Involvement of the ocular mucous membrane can be particularly hazardous. Visceral organ involvement may include liver, kidney, and lung.

When EM has progressed to the stage of bullous formation and mucosal and visceral involvement (although not necessarily all three organ systems), the term *Stevens-Johnson syndrome* is applied. SJS is often accompanied by fever and severe malaise. SJS is a severe and often fatal variant of EM. It is characterized by high fever, extensive purpura, bullae, ulcers of the mucous membrane and, after 2 or 3 days, ulcers of the skin. Eye involvement can result in blindness.[2]

Toxic epidermal necrolysis (Lyell's syndrome) is the progression of the cutaneous lesions of SJS to the degree that sloughing of the skin occurs equivalent to a third-degree burn.

IMMUNOPATHOGENESIS

Stevens-Johnson syndrome is an immunologically mediated disease secondary in most cases to an immunologic hypersensitivity reaction to a drug or viral macromolecule. Some evidence for this concept is presented in Table 16-1.[3-6] That the immune system recognizes the drug–cell complex as foreign and rejects these drug–cell complexes is entirely logical. Thus, SJS may be considered a host-versus-host reaction involving skin, mucous membrane, and viscera. Corticosteroids act to suppress the immunologically mediated inflammation until the drug or its metabolite is eliminated from the body of the host. This explains why complete recovery can be expected in all patients with SJS in whom the diagnosis is made early, the offending drug stopped, and corticosteroids used promptly and in sufficient doses.

CLINICAL FEATURES

Herpes simplex virus may result in SJS or EM, and protocols for control of the herpes simplex with acyclovir and prevention of progression to SJS to corticosteroids have been published.[7]

Oral herpes simplex lesions may be followed by EM. These can be controlled by acyclovir and temporary early prednisone therapy, 30 to 50 mg/day for 3 to 5 days.

SJS may be difficult to diagnose, and infection is a serious consideration in some cases. An example of SJS initially thought to be sepsis is reviewed by Cheriyan and colleagues.[8]

TABLE 16-1. *Pathogenesis of Stevens-Johnson syndrome and erythema multiforme: evidence for an immunologic mechanism*

SJS follows the administration of nontoxic drugs associated with immunologic drug reactions, such as sulfa, dilantin, and penicillin or its derivatives.

SJS may follow herpes simplex lesions.

Associations between HLA-B15 and EM and between HLA-B12 and SJS have been noted.[3]

Supernatants from sera in patients with EM demonstrate an increase in macrophage-aggregating activity.[4]

The presence of lymphocytes, basophils, and interstitial fibrin suggests a role for cell-mediated immunity in the pathogenesis.[5]

Granular IgM and C3 can be found in the upper dermal vessels, and granular C3 can be found along the dermoepidermal junction.[3,6]

Graft-versus-host disease, known to have an immunologic pathogenesis, has much in common with SJS both clinically and immunologically.

TABLE 16-2. *Diagnosis of Stevens-Johnson syndrome*

The prevalence of SJS is so limited that most physicians see few cases, therefore:

Consider SJS when there is an erythematous multiform dermatitis.

Look for vesicles and watch for bullous formation.

There is no diagnostic test.

Look immediately for involvement of any mucosal surface.

Evaluate drug therapies, current or recent, especially sulfa, dilantin, and penicillins. Stop the drug.

Evaluate liver, renal, and pulmonary status.

Start corticosteroids. For major, severe cases, give 60 mg of methylprednisolone every 6 hours. Observe effect:

    Progression of lesions ceases within 24 hours, or within 48 hours at the latest.

    Improvement is obvious 3 to 4 days after initiation of corticosteroids provided the dose is sufficient.

    An exacerbation occurs if corticosteroids are reduced too rapidly. This has diagnostic value. Resume high-dose corticosteroids.

    After complete resolution of cutaneous, mucosal, and visceral lesions, begin cautious reduction of daily corticosteroids and then convert to alternate-day prednisone with further *cautious* reduction and discontinuation.

DIAGNOSIS AND MANAGEMENT

The diagnosis of SJS is being made earlier, particularly by infectious disease physicians and emergency service physicians. The offending drug is stopped, and corticosteroids are initiated immediately. Emergency admission to the hospital is often necessary. Some patients with SJS can be treated as outpatients if the diagnosis is made early, SJS is of moderate severity, and corticosteroids are started immediately. A summary of diagnostic features is shown in Table 16-2.

Erythema multiforme is mild, may be self-limiting, and requires only antihistamine therapy. Progressive SJS requires the use of corticosteroids. Toxic epidermal necrolysis is a seri-

TABLE 16-3. *Management Protocols for Stevens-Johnson syndrome*

Rapid assessment of severity

    Extent and severity of dermatitis. Are vesicles and bullae present?

    Extent and severity of mucosal lesions: Ophthalmology consult for eyes. Are ulcers present on any mucosal surface?

    Is there liver, renal, or pulmonary involvement?

    Duration of SJS: days or weeks?

Stop most likely offending drug.

Start corticosteroids immediately.

    Mild case: give 60 to 80 mg prednisone immediately. If treated as outpatient, have daily contact with patient.

    Moderate or severe case: give loading dose of 60 to 80 mg methylprednisolone (Solu-Medrol) intravenously, admit to hospital, continue steroid dose every 6 hours.

    Continue treatment until major improvement has occurred.

    Do not reduce corticosteroids too rapidly.

If lesions are related to herpes simplex virus, treat as above, with addition of acyclovir.

ous disease in which the antiinflammatory action of corticosteroids cannot reverse the cutaneous lesions because the skin is already lost. Management suggestions for SJS are given in Table 16-3.

CONTROVERSY ABOUT THE USE OF CORTICOSTEROIDS

When we prepared our initial report on the successful use of corticosteroids for SJS, we also reviewed our experience with consulting physicians[1] and the statements about the use of corticosteroids in SJS in three textbooks of medicine, four textbooks of pediatrics, and three textbooks of dermatology.[1] Table 16-4 provides an updated review of statements regarding the management of SJS with corticosteroids.[9–16]

In our first study on the use of corticosteroids in 13 patients with SJS, all patients completely recovered from the SJS; one patient had persisting renal disease.[1] In our second series of 15 patients, corticosteroid use clearly benefited every patient.[17]

TABLE 16-4. *Review of statements regarding use of corticosteroids in erythema multiforme and Stevens-Johnson syndrome in representative textbooks of medicine, pediatrics, and dermatology*

Specialty	Reference	Relevant comments
Cecil Textbook of Medicine[9]	Medicine	"The value of systemic corticosteroids in SJS is controversial." (p 2310) "Systemic steroids are used in life threatening diseases (such as erythema multiforme) known to be responsive to corticosteroids in initial high doses—80 to 100 mg daily." (p 2295)
Current Medical: Diagnosis and Treatment[10]	Medicine	"Although there are no good data to support the use of corticosteroids in EM major, they are still often prescribed. If corticosteroids are to be tried in more severe cases, they should be used early, before blistering occurs, and in moderate doses (prednisone, 60–80 mg)." (p 116)
Nelson Textbook of Pediatrics[11]	Pediatrics	"Systemic steroids are not necessary." (p 1641)
Rudolph's Pediatrics[12]	Pediatrics	"Although the use of systemic corticosteroids in treatment of EM is controversial, no studies have clearly demonstrated their efficacy. It is likely that they are efficacious only in the early evolving stages of disease." (p 903)
Primary Pediatric Care[13]	Pediatrics	"Use of systemic steroids is more controversial. Clearly, a prospective study is needed to determine its benefit." (p 1236)
Pediatric Primary Care: A Problem Oriented Approach[14]	Pediatrics	"Severe involvement may require corticosteroids to treat systemic effects. Given early a short course of prednisone can even obliterate the development of EM." (p 414)
Principles and Practice of Pediatrics[15]	Pediatrics	"Use of systemic steroids remains controversial." (p 938)
Andrew's Diseases of the Skin[16]	Dermatology	"Despite Rasmussen's study indicating little benefit from corticosteroid therapy, we believe that treatment of choice is early vigorous steroid therapy with 1.5 to 2 mg of prednisone per kg body weight per day." (p 137)

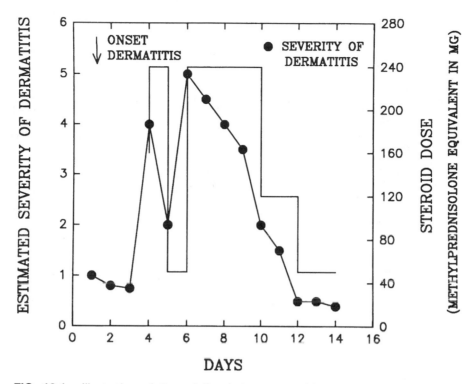

FIG. 16-1. Illustration of the relation between steroid dose and dermatitis in a patient with Stevens-Johnson syndrome. (Patterson R, Miller M, Kaplan M, et al. Effectiveness of early therapy with corticosteroids in Stevens-Johnson syndrome: experience with 41 cases and a hypothesis regarding pathogenesis. Ann Allergy 1994;73:27.)

We continued our prospective study and continued to publish our series because the controversy about the use of corticosteroids continued, although we believed efficacy had clearly been demonstrated in the initial 28 patients. The next publication[18] brought the total cases to 41 patients treated successfully. Further, we clearly documented the successful effect of steroids in patients with SJS in whom there was an exacerbation of SJS when the steroid dose was reduced too rapidly, with control when the steroid dose was again increased. An example of such a case is shown in Figure 16-1.[18]

Finally, we have extended our published series to a total of 54 cases and have demonstrated successful management of SJS in every case.19 Six successful unpublished cases bring the total to over 60 cases.

Some dermatologists still oppose the use of corticosteroids. The citations they use in support of their opposition are the studies of Rasmussen[20] and Nethercott and Choi.[21] Both these studies are retrospective record analyses, and it is not apparent that the authors saw any of the patients in either series, in contrast to our series, in which every patient was seen by one or more of the authors. We have been asked why we did not do a controlled study of corticosteroid use in some patients and no corticosteroids in others. The answer is obvious: the effectiveness of corticosteroids in SJS is so well documented in all of our series that we would consider such a study unethical. Some patients not treated with corticosteroids would progress to toxic epidermal necrosis, scarring of skin, or a fatal outcome.

REFERENCES

1. Patterson R, Dykewicz M, Gonzazles A, et al. Erythema multiforme and Stevens-Johnson syndrome descriptive and therapeutic controversy. Chest 1990;98:331.
2. Sauer GC. Erythema multiforme, In: Sauer GC, ed. Manual of skin diseases. 4th ed. Philadelphia: JB Lippincott, 1980:98.
3. Soter NA, Wuepper KD. Erythema multiforme and Stevens-Johnson syndrome. In: Samter M, Talmage DW, Frank MM, Austen KF, Claman HN, eds. Immunological diseases. 4th ed. Boston: Little, Brown, 1988:1257.
4. Krueger GG, Weston WL, Thorne EG, Mandel MJ, Jacobs RJ. A phenomenon of macrophage aggregation activity in sera of patients with exfoliative erythroderma, erythema multiforme, and erythema nodosum. J Invest Dermatol 1973;60:282.
5. Tonnesen MG, Harrist TJ, Wintroub BU, Mihm MC, Soter NA. Erythema multiforme: microvascular damage and infiltration of lymphocytes and basophils. J Invest Dermatol 1983;80:282.
6. Huff JC, Weston WL, Tonnesen MG. Erythema multiforme: a clinical review of characteristics, diagnostic criteria and causes. J Am Acad Dermatol 1983;8:763.
7. Detjen PF, Patterson RP, Noskin GA, Phair JP, Loyd SO. Herpes simplex virus associated with recurrent Stevens-Johnson syndrome: a management strategy. Arch Intern Med 1992;152:1513.
8. Cheriyan S, Rosa RM, Patterson R. Stevens-Johnson syndrome presenting as intravenous line sepsis. Allergy Proc 1995;16:85.
9. Parker F. Skin diseases. In: Wyngaarden JB, Smith LH, Bennett JC, eds. Cecil textbook of medicine. 19th ed. Philadelphia: WB Saunders, 1992;2280.
10. Goldstein SM, Odom RB. Erythema multiforme. In: Tierney LM Jr, McPhee SJ, Papadakis MA, eds. Current medical diagnosis and treatment. 34th ed. Norwalk, CT: Appleton & Lange, 1995:115.
11. Esterly NB. Vesiculobullous disorders. In: Behrman RE, Kliegman RM, Nelson WE, Vaughan III VC, eds. Nelson textbook of pediatrics. 14th ed. Philadelphia: WB Saunders, 1992:1638.
12. Frieden IJ. Hypersensitivity reactions. In: Rudolph AM, Hoffman JIE, Rudolph CD, eds. Rudolph's pediatrics. 19th ed. Norwalk, CT: Appleton & Lange, 1991:901.
13. Lookingbill DP. Erythema multiforme. In: Hoekelman RA, Friedman SB, Nelson NM, Seidel HM, eds. Primary pediatric care. 2nd ed. St Louis: Mosby Year Book Medical Publishers, 1992:1235.
14. Allen HB, Honig PJ. Erythema multiforme. In: Schwartz MW, Charney EB, Curry TA, Ludwig S, eds. Pediatric primary care: a problem-oriented approach. 2nd ed. Chicago: Mosby Year Book Medical Publishers, 1990;414.
15. Tunnessen Jr WW. Erythema multiforme. In: Oski FA, DeAngelis CD, McMillan JA, Feigin RD, Warshaw JB, eds. Principles and practice of pediatrics. 2nd ed. Philadelphia: JB Lippincott, 1994:938.
16. Arnold Jr HL, Odom RB, James WD. Stevens-Johnson syndrome. In: Arnold Jr HL, Odom RB, James WD, eds. Andrew's diseases of the skin. 8th ed. Philadelphia: WB Saunders, 1990;136.
17. Patterson R, Grammer LC, Greenberger PA, et al. Stevens-Johnson syndrome (SJS): effectiveness of corticosteroids in management and recurrent SJS. Allergy Proc 1992;13:89.
18. Patterson R, Miller M, Kaplan M, et al. Effectiveness of early therapy with corticosteroids in Stevens-Johnson syndrome: experience with 41 cases and a hypothesis regarding pathogenesis. Ann Allergy 1994;73:27.
19. Cheriyan S, Patterson R, Greenberger PA, Grammer LC, Latall J. The outcome of Stevens-Johnson syndrome treated with corticosteroids. Allergy Proc 1995;16:151.
20. Rasmussen JE. Erythema multiforme in children: response to treatment with systemic corticosteroids. Br J Dermatol 1976;95:181.
21. Nethercott JR, Choi BCK. Erythema multiforme (Stevens-Johnson syndrome): chart review of 123 hospitalization patients. Dermatologica 1985;171:383.

Allergic Diseases, 5th Edition,
edited by Roy Patterson, Leslie Carroll Grammer, and
Paul A. Greenberger. Lippincott–Raven Publishers, Philadelphia, © 1997.

17

Drug Allergy

Richard D. DeSwarte and Roy Patterson

*R.D. DeSwarte and R. Patterson: Division of Allergy-Immunology,
Northwestern University Medical School, Chicago, IL 60611.*

Pearls for Practitioners
Roy Patterson

- This chapter on drug allergy is the fifth revision of the initial chapter, which was recognized by many in the field 25 years ago the best and most definitive chapter on drug allergy ever written. Its comprehensive stature continues in this edition. Recommendations for use of this chapter include:
  1. Study of the classification of drug reactions by all physicians.
  2. Use of the chapter as a reference source by all primary care physicians.
- A patient listing more than three or more drugs of different classes or causes of allergy may have been misinformed about some or even all of them.
- Test dosing is the cautious administration of small and then increasing doses of a drug to determine if a reaction occurs. It is not desensitization.
- Desensitization is the neutralization of the antibody by small but increasing doses of of a drug. It is dangerous.
- Skin testing with low-molecular-weight drugs is rarely useful, except for penicillin.
- As high-molecular-weight biologic agents come into increasing use, expect to see more allergic-type reactions. We saw this with foreign serum years ago.
- The term *drug allergy* should be limited to reactions for which there is a proven or a presumptive immunologic mechanism.
- When Stevens-Johnson syndrome occurs, look for a drug as a cause, stop the drug, and start high-dose corticosteroids as soon as possible.
- IgE-mediated reactions to local anesthetics do not occur. Prick testing and subcutaneous test dosing demonstrate safety of a local anesthetic. Intracutaneous tests give false-positive reactions. Do not use a local anesthetic with epinephrine. Test dosing with local anesthetics is frequently associated with hysterical reactions.

In the last edition of this text, the subject of drug allergy was extensively reviewed.[1] Although a reasonably comprehensive overview of this important topic is given in this edition, an effort was made to focus more sharply on clinically applicable information. A more concise, practical review has been published elsewhere.[2] Other reviews of drug allergy are also recommended.[3,4]

Although specific recommendations are suggested regarding drug challenges and desensitization protocols, it is advisable, when possible, for those inexperienced in such matters to consult with physicians who regularly evaluate and manage hypersensitivity phenomena.

EPIDEMIOLOGY

A consequence of the rapid development of new drugs to diagnose and treat human illness has been the increased incidence of adverse reactions to these agents, which may produce additional morbidity and, on occasion, mortality. Their occurrence violates a basic principle of medical practice, primum non nocere (above all do no harm). It is a sobering fact that adverse drug reactions are responsible for most iatrogenic illnesses. This should serve to remind physicians not to select potent and often unnecessary drugs to treat inconsequential illnesses. Many patients have come to expect drug treatments for the most trivial of symptoms. On the other hand, a physician should not deprive a patient of necessary medication for fear of a reaction. Fortunately, most adverse reactions are not severe, but the predictability of seriousness is usually not possible in the individual case or with the individual drug.

An *adverse drug reaction* may be defined as any undesired and unintended response that occurs at doses of an appropriate drug given for the therapeutic, diagnostic, or prophylactic benefit of the patient. The reaction should appear within a reasonable time after administration of the drug. This definition excludes therapeutic failure, which the patient may perceive as an adverse drug reaction. A *drug* may be defined as any substance used in diagnosis, therapy, and prophylaxis of disease.

Although the exact incidence of adverse drug reactions is unknown, some estimates of their magnitude are available. Reported estimates of the incidence of adverse drug reactions leading to hospitalization vary, but one study based on a computerized surveillance system determined that 2% were due to such.[5] As many as 15% to 30% of medical inpatients experience an adverse drug reaction.[6] Drug-attributed deaths occur in 0.01% of surgical inpatients and in 0.10% of medical inpatients.[7,8] Most of these fatalities occurred among patients who were terminally ill.[9] Most deaths were due to a small number of drugs that are known to be toxic.

Information regarding outpatient adverse drug events is scant by comparison because most are not reported to pharmaceutical companies and appropriate national registries. Such surveys are complicated by the problem of differentiating between signs and symptoms attributable to the natural disease and those related to its treatment. Adverse drug reactions mimic virtually every disease, including the disease being treated. The challenge of monitoring adverse drug reactions is further complicated by multiple drug prescribing and the frequent use of nonprescription medications. Despite these limitations, such monitoring did identify the excess drug-induced skin rash after ampicillin therapy.

Although most drug safety information is obtained from clinical trials before drug approval, premarketing studies are narrow in scope and cannot uncover adverse drug reactions in all patient populations. Adverse effects that occur over time or that occur in fewer than 1 in 1000 cases (e.g., drug hypersensitivity) will not be detected until used by large numbers of patients after drug approval.[10]

Thus, postmarketing surveillance is essential to the discovery of unexpected adverse drug effects. One estimate, however, is that only 1% of adverse drug reactions are voluntarily reported to pharmaceutical companies and the Food and Drug Administration (FDA).[11] In an attempt to ensure the timely collection of adverse drug reactions, the FDA introduced a simplified medical products reporting program in 1993, called MedWatch.[12] Although the FDA had an adverse drug reaction reporting system in place before MedWatch, it was awkward to use and understandably discouraged health professionals' participation. Using MedWatch, the reporting person does not have to prove an association between the drug and the adverse reaction. When reported, the information becomes part of a large data base and can be investigated further. A simple, self-addressed, one-page form is available and can be sent by mail, fax, or computer modem. This form can be obtained directly from the FDA and is also available in hospital pharmacies, *The Physicians' Desk Reference*, and the *FDA Medical Bulletin*. The FDA can also provide a copy of their new *FDA Desk Guide to Adverse Event and Product Problem Reporting*. Table 17-1 summarizes how to report adverse drug reactions to MedWatch.

Such voluntary reporting led to the observation that ventricular arrhythmias, such as torsades de pointes, may occur when terfenadine was administered with erythromycin or ketoconazole.[13]

Most adverse drug reactions do not have an allergic basis. The following discussion focuses on those reactions that are, or possibly could be, mediated by immunologic mechanisms. Allergic drug reactions account for 6% to 10% of all observed adverse drug reactions. The risk of an allergic reaction is about 1% to 3% for most drugs.

About 5% of adults may be allergic to one or more drugs. As many as 15%, however, believe themselves to be or have been incorrectly labeled as being allergic to one or more drugs and, therefore, may be denied treatment with an essential medication. At times, it may be imperative to establish the presence or absence of allergy to a drug when its use is necessary and when there are no safe alternatives. Although most patients with histories of reacting to a drug could safely receive that drug again, the outcome could be serious if the patient is truly allergic. Hence, a suspicion of drug hypersensitivity must be evaluated carefully.

CLASSIFICATION OF ADVERSE DRUG REACTIONS

Before proceeding with a detailed analysis of drug hypersensitivity, it is appropriate to attempt to place it in perspective with other adverse drug reactions. Patients often, and physicians occasionally, should carefully analyze adverse drug reactions to determine their nature because this influences future use. For example, a drug-induced side effect may be corrected by simply reducing the dose. On the other hand, an allergic reaction to a drug may mean that the drug cannot be used or may require special considerations before future administration.[14]

Adverse drug reactions can be divided into two major groups: (1) *predictable adverse reactions*, which are (a) often dose dependent, (b) related to the known pharmacologic actions of the drug, (c) occur in otherwise normal patients, and (d) account for 80% or more of adverse drug effects; and (2) *unpredictable adverse reactions*, which are (a) usually dose independent, (b) usually unrelated to the drug's pharmacologic actions, and (c) often related to the patient's immunologic responsiveness or, on occasion, to genetic differences in susceptible patients.

TABLE 17-1. *Reporting adverse reactions to MedWatch*

By Mail
Use postage-paid MedWatch form 3500

By Telephone
1-800-FDA-1088 to report by phone, to receive copies of form 3500 or a copy of the *FDA Desk Guide for Adverse Event and Product Problem Reporting*

1-800-FDA-0178 to FAX report

1-800-FDA-7737 to report by computer modem

1-800-FDA-7967 for a Vaccine Adverse Event Reporting System (VAERS) form for vaccines

Not included in this classification are those reactions that are unrelated to the drug itself, but are attributable to events associated with and during its administration. Such events are often mistakenly ascribed to the drug, and the patient is inappropriately denied that agent in the future. Particularly after parenteral administration of a drug, *psychophysiologic reactions* in the form of hysteria, hyperventilation, or vasovagal response may ensue. Some of these reactions may be manifestations of underlying psychiatric disorders.[15] Even anaphylactoid symptoms have been observed in placebo-treated patients.[16] Another group of signs and symptoms is considered *coincidental reactions.* They are a result of the disease under treatment and may be incorrectly attributed to the drug, for example, the appearance of viral exanthems and even urticaria during the course of treatment with an antibiotic.

Although it may be difficult to characterize a particular drug reaction, a helpful classification is shown in Table 17-2, followed by a brief description of each.

Overdosage: Toxicity

The toxic effects of a drug are directly related to the systemic or local concentration of the drug in the body. Such effects are usually predictable on the basis of animal experimentation and may be expected in any patient, provided a threshold level has been exceeded. Each drug tends to have its own characteristic toxic effects. Overdosage may result from an excess dose taken accidentally or deliberately. It may be due to accumulation as a result of some abnormality in the patient that interferes with normal metabolism and excretion of the drug. The toxicity of morphine is enhanced in the presence of liver disease (inability to detoxify the drug) or myxedema (depression of metabolic rate). The toxicity of chloramphenicol in infants is due to immaturity of the glucuronide-conjugating system, allowing a toxic concentration to accumulate. In the presence of renal failure, drugs such as the aminoglycosides, normally excreted by this route, may accumulate and produce toxic reactions.

TABLE 17-2. *Classification of adverse drug reactions*

Predictable Adverse Reactions Occurring in Normal Patients

Overdosage: toxicity

Side effects

   Immediate expression

   Delayed expression

Secondary or indirect effects

   Drug related

   Disease associated

Drug–drug interactions

Unpredictable Adverse Reactions Occurring in Susceptible Patients

Intolerance

Idiosyncratic reactions

Allergic (hypersensitivity) reactions

Pseudoallergic reactions

Side Effects

Side effects are the most frequent adverse drug reactions. They are therapeutically undesirable, but often unavoidable, pharmacologic actions occurring at usual prescribed drug dosages. A drug frequently has several pharmacologic actions, and only one of those may be the desired therapeutic effect. The others may be considered side effects. The first-generation antihistamines commonly cause adverse central nervous system effects, such as sedation. Anticholinergic side effects include dry mouth, blurred vision, and urinary retention.

Other side effects may be delayed in expression and include teratogenicity and carcinogenicity. Methotrexate, which has been used in some steroid-dependent asthmatic patients, is teratogenic and should not be used during pregnancy. Immunosuppressive agents can alter host immunity and may predispose the patient to malignancy.[17]

Secondary or Indirect Effects

Secondary effects are indirect, but not inevitable, consequences of the drug's primary pharmacologic action. They may be interpreted as the appearance of another naturally occurring disease, rather than being associated with administration of the drug. Some appear to be due to the drug itself creating an ecologic disturbance and permitting the overgrowth of microorganisms. In the presence of antimicrobial (notably ampicillin, clindamycin, or cephalosporins) exposure, *Clostridium difficile* can flourish in the gastrointestinal tract in an environment where there is reduced bacterial competition. Toxins produced by this organism may result in the development of pseudomembranous colitis.[18]

Antimicrobial agents may be associated with another group of reactions that may mimic hypersensitivity but that appear to be disease associated. The Jarisch-Herxheimer phenomenon involves the development of fever, chills, headache, skin rash, edema, lymphadenopathy, and often an exacerbation of preexisting skin lesions. The reaction is believed to result from the release of microbial antigens, endotoxins, or both.[19] This has usually followed penicillin treatment of syphilis and leptospirosis, but also has been observed during treatment of parasitic and fungal infections. With continued treatment, the reaction subsides, thus confirming it is not an allergic response. Unfortunately, treatment is often discontinued and the drug blamed for the reaction. Other examples include the high incidence of skin rash in patients with the Epstein-Barr virus treated with ampicillin and among acquired immunodeficiency syndrome (AIDS) patients treated with trimethoprim-sulfamethoxazole (TMP-SMX).

Drug–Drug Interactions

A drug–drug interaction is generally regarded as the modification of the effect of one drug by prior or concomitant administration of another. Fortunately, drug–drug interactions of major clinical consequence are relatively infrequent.[20] In addition, not all drug interactions are harmful, and some may be used to clinical advantage.

As the number of drugs taken concurrently increases, the greater is the likelihood of an adverse drug interaction. When an interaction is reported, an average of between four and eight drugs are being taken by the patient. Therefore, the largest risk group is the elderly, who often receive polypharmacy. The danger of an interaction also escalates when several physicians are treating a patient, each for a separate condition. It is the physician's responsibility to determine what other medications the patient is taking, even nonprescription drugs.

Several widely prescribed agents used to treat allergic rhinitis and asthma interact significantly with other drugs. The second-generation antihistamines, terfenadine and astemizole, are metabolized by cytochrome P-450 mixed-function oxidase enzymes. They should not be used in combination with drugs that inhibit this enzyme system, such as the imidazole antifungals ketoconazole and itraconazole, or the macrolide antibiotics erythromycin and Clarithromycin. The resultant increased concentrations of the antihistamines may cause prolongation of the QT interval, sometimes producing torsades de pointes or other serious cardiac arrhythmias.[13] Although plasma concentrations of loratadine increased with concomitant administration of ketoconazole, this did not cause prolongation of the QT interval and the risk of torsades de pointes.[21]

An excellent review of other adverse drug interactions can be found in a loose-leaf publication authored by Hansten and Horn.[22]

Intolerance

A characteristic pharmacologic effect of a drug is quantitatively increased, and often is produced, by an unusually small dose of medication. Most patients develop tinnitus on large doses of salicylates and quinine, but few experience it after a single average dose or a smaller dose than usual. This untoward effect may be genetically determined and appears to be a function of the recipient, or it may occur in patients lying at the extremes of dose–response curves for pharmacologic effects.

Although intolerance usually implies a quantitatively increased pharmacologic effect occurring among susceptible patients, *idiosyncratic* and *allergic reactions* are qualitatively aberrant and inexplicable in terms of the normal pharmacology of the drug given in usual therapeutic doses.

Idiosyncratic Reactions

Idiosyncrasy is a term used to describe a qualitatively abnormal, unexpected response to a drug, differing from its pharmacologic actions and thus resembling hypersensitivity. This reaction does not involve a proven, or even suspected, allergic mechanism.

The most familiar example of an idiosyncratic reaction is the hemolytic anemia that occurs commonly in African and Mediterranean populations and in 10% to 13% of African-American males (sex-linked dominant) exposed to oxidant drugs or their metabolites. About 25% of African-American females are carriers, and of these, only 20% have a sufficiently severe expression of the deficiency to be clinically important. A more severe form of the deficiency occurs in whites, primarily among those of Mediterranean origin. The erythrocytes of such patients lack the enzyme glucose-6-phosphate dehydrogenase (G6PD) that is essential for aerobic metabolism of glucose and, consequently, cellular integrity.[23] Although the original observations of this phenomenon were among susceptible patients receiving primaquine, more than 50 drugs are known that induce hemolysis in G6PD-deficient patients. Clinically, the three classes of drugs most important in terms of their hemolytic potential are sulfonamides, nitrofurans, and water-soluble vitamin K analogues. If G6PD deficiency is suspected, simple screening tests dependent on hemoglobin oxidation, dye reduction, or fluorescence generation provide supporting evidence.

The study of genetic G6PD deficiency and other genetic defects leading to adverse drug reactions has been termed *pharmacogenetics.*[24]

Allergic Reactions

Allergic drug reactions occur in only a small number of patients, are unpredictable and quantitatively abnormal, and are unrelated to the pharmacologic action of the drug. Unlike idiosyncrasy, allergic drug reactions are the result of an immune response to a drug after previous expose to the same drug or to an immunochemically related substance that had resulted in the formation of specific antibodies, or of sensitized T-lymphocytes, or both. Ideally, the term *drug allergy* or *hypersensitivity* should be restricted to those reactions proven, or more often presumed, to be the result of an immunologic mechanism.

The establishment of an allergic mechanism should be based on the demonstration of specific antibodies, sensitized lymphocytes, or both. This is not often possible for many reactions ascribed to drug allergy. The diagnosis is usually based on clinical observations and, in selected instances, reexposure to the suspected agent under controlled circumstances. Even in the absence of direct immunologic evidence, an allergic drug reaction often is suspected when certain clinical and laboratory criteria are present (Table 17-3). Obviously, none of these is absolutely reliable.[25]

Immediate reactions occurring within minutes often include manifestations of anaphylaxis. Accelerated reactions taking place after 1 hour to 3 days frequently are manifested as urticaria and angioedema and occasionally as other rashes, especially exanthems, and fever. Delayed or late reactions do not appear until 3 days or longer after drug therapy is initiated and commonly include a diverse group of skin rashes, drug fever, and serum sickness–like reactions; less commonly seen are hematologic, pulmonary, hepatic, and renal reactions, vasculitis, and a condition resembling lupus erythematosus.

Because clinical criteria are often inadequate, specific immunologic testing is desirable. Until this is accomplished, the relation can be considered only presumptive. With few exceptions, safe, reliable in vivo tests and simple, rapid, predictable in vitro tests for the absolute diagnosis of drug allergy are unavailable. The most conclusive test is cautious readministration of the suspected drug, but usually the risk is not justified.

TABLE 17-3. *Clinical criteria of allergic drug reactions*

Allergic reactions occur in only a small percentage of patients receiving the drug and cannot be predicted from animal studies.

The observed clinical manifestations do not resemble known pharmacologic actions of the drug.

In the absence of prior exposure to the drug, allergic symptoms rarely appear before 1 week of continuous treatment. After sensitization, even years previously, the reaction may develop rapidly on reexposure to the drug. As a rule, drugs used with impunity for several months or longer are rarely the culprits. This temporal relation is often the most vital information in determining which of many drugs being taken should be considered most seriously as the cause of a suspected drug hypersensitivity reaction.

The reaction may resemble other established allergic reactions, such as anaphylaxis, urticaria, asthma, and serum sickness–like reactions. However, a variety of skin rashes (particularly exanthems), fever, pulmonary infiltrates with eosinophilia, hepatitis, acute interstitial nephritis, and lupus syndrome have been attributed to drug hypersensitivity.

The reaction may be reproduced by small doses of the suspected drug or other agents possessing similar or cross-reacting chemical structures.

Eosinophilia may be suggestive if present.

Rarely, drug-specific antibodies or T lymphocytes have been identified that react with the suspected drug or relevant drug metabolite.

As with adverse drug reactions in general, the reaction usually subsides within several days after discontinuation of the drug.

Pseudoallergic Reactions

Pseudoallergy refers to an immediate generalized reaction involving mast cell mediator release by an immunoglobulin E (IgE) independent mechanism.[26] Although the clinical manifestations often mimic or resemble IgE-mediated events (anaphylaxis), the initiating event does not involve an interaction between the drug or drug metabolites and drug-specific IgE antibodies. A differential point is that these reactions may occur in patients without previous exposure to these substances.

Such reactions appear to result from nonimmunologic activation of effector pathways. Certain drugs, such as opiates, vancomycin, polymyxin B, and d-tubocurarine, may directly release mediators from mast cells, resulting in urticaria, angioedema, or even a clinical picture resembling anaphylaxis.

Overview

The classification of adverse drug reactions presented here must be considered tentative. At times, it may be impossible to place a particular drug reaction under one of these headings. However, the common practice of labeling any drug reaction as *allergic* should be discouraged.

IMMUNOCHEMICAL BASIS OF DRUG ALLERGY

Drugs as Immunogens

The allergenic potential of drugs is largely dependent on their chemical properties. Increases in molecular size and complexity are associated with an increased ability to elicit an immune response. Hence, large-molecular-weight drugs, such as heterologous antisera, chymopapain, streptokinase, L-asparaginase, and insulin, are complete antigens that can induce immune responses and elicit hypersensitivity reactions. Immunogenicity is weak or absent when substances have a molecular weight less than 4000 daltons.[27]

Most drugs are simple organic chemicals of low molecular weight, usually less than 1000 daltons. For such low-molecular-weight drugs to become immunogenic, the drug or a drug metabolite must be bound to a macromolecular carrier, often by covalent bonds, for effective antigen processing. The simple chemical (hapten), nonimmunogenic by itself, becomes immunogenic in the presence of the carrier macromolecule and now directs the specificity of the response.

β-Lactam antibiotics are highly reactive with proteins and can directly haptenate carrier macromolecules. Most drugs, however, are not sufficiently reactive to form a stable immunogenic complex. Haptens derived from most drugs likely are *reactive metabolites* of the parent compound, which then bind to carrier macromolecules to become immunogenic. This requirement for metabolic processing may help to explain the low incidence of drug allergy; the predisposition of certain drugs to cause sensitization because they are prone to form highly reactive metabolites; and the inability of skin testing and other immunologic tests with the unaltered drug to predict or identify the reaction as being allergic in nature.

Penicillin allergy has received most attention as a model of drug haptenization.[28] Unfortunately, relevant drug haptens have not been identified for most allergic drug reactions. Studies of human IgE and IgG to sulfonamides have established the N^4-sulfonamidoyl determinant to be the major sulfonamide haptenic determinant.[29]

An antigen must have multiple combining sites (multivalent) to elicit hypersensitivity reactions. This requirement permits bridging of IgE and IgG antibody molecules or antigen receptors on lymphocytes. Conjugation of the free drug or metabolite (hapten) with a macromolecular carrier to form a multivalent hapten–carrier conjugate is necessary to initiate an immune response and elicit a hypersensitivity reaction. The univalent ligand (free drug or metabolite), in large excess, may inhibit the response by competing with the multivalent conjugates for the same receptors. Therefore, the relative concentration of each determines the frequency, severity, and rate of allergic drug reactions. Also, removal of haptens from carrier molecules by plasma enzymes (dehaptenation) influences the likelihood of such reactions.[30]

Finally, some low-molecular-weight drugs, such as quaternary ammonium muscle relaxants and aminoglycosides, have enough distance between determinants to act as bivalent antigens without requiring conjugation to a carrier.[31]

Immunologic Response to Drugs

Drugs often induce an immune response, but only a small number of patients actually experience clinical hypersensitivity reactions. For example, most patients exposed to penicillin and insulin develop demonstrable antibodies; however, in most instances, these do not result in allergic reactions or reduced effectiveness of the drug.

Mechanisms of Drug-Induced Immunopathology

An immunologic response to any antigen may be diverse and the attendant reactions complex. Drugs are no exception and have been associated with all of the immunologic reactions proposed by Coombs and Gell.[32] It is likely that more than one mechanism contributes to a particular reaction, but often one predominates. Table 17-4 is an attempt to provide an overview of the immunopathology of allergic drug reactions based on the original Gell and Coombs classification.

Penicillin alone has been associated with many of these reactions. Anaphylaxis and urticaria after penicillin administration are examples of type I reactions. The hemolytic anemia associated with high-dose penicillin therapy is a type II reaction. A serum sickness–like

TABLE 17-4. *Immunopathology of allergic reactions to drugs*

Gell and Coombs Classification	Immunoreactants	Clinical presentation
Type I	Mast cell-mediated immediate generalized reactions IgE dependent (anaphylactic) IgE independent (pseudoallergy)	Anaphylaxis, urticaria, angioedema, asthma, rhinitis
Type II	Antibody-mediated cytotoxic reactions; IgG and IgM antibodies; complement often involved	Immune cytopenias Some organ inflammation
Type III	Immune complex-mediated reactions; complement involved	Serum sickness, vasculitis
Type IV	T-lymphocyte–mediated reactions; lymphokines	Contact dermatitis; some exanthems; some organ inflammation

reaction, now most commonly associated with penicillin treatment, is a type III reaction. Finally, the contact dermatitis that occurred when penicillin was used topically in the past is an example of a type IV reaction.

RISK FACTORS FOR DRUG ALLERGY

Several factors have been identified that may influence the induction of drug-specific immune responses and the elicitation of clinical reactions to these agents[33,34] (Table 17-5).

Drug- and Treatment-Related Factors

Nature of the Drug

Macromolecular drugs, such as heterologous antisera and insulin, are complex antigens and have the potential to sensitize any patient. As noted earlier, most drugs have molecular weights under 1000 daltons and are not immunogenic by themselves. Immunogenicity is determined by the potential of the drug or, more often, a drug metabolite to form conjugates with carrier proteins.

β-Lactam antibiotics, aspirin (acetylsalicylic acid, ASA) and nonsteroidal antiinflammatory drugs (NSAIDs), and sulfonamides account of 80% of allergic or pseudoallergic reactions.

Drug Exposure

Cutaneous application of a drug is generally considered to be associated with the greatest risk of sensitizing patients.[34] In fact, penicillin, sulfonamides, and antihistamines are no longer used topically because of this potential. The adjuvant effect of some intramuscular prepara-

TABLE 17-5. *Risk factors for drug allergy*

Drug and Treatment-Related Factors	
Nature of the drug Immunologic reactivity	*Drug exposure* Route of administration
Nonimmunologic activity	Dose, duration, and frequency of treatment
Patient-Related Factors	
Age and gender *Genetic factors* Role of atopy	*Concurrent medical illness* Asthma
Acetylator status	Cystic fibrosis
HLA type	Epstein-Barr viral infection
Familial drug allergy	HIV-infected patients
Prior drug reactions Persistence of drug immune response	*Concurrent medical therapy* β-Adrenergic–blocking agents
Cross-sensitization	
Multiple drug allergy syndrome	

tions may increase the risk of sensitization; for example, the incidence of reactions to benzathine penicillin is higher than that of other penicillin preparations. The intravenous route may be the least likely to sensitize patients.

Once a patient is sensitized, the difference in reaction rates between oral and parenteral drug administration is likely related to the rate of drug administration. Anaphylaxis is less common after oral administration of a drug, although severe reactions have occurred. For other allergic drug reactions, the evidence supporting oral administration is less clear.

The dose and duration of treatment appear to affect the development of a drug-specific immunologic response. In drug-induced lupus erythematosus, the dose and duration of hydralazine therapy are important factors. Penicillin-induced hemolytic anemia follows high sustained levels of drug therapy.

There is little evidence that the frequency of drug administration affects the likelihood of sensitization.[34] Frequent courses of treatment, however, are more likely to elicit an allergic reaction. The longer the intervals between therapy, the less likely is an allergic reaction.

Patent-Related Factors

Age and Gender

Generally, children appear less likely to become sensitized to drugs than adults; however, serious allergic drug reactions do occur in children. Some confusion may arise in that the rash associated with a viral illness in children may incorrectly be ascribed to an antibiotic being administered as treatment.

Genetic Factors

Allergic drug reactions occur in only a small percentage of patients treated with a given drug. Many factors, both genetic and environmental, probably are involved in determining which patients in a large random population will develop an allergic reaction to a given drug.

Patients with histories of allergic rhinitis, asthma, or atopic dermatitis (the *atopic constitution*) are not at increased risk of being sensitized to drugs compared with the general population.[34] Also, it appears that atopic patients are more likely to develop pseudoallergic reactions, especially to radiographic contrast media.[35]

The rate of metabolism of a drug may influence the prevalence of sensitization. Patients who are genetically *slow acetylators* are more likely to develop drug-induced lupus erythematosus associated with the administration of hydralazine and procainamide.[36,37] Adverse reactions to sulfonamides may be more severe among slow acetylators.[38]

Specific HLA genes have been associated with the risk of developing drug allergy. The susceptibility for drug-induced nephropathy in patients with rheumatoid arthritis treated with gold salts or penicillamine is associated with the HLA-DRw3 and HLA-B8 phenotypes.[39] In addition, specific HLA genes have been associated with hydralazine-induced lupus erythematosus, levamisole-induced agranulocytosis, and sulfonamide-induced toxic epidermal necrolysis (TEN).[40]

The possibility of *familial drug allergy* has been reported.[41] Among adolescents whose parents had sustained an allergic reaction to antibiotics, 25.6% experienced an allergic reaction to an antimicrobial agent, whereas only 1.7% reacted when their parents tolerated antibiotics without an allergic reaction.

Prior Drug Reactions

Undoubtedly, the most important risk factor is a history of a prior reaction to a drug being considered for treatment or one that may be immunochemically similar. Drug hypersensitivity, however, might not persist indefinitely. It is well established that, after an allergic reaction to penicillin, the half-life of antipenicilloyl IgE antibodies in serum ranges from 55 days to an indeterminate long interval in excess of 2000 days.[34]

Cross-sensitization between drugs may occur. The likelihood of cross-reactivity among the various sulfonamide groups (antibacterials, sulfonylureas, diuretics) has not been resolved. There is little supporting evidence in the medical literature that cross-sensitization is a significant problem. Patients who have demonstrated drug hypersensitivity in the past appear to have an increased tendency to develop sensitivity to new drugs. Penicillin-allergic patients have about a 10-fold increased risk of having an allergic reaction to non–β-lactam antimicrobial drugs.[42,43] The reactions were not restricted to immediate-type hypersensitivity. Fifty-seven percent reacted to a sulfonamide. With the exception of the aminoglycosides, reaction rates were much higher than expected in all other antibiotic classes, including erythromycin. Among children with multiple antibiotic sensitivities by history, 26% had positive penicillin skin tests.[44] These observations suggest that such patients are prone to react to haptenating drugs during an infection.[45] Obviously, such patients present difficult clinical management problems.

Concurrent Medical Illness

Although asthmatic patients do not appear to be at increased risk for drug-induced anaphylaxis, the outcome is more often unfavorable.[33,34] Children with cystic fibrosis are more likely to experience allergic drug reactions, especially during drug desensitization.[46]

Maculopapular rashes after the administration of ampicillin occur more frequently during Epstein-Barr viral infections and among patients with lymphatic leukemia.[47]

Immune deficiency is associated with an increased frequency of adverse drug reactions, many of which appear of be allergic in nature. Patients who are immunosuppressed may become deficient in suppressor T lymphocytes that regulate IgE antibody synthesis.

Much attention has been given to adverse drug reactions, in particular hypersensitivity, which occurs with a much higher frequency among patients infected with the human immunodeficiency virus (HIV) than in patients who are HIV-seronegative.[48,49] A retrospective study comparing *Pneumocystis carinii* pneumonia (PCP) in patients with AIDS to a similar pneumonia in patients with other underlying immunosuppressive conditions reported adverse reactions to TMP-SMX in 65% of AIDS patients compared with 12% of patients with other immunosuppressive diseases, suggesting the abnormality may be due to the HIV infection.[50] TMP-SMX has been associated with rash, fever, and hematologic disturbances and, less frequently, with more severe reactions such as Stevens-Johnson syndrome, TEN, and anaphylactic reactions. Also, pentamidine, antituberculosis regimens containing isoniazid and rifampin, amoxicillin-clavulanate, and clindamycin have been associated with an increased incidence of adverse drug reactions, some of which may involve an allergic mechanism. It also appears that progression of HIV disease to a more advanced stage confers an increased risk of hypersensitivity reactions.[48]

Concurrent Medical Therapy

Some medications may alter the risk and severity of reactions to drugs. Patients treated with β-adrenergic blocking agents, even timolol maleate ophthalmic solution, may be more susceptible to, and may prove more refractory to, treatment of drug-induced anaphylaxis.[51]

CLINICAL CLASSIFICATION OF ALLERGIC REACTIONS TO DRUGS

A useful classification is based primarily on the clinical presentation or manifestations of such reactions. The presumption of allergy is based on clinical criteria cited earlier (see Table 17-3).

Table 17-6 provides an overview of a clinical classification based on organ systems involved, namely, generalized multisystem involvement and predominantly organ-specific responses.

What follows is a brief discussion of each of these clinical entities, including a list of most commonly implicated drugs. Detailed lists of implicated drugs appear in periodic literature reviews.[52,53]

TABLE 17-6. *Clinical classification of allergic reactions to drugs*

Generalized or Multisystem Involvement

Immediate generalized reactions

  Anaphylaxis (IgE-mediated reactions)

  Anaphylactoid reactions (IgE-independent reactions)

Serum sickness and serum sickness–like reactions

Reactions Predominantly Organ Specific

*Dermatologic manifestations**

Pulmonary manifestations

  Asthma

  Pulmonary infiltrates with eosinophilia

  Pneumonitis and fibrosis

  Noncardiogenic pulmonary edema

Hematologic manifestations

  Eosinophilia

  Thrombocytopenia

  Hemolytic anemia

  Agranulocytosis

Drug fever

Drug-induced autoimmunity

  Reactions simulating systemic lupus erythematosus

  Other reactions

Hypersensitivity vasculitis

Hepatic manifestations

  Cholestasis

  Hepatocellular damage

  Mixed pattern

Renal manifestations

  Glomerulitis

  Nephrotic syndrome

  Acute interstitial nephritis

Lymphoid system manifestations

  Pseudolymphoma

  Infectious mononucleosis-like syndrome

Cardiac manifestations

Neurologic manifestations

*A separate listing of dermatologic manifestations is included in that section (see Table 17-8).

Generalized or Multisystem Involvement

Immediate Generalized Reactions

The acute systemic reactions are among the most urgent of drug-related events. Greenberger[54] has used the term *immediate generalized reactions* to underscore the fact that many are not IgE mediated. The term drug-induced *anaphylaxis* should be reserved for a systemic reaction proven to be IgE mediated. Drug-induced *anaphylactoid reactions* are clinically indistinguishable from anaphylaxis but occur through IgE-independent mechanisms. Both ultimately result in the release of potent vasoactive and inflammatory mediators from mast cells and basophils.

In a series of 32,812 continuously monitored patients, such reactions occurred in 12 patients (0.04%), and there were 2 deaths.[55] Because anaphylaxis is more likely to be reported when a fatality occurs, its prevalence may be underestimated. Drug-induced anaphylaxis does not appear to confer increased risk of such generalized reactions to allergens from other sources.[56]

Most reactions occur within 30 minutes, and death may ensue within minutes. Anaphylaxis occurs most commonly after parenteral administration, but it has also followed oral, percutaneous, and respiratory exposure. Symptoms usually subside rapidly with appropriate treatment but may last 24 hours or longer, and recurrent symptoms may appear several hours after apparent resolution of the reaction. As a rule, the severity of the reaction decreases with increasing time between exposure to the drug and onset of symptoms. Death is usually due to cardiovascular collapse or respiratory obstruction, especially laryngeal or upper airway edema. Although most reactions do not terminate fatally, the potential for mortality must be borne in mind, and the attending physician must respond immediately with appropriate treatment.

Table 17-7 summarizes most agents frequently associated with immediate generalized reactions. In some situations, drugs, such as general anesthetic agents and vancomycin, which are primarily direct mast cell–mediator releasers, can produce an IgE-mediated reaction.[31,57] This distinction has clinical relevance in that IgE-independent reactions may be prevented or modified by pretreatment with corticosteroids and antihistamines, whereas such protection from drug-induced IgE-mediated reactions is less likely. In the latter situation, when the drug is medically necessary, desensitization is an option.

TABLE 17-7. *Drugs implicated in immediate generalized reactions*

Anaphylaxis (IgE mediated)	Anaphylactoid reactions (IgE independent)
β-Lactam antibiotics	Radiocontrast material
Allergen extracts	Aspirin
Heterologous antisera	Nonsteroidal antiinflammatory drugs
Insulin	Dextran and iron dextran
Vaccines (egg-based)	Anesthetic drugs
Streptokinase	Induction agents†
Chymopapain	Muscle relaxants†
L-Asparaginase	Protamine†
Cisplatin	Vancomycin†
Carboplatinum	Ciprofloxacin
Latex*	Paclitaxel

*Not a drug per se, but often an important consideration in a medical setting.
†Some reactions may be mediated by IgE antibodies.

The β-lactam antibiotics, notably penicillin, are by far the most common causes of drug-induced anaphylaxis. Essentially all β-lactam anaphylactic reactions are IgE mediated. Immediate generalized reactions to other antibiotics occur but are relatively uncommon. Anaphylactoid reactions have been observed after the administration of ciprofloxacin and norfloxacin.[58]

Cancer chemotherapeutic agents have been associated with hypersensitivity reactions, most commonly type I immediate generalized reactions.[59] L-asparaginase has the highest risk for such reactions. Serious anaphylactic reactions with respiratory distress and hypotension occur in about 10% of patients treated. It is likely that most of these reactions are IgE mediated. Skin testing appears to be of no value in predicting a reaction because there are both false-positive and false-negative results. Therefore, the physician must be prepared to treat anaphylaxis with each dose. For patients who react to L-asparaginase derived from *Escherichia coli*, an asparaginase derived from *Erwinia chyoanthermia* (a plant pathogen) or a modified asparaginase (pegaspargase) may be a clinically effective substitute. Cisplatin and carboplatin are second only to L-asparaginase in producing such reactions. Skin testing with these agents appears to have predictive value, and desensitization has been successful, when these drugs are medically necessary.[60] The initial use of paclitaxel (Taxol) to treat ovarian and breast cancer was associated with a 10% risk of anaphylactoid reactions. With premedication and lengthening of the infusion time, however, the risk is significantly reduced.[61] All other antitumor drugs, except altretamine, the nitrosoureas, and dactinomycin, have occasionally been associated with hypersensitivity reactions.[59] Some appear to be IgE mediated, but most are probably IgE independent.

Anaphylactic and anaphylactoid reactions occurring during the perioperative period have received increased attention. The evaluation and detection of these reactions is complicated by the use of multiple medications and the fact that patients are often unconscious and draped, which may mask the early signs and symptoms of an immediate generalized reaction.[62] During anesthesia, the only feature observed may be cardiovascular collapse or airway obstruction. Cyanosis due to oxygen desaturation may be noted. One large multicenter study indicated that 70% of cases were due to muscle relaxants, while 12% were due to latex.[63] Other agents, such as intravenous induction drugs, plasma volume expanders (dextran), and opioid analgesics, also require consideration. With the increased use of cardiopulmonary bypass surgery, the incidence of protamine-induced immediate life-threatening reactions has risen.[64] Anaphylaxis to ethylene oxide–sterilized devices has been described; hence, such devices used during anesthesia could potentially cause anaphylaxis.[65]

Psyllium seed is an active ingredient of several bulk laxatives and has been responsible for asthma after inhalation and anaphylaxis after ingestion, particularly in atopic subjects.[66] Anaphylactoid reactions after intravenous fluorescein may be modified by pretreatment with corticosteroids and antihistamines.[67] Of patients reacting to iron-dextran, 0.6% had a life-threatening anaphylactoid reaction.[68] Anaphylactoid reactions may also be caused by blood and blood products through the activation of complement and the production of anaphylatoxins. Adverse reactions to monoclonal antibodies include immediate generalized reactions, but the mechanism for such remains unclear.[69]

Virtually all drugs, including corticosteroids, tetracycline, cromolyn, erythromycin, and cimetidine, have been implicated in such immediate generalized reactions. These infrequent reports, however, should not be a reason to withhold essential medication.

Serum Sickness and Serum Sickness–like Reactions

Serum sickness results from the administration of heterologous (often equine) antisera and is the human equivalent of immune complex–mediated serum sickness observed in experimental animals.[70] A serum sickness–like illness has been attributed to a number of nonprotein drugs, notably the β-lactam antibiotics. These reactions are usually self-limiting, and the outcome favorable, but H_1 blockers and prednisone may be needed.

With effective immunization procedures, antimicrobial therapy, and the availability of human antitoxins, the incidence of serum sickness has declined. Heterologous antisera are still used to counteract potent toxins, such as snake venom, black widow and brown recluse spider venom, botulism, and gas gangrene toxins, as well as to treat diphtheria and rabies. Equine and murine antisera, used as antilymphocyte or antithymocyte globulins and as monoclonal antibodies for immunomodulation and cancer treatment, may cause serum sickness.[71] Serum sickness has also been reported in patients receiving streptokinase.[72]

β-Lactam antibiotics are considered to be the most common nonserum causes of serum sickness–like reactions; however, a literature review did not support this assertion.[73] In fact, such reactions appear to be infrequent, with an incidence of 1.8 per 100,000 prescriptions of cefaclor and 1 per 10 million prescriptions for amoxicillin and cephalexin.[74] Other drugs occasionally incriminated include ciprofloxacin, metronidazole, streptomycin, sulfonamides, allopurinol, carbamazepine, hydantoins, methimazole, phenylbutazone, propanolol, and thiouracil. The criteria for diagnosis, however, may not be uniform for each drug.

The onset of serum sickness typically begins 6 to 21 days after administration of the causative agent. The latent period reflects the time required for the production of antibodies. The onset of symptoms coincides with the development of immune complexes. Among previously immunized patients, the reaction may begin within 2 to 4 days after administration of the inciting agent. The manifestations include fever and malaise, skin eruptions, joint symptoms, and lymphadenopathy.

Laboratory abnormalities include an elevated erythrocyte sedimentation rate. Leukopenia, resulting from decreased neutrophils, may be present during the acute phase. Plasmacytosis may occasionally be present; in fact, serum sickness is one of the few illnesses in which plasma cells may be seen in the peripheral blood.[75] The urinalysis may reveal slight proteinuria, hyaline casts, hemoglobinuria, and microscopic hematuria. Nitrogen retention is rare.

Serum concentrations of C3, C4, and total hemolytic complement are depressed, providing some evidence that an immune complex mechanism is operative. Immune complex and elevated plasma concentrations of C3a and C5a anaphylatoxins have been documented.[76]

The prognosis for complete recovery is excellent. The symptoms may be mild, lasting only a few days, or severe, persisting for several weeks or longer.

Antihistamines control urticaria. If symptoms are severe, corticosteroids (e.g., prednisone, 40 mg/day for 1 week and then tapered) are indicated. Corticosteroids, however, do not prevent serum sickness in patients receiving antithymocyte globulin.[71] Skin testing with foreign antisera is routinely performed to avoid anaphylaxis with future use of foreign serum.

Drug Fever

Fever is a well-known drug hypersensitivity reaction. An immunologic mechanism is often suspected. Fever may be the sole manifestation of drug hypersensitivity and is particularly perplexing in a clinical situation in which a patient is being treated for an infection.

The height of the temperature does not distinguish drug fever, and there does not appear to be any fever pattern typical of this entity. Although a distinct disparity between the recorded febrile response and the relative well-being of the patient has been emphasized, these patients may have high fever and shaking chills. A skin rash is occasionally present and tends to support the diagnosis of a drug reaction.

Laboratory studies usually reveal leukocytosis with a shift to the left, thus mimicking an infectious process. Mild eosinophilia may be present. An elevated erythrocyte sedimentation rate and abnormal liver function tests are present in most cases.

The most consistent feature of drug fever is prompt defervescence, usually within 48 to 72 hours after withdrawal of the offending agent. Subsequent readministration of the drug produces fever, and occasionally chills, within a matter of hours.

In general, the diagnosis of drug fever is usually one of exclusion after eliminating other potential causes of the febrile reaction. Prompt recognition of drug fever is essential. If not appreciated, patients may be subjected to multiple diagnostic procedures and inappropriate treatment. Of greater concern is the possibility that the reaction may become more generalized with resultant tissue damage. Tissues from patients who died during drug fever show arteritis and focal necrosis in many organs, including myocardium, lung, and liver.

Drug-Induced Autoimmunity

Drug-Induced Lupus Erythematosus

Drug-induced lupus erythematosus is the most familiar drug-induced autoimmune disease, in part because systemic lupus erythematosus (SLE) remains the prototype of autoimmunity. Drug-induced lupus erythematosus is termed *autoimmune* because of its association with the development of antinuclear antibodies (ANAs). These same autoantibodies, however, are found frequently in the absence of frank disease. An excellent review of drug-induced autoimmunity appears elsewhere.[77]

Convincing evidence for drug-induced lupus erythematosus first appeared in 1953 after the introduction of hydralazine for treatment of hypertension.[78] Procainamide-induced lupus was first reported in 1962 and is now the most common cause of drug-induced lupus erythematosus in the United States.[79] These drugs have also been the best studied. Other agents for which there has been definite proof of an association include isoniazid, chlorpromazine, methyldopa, and quinidine. Another group of drugs that are probably associated with the syndrome include many anticonvulsants, β-blockers, antithyroid drugs, penicillamine, sulfasalazine, and lithium.

The incidence of drug-induced lupus erythematosus is not precisely known. In a survey of patients with lupus erythematosus seen in a private practice, 3% had drug-induced lupus.[80] Patients with idiopathic SLE do not appear to be at increased risk from drugs implicated in drug-induced lupus erythematosus.[81]

Fever, malaise, arthralgia, myalgia, pleurisy, and slight weight loss may appear acutely in a patient receiving an implicated drug. Pleuropericardial manifestations, such as pleurisy, pleural effusions, pulmonary infiltrates, pericarditis, and pericardial effusions, are more often seen in patients taking procainamide. Unlike idiopathic SLE, the classic butterfly malar rash, discoid lesions, oral mucosal ulcers, Raynaud's phenomenon, alopecia, and renal and central nervous system disease are unusual in drug-induced lupus erythematosus. Glomerulonephritis has occasionally been reported in hydralazine-induced lupus. As a rule, drug-induced lupus erythematosus is a milder disease than idiopathic SLE. Because many clinical features are nonspecific, the presence of ANAs is essential in the diagnosis of drug-induced disease.

Clinical symptoms usually do not appear for many months after institution of drug treatment. Clinical features of drug-induced lupus erythematosus usually subside within days to weeks once the offending drug is discontinued. Occasionally, symptoms may persist or recur over several months before disappearing. ANAs often disappear in a few weeks to months, but may persist for a year or longer.

Mild symptoms may be managed with NSAIDs; more severe disease may require corticosteroid treatment.

If no satisfactory alternative drug is available, and treatment is essential, the minimum effective dose of the drug and corticosteroids may be given simultaneously with caution and careful observation. With respect to procainamide, drug-induced lupus can be prevented by giving N-acetylprocainamide, the major acetylated metabolite of procainamide. In fact, remission of procainamide-induced lupus has occurred when patients were switched to N-acetylprocainamide therapy.[82,83]

Finally, there are no data to suggest that the presence of ANAs necessitates discontinuance of the drug in symptom-free patients. The low probability of clinical symptoms in seroreactors and the fact that major organs are usually spared in drug-induced lupus erythematosus support this recommendation.[84]

Other Drug-Induced Autoimmune Disorders

In addition to drug-induced lupus erythematosus, D-penicillamine has been associated with several other autoimmune syndromes, such as myasthenia gravis, polymyositis and dermatomyositis, pemphigus and pemphigoid, membranous glomerulonephritis, Goodpasture's syndrome, and immune cytopenias.[77] By binding to cell membranes as a hapten, penicillamine could induce an autologous T-cell reaction, B-cell proliferation, autoantibodies, and autoimmune disorders.[85]

Hypersensitivity Vasculitis

Vasculitis is characterized by inflammation and necrosis of blood vessels. Organs or systems with a rich supply of blood vessels are most often involved. Thus, the skin is often involved in vasculitic syndromes. In the systemic necrotizing vasculitis group (polyarteritis nodosa, allergic granulomatosis of Churg-Strauss syndrome) and granulomatous vasculitides (Wegener's granulomatosis, lymphomatoid granulomatosis, giant cell arteritides), cutaneous involvement is not as common a presenting feature as is seen in hypersensitivity vasculitis (HSV). Also, drugs do not appear to be implicated in the systemic necrotizing and granulomatous vasculitic syndromes.

Drugs appear to be responsible for or associated with a significant number of cases of HSV.[86] HSV can occur at any age, but the average age of onset is in the fifth decade.[87] The older patient is more likely to be taking medications that have been associated with this syndrome, for example, diuretics and cardiac drugs. Other frequently implicated agents include penicillin, sulfonamides, thiouracils, hydantoins, iodides, and allopurinol. Allopurinol administration, particularly in association with renal compromise and concomitant thiazide therapy, has produced a vasculitic syndrome manifested by fever, malaise, rash, hepatocellular injury, renal failure, leukocytosis, and eosinophilia. The mortality rate approaches 25%.[88] In many cases of HSV, no cause is ever identified. Fortunately, idiopathic cases tend to be self-limiting.

The most common clinical feature of HSV is palpable purpura, and the skin may be the only site where vasculitis is recognized. The lesions occur in recurrent crops of varying size and numbers and are usually distributed in a symmetric pattern on the lower extremities and sacral area. Fever, malaise, myalgia, and anorexia may accompany the appearance of skin lesions. Usually, only cutaneous involvement occurs in drug-induced HSV, but glomerulitis, arthralgia or arthritis, abdominal pain and gastrointestinal bleeding, pulmonary infiltrates, and peripheral neuropathy are occasionally present.

The diagnosis of HSV is established by skin biopsy of a lesion demonstrating characteristic neutrophilic infiltrate of the blood vessel wall terminating in necrosis, leukocytoclasis (nuclear dust or fragmentation of nuclei), fibrinoid changes, and extravasation of erythrocytes. This inflammation involves small blood vessels, predominantly postcapillary venules.

When a patient presents with palpable purpura and has started a drug within the previous few months, consideration should be given to stopping that agent.

Generally, the prognosis for HSV is excellent, and elimination of the offending agent, if one exists, usually suffices for therapy. For a minority who have persistent lesions or significant involvement of other organ systems, corticosteroids are indicated.

Predominantly Organ-Specific Reactions

Dermatologic Manifestations

Cutaneous eruptions are the most frequent manifestations of adverse drug reactions and occur in 2% to 3% of hospitalized inpatients.[89] The offending drug could be easily identified in most cases and in one study was confirmed by drug challenges in 62% of patients.[90]

Frequently implicated agents include β-lactam antibiotics (especially ampicillin and amoxicillin), sulfonamides (especially TMP-SMX), NSAIDs, anticonvulsants, and central nervous system depressants.[91]

Drug eruptions are most often exanthematous or morbilliform. Most are of mild or moderate severity, often fade within a few days, and pose no threat to life or subsequent health. On rare occasions, such drug eruptions may be severe or even life-threatening, for example, Stevens-Johnson syndrome and TEN. Some more typical features of a drug-induced eruption include an acute onset within 1 to 2 weeks after drug exposure, symmetric distribution, predominant truncal involvement, brilliant coloration, and pruritus.

Features that suggest a serious reaction include the presence of urticaria, blisters, mucosal involvement, facial edema, ulcerations, palpable purpura, fever, lymphadenopathy, and eosinophilia.[92] The presence of these usually necessitates prompt withdrawal of the offending drug.

Table 17-8 provides a list of recognizable cutaneous eruptions frequently induced by drugs, in which an allergic mechanism is likely or suspected.

Exanthematous or Morbilliform Eruptions

These are the most common drug-induced eruptions and may be difficult to distinguish from viral exanthems. The rash may be predominantly erythematous, maculopapular, or morbilliform (measles-like), and often begins on the trunk or in areas of pressure (e.g., the backs of bedridden patients). Pruritus is variable or minimal. Occasionally, pruritus may be an early symptom, preceding the development of cutaneous manifestations. Gold salts and sulfonamides have been associated with pruritus as an isolated feature. This rash rarely progresses to overt exfoliation, although this is possible.[93]

Usually, this drug-induced eruption appears within a week after institution of treatment. Unlike the generally benign nature of this adverse drug reaction, a syndrome with a similar rash and fever, often with hepatitis, arthralgia, lymphadenopathy, and eosinophilia, has been

TABLE 17-8. *Drug-induced cutaneous manifestations*

Most Frequent

Exanthematous or morbilliform eruptions

Urticaria and angioedema

Contact dermatitis*

    Allergic eczematous contact dermatitis

    Systemic eczematous contact-type dermatitis

Less Frequent

Fixed drug eruptions

Erythema multiforme–like eruptions

    Stevens-Johnson syndrome

Generalized exfoliative dermatitis

Photosensitivity

Uncommon

Purpuric eruptions

Toxic epidermal necrolysis (Lyell's syndrome)

Erythema nodosum

---

*Contact dermatitis is still listed among the top three, but there is evidence that this problem may be decreasing with the purposeful avoidance of topical sensitizers.

termed *hypersensitivity syndrome.*[92] It has a relatively late onset (2 to 6 weeks after onset of treatment), evolves slowly, and may be difficult to distinguish from drug-induced vasculitis. Anticonvulsants, sulfonamides, and allopurinol are the most frequent causes of hypersensitivity syndrome. Recovery is usually complete, but the rash and hepatitis may persist for weeks.

Urticaria and Angioedema

Urticaria with or without angioedema is the second most common drug-induced eruption. It may occur alone or may be part of an immediate generalized reaction, such as anaphylaxis or serum sickness. An allergic IgE-mediated mechanism is often suspected, but it may be the result of a pseudoallergic reaction. A study found that β-lactam antibiotics (through an allergic mechanism) accounted for one third of cases, and NSAIDs (through a pseudoallergic mechanism) accounted for another third of drug-induced urticarial reactions.[94]

Often, urticaria appears shortly after drug therapy is initiated, but its appearance may be delayed for many days. Usually, individual urticarial lesions do not persist much longer than 24 hours, but new lesions may continue to appear in different areas of the body for 1 to 2 weeks. If the individual lesions last longer than 24 hours, or the rash persists for much longer than 2 weeks, the possibility of another diagnosis such as urticarial vasculitis should be considered. A drug-related cause should be considered in any patient with chronic urticaria, which is defined as lasting more than 6 weeks.

Angioedema most often is associated with urticaria, but it may occur alone. Angiotensin-converting enzyme (ACE) inhibitors are responsible for most cases of angioedema that require hospitalization.[95] The risk for angioedema is estimated to be between 0.1% and 0.2% in patients receiving such therapy.[96] The angioedema commonly involves the face and oropharyngeal tissues and may result in acute airway obstruction necessitating emergency intervention. Most episodes occur within the first week of therapy, but occasional reports have been made of angioedema appearing as long as 2 years after initiation of treatment.[97] The mechanism of angioedema is probably ACE inhibitor potentiation of bradykinin.[98] Treatment with epinephrine, antihistamines, and corticosteroids may be ineffective, and the physician must be aware of the potential for airway compromise and the possible need for early surgical intervention. When angioedema follows the use of any one of these agents, treatment with any ACE inhibitor should be avoided.

Allergic Contact Dermatitis

Allergic contact dermatitis is produced by medications or by components of the drug delivery system applied topically to the skin, and is an example of a type IV cell-mediated immune reaction (see Table 17-4). After topical sensitization, the contact dermatitis may be elicited by subsequent topical application. The appearance of the skin reaction and diagnosis by patch testing are similar to those for allergic contact dermatitis from other causes. The diagnosis should be suspected when the condition for which the topical preparation is being applied fails to improve or worsens.

Patients at increased risk for the development of allergic contact dermatitis include those with stasis dermatitis, leg ulcers, perianal dermatitis, and hand eczema.[99]

Common offenders include neomycin, benzocaine, and ethylenediamine. Less common sensitizers include paraben esters, thimerosal, antihistamines, bacitracin, and, rarely, sunscreens and topical corticosteroids.[100]

Neomycin is the most widely used topical antibiotic and has become the most sensitizing of all antibacterial preparations. Other aminoglycosides (e.g., streptomycin, kanamycin, gentamicin, tobramycin, amikacin, and netilmicin) may cross-react with neomycin, but this is not absolute.[101] Neomycin-allergic patients may develop a systemic contact-type dermatitis when exposed to some of these drugs systemically. Many neomycin-allergic patients also react to bacitracin. In addition to neomycin, other topical antibiotics that are frequent sensitizers include penicillin, sulfonamides, chloramphenicol, and hydroxyquinolones. For this reason, they are seldom used in the United States.

Benzocaine, a paraaminobenzoic acid (PABA) derivative, is the most common topical anesthetic associated with allergic contact dermatitis. It is found in many nonprescription preparations, such as sunburn and poison ivy remedies, topical analgesics, throat lozenges, and hemorrhoid preparations. Benzocaine-sensitive patients may show cross-reactivity with other local anesthetics that are based on PABA esters, such as procaine, butacaine, and tetracaine. Suitable alternatives are the local anesthetics based on an amide structure, such as lidocaine, mepivacaine, and bupivacaine. These patients may also react to other paraamino compounds, such as some hair dyes (paraphenylenediamine), PABA-containing sunscreens, aniline dyes, and sulfonamides.

Ethylenediamine, a stabilizer used in some antibiotics- corticosteroid-, and nystatin-containing combination creams, is a common sensitizer. Once sensitized to ethylenediamine topically, a patient may experience widespread dermatitis after the systemic administration of medicaments that contain ethylenediamine, such as aminophylline, hydroxyzine, and tripelennamine.[102]

Among the less frequent topical sensitizers, paraben esters, used as preservatives in topical corticosteroid creams, were thought to be important; however, a study failed to support this assertion.[103] Thimerosal (Merthiolate) is used topically as an antiseptic and also as a preservative. In one study, 7.5% of patients had a positive patch test to this material. Not all such patients are allergic to mercury; many react to the thiosalicylic moiety. Local and even systemic reactions have been ascribed to thimerosal used as a preservative in some vaccines.[104] Systemic administration of antihistamines is rarely, if ever, associated with an allergic reaction; however, topical antihistamines are potential sensitizers, and their use should be avoided. Most instances of allergic contact dermatitis attributed to topical corticosteroids are due to the vehicle, not to the steroid. Patch testing with the highest concentration of the steroid ointment may help identify whether the steroid or the vehicle constituent is responsible. Some attention has already been focused on systemic eczematous contact-type dermatitis.

In summary, physicians should attempt to avoid or minimize the use of common sensitizers, such as neomycin and benzocaine, in the treatment of patients with chronic dermatoses, such as stasis dermatitis and hand eczema. A more comprehensive review of drug-induced allergic contact dermatitis is found elsewhere.[105]

Fixed Drug Eruptions

Fixed drug eruptions, in contrast to most other drug-induced dermatoses, are considered to be pathognomonic of drug hypersensitivity. The term *fixed* relates to the fact that these lesions tend to recur in the same sites each time the specific drug is administered. On occasion, the dermatitis may flare with antigenically related and even unrelated substances.

The characteristic lesion is well delineated, is round or oval, and varies in size from a few millimeters to 25 to 30 cm. Edema appears initially, followed by erythema, which then darkens to become a deeply colored, reddish-purple, dense raised lesion. On occasion, the lesions may be eczematous, urticarial, vesiculobullous, hemorrhagic, or nodular. Mucous membrane involvement, particularly the oral mucous membranes and penis, occasionally has been observed. Usually, a solitary lesion is present, but they may be more numerous, and additional lesions may develop with subsequent administration of the drug. The length of time from reexposure to the drug and the onset of symptoms is 0.5 to 8 hours (mean, 2.1 hours). Lesions usually resolve within 2 to 3 weeks after drug withdrawal, leaving transient desquamation and residual hyperpigmentation.

The mechanism is unknown, but antibody-dependent cellular cytotoxicity may result in keratinocyte damage.[106] Commonly implicated drugs include phenolphthalein, barbiturates, sulfonamides, tetracycline, and NSAIDs.

Treatment is usually not required after the offending drug has been withdrawn because most fixed drug eruptions are mild and not associated with significant symptoms. Corticosteroids may decrease the severity of the reaction without changing the course of the dermatitis.[100]

Erythema Multiforme–like Eruptions

A useful classification for this heterogeneous syndrome has been suggested.[107] It is often a benign cutaneous illness with or without minimal mucous membrane involvement and has been designated *erythema multiforme minor* (EM minor). A more severe cutaneous reaction with marked mucous membrane (at least two mucosal surfaces) involvement and constitutional symptoms has been termed *erythema multiforme major* (EM major). The eponym *Stevens-Johnson syndrome* has become synonymous with EM major. In addition, some have considered TEN to represent the most severe form of this disease process, but others believe it should be considered as a separate entity.

EM minor is a mild, self-limiting cutaneous illness characterized by the sudden onset of symmetric erythematous eruptions on the dorsa of the hands and feet and on the extensor surfaces of the forearms and legs; palms and soles are commonly involved. Lesions rarely involve the scalp or face. Truncal involvement is usually sparse. The rash is minimally painful or pruritic. It is a relatively common condition in young adults 20 to 40 years of age and is often recurrent in nature. Mucous membrane involvement is usually limited to the oral cavity. Typically, the lesions begin as red, edematous papules that may resemble urticaria. Some lesions may develop concentric zones of color change, producing the pathognomonic target or "iris" lesions. The rash usually resolves in 2 to 4 weeks, leaving some residual postinflammatory hyperpigmentation but no scarring or atrophy. Constitutional symptoms are minimal or absent. The most common cause is believed to be herpes simplex virus, and oral acyclovir has been used to prevent recurrence of EM minor.[108]

Most instances of drug-induced EM result in more severe manifestations, classified as EM major or Stevens-Johnson syndrome. This bullous-erosive form is often preceded by constitutional symptoms of high fever, headache, and malaise. Mucous involvement of mucosal surfaces is a more prominent and consistent feature than cutaneous lesions. The cutaneous involvement is more extensive than EM minor, and there is often more pronounced truncal involvement. Painful oropharyngeal mucous membrane lesions may interfere with nutrition. The vermilion border of the lips becomes denuded and develops serosanguinous crusts, a typical feature of this syndrome. Eighty-five percent of patients develop conjunctival lesions, ranging from hyperemia to extensive pseudomembrane formation. Serious ocular complications include the development of keratitis sicca, corneal erosions, uveitis, and even bulbar perforation. Permanent visual impairment occurs in about 10% of patients. Mucous membrane involvement of the nares, anorectal junction, vulvovaginal region, and urethral meatus is less common. The epithelium of the tracheobronchial tree and esophagus may be involved, leading to stricture formation. EM major has a more protracted course, but most cases heal within 6 weeks. [107] The mortality rate approaches 10% among patients with extensive disease. Sepsis is a major cause of death. Visceral involvement may include liver, kidney, or pulmonary disease.

The pathogenesis of this disorder is uncertain, but the histopathologic features suggest an immune mechanism. Deposition of C3, IgM, and fibrin can be found in the upper dermal blood vessels.[109] Unlike immune complex–mediated cutaneous vasculitis, however, in which the cell infiltrate is mostly polymorphonuclear leukocytes, a mononuclear (mostly lymphocytes) cell infiltrate is present around the upper dermal blood vessels.[110] The presence of activated lymphocytes, mainly CD8+ cells, suggests a cell-mediated cytotoxic reaction against epidermal cells.[111] A drug or drug metabolite may bind to the cell surface, after which the patient develops lymphocyte reactivity directed against the drug–cell complex.

Drugs are the most common cause of Stevens-Johnson syndrome, accounting for at least half of cases.[92] Drugs most frequently associated with this syndrome and with TEN include sulfonamides (especially TMP-SMX), anticonvulsants (notably carbamazepine), barbiturates, phenylbutazone, piroxicam, allopurinol, and the aminopenicillins. Occasional reactions have followed the use of cephalosporins, fluoroquinolones, vancomycin, antituberculous drugs, and NSAIDs. Typically, symptoms begin 1 to 3 weeks after initiation of therapy.

Although there is some disagreement, based on a series of 54 patients, early management of Stevens-Johnson syndrome with high-dose corticosteroids (160 to 240 mg/day methylprednisolone) should be implemented.[112] Corticosteroids hastened recovery, produced no major side effects, and were associated with 100% survival and full recovery with no significant residual complications. This recommendation does not apply to the management of TEN.

Drug challenges to establish whether a patient can safely tolerate a drug after a suspected reaction should not be considered with serious adverse reactions such as Stevens-Johnson syndrome, TEN, and exfoliative dermatitis.

Generalized Exfoliative Dermatitis

Exfoliative dermatitis is a serious and potentially life-threatening skin disease characterized by erythema and extensive scaling in which the superficial skin is shed over virtually the entire body. Even hair and nails are lost. Fever, chills, and malaise are often prominent, and there is a large extrarenal fluid loss. Secondary infection frequently develops, and on occasion glomerulitis develops. Fatalities occur most often in elderly or debilitated patients. Laboratory tests and skin biopsy are helpful only to rule out other causes, such as psoriasis or cutaneous lymphoma. High-dose systemic corticosteroids and careful attention to fluid and electrolyte replacement are essential.

Exfoliative dermatitis may occur as a complication of preexisting skin disorders (e.g., psoriasis, seborrheic dermatitis, atopic dermatitis, and contact dermatitis); in association with lymphomas, leukemias, and other internal malignancies; or as a reaction to drugs. At times, a predisposing cause is not evident. The drug-induced eruption may appear abruptly or may follow an apparently benign, drug-induced exanthematous eruption. The process may continue for weeks or months after withdrawal of the offending drug.

Many drugs have been implicated in the development of exfoliative dermatitis, but the most frequently encountered are sulfonamides, penicillins, barbiturates, carbamazepine, phenytoin, phenylbutazone, allopurinol, and gold salts.[113]

No immunologic mechanism has been identified. The diagnosis is based on clinical grounds, the presence of erythema followed by scaling, and drug use compatible with this cutaneous reaction. The outcome is usually favorable if the causative agent is identified and then discontinued and corticosteroids initiated. An older study, however, had a 40% mortality rate, reminding us of the potential seriousness of this disorder.[114]

Photosensitivity

Photosensitivity reactions are produced by the interaction of a drug present in the skin and light energy. The drug may be administered topically, orally, or parenterally. Although direct sunlight (ultraviolet spectrum 2800 to 4500 nm or 280 to 450 mm) is usually required, filtered or artificial light may produce reactions. African Americans have a lower incidence of drug photosensitivity, presumably because of greater melanin protection. The eruption is limited to light-exposed areas, such as the face, the V area of the neck, the forearms, and the dorsa of the hands. Often, a triangular area on the neck is spared because of shielding by the mandible. The infranasal areas and the groove of the chin are also spared. Although symmetric involvement is usual, unilateral distribution may result from activities such as keeping an arm out of the window while driving a car.

Photosensitivity can occur as a phototoxic nonimmunologic phenomenon or, less frequently, as a photoallergic immunologic reaction. Differential features are shown in Table 17-9.

Phototoxic reactions are nonimmunologic, occurring in a significant number of patients on first exposure when adequate light and drug concentrations are present. The drug absorbs light, and this oxidative energy is transferred to tissues, resulting in damage. The light absorption spectrum is specific for each drug. Clinically, the reaction resembles an exaggerated sunburn developing within a few hours after exposure; on occasion, vesiculation occurs. Hyperpigmentation remains in the area. Most phototoxic reactions are prevented if the light is filtered through ordinary window glass. Tetracycline and amiodarone are two of the many agents implicated in phototoxic reactions.[115]

Photoallergic reactions, in contrast, generally go through an eczematous phase and more closely resemble contact dermatitis. Here, the radiant energy presumably alters the drug to form reactive metabolites that combine with cutaneous proteins to form a complete antigen,

TABLE 17-9. *Differential features of photosensitivity*

Feature	Phototoxic	Photoallergic
Incidence	Common	Uncommon
Clinical picture	Sunburn like	Eczematous
Reaction possible with first drug exposure	Yes	Requires sensitization period of days to months
Onset	4–8 h after exposure	12–24 h after exposure once sensitized
Chemical alteration of drug	No	Yes
Ultraviolet range	2800–3100 nm	3200–4500 nm
Drug dosages	Dose related	Dose-independent once sensitized
Immunologic mechanism	None	T-cell mediated
Flares at distant previously involved sites	No	May occur
Recurrence from exposure to ultraviolet light alone	No	May occur in persistent eruptions

to which a T-cell–mediated immunologic response is directed. Such reactions occur in only a small number of patients exposed to the drug and light. The sensitization period may be days or months. The concentration of drug required to elicit the reaction can be very small, and there is cross-reactivity with immunochemically related substances. Flare-ups may occur at lightly covered or unexposed areas and at distant, previously exposed sites. The reaction may recur over a period of days or months after light exposure, even without further drug administration. As a rule, longer ultraviolet light waves are involved, and window glass does not protect against a reaction. The photoallergic reaction may be detected by a positive photopatch test, which involves application of the suspected drug as an ordinary patch test for 24 hours, followed by exposure to a light source. Drugs implicated include the sulfonamides (antibacterials, hypoglycemics, diuretics), phenothiazines, NSAIDs, and griseofulvin.[116]

Purpuric Eruptions

Purpuric eruptions may occur as the sole expression of drug allergy, or they may be associated with other severe eruptions, notably EM. Purpura caused by a drug hypersensitivity may be due to thrombocytopenia.

Simple, nonthrombocytopenic purpura has been described with sulfonamides, barbiturates, gold salts, carbromal, iodides, antihistamines, and meprobamate. Phenylbutazone has produced both thrombocytopenic and nonthrombocytopenic purpura. The typical eruption is symmetric and appears around the feet and ankles or on the lower part of the legs, with subsequent spread upward. The face and neck usually are not involved. The eruption is composed of small, well-defined macules or patches of a reddish brown color. The lesions do not blanch on pressure and often are pruritic. With time, the dermatitis turns brown or grayish brown, and pigmentation may persist for a relatively long period. The mechanism of simple purpura is unknown.

A severe purpuric eruption, often associated with hemorrhagic infection and necrosis with large sloughs, has been associated with coumarin anticoagulants. Although originally thought to be an immune-mediated process, it is now thought to be the result of an imbalance between procoagulant and fibrinolytic factors.[117,118]

Toxic Epidermal Necrolysis

Toxic epidermal necrolysis (Lyell's syndrome) induced by drugs is a rare, fulminating, potentially lethal syndrome characterized by the sudden onset of widespread blistering of the skin, extensive epidermal necrosis, and exfoliation of the skin associated with severe constitutional symptoms. It has been suggested that TEN may represent the extreme manifestation of EM major, but this position has been contested by others who cite the explosive onset of widespread blistering, the absence of target lesions, the epidermal necrosis without dermal infiltrates, and the paucity of immunologic deposits in the skin in TEN.[119]

TEN usually affects adults and is not to be confused with the staphylococcal scalded-skin syndrome seen in children. The latter is characterized by a staphylococcus-elaborated epidermolytic toxin, a cleavage plane high in the epidermis, and response to appropriate antimicrobial therapy. Features of TEN include keratinocyte necrosis and cleavage at the basal layer with loss of the entire epidermis.[120] In addition, the mucosa of the respiratory and gastrointestinal tracts may be affected.

These patients are seriously ill with high fever, asthenia, skin pain, and anxiety. Marked skin erythema progresses for 1 to 3 days to the formation of huge bullae, which peel off in sheets, leaving painful denuded areas. Detachment of more than 30% of the epidermis is expected, whereas less than 10% detachment is compatible with the Stevens-Johnson syndrome.[121] A positive Nikolsky's sign (i.e., dislodgement of the epidermis by lateral pressure) is present on erythematous areas. Mucosal lesions, including painful erosions and crusting, may be present on any surface. The complications of TEN and extensive thermal burns are similar. Unlike in Stevens-Johnson syndrome, high-dose corticosteroids are of no benefit.[112] Mortality may be reduced from an overall rate of 50% to less than 30% by early transfer to a burn center.[122]

The drugs most frequently implicated in TEN include sulfonamides (20% to 28%, especially TMP-SMX), allopurinol (6% to 20%), barbiturates (6%), carbamazepine (5%), phenytoin (18%), and NSAIDs (especially oxyphenbutazone, 18%; piroxicam, isoxicam, and phenylbutazone, 8% each).[123,124]

TEN probably is an immunologically mediated disease because of its association with graft-versus-host disease, reports of immunoreactants in the skin, drug-dependent antiepidermal antibodies in some cases, and altered lymphocyte subsets in peripheral blood and the inflammatory infiltrate.[119] An increased expression of HLA-B12 has been reported in TEN cases.[125]

Erythema Nodosum

Erythema nodosum–like lesions are usually bilateral, symmetric, ill-defined, warm, tender, subcutaneous nodules involving the anterior aspects (shins) of the legs. The lesions are usually red, sometimes resemble a hematoma, and may persist for a few days to several weeks. They do not ulcerate or suppurate and usually resemble contusions as they involute. Mild constitutional symptoms of low-grade fever, malaise, myalgia, and arthralgia may be present. The lesions are seen with streptococcal infections, tuberculosis, leprosy, deep fungal infections, cat scratch fever, lymphogranuloma venereum, sarcoidosis, ulcerative colitis, and other illnesses.

There is some disagreement about whether drugs may cause erythema nodosum. Because the cause of this disorder is unclear, its occurrence simultaneously with drug administration may be more coincidental than causative. Drugs most commonly implicated include sulfonamides, bromides, and oral contraceptives. Several other drugs, such as penicillin, barbiturates, and salicylates, are often suspected but seldom proved as causes of erythema nodosum. Treatment with corticosteroids is effective but is seldom necessary after withdrawal of the offending drug.

Pulmonary Manifestations

Bronchial Asthma

Pharmacologic agents are a common cause of acute exacerbations of asthma, which on occasion, may be severe or even fatal. Drug-induced bronchospasm most often occurs in patients with known asthma but may unmask subclinical reactive airways disease. It may occur as a result of inhalation, ingestion, or parenteral administration of a drug.

Although asthma can occur in drug-induced anaphylaxis or anaphylactoid reactions, bronchospasm is usually not a prominent feature; laryngeal edema is far more common and is a potentially more serious consideration.

Airborne exposure to drugs during manufacture and during final preparation in the hospital or at home has resulted in asthma. Parents of children with cystic fibrosis have developed asthma after inhalation of pancreatic extract powder in the process of preparing their children's meals.[126] Occupational exposure to some of these agents has caused asthma in nurses (e.g., psyllium in bulk laxatives)[127] and in pharmaceutical workers after exposure to various antibiotics.[128] Spiramycin used in animal feed has resulted in asthma among farmers, pet shop owners, and laboratory animal workers who inhale dusts from these products.

NSAIDs account for more than two thirds of drug-induced asthmatic reactions; ASA is responsible for more than half of these.[129]

Both oral and ophthalmic preparations that block β-adrenergic receptors may induce bronchospasm among patients with asthma or subclinical bronchial hyperreactivity. This usually occurs immediately after initiation of treatment but can occur after several months or years of therapy. Metoprolol, atenolol, and labetalol are less likely to cause bronchospasm than are propranolol, nadolol, and timolol.[130] Timolol has been associated with fatal bronchospasm in patients using this opthalmic preparation for glaucoma. Occasional subjects without asthma have developed bronchoconstriction after treatment with β-blocking drugs.[131] Also, β-blockers may increase the occurrence and magnitude of immediate generalized reactions to other agents.[51]

Cholinesterase inhibitors, such as echothiophate ophthalmic solution used to treat glaucoma and neostigmine or pyridostigmine used for myasthenia gravis, have produced bronchospasm. For obvious reasons, methacholine is no longer used in the treatment of glaucoma.

Although ACE inhibitors have been reported to cause acute bronchospasm and to aggravate chronic asthma,[132] a harsh, at times disabling, cough is a more likely side effect that may be confused with asthma. This occurs in 10% to 25% of patients taking these drugs, usually within the first 8 weeks of treatment, although it may develop within days or may not appear for up to 1 year.[133] Switching from one agent to another is of no benefit. The cough typically resolves within 1 to 2 weeks after discontinuing the medication; persistence longer than 4 weeks should trigger a more comprehensive diagnostic evaluation. The mechanism of ACE inhibitor-induced cough is unclear. Early results suggested that cough may not be a problem with a new class of antihypertensive agents that are direct angiotensin II receptor antagonists, such as losartan.[134] Also, ACE inhibitors may cause angioedema and may be a source of cough and dyspnea.[135]

Sulfites and metabisulfites can provoke bronchospasm in a subset of asthmatic patients. The incidence is probably low, but this may be more prevalent among steroid-dependent patients.[136] These agents are used as preservatives to reduce microbial spoilage of foods, as inhibitors of enzymatic and nonenzymatic discoloration of foods, and as antioxidants that are often found in bronchodilator solutions. The mechanism responsible for sulfite-induced asthmatic reactions may be the result of the generation of sulfur dioxide, which is then inhaled. Sulfite-sensitive asthmatic patients, however, are not more sensitive to inhaled sulfur dioxide than other asthmatic patients.[137] The diagnosis of sulfite sensitivity can be established on the basis of sulfite challenge. There is no cross-reactivity between sulfites and ASA. [138] Bronchospasm in these patients can be treated with metered-dose inhalers or nebulized bronchodilator solutions containing negligible amounts of metabisulfites. Although epinephrine contains sulfites, its use in an emergency situation even among sulfite-sensitive asthmatic patients should not be discouraged.[137]

Pulmonary Infiltrates With Eosinophilia

An immunologic mechanism is probably operative in two forms of drug-induced acute lung injury, namely hypersensitivity pneumonitis and pulmonary infiltrates associated with peripheral eosinophilia.

Pulmonary infiltrates with peripheral eosinophilia has been associated with the use of a number of drugs, including sulfonamides, penicillin, NSAIDs, methotrexate, carbamazepine, nitrofurantoin, phenytoin, cromolyn sodium, imipramine, and L-tryptophan.[139] Although a nonproductive cough is the main symptom, headache, malaise, fever, nasal symptoms, dyspnea, and chest discomfort may occur. Many patients develop a maculopapular rash. The chest radiograph may show diffuse or migratory focal infiltrates. Peripheral blood eosinophilia is usually present. Pulmonary function testing reveals restriction with decreased DLCO. A lung biopsy demonstrates interstitial and alveolar inflammation consisting of eosinophils and mononuclear cells. The outcome is usually excellent, with rapid clinical improvement on drug cessation and corticosteroid therapy. Usually, the patient's pulmonary function is restored with little residual damage.

Nitrofurantoin may also induce an acute syndrome, in which peripheral eosinophilia is present in about one third of patients. This reaction differs from the drug induced syndrome just described because tissue eosinophilia is not present, and the clinical picture frequently includes the presence of a pleural effusion.[140] Adverse pulmonary reactions occur in less than 1% of those taking the drug. Typically, the onset of the acute pulmonary reaction begins a few hours to 7 to 10 days after commencement of treatment. Typical symptoms include fever, dry cough, dyspnea (occasional wheezing), and, less commonly, pleuritic chest pain. A chest radiograph may show diffuse or unilateral involvement, with an alveolar or interstitial process that tends to involve lung bases. A small pleural effusion, usually unilateral, is seen in about one third of patients. With the exception of drug-induced lupus, nitrofurantoin is one of only a few drugs producing an acute drug-induced pleural effusion. Knowledge of this reaction can prevent unnecessary hospitalization for suspected pneumonia. Acute reactions have a mortality rate of less than 1%. On withdrawal of the drug, resolution of the chest radiograph findings occurs within 24 to 48 hours.

Although the acute nitrofurantoin-induced pulmonary reaction is rarely fatal, a chronic reaction, which is uncommon, has a higher mortality rate of 8%. Cough and dyspnea develop insidiously after 1 month or often longer of treatment. The chronic reaction mimics idiopathic pulmonary fibrosis clinically, radiologically, and histologically. Although somewhat controversial, if no improvement occurs after the drug has been withdrawn for 6 weeks, prednisone, 40 mg/day, should be given and continued for 3 to 6 months.[139]

Of the cytotoxic chemotherapeutic agents, methotrexate is the most common cause of a noncytotoxic pulmonary reaction in which peripheral blood, but not tissue, eosinophilia may be present.[141] This drug has also been used to treat nonmalignant conditions, such as psoriasis, rheumatoid arthritis, and asthma. Symptoms usually begin within 6 weeks after initiation of treatment. Fever, malaise, headache, and chills may overshadow the presence of a nonproductive cough and dyspnea. Eosinophilia is present in 40% of cases. The chest radiograph demonstrates a diffuse interstitial process, and 10% to 15% of patients develop hilar adenopathy or pleural effusions. Recovery is usually prompt on withdrawal of methotrexate, but the condition can occasionally be fatal. The addition of corticosteroid therapy may hasten recovery time. Although an immunologic mechanism has been suggested, some patients who have recovered may be able to resume methotrexate without adverse sequelae. Bleomycin and procarbazine, chemotherapeutic agents usually associated with cytotoxic pulmonary reactions, have occasionally produced a reaction similar to that of methotrexate.

Pneumonitis and Fibrosis

Slowly progressive pneumonitis or fibrosis is usually associated with cytotoxic chemotherapeutic drugs, such as bleomycin. Some drugs, such as amiodarone, may produce a clinical picture similar to hypersensitivity pneumonitis without the presence of eosinophilia. In many cases, this category of drug-induced lung disease is often dose dependent.

Amiodarone, an important therapeutic agent in the treatment of many life-threatening arrhythmias, has produced an adverse pulmonary reaction in about 6% of patients, and 5% to 10% of these reactions are fatal.[142] Symptoms rarely develop in a patient receiving less than 400 mg/day for less than 2 months. The clinical presentation is usually subacute with initial symptoms of nonproductive cough, dyspnea, and occasionally low-grade fever. The chest radiograph reveals an interstitial or alveolar process. Pulmonary function studies demonstrate a restrictive pattern with a diffusion defect. The sedimentation rate is elevated, but there is no eosinophilia. Histologic findings include the intraalveolar accumulation of foamy macrophages, alveolar septal thickening, and occasional diffuse alveolar damage.[143] Amiodarone has the unique ability to stimulate the accumulation of phospholipids in many cells, including type II pneumocytes and alveolar macrophages. It is unclear whether this causes interstitial pneumonitis, which is present in most patients receiving this drug without any adverse pulmonary reactions. Although an immunologic mechanism has been suggested, the role of hypersensitivity in amiodarone-induced pneumonitis remains speculative.[144] Most patients recover completely after cessation of therapy, although the addition of corticosteroids may be required. Further, when the drug is absolutely required to control a potentially fatal cardiac arrhythmia, patients may be able to continue treatment at the lowest dose possible when corticosteroids are given concomitantly.[145]

Gold-induced pneumonitis is subacute in onset, occurring after a mean duration of therapy of 15 weeks and a mean cumulative dose of 582 mg.[146] Exertional dyspnea is the predominant symptom, although a nonproductive cough and fever may be present. Radiographic findings include interstitial or alveolar infiltrates, while pulmonary function testing reveals findings compatible with a restrictive lung disorder. Peripheral blood eosinophilia is rare. Bronchoalveolar lavage usually shows intense lymphocytosis. The condition is usually reversible after discontinuation of the gold injections, but corticosteroids may be required to reverse the process. Although this pulmonary reaction is rare, it must not be confused with rheumatoid lung disease.

Drug-induced chronic fibrotic reactions are probably nonimmunologic in nature, but their exact mechanism is unknown. Cytotoxic chemotherapeutic agents (azathioprine, bleomycin sulfate, busulfan, chlorambucil, cyclophosphamide, hydroxyurea, melphalan, mitomycin, nitrosoureas, and procarbazine hydrochloride) may induce pulmonary disease that is manifested clinically by the development of fever, nonproductive cough, and progressive dyspnea of gradual onset after treatment for 2 to 6 months or, rarely, years.[147] It is essential to recognize this complication because such reactions may be fatal and could mimic other diseases, such as opportunistic infections. The chest radiograph reveals an interstitial or intraalveolar pattern, especially at the lung bases. A decline in carbon monoxide–diffusing capacity may even precede chest radiograph changes. Frequent early histologic findings include damage to type I pneumocytes, which are the major alveolar lining cells, and atypia and proliferation of type II pneumocytes. Mononuclear cell infiltration of the interstitium may be seen early, followed by interstitial and alveolar fibrosis, which may progress to honeycombing. The prognosis is often poor, and the response to corticosteroids is variable. Even those who respond to treatment may be left with clinically significant pulmonary function abnormalities. Although an immunologic mechanism has been suspected in some cases,[148] it is generally believed that these drugs induce the formation of toxic oxygen radicals that produce lung injury.

Noncardiogenic Pulmonary Edema

Another acute pulmonary reaction without eosinophilia is drug-induced noncardiogenic pulmonary edema. This develops rapidly, and may even begin with the first dose of the drug. The chest radiograph is similar to that seen with congestive heart failure. Hydrochlorothiazide is the only thiazide associated with this reaction.[149] Most of the drugs associated with this reaction are illegal (e.g., cocaine, heroin, and methadone).[150,151] Salicylate-induced noncardiogenic pulmonary edema can occur when the blood salicylate level is more than 40 mg/dL.[152] In most cases, the reaction resolves rapidly after the drug is stopped. Some cases, however, may follow the clinical course of acute respiratory distress syndrome, notably with chemotherapeutic agents such as mitomycin C or cytosine arabinoside and rarely 2 hours after injection of radiographic contrast material.[153] The mechanism is unknown.

Hematologic Manifestations

Many instances of drug-induced thrombocytopenia and hemolytic anemia have been unequivocally shown by in vitro methods to be mediated by immunologic mechanisms. There is less certainty regarding drug-induced agranulocytosis. These reactions usually appear alone, without other organ involvement. The onset is usually abrupt, and recovery is expected within 1 to 2 weeks after drug withdrawal.

Eosinophilia

Eosinophilia may be the sole manifestation of drug hypersensitivity.[154] More commonly, it is associated with other manifestations of drug allergy. Its recognition is useful because it may give early warning of hypersensitivity reactions that could produce permanent tissue damage or even death. Eosinophilia alone, however, is not sufficient reason to discontinue treatment. In fact, some drugs, such as digitalis, may regularly produce eosinophilia, yet hypersensitivity reactions to this drug are rare.

Drugs that may be associated with eosinophilia in the absence of clinical disease include gold salts, allopurinol, aminosalicylic acid, ampicillin, tricyclic antidepressants, capreomycin sulfate, carbamazepine, digitalis, phenytoin, sulfonamides, vancomycin, and streptomycin. No common chemical or pharmacologic feature of these agents appears to account for the development of eosinophilia. Although the incidence of eosinophilia is probably less than 0.1% for most drugs, gold salts have been associated with marked eosinophilia in up to 47% of patients with rheumatoid arthritis, and may be an early sign of an adverse reaction.[155] Drug-induced eosinophilia does not appear to progress to a chronic eosinophilia or hypereosinophilic syndrome. In the face of a rising eosinophil count, however, discontinuing the drug may prevent further problems.

Thrombocytopenia

Thrombocytopenia is a well-recognized complication of drug therapy. The usual clinical manifestations are widespread petechiae and ecchymoses and occasionally gastrointestinal bleeding, hemoptysis, hematuria, and vaginal bleeding. Fortunately, intracranial hemorrhage is rare. On occasion, there may be associated fever, chills, and arthralgia. Bone marrow examination shows normal or increased numbers of normal-appearing megakaryocytes. With the exception of gold-induced immune thrombocytopenia, which may continue for months because of the persistence of the antigen in the reticuloendothelial system, prompt recovery within 2 weeks is expected on withdrawal of the drug.[156] Fatalities are relatively infrequent. Readministration of the drug, even in minute doses, may produce an abrupt recrudescence of severe thrombocytopenia, often within a few hours.

Although many drugs have been reported to cause immune thrombocytopenia, the most common offenders in clinical practice are quinidine, the sulfonamides (antibacterials, sulfonylureas, thiazide diuretics), gold salts, and heparin.

The mechanism of drug-induced immune thrombocytopenia is thought to be the "innocent bystander" type. Shulman[157] suggested the formation of an immunogenic drug–plasma protein complex to which antibodies are formed. This antibody–drug complex then reacts with the platelet (the innocent bystander), thereby initiating complement activation with subsequent platelet destruction. Other studies indicate that quinidine antibodies react with a platelet membrane glycoprotein in association with the drug.[158] Patients with HLA-DR3 appear to be at increased risk of developing gold-induced thrombocytopenia.

Because heparin has had more widespread clinical use, the incidence of heparin-induced thrombocytopenia is about 5%.[159] Some of these patients simultaneously develop acute thromboembolic complications. A heparin-dependent IgG antibody has been demonstrated in the serum of these patients. A low-molecular-weight heparinoid can be substituted for heparin in patients who previously developed heparin-induced thrombocytopenia.[160]

The diagnosis is often presumptive, and the platelet count usually returns to normal within 2 weeks (longer if the drug is slowly excreted) after the drug is discontinued. Many in vitro tests are available at some centers to demonstrate drug-related platelet antibodies. A test dose of the offending drug is probably the most reliable means of diagnosis, but this involves significant risk and is seldom justified.

Treatment involves stopping the suspected drugs, and observing the patient carefully for the next few weeks. Corticosteroids do not shorten the duration of thrombocytopenia but may hasten recovery owing to their capillary protective effect. Platelet transfusions should not be given because transfused platelets are destroyed rapidly and may produce additional symptoms.

Hemolytic Anemia

Drug-induced immune hemolytic anemia may develop through three mechanisms: (1) immune complex, (2) hapten or drug adsorption, and (3) autoimmune induction.[77] Another mechanism involves nonimmunologic adsorption of protein to the red blood cell membrane, which results in a positive Coombs' test but seldom causes hemolytic anemia. Hemolytic anemia after drug administration accounts for about 16% to 18% of acquired cases.

The *immune complex mechanism* accounts for most cases of drug-induced immune hemolysis. The antidrug antibody binds to a complex of drug and a specific blood group antigen, for example Kidd, Kell, Rh, or Ii, on the red-cell membrane.[161] Drugs implicated include quinidine, chlorpropamide, nitrofurantoin, probenecid, Rifampicin, and streptomycin. Many of these drugs have also been associated with immune complex–mediated thrombocytopenia. The serum antidrug antibody is often IgM, and the direct Coombs' test is usually positive.

Penicillin is the prototype of a drug that induces a hemolytic anemia by the *hapten or drug absorption mechanism.*[162] Penicillin normally binds to proteins on the red-cell membrane; and among patients who develop antibodies to the drug hapten on the red cell, a hemolytic anemia may occur. In sharp contrast to immune complex–mediated hemolysis, penicillin-induced hemolytic anemia occurs only with large doses of penicillin, at least 10 million units/day intravenously. Anemia usually develops after 1 week of therapy, more rapidly in patients with preexisting penicillin antibodies. The antidrug antibody is IgG, and the red blood cells are removed by splenic sequestration independent of complement. About 3% of patients receiving high-dose penicillin therapy develop a positive Coombs' test, only some of whom actually develop hemolytic anemia. The anemia usually abates promptly, but mild hemolysis may persist for several weeks. Other drugs occasionally associated with hemolysis by this mechanism include cisplatin and tetracycline.

Methyldopa is the most common cause of an *autoimmune drug-induced hemolysis.* A positive Coombs' test develops in 11% to 36% of patients, depending on drug dosage, after 3 to 6 months of treatment.[163] Less than 1% of patients, however, develop hemolytic anemia. The IgG autoantibody has specificity for antigens related to the Rh complex. The mechanism of autoantibody production is not clear. Hemolysis usually subsides within 1 to 2 weeks after the drug is stopped, but the Coombs' test may remain positive for up to 2 years. These drug-induced antibodies react with normal red blood cells. Because only a small number of patients actually develop hemolysis, a positive Coombs' test alone is not sufficient reason to discontinue the medication. Several other drugs have induced autoimmune hemolytic disease, including levodopa, mefenamic acid, procainamide, and tolmetin.

A small number of patients treated with cephalothin develop a positive Coombs' test due to *nonspecific adsorption of plasma proteins* onto red-cell membranes. This does not result in hemolytic anemia but may provide confusion in blood bank serology.

Finally, several other drugs have been associated with hemolytic disease, but the mechanism is unclear. Such agents include chlorpromazine, erythromycin, ibuprofen, isoniazid, mesantoin, paraaminosalicylic acid, phenacetin, thiazides, and triamterene.

Agranulocytosis

Most instances of drug-induced neutropenia are due to bone marrow suppression, but it can also be mediated by immunologic mechanisms.[164] The process usually develops 6 to 10 days after initial drug therapy; readministration of the drug after recovery may result in a hyperacute fall in granulocytes within 24 to 48 hours. Patients frequently develop high fever, chills, arthralgia, and severe prostration. The granulocytes disappear within a matter of hours, and this may persist 5 to 10 days after the offending drug is stopped. The role of drug-induced leukoagglutinins in producing the neutropenia has been questioned because these antibodies have also been found in patients who are not neutropenic. The exact immunologic mechanism by which some drugs induce neutropenia is unknown.[165] Although many drugs have been incriminated, sulfonamides, sulfasalazine, propylthiouracil, quinidine, procainamide, phenytoin, phenothiazines, semisynthetic penicillins, cephalosporins, and gold are the more commonly reported offenders. After withdrawal of the offending agent, recovery is usual within 1 to 2 weeks, although it may require many weeks or months. Treatment includes the use of antibiotics and other supportive measures. The value of leukocyte transfusions is unclear.

Hepatic Manifestations

The liver is especially vulnerable to drug-induced injury owing to its location, whereby high concentrations of drugs are presented to the liver after ingestion. The liver also has a prominent role in the biotransformation of drugs to potentially toxic reactive metabolites. These reactive metabolites may induce tissue injury through inherent toxicity, or possibly on an immunologic basis.[166] Drug-induced hepatic injury may mimic any form of acute or chronic hepatobiliary disease, but these hepatic reactions are more commonly associated with acute injury.

Some estimates of the frequency of liver injury due to drugs follow:[167]

- More than 2%: aminosalicylic acid, troleandomycin, dapsone, chenodeoxycholate
- 1% to 2%: Lovastatin, cyclosporine, dantrolene
- 1%: Isoniazid, amiodarone
- 0.5% to 1%: Phenytoin, sulfonamides, cholopromazine
- 0.1% to 0.5%: Gold salts, salicylates, methyldopa, chlorpropamide, erythromycin estolate
- Less than 0.01%: ketoconazole, contraceptive steroids
- Less than 0.001%: hydralazine, halothane
- Less than 0.0001%: penicillin, enflurane, cimetidine

Drug-induced liver injury due to intrinsic toxicity of the drug or one of its metabolites is becoming less common. Such toxicity is often predictable because it is frequently detected in animal studies and during the early phases of clinical trials. A typical example of a drug producing such hepatotoxicity is a massive dose of acetaminophen.[168] The excess acetaminophen is shunted into the cytochrome P-450 system pathway, resulting in excess formation of the reactive metabolite that binds to subcellular proteins, which in turn leads to cellular necrosis.

Although there is little direct evidence that an immunologic mechanism (hepatocyte-specific antibodies or sensitized T lymphocytes) is operative in drug-induced hepatic injury, these reactions are often associated with other hypersensitivity features. Injury attributed to hypersensitivity is suspected when there is a variable sensitization period of 1 to 5 weeks; when the hepatic injury is associated with clinical features of hypersensitivity (fever, skin rash, eosinophilia, arthralgia, and lymphadenopathy); when histologic features reveal an eosinophil-rich inflammatory exudate or granulomas in the liver; when hepatitis-associated antigen is absent; and when there is prompt recurrence of hepatic dysfunction after the readministration of small doses of the suspected drug (not usually recommended). After withdrawal of the offending drug, recovery is expected unless irreversible cell damage has occurred. Such liver injury may take the form of cholestatic disease, hepatocellular injury or necrosis, or a mixed pattern.

Drug-induced cholestasis is most often manifested by icterus, but fever, skin rash, and eosinophilia may also be present. The serum alkaline phosphatase levels are often elevated at 2 to 10 times normal, whereas the serum aminotransferases are only minimally increased. Occasionally, antimitochondrial antibodies are present. Liver biopsy reveals cholestasis, slight periportal mononuclear and eosinophilic infiltration, and minimal hepatocellular necrosis. After withdrawal of the offending drug, recovery may take several weeks. Persistent reactions may mimic primary biliary cirrhosis; but antimitochondrial antibodies are usually not present. The most frequently implicated agents are the phenothiazines (particularly chlorpromazine) and the estolate salt of erythromycin; less frequently implicated are nitrofurantoin and the sulfonamides.[169]

Drug-induced hepatocellular injury mimics viral hepatitis but has a higher morbidity rate. Ten to 20% of patients with fulminant hepatic failure have drug-induced injury. The serum aminotransferases are increased, and icterus may develop; the latter is associated with a higher mortality rate. The histologic appearance of the liver is not specific for drug-induced injury. Drugs commonly associated with hepatocellular damage are halothane, isoniazid, phenytoin, methyldopa, nitrofurantoin, allopurinol, and sulfonamides. Damage from isoniazid is due to metabolism of the drug to a toxic metabolite, acetylhydrazine.[170]

Only halothane-induced liver injury has reasonably good support for an immune-mediated process, primarily on the basis of finding circulating antibodies that react with halothane-induced hepatic neoantigen in a significant number of patients with halothane-induced hepatitis.[171] In the United States, enflurane and isoflurane have largely replaced halothane (except in children), and the incidence of hepatic injury appears to be less. Cross-reacting antibodies, however, have been identified in some patients.[172]

Mixed-pattern disease denotes instances of drug-induced liver disease that do not fit exactly into acute cholestasis or hepatocellular injury. There may be moderate abnormalities of serum aminotransferases and alkaline phosphatase levels with variable icterus. Among patients with phenytoin-induced hepatic injury, the pattern may resemble infectious mononucleosis with fever, lymphadenopathy, lymphoid hyperplasia, and spotty necrosis. Granulomas in the liver with variable hepatocellular necrosis are a hallmark of quinidine-induced hepatitis.[173] Other drugs associated with hepatic granulomas are sulfonamides, allopurinol, carbamazepine, methyldopa, and phenothiazines.

Drug-induced chronic liver disease is rare but may also mimic any chronic hepatobiliary disease. Drug-induced chronic active hepatitis has been associated with methyldopa, isoniazid, and nitrofurantoin.[174] Some of these patients may develop antinuclear and smooth muscle antibodies. Also, the chronic liver injury may not improve after the withdrawal of the offending drug.

Renal Manifestations

The kidney is especially vulnerable to drug-induced toxicity because it receives, transports, and concentrates within its parenchyma a variety of potentially toxic substances. Tubular necrosis may follow drug-induced anaphylactic shock or drug-induced immunohemolysis. Immune drug-induced renal disease is rare, but glomerulitis, nephrotic syndrome, and acute interstitial nephritis (AIN) occasionally have been ascribed to drug hypersensitivity.

Glomerulitis is a prominent feature of experimental serum sickness but is rarely of clinical significance in drug-induced, serum sickness–like reactions in humans. In all probability, it is a transient, completely reversible phenomenon that completely subsides once the offending drug has been discontinued. Although spontaneously occurring SLE frequently is associated with glomerulonephritis, drug-induced SLE rarely manifests significant renal involvement. As a rule, cutaneous involvement is the prominent feature of drug-induced vasculitis, but occasionally glomerulonephritis is present. Chronic glomerulonephritis was described in a patient with Munchausen's syndrome who repeatedly injected herself with diphtheria–pertussis–tetanus vaccine.[175] Among heroin addicts, there is a 10% incidence of chronic glomerulonephritis at autopsy. This may be due to immune complexes developing as a result of an immune response to contaminants acquired in the street processing of the drug.[176] A case of Goodpasture's syndrome (pulmonary hemorrhage and progressive glomerulonephritis) was associated with D-penicillamine treatment of Wilson's disease—the first case report of a drug implicated in the cause of this syndrome.[177]

Nephrotic syndrome induced by drugs occurs primarily from immunologic processes that result in membranous glomerulonephritis. This has been more commonly associated with heavy metals (especially gold salts), captopril, heroin, NSAIDs, penicillamine, and probenecid; it is less commonly associated with anticonvulsants (mesantoin, trimethadione, paramethadione), sulfonylureas, lithium, ampicillin, Rifampicin, and methimazole. An immune complex mechanism is probably responsible for this drug-induced nephropathy.[178,179] Proteinuria usually resolves when these agents are discontinued.

AIN, thought to be due to drug hypersensitivity, has been recognized with many agents.[180] More frequently reported drugs include the β-lactam antibiotics (especially methicillin), NSAIDs, Rifampicin, sulfonamide derivatives, captopril, allopurinol, methyldopa, anticonvulsants, cimetidine, and ciprofloxacin. Drug-induced AIN should be suspected when acute renal insufficiency is associated with fever, skin rash, arthralgia, eosinophilia, mild proteinuria, microhematuria, and eosinophiluria beginning days to weeks after initiation of therapy. NSAID-induced AIN usually develops in elderly patients on long-term therapy and is often associated with massive proteinuria and rapidly progressive renal failure.[181] Although the pathogenesis of this drug-induced nephropathy is uncertain, a number of immunologic findings have been documented in methicillin-induced AIN.[182] These include the detection of penicilloyl haptenic groups and immunoglobulin deposition along glomerular and tubular basement membranes, circulating antitubular basement membrane antibodies, a positive delayed skin test reaction to methicillin, and a positive lymphocyte transformation test to methicillin. Also, the lymphocytes infiltrating the renal interstitium are cytotoxic T cells. The prognosis is excellent after discontinuation of the drug, with full recovery expected within 12 months. After recovery, the offending drug and chemically related drugs should be avoided because there have been several cases of cross-reactivity between methicillin and another β-lactam drug, and between various NSAIDs.

Lymphoid System Manifestations

Lymphadenopathy is a common feature of the serum sickness syndrome and may be present in drug-induced SLE. Lymphadenopathy associated with prolonged treatment with anticonvulsants, notably phenytoin, is a rare but well-established disorder that may clinically and pathologically mimic a malignant lymphoma.[183] Cervical lymphadenopathy is most frequent but may be generalized; hepatomegaly and splenomegaly are uncommon. Other features may include fever, a morbilliform or erythematous skin rash, and eosinophilia. Rarely, arthritis and jaundice are present. The pathogenesis of this syndrome is unknown, but phenytoin may induce immunosuppression, which then leads to lymphoreticular malignancies. The reaction usually subsides within several weeks after the drug is stopped and reappears promptly on readministration of the offending drug. Not all patients recover after drug withdrawal, and some develop Hodgkin's disease and lymphoma.[184]

An infectious mononucleosis-like syndrome has been described with phenytoin, aminosalicylic acid, and dapsone.[185]

Cardiac Manifestations

Hypersensitivity myocarditis is rarely identified as a clinical entity. Although endomyocardial biopsy has suggested hypersensitivity myocarditis, reported cases are usually diagnosed at autopsy.[186] Many drugs have been implicated, but the main offenders are the sulfonamides, methyldopa, and penicillin and its derivatives. Many of these drugs have also been associated with HSV. In most cases diagnosed at autopsy, the patients died suddenly and unexpectedly while being treated for an unrelated and nonlethal illness.[187]

The diagnosis should be considered when new electrocardiographic changes appear in association with unexpected tachycardia, mildly elevated cardiac enzymes, and cardiomegaly in a patient with an allergic drug reaction, usually with evidence of eosinophilia.[188] Confirmation is usually obtained a biopsy specimen of the endomyocardium that demonstrates diffuse interstitial infiltrates rich with eosinophils.

Because cellular necrosis in hypersensitivity myocarditis is less prominent than in other forms of myocarditis, permanent cardiac damage is less if the entity is recognized and the offending drug eliminated. Most patients recover in a few days or a few weeks. Aggressive treatment with corticosteroids, immunosuppressives, or both may be necessary if the myocarditis is severe and persistent.

The diagnosed cases probably represent only the a fraction of the true number, with many cases presumably self-limiting and unrecognized. This reaction should not be confused with other types of chronic eosinophilic myocardiopathy, which often lead to permanent cardiac damage and impairment of function.

Neurologic Manifestations

An allergic cause of drug-induced damage to the central and peripheral nervous system is unusual. Postvaccinal encephalomyelitis does resemble experimental encephalomyelitis in animals. A peripheral neuritis has been reported in patients receiving gold salts, colchicine, nitrofurantoin, and sulfonamides, but such reactions have not been analyzed sufficiently to implicate an immunologic mechanism, although this has been suggested.

EVALUATION OF PATIENTS WITH SUSPECTED DRUG HYPERSENSITIVITY

The investigation and identification of a drug responsible for a suspected allergic reaction depends largely on circumstantial evidence and the clinical skills of the physician. Absolute proof that a drug is the actual offender is usually lacking because, with few exceptions, conventional methods to diagnose allergic disorders are either unavailable or unreliable.

A knowledge of the clinical criteria (see Table 17-3) and clinical manifestations (see previous section) ascribed to drug hypersensitivity is helpful in evaluation. None of these clinical manifestations is unique for drug allergy, but physicians should consider this treatable condition along with other diagnostic possibilities.

The complexity and heterogeneity of immune responses induced by drugs, the variety of immunologic tests needed for their detection, and the fact that the relevant drug antigens in most cases cannot be prepared in vitro, but are the result of complex metabolic interactions occurring in vivo, have largely prevented the development of clinically applicable in vivo and in vitro diagnostic tests.

Table 17-10 provides an overview of useful approaches available to evaluate and diagnose allergic drug reactions.

Detailed History

The most important consideration in the evaluation of patients for possible drug allergy is a suspicion by the physician that an unexplained symptom or sign may be due to a drug being administered.

Next in importance is obtaining a complete history of *all* drugs taken within the past month or so as well as a history of any drug reactions. It is helpful to be aware of those drugs most frequently implicated in allergic reactions (Table 17-11).

The clinical features of the reaction may suggest drug hypersensitivity, although morphologic changes associated with drug allergy are often protean in nature and usually not agent

TABLE 17-10. *Overview of methods used to evaluate patients with suspected drug hypersensitivity*

Detailed history*: basis for diagnosis in most cases

  Consider the possibility

  Complete history of *all* drugs taken and any prior reactions

  Compatible clinical manifestations

  Temporal eligibility

In vivo testing: Clinically indicated in some cases

  Cutaneous tests for IgE-mediated reactions*

  Patch tests

  Incremental provocative test dosing*

In vitro testing: Rarely helpful clinically

  Drug-specific IgE antibodies (radioallergosorbent test)

  Drug-specific IgG and IgM antibodies

  Lymphocyte blast transformation

  Others, including mediator release, complement activation, immune complex detection

Withdrawal of the suspected drug*: Presumptive evidence if symptoms clear

  Eliminate any drug not clearly indicated

  Use alternate agents if possible

*These methods are the most available and useful in evaluating allergic drug reactions.

specific. It is helpful to know whether the presenting manifestations have been reported as features of a reaction to the drug being taken.

The history should establish temporal eligibility of the suspected drug. Unless the patient has been sensitized to the same or a cross-reacting drug, there should be an interval between initiation of treatment and the subsequent reaction. For most medications, this interval is rarely less than 1 week, and reactions generally appear within 1 month after initiation of therapy. It is unusual for a drug taken for long periods to be incriminated. This information has proved especially useful in deciding which drug is the likely offender when patients are receiving multiple medications. It is helpful to construct a graph denoting times when drugs were added and discontinued, along with the time of onset of clinical manifestations. For patients previously sensitized to a drug, allergic reactions may occur within minutes or hours after institution of therapy.

In Vivo Testing

In vivo testing for drug hypersensitivity involves skin testing or cautious readministration of the suspected agent (test dosing). Such an approach may be clinically indicated in selected cases.

Immediate Wheal-and-Flare Skin Tests

Prick (puncture) and intradermal cutaneous tests for IgE-mediated drug reactions may be helpful in some clinical situations. Tests must be performed in the absence of medications that interfere with the wheal-and-flare response, such as antihistamines and tricyclic antidepressants. Positive (histamine) and negative (diluent) controls should be used. For safety, prick tests must be negative before proceeding with intradermal tests. A wheal without surrounding erythema is clinically insignificant.[189]

TABLE 17-11. *Drugs frequently implicated in allergic drug reactions*

Drugs	Reactions
Aspirin and nonsteroidal antiinflammatory drugs	Iodinated contrast media
β-Lactam antibiotics	Antihypertensive agents (ACE inhibitors, methyldopa)
Sulfonamides (antibacterials, hypoglycemics, diuretics)	Antiarrythmia drugs (procainamide, quinidine)
Antituberculous drugs (isoniazid, rifampin)	Heavy metals (gold salts)
Nitrofurans	Organ extracts (insulin, other hormones)*
Anticonvulsants (hydantoin, carbamazepine)	Antisera (antitoxins, monoclonal antibodies)*
Anesthetic agents (muscle relaxants, thiopental)	Enzymes* (L-asparaginase, streptokinase, chymopapain)*
Allopurinol	Vaccines (egg-based)*
Antipsychotic tranquilizers	Latex*†
Cisplatin	

*These are complete antigens.
†Not a drug per se, but frequently present in a medical setting.

For large-molecular-weight agents that have multiple antigenic determinants, such as foreign antisera, hormones (e.g., insulin), enzymes, egg-containing vaccines, and latex, positive immediate wheal-and-flare skin test reactions identify patients at risk for anaphylaxis. With low-molecular-weight drugs, skin testing has a role in the evaluation of IgE-mediated reactions to β-lactam antibiotics, and at times has been helpful in the detection of IgE antibodies to muscle relaxants, aminoglycosides, and sulfamethoxazole.

Some reports have been made of immediate wheal-and-flare skin tests to other drugs implicated in immediate generalized reactions, but their significance is uncertain. This should not deter the physician, however, from attempting such with dilute solutions of the suspected drug.[190] It is theoretically possible that a drug may bind to large-molecular-weight carriers at the skin test site, thus permitting the required IgE-antibody crosslinking for mast cell mediator release and the attendant wheal-and-flare response. When such testing is attempted with drugs that have not been previously validated, normal controls must also be tested to eliminate the possibility of false-positive responses. A positive skin test suggests that the patient may be at risk for an IgE-mediated reaction; however, a negative skin test reaction does not eliminate that possibility.

Patch Tests

Patch and photopatch tests are of value in cases of contact dermatitis to topically applied medicaments, even if the eruption was provoked by systemic administration of the drug. In photoallergic reactions, the patch test may become positive only after subsequent exposure to an erythemic dose of ultraviolet light (photopatch testing).

The value of the patch test as a diagnostic tool in systemic drug reactions is unclear. Some patients who have developed maculopapular or eczematous rashes after the administration of carbamazepine, practolol, and diazepam have consistently demonstrated positive patch tests to these drugs.[191]

Incremental Provocative Test Dosing

Direct challenge of the patient with a test dose of the drug (provocative test dosing) remains the only absolute method to establish or exclude an etiologic relation between most suspected drugs and the clinical manifestations produced. In certain situations, it is essential to determine whether a patient reacts to a drug, especially if there are no acceptable substitutes. Provocative testing only to satisfy the patient's curiosity or physician's academic interest is not justified. The procedure is potentially dangerous and is inadvisable without appropriate consultation and considerable experience in management of hypersensitivity phenomena. In fact, in one large series, patients were rechallenged with a drug suspected of producing a cutaneous reaction, and the recurrence rate was 86%, 11% of which were severe reactions.[91]

The principle of incremental test dosing, also known as *graded challenge,* is to administer sufficiently small doses that would not cause a serious reaction initially, and to increase by safe increments (usually 2- to 10-fold) over a matter of hours or days until a therapeutic dose is achieved.[2] Generally, the initial starting dose is 1% of the therapeutic dose; 100- to 1000-fold less if the previous reaction was severe. If the prior reaction was acute (e.g., anaphylaxis), the increased doses may be given at 15- to 30-minute intervals, with the entire procedure completed in 4 hours or less. When the previous reaction was delayed (e.g., morbilliform dermatitis), the interval between doses may be 24 to 48 hours and requires several weeks or longer for completion. Such slow test dosing may not be feasible in urgent situations, such as the need for TMP-SMX in AIDS patients with life-threatening pneumocystis pneumonia. If a reaction occurs during test dosing, a decision must be made whether the drug should be terminated or desensitization attempted.

Test dosing should not be confused with desensitization.[192] With respect to test dosing, the probability of a true allergic reaction is low, but the clinician is concerned about the possibility of such a reaction. It is likely that many of these patients could have tolerated the drug without significant risk, but for safety, reassurance, and medicolegal concerns, this cautious administration has merit. Desensitization is the procedure employed to administer a drug to a patient in whom true allergy has been reasonably well established.

Before proceeding with drug challenges, informed consent must be obtained and the information recorded in the medical record. It is advisable to explain the risks of giving as well as withholding the drug. Appropriate specialty consultation to underscore the need for the drug is desirable, if available. Hospitalization may be required, and emergency equipment to treat anaphylaxis must be available. The drug challenge is performed immediately before treatment, not weeks or months in advance of therapy. Also, prophylactic treatment with antihistamines and corticosteroids before drug challenges is not recommended because these may be needed for treatment of reactions if they occur at low doses.

Drug rechallenges should not be considered when the previous reaction resulted in EM major (Stevens-Johnson syndrome), TEN, exfoliative dermatitis, and drug-induced immune cytopenia.

In Vitro Testing

Testing in vitro to detect drug hypersensitivity has the obvious advantage of avoiding the dangers inherent in challenging patients with the drug. Although the demonstration of the drug-specific IgE is usually considered significant, the presence of other drug-specific immunoglobulin classes or cell-mediated allergy correlates poorly with a clinical adverse reaction. Drug-specific immune responses occur more frequently than clinical allergic drug reactions.

Drug-Specific IgE Antibodies

The in vitro detection of drug-specific IgE antibodies is generally less sensitive than skin testing with the suspected agent. Further, this approach, as was true for skin testing with drugs, is hampered by the lack of information regarding relevant drug metabolites that are immunogenic.

A solid-phase radioimmunoassay, the radioallergosorbent test (RAST), has been validated mainly for the detection of IgE antibodies to the major determinant of penicillin (penicilloyl), and correlates reasonably well with skin tests using penicilloyl-polylysine (PPL). A RAST test for penicillin minor determinant mixture (MDM) sensitivity remains elusive. In addition to penicillin, specific IgE antibodies have been detected in the sera of patients who sustained generalized immediate reactions to other β-lactam antibiotics, sulfamethoxazole, trimethoprim, sodium aurothiomalate, muscle relaxants, insulin, chymopapain, and latex.[193] If positive, these tests may be helpful in identifying patients at risk; if negative, they do not exclude the possibility.

Drug-Specific IgG and IgM Antibodies

With the exception of drug-induced immune cytopenias, there is often little correlation between the presence of drug-specific IgG and IgM antibodies and other drug-induced immunopathologic reactions. The presence of IgG antibodies to protamine in diabetic patients treated with NPH insulin increased the risk of immediate generalized reactions to protamine sulfate.[194]

Drug-induced immune cytopenias afford an opportunity to test affected cells in vitro. Such testing should be performed as soon as the suspicion arises because the antibodies may disappear rapidly after withdrawal of the drug. For drug-induced immune hemolysis, a positive Coombs' test is a useful screening procedure and may be followed by tests for drug-specific antibodies if available. Antiplatelet antibodies are best detected by the complement fixation test and the liberation of platelet factor 3. In vitro tests for drug-induced immune agranulocytosis are often disappointing because leukoagglutinins disappear rapidly and are occasionally present in neutropenic conditions in which no drug is involved.

Lymphocyte Blast Transformation

T-lymphocyte–mediated reactions (delayed hypersensitivity) have been suspected in some patients with drug allergy. Lymphocyte blastogenesis (lymphocyte transformation test) has been suggested as an in vitro diagnostic test for such reactions. This test detects in vitro proliferation of the patient's lymphocytes in response to drugs.[195] A variation on this assay measures the T-lymphocyte cytokine production rather than proliferation.[196] There is disagreement regarding the value of this procedure in the diagnosis of drug allergy. Because there appears to be a high incidence of false-negative and false-positive results, however, these tests have little clinical relevance.[197]

Other Tests

The measurement of mast cell mediator release during drug-induced anaphylaxis or anaphylactoid reactions appears promising. Tryptase is a neutral protease that is specifically released by mast cells and that remains in the serum for at least 3 hours after the reaction.[198] It is a relatively stable protein that may be measured in stored serum samples. After a reaction, several serum samples should be obtained during the first 8 to 12 hours. A positive test for tryptase is helpful, but a negative result does not rule out an immediate generalized reaction.

Complement activation and immune complex assays may be helpful in the evaluation of drug-induced serum sickness–like reactions. Immunoglobulins and complement have been demonstrated in drug-induced immunologic nephritis, but it is often unclear whether the drugs themselves are present in the immune complexes.[199]

Withdrawal of the Suspected Drug

With a reasonable history suggesting drug allergy, and the usual lack of objective tests to support the diagnosis, further clinical evaluation involves withdrawal of the suspected drug followed by prompt resolution of the reaction, often within a few days or weeks. This is presumptive evidence of drug allergy and usually suffices for most clinical purposes.

Typically, patients are taking several medications. Those drugs that are not clearly indicated should be stopped. For drugs that are necessary, an attempt should be made to switch to alternative, non–cross-reacting agents. After the reaction subsides, resumption of treatment with the drug least likely to have caused the problem may be considered, if that drug is sufficiently important.

In some circumstances, it would be detrimental to discontinue a drug when there is no suitable alternative available. The physician must then consider whether the drug reaction or the disease poses a greater risk. If the reaction is mild and does not appear to be progressive, it may be desirable to treat the reaction symptomatically and continue therapy. For example, in patients treated with a β-lactam antibiotic, the appearance of urticaria may be managed with antihistamines or low-dose prednisone. Anaphylaxis has not developed in this setting[3]; however, interruption of therapy for 24 to 48 hours may result in anaphylaxis if treatment is resumed.

PATIENT MANAGEMENT CONSIDERATIONS: TREATMENT, PREVENTION, AND REINTRODUCTION OF DRUGS

Treatment of Allergic Drug Reactions

General Principles

Withdrawal of the suspected drug is the most helpful diagnostic maneuver; it is also the treatment of choice. Frequently, no additional treatment is necessary, and the clinical manifestations often subside within a few days or weeks without significant morbidity. If the reaction is not severe, and more than one drug is a candidate, withdrawal of one drug at a time may clarify the situation.

Clinical situations can occur in which continued use of the suspected drug is essential. The risk of continuing the drug may be less than the risk of not treating the underlying disease, particularly if no suitable alternative drug is available. Careful observation of the patient to detect any progression of the reaction, such as a morbilliform rash becoming exfoliative, and use of allergy suppressants, such as antihistamines and prednisone, may permit completion of the recommended course of therapy.

Some physicians may elect to "treat through" milder reactions, but this is not without risk and should be attempted by physicians with experience. There are also situations in which a manifestation, often cutaneous, appears during the treatment but is due to the basic illness and not to the drug.

Symptomatic Treatment

Pharmacologic management of allergic drug reactions is aimed at alleviating the manifestations until the reaction subsides. For mild reactions, therapy is usually not required. Treatment of more severe reactions depends on the nature of the skin eruption and the degree of systemic involvement.

Drug-induced anaphylaxis and anaphylactoid reactions, urticaria, angioedema, and asthma are treated in a manner described in other chapters in this text dealing with these entities.

For most patients with drug-induced serum sickness or serum sickness–like reactions, treatment with antihistamines is all that is required. More severe manifestations require treatment with prednisone, 40 to 60 mg/day to start, with tapering over 7 to 10 days. Occasionally, plasmapheresis is used to remove immune reactants.

The treatment of Stevens-Johnson syndrome includes high-dose corticosteroid therapy.[112] For milder ambulatory cases, a minimum of 80 mg/day of prednisone is advised. Severe cases require hospitalization and 60 mg of intravenous methylprednisolone every 4 to 6 hours until the lesions show improvement. For TEN, corticosteroids do not suppress the severe cutaneous involvement, and these patients are most efficiently managed in a burn unit. Sepsis is the principal cause of death in affected patients.

For other drug-induced immune reactions, such as drug fever, drug-induced lupus and vasculitis, and reactions involving circulating blood elements and solid organs, corticosteroids accelerate resolution of these adverse drug effects.

Prevention of Allergic Drug Reactions

Drug Considerations

The best way to reduce the incidence of allergic drug reactions is to prescribe only those medications that are clinically essential. Of 30 penicillin anaphylactic deaths, only 12 patients had clear indication for penicillin administration.[200] A survey of patients with allopurinol hypersensitivity syndrome revealed that the drug was given correctly in only 14 of 72 cases, and there were 17 deaths.[201] Also, using many drugs when fewer would be adequate can complicate identification of the offending drug should a reaction occur. The use of drugs in Scotland is about half that in the United States, and the incidence of adverse drug reactions is considerably less.[202]

The physician must be well informed regarding adverse reactions to drugs.

Patient Considerations

The patient or a responsible person must be questioned carefully about a previous reaction to any drug about to be prescribed, and information should also be obtained about all other drugs previously taken. If available, a review of patients' medical records may uncover essential information regarding prior drug reactions. Unfortunately, studies have demonstrated that many health care professionals do not obtain adequate drug histories and document them in the medical record. Such incomplete documentation did not appear to be related to patients' inability to provide accurate information.[203] Failure to follow these simple procedures may not only harm patients but also may result in significant malpractice claims.[204]

Although overdiagnosis may be a problem, it is generally advisable to accept what the patient believes or has been advised without the need for further documentation. Fortunately, alternative, non–cross-reacting agents are available for most clinical situations. In some situations, however, the physician may choose an alternative drug when there is a chance of cross-reactivity, for example, by selecting a cephalosporin in a penicillin-allergic patient to avoid using a more toxic drug, such as an aminoglycoside.

Drug-induced immunologic responses occur in only a small proportion of patients, and even a smaller number express clinical hypersensitivity reactions.

Available Screening Tests

For acute generalized reactions, immediate wheal-and-flare skin tests are sensitive indicators for the detection of specific IgE antibodies to proteins. Skin testing is mandatory before administration of foreign antisera to reduce the likelihood of anaphylaxis (not serum sickness).

Immediate wheal-and-flare skin tests with nonprotein, haptenic drugs have been validated for penicillin, thus permitting identification of patients with histories of penicillin allergy who are no longer at significant risk for readministration of this agent. For other haptenic drugs, such testing may detect drug-specific IgE antibodies when positive at concentrations that do not result in false-positive reactions in normal subjects. Negative skin tests, however, do not eliminate the possibility of clinically significant allergic sensitivity.

None of the available in vitro tests for assessment of drug hypersensitivity qualifies as a screening procedure. Obviously, the simplicity, rapidity, and sensitivity of skin testing makes it a logical choice for clinical purposes.

Methods of Drug Administration

Although there is some disagreement,[34] the oral route of drug administration is perhaps preferable to parenteral administration because it is less apt to sensitize the patient and because allergic reactions are less frequent and generally less severe. Topical use of drugs carries the highest risk of sensitization. For drugs given parenterally, an extremity should be used if possible to permit placement of tourniquet should a reaction occur. In addition, patients should be kept under observation for 30 minutes after parenteral administration of a drug. If the patient is likely to develop a vasovagal reaction after an injection, the drug may be given while the patient is sitting or in a recumbent position.

Prolonged exposure to a drug increases the likelihood of sensitization. The frequency of drug usage increases the chance of eliciting an allergic response. The risk of a reaction appears to be greater during the first few months after a preceding course of treatment.

Follow-Up After an Allergic Drug Reaction

The responsibility to a patient who has sustained an adverse drug reaction does not end with discontinuation of the agent and subsequent management of the reaction. The patient or responsible person must be informed of the reaction and advised how to avoid future exposure to the suspected agent. It is also helpful to mention alternative drugs that may be useful in the future. The patient should be educated regarding the importance of alerting other treating physicians about drugs being taken and about any past adverse drug reactions.

All medical records must prominently display this information in a conspicuous location. The patient could carry a card[205] or wear an identification tag or bracelet (MedicAlert Emblems, Turlock, California 95380) noting those drugs to be avoided.

Reintroduction of Drugs to Patients With Histories of Previous Reactions

If the patient has had a previous documented or suspected allergic reaction to a medication and now requires its use, the physician must consider the risks and benefits of readministration of that drug. When there are no acceptable alternatives available (which is rare these days), if the alternative drug produces unacceptable side effects, or if the alternative drug is less effective, cautious reintroduction of that medication may be considered. Physicians with an interest in hypersensitivity phenomena have evolved a number of management strategies that permit many patients to receive appropriate drug therapy safely or to undergo an essential diagnostic evaluation.[2] These procedures include premedication protocols, desensitization schedules, and test dosing regimens (Fig. 17-1)

Because these approaches constitute reintroduction of an agent previously implicated in an allergic reaction, and thereby carry a risk of a potentially severe, even fatal, reaction, consultation should be obtained from the appropriate specialist to underscore the necessity of the drug and its subsequent readministration. The medical record must contain that information in writing as well as informed consent from the patient or other responsible person. Informed consent must include a statement of potential risks of the procedure as well as risks of withholding the treatment. Further, the medical setting should provide arrangements for emergency treatment of an acute reaction. Ideally, patients should not be receiving β-blocking drugs (even timolol ophthalmic solution); and asthma, if present, must be under optimal control.

Desensitization is best performed by an experienced allergist. Medical supervision is required throughout the procedure. Patients are often frightened by the risks of these proce-

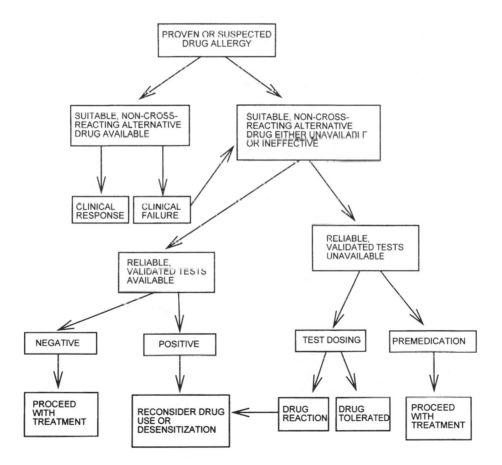

FIG. 17-1. This algorithm provides guidelines for the reintroduction of drugs to a patient with a history of a previous drug reaction.

dures, and symptoms of anxiety may make evaluation difficult. The physician must quickly decide whether to continue or abandon the procedure. In general, the presence of symptoms without objective findings suggests that the reaction may be hysterical, and treatment should be continued.

Premedication

The prophylactic administration of antihistamines and corticosteroids alone or in combination with β-adrenergic agonists has been effective in reducing the incidence and severity of anaphylactoid reactions to radiocontrast media (RCM) among patients with previous histories of such reactions. A similar approach has been used to minimize the likelihood of an anaphylactoid reaction after the administration of intravenous muscle relaxants, opiates, iron dextran, and protamine.[2,206] Drug-induced anaphylactoid events and possibly other situations in which the mechanisms of the reactions are unknown may be susceptible to modification by such pretreatment regimens.

Such premedication protocols are ineffective in blocking drug-induced IgE-mediated anaphylaxis. For this reason, prophylactic therapy before desensitization or test dosing to drugs is not recommended.[2] It is preferable to treat rather than mask a mild reaction occurring at low doses of the drug, rather than risk a more serious reaction at higher doses, which may be more difficult to manage.

Desensitization

Among patients with histories of an immediate generalized reaction to a drug, most likely IgE mediated, desensitization involves the conversion from a highly sensitive state to one in which the drug is tolerated. Ideally, the term *desensitization* should be reserved for reactions that have an established immunologic basis, and the cautious reaction with, and elimination of, IgE antibody is the goal.

Acute desensitization with agents causing IgE-mediated reactions involves the administration of gradually increasing doses of the drug over several hours (e.g., penicillin) or days (e.g., insulin), often starting with amounts as low as $\frac{1}{10,000}$ to $\frac{1}{1,000}$ of the therapeutic dose. The initial desensitizing dose may be based on the results of skin testing or test dosing. This process is accomplished with the agent that is required for treatment. Both oral and parenteral routes have been used for desensitization. The choice of route depends on the clinical condition, the drug being given, and the experience or preference of the attending physician. The intravenous dose is then doubled every 15 minutes while carefully monitoring the patient. Using such a protocol, anaphylaxis has not been reported during desensitization or with continued uninterrupted treatment using a reduced dose. Mild, transient signs and symptoms, however, notably rash or pruritus, occur in about one third of patients during desensitization. These mild reactions may subside spontaneously; they usually respond to symptomatic treatment, dosage adjustment, or both. If therapy is interrupted, anaphylactic sensitivity may return within 48 hours of stopping the drug. Thus, continuation of an agent, such as insulin, after desensitization is appropriate.

This approach has been used successfully to permit treatment with β-lactam antibiotics among patients with histories of penicillin allergy who test positive for the major and minor haptenic determinants of penicillin, among diabetics with systemic insulin allergy, and among patients with positive skin tests to heterologous antisera. Desensitization to these IgE-mediated reactions renders mast cells specifically unresponsive to only the drug antigen used for desensitization. In many patients, successful desensitization is accompanied by a marked decrease or disappearance of the cutaneous wheal-and-flare response. Similar changes in skin test responses have been reported after successful desensitization to aminoglycosides and vancomycin.[207,208]

As noted earlier, the term desensitization has also been used in its broadest sense to describe a state of unresponsiveness to a drug that is accomplished by repeated and increasing exposure to that agent. Similar to acute desensitization for IgE-mediated reactions, these patients have had undeniable reactions to these drugs in the past. Protocols have been described for the cautious administration of ASA, sulfonamides (especially TMP-SMX and sulfasalazine), allopurinol,[209] and others. Unlike desensitization to IgE-mediated reactions, these protocols are often more cumbersome and may require days or even weeks to complete.

Finally, desensitization is a potentially hazardous procedure best left to physicians experienced in managing hypersensitivity phenomena.

Test Dosing

In situations in which a drug is needed and the history of a previous reaction to that agent is vague, and in which the possibility of true allergy is low or the drug itself is an unlikely cause of such a reaction, test dosing or graded challenge is a method used to clarify the situation and safely determine whether the drug may be administered. A common example is a patient who has been advised to avoid all "caines" and now requires a local anesthetic. True systemic allergy to local anesthetics is rare. Test dosing provides reassurance to the patient, physician, or dentist that this agent can be given safely.

The principle of test dosing is to select a dose of the drug below that which would potentially cause a serious reaction, and then to proceed with relatively large incremental increases to full therapeutic doses. Using this technique, the physician can determine whether a reaction occurs before proceeding to the next dose. If a reaction occurs, it can be easily treated. If the drug is necessary, a desensitization protocol may then be considered.

The starting dose, incremental increase, and interval between challenges depend on the drug and the urgency of reaching therapeutic doses. For oral drugs, a usual starting dose is 0.1 or 1 mg, and then proceeds to 10 mg, 50 mg, 100 mg, and 200 mg. For parenteral drugs, the initial dose is less, for example, 0.01 or 0.001 mg. When the suspected reaction was immediate, a 30-minute interval between doses is appropriate, and the procedure is usually completed in 3 to 5 hours or less. For late-onset reactions, such as a dermatitis, the dosing interval may be as long as 24 to 48 hours, with the procedure requiring 1 to 2 weeks or longer. Although there is always the possibility of a severe reaction, the risk of test dosing is low.[192]

SPECIAL CONSIDERATIONS FOR PROVEN OR SUSPECTED ALLERGIC REACTIONS TO INDIVIDUAL DRUGS

Specific recommendations as they pertain to important drugs commonly used in clinical practice are discussed next. For each agent, relevant background information is provided. Additional information about those drugs can be found in the last edition of this text[1] and elsewhere.[3,4,54,62,210]

Table 17-12, based on Patterson,[2] summarizes useful strategies for agents.

TABLE 17-12. *Examples of useful evaluation techniques and management strategies for selected drugs and agents*

Drugs or agents	Skin tests of value	Useful premedication	Test dosing indicated	Desensitization if essential	Additional comments
Immediate Generalized Reactions (IgE Mediated)					
β-Lactam antibiotics	√		See comments	√	Test dose in absence of penicillin minor determinant mixture or validated cephalosporin skin tests
Insulin	√			√	Use least reactive insulin by skin test for desensitization
Immune sera	√			√	Risky in atopic patients allergic to horse dander
Egg-containing vaccines	√			√	May be unnecessary for MMR vaccine
Tetanus toxoid	√			√	If serum antitoxin levels adequate, desensitization not required
Latex	See comments				No standardized skin test available Avoidance is only effective treatment
Protamine		See comments			No studies to validate premedication
Streptokinase	√				Substitute urokinase or tissue plasminogen activator
Chymopapain	√				Consider laminectomy
Immediate Generalized Reactions (IgE Independent)					
Aspirin and nonsteroidal antiinflammatory drugs			√	See comments	Term *desensitization* used, although reaction is not IgE mediated
Contrast media		√			Also useful for nonvascular studies; lower osmolality media a better choice
Opioid analgesics			√		Pentazocine or fentanyl are less active histamine releasers
Cancer chemotherapy		√			Slow infusion and premedication has been useful
Allergy Presumed Mechanism Unclear					
Sulfonamides			√	See comments	Term *desensitization* often used, but reaction is usually not–IgE dependent
Local anesthetics			√		True systemic reactions are rare; reassurance is primary goal.
Anticonvulsants			√		A potentially dangerous procedure
Other rarely incriminated drugs or agents			√		Seek consultation with experienced allergist

Patterson R, DeSwarte RD, Greenberger PA, Grammer LC, Brown JE, Choy AC. Drug allergy and protocols for management of drug allergies. Allergy Proc 1994;15:239.

Penicillins and Other β-Lactam Antibiotics

Background

β-Lactam antibiotic hypersensitivity deserves special consideration because of its medical importance. Penicillin has been extensively studied and has become a prototype for the study of allergic drug reactions. About 10% of hospitalized patients claim a history of penicillin allergy. Clinical experience, however, indicates that many of these patients have been incorrectly labeled as allergic to penicillin[211] and are therefore denied this useful, remarkably nontoxic agent. The reasons for this discrepancy are either a previously incorrect diagnosis or the frequently evanescent nature of penicillin allergy. After an acute allergic reaction, there is a time-dependent decline in the rate of positive skin tests to penicillin of about 10% per year to less than 20% by 10 years.[212] Some patients, however, maintain penicillin-specific IgE antibody indefinitely. It is therefore highly desirable to predict which patients are at risk for a penicillin reaction, and this is now possible.

The overall prevalence of β-lactam allergy is estimated to be about 2% per course of treatment.[213] The most frequent manifestations are cutaneous, notably morbilliform and urticarial eruptions; the most serious is anaphylaxis. In an older, often quoted study, penicillin-induced anaphylaxis occurred in about 0.01% to 0.05% (1 per 5000 to 10,000) of patient treatment courses, with a fatal outcome in 0.0015% to 0.002% (1 death per 50,000 to 100,000 treatment courses).[214] This would translate to 400 to 800 deaths per year in the United States. A more recent report indicated only 16 deaths attributed to penicillin-induced anaphylaxis during 1981.[215] This probably reflects an increased use of other β-lactam antibiotics, notably the cephalosporins, which cause anaphylaxis less frequently.

An atopic background (allergic rhinitis, asthma, atopic dermatitis) does not predispose a patient to the development of penicillin hypersensitivity, but once sensitized, these patients are at increased risk of severe or fatal anaphylactic reactions.[216] Also, atopic patients with *Penicillium* mold allergy can receive penicillin unless specifically allergic to penicillin.

Patients with histories of prior penicillin reactions have a four- to six-fold increased risk of subsequent reactions to β-lactam antibiotics. The administration of this drug causes acute reactions in about two thirds of penicillin-allergic patients, life-endangering anaphylaxis in 5% to 10%, and fatal anaphylaxis in 0.2% to 0.5%.[217]

Although this discussion focuses primarily on the evaluation of and strategies to deal with IgE-mediated reactions, this group of agents has been associated with other adverse, IgE-independent events that are briefly noted here and that have been extensively reviewed elsewhere.[213] *Immediate reactions* occur within the first hour after administration of the β-lactam drug, are IgE mediated, and may present an immediate threat to life. *Accelerated reactions* develop 1 to 72 hours after drug administration, are usually IgE mediated, usually present as urticaria and angioedema, and are rarely life-endangering. *Delayed or late reactions* occur after 3 days, are IgE independent, and usually present as benign morbilliform skin eruptions. Exfoliative dermatitis and the Stevens-Johnson syndrome may occur. Late noncutaneous reactions include serum sickness–like reactions and drug fever. Unusual late reactions are immune cytopenias, AIN, pulmonary infiltrates with eosinophilia, and HSV.

In general, these adverse events are common to all β-lactam antibiotics. Compared with the natural penicillins (penicillin G, penicillin V), anaphylaxis is less common with the penicillinase-resistant penicillins (methicillin, nafcillin, dicloxacillin), the aminopenicillins (ampicillin, amoxicillin), the extended spectrum penicillins (carbenicillin, ticarcillin, mezlocillin, azlocillin, piperacillin), and the cephalosporins.

Individual β-lactam antibiotics have been associated more commonly with certain types of reactions. Ampicillin and amoxicillin therapy is associated with a higher incidence (about

10%) of usually nonpruritic maculopapular rash than are other penicillins (about 2%).[218] The rash usually appears after at least 1 week of therapy, initially develops on the knees and elbows, and then spreads symmetrically to cover the entire body.[93] If the patient has infectious mononucleosis, the incidence approaches 90%. The incidence of this cutaneous reaction is also increased in patients with human immunodeficiency virus infection, cytomegalovirus infection, chronic lymphatic leukemia, and hyperuricemia.[219] This eruption does not appear to be allergic, but if there is an urticarial component, it may represent true IgE-mediated penicillin allergy, and rechallenge could result in a severe immediate generalized allergic reaction.

Cephalosporins produce reactions similar to those described for penicillins. The more common reactions include maculopapular or morbilliform skin eruption, drug fever, and a positive Coombs' test (clinical hemolysis unusual). Less common reactions are urticaria, serum sickness–like reactions (especially with cefaclor in children),[74] and anaphylaxis. Drug-induced cytopenias and AIN are rare. Compared with the first-generation (e.g., cephalothin, cefazolin, cephalexin, cefadroxil, cefaclor) and second-generation (e.g., cefamandole, cefuroxime, cefuroxime axetil) cephalosporins, the third-generation (e.g., cefotaxamine, ceftizoxime, ceftriaxone, ceftazidime, cefixime) cephalosporins have a lower incidence of immediate, presumably IgE mediated, generalized allergic reactions.[220]

Some degree of cross-reactivity among the different classes of β-lactam antibiotics is well established. Since the semisynthetic penicillins contain the same 6-aminopenicillanic acid nucleus as natural penicillin G, it is not surprising that cross-allergenicity between these agents exists, albeit to various degrees. Patients have been identified who have reacted to ampicillin and amoxicillin, but not to penicillin.[221,222] This probably is related to hypersensitivity to the side chains that differentiate the antibiotic from the parent compound. The incidence and clinical significance of these side-chain–specific reactions is unknown. If a patient reports a history of penicillin allergy, however, it is prudent to assume that the patient is allergic to all penicillins.[223]

Cephalosporins share a common β-lactam ring with penicillin but have a six-membered dihydrothiazine ring instead of the five-membered thiazolidine ring of the penicillin molecule. Shortly after the introduction of the cephalosporins into clinical use, allergic reactions, including anaphylaxis, were reported, and the question of cross-reactivity between cephalosporins and penicillins was raised.[224] This issue has not been completely resolved. Significant in vitro cross-reactivity has been demonstrated.[225] Fortunately, clinically relevant cross-reactivity between penicillin and the cephalosporins (especially second- and third-generation agents) is small, but the exact incidence remains a matter of considerable uncertainty. A literature review of patients with histories of penicillin allergy challenged with cephalosporins revealed allergic reactions in 5.6% of patients with positive penicillin skin tests, compared with 1.7% among those with negative penicillin skin tests.[213] A more recent review suggests that penicillin-allergic patients who are identified by either histories or positive penicillin skin tests are not at higher risk than the general population and may be safely treated with cephalosporin antibiotics.[226] Until this issue is completely resolved, cautious administration of cephalosporins to penicillin-allergic patients is advised.

Primary cephalosporin allergy, including anaphylaxis, has occasionally been reported in both penicillin-allergic and penicillin-nonallergic patients, but the exact incidence is unknown.[227] Most investigators have studied tolerance to the cephalosporins in penicillin-allergic patients, but little information is available regarding tolerance to other β-lactam antibiotics in patients with primary cephalosporin allergy. Such studies are limited by the lack of reliable cephalosporin haptenic determinants for skin testing. It appears that antibodies directed against unique side chains rather than to the common ring structure are more important in the immune response to cephalosporins.[228] This would explain the low cross-reactivity among different cephalosporins, which share the same nucleus but have different side chains.[229] It may also help to explain the low cross-reactivity between cephalosporins and penicillins, which share the same β-lactam ring in the nucleus but have different side chains. Until better information is available, it is best to avoid the use of β-lactam antibiotics in cephalosporin-allergic patients; if absolutely indicated, cautious administration is advised.

The carbapenems (imipenem), monobactams (aztreonam), and carbacephems (loracarbef) are three new classes of antibiotics that possess β-lactam ring structures. There is significant cross-reactivity between penicillin and imipenem.[230] Aztreonam is the prototypical monobactam antibiotic. It is weakly immunogenic and may be administered safely to most, if not all, patients allergic to other β-lactam antibiotics.[231] The antibodies generated are specific to the side chain rather than the β-lactam ring. Ceftazidime, however, a third-generation cephalosporin, shares an identical side chain. It may be prudent not to use ceftazidime in subjects allergic to aztreonam. Loracarbef, a carbacephem, structurally resembles cefaclor, but the degree of cross-reactivity with penicillins and cephalosporins is unknown. It is best to avoid its use among patients allergic to β-lactam antibiotics. Finally, clavulanic acid is also a β-lactam antibiotic with weak antibacterial activity, but a potent inhibitor of β-lactamase. It is often combined with amoxicillin to enhance antimicrobial activity. Two immediate generalized allergic reactions have been attributed to clavulanic acid.[232]

Diagnostic Testing

Although obtaining a past history of penicillin allergy is essential, the physician cannot completely rely on that information to predict who is allergic. The history may be inaccurate, and many patients lose their sensitivity over time. The failure to elicit this information has resulted in several fatalities after the administration of these drugs to patients with good histories of β-lactam hypersensitivity.[233] To help clarify this situation, when the drug is essential, skin testing with penicillin has been useful to identify those patients at risk for anaphylaxis and other, milder IgE-mediated reactions. When appropriate skin testing reagents are either unavailable or have not been validated, test dosing with the desired β-lactam antibiotic is recommended.

Benzylpenicillin has a molecular weight of 300 and is metabolized in large part (about 95%) into a penicilloyl hapten moiety. This metabolite is referred to as the *major determinant* and has been conjugated to poly-D-lysine to form PPL, which is commercially available as Pre-Pen (Schwarz Pharma, Kremers-Urban, Milwaukee, WI) for skin testing. Other penicillin metabolites, including benzylpenicillin, constitute 5% or less of administered penicillin and are collectively referred to as the *MDM*. They are minor in name only, being responsible for most penicillin anaphylactic reactions. Unlike PPL, a standardized MDM is not commercially available for skin testing. Therefore, a fresh solution of benzylpenicillin (10,000 U/mL) has been used for skin testing purposes. Skin testing with both PPL and freshly prepared benzylpenicillin (as the sole minor determinant) should detect up to 97% of potential reactors. Almost all patients (99%) with negative skin tests to PPL and MDM reagents can safely be treated with penicillin.[234] In fact, penicillin-induced anaphylaxis has not been reported in patients with negative skin tests. Among patients with positive skin tests receiving penicillin, the risk of an immediate generalized allergic reaction is 10% in patients with negative histories and 50% to 70% in patients with positive histories.[216]

In general, skin testing with benzylpenicillin is also predictive of reactions to other β-lactam antibiotics;[235] however, there are patients with reactions to ampicillin, amoxicillin, and cephalosporin side chains that may not be detected by such testing.[221,222] Although skin testing with the β-lactam antibiotic of therapeutic choice has been advocated to detect additional potential reactors, skin test reagents prepared from other penicillins, cephalosporins, imipenem, and aztreonam have not been standardized, and the results are not validated.[213,236] A positive skin test using these materials suggests the potential for an IgE-mediated reaction, but a negative test does not eliminate this concern. The incidence of such reactions to other β-lactam antibiotics when skin tests are negative to standard penicillin reagents is unknown but is probably small.[237]

In practice, penicillin skin testing to evaluate the potential for or risk of an IgE-mediated reaction should be reserved for patients with histories suggesting penicillin allergy when administration of the drug is essential. Such testing is of no value in predicting the occurrence of non–IgE-mediated reactions and is contraindicated when the previous reaction was Stevens-Johnson syndrome, TEN, or exfoliative dermatitis. Elective penicillin skin testing followed by an oral challenge and a subsequent 10-day course of treatment with penicillin or amoxicillin in patients with negative skin tests has been recommended, particularly for children with a history suggesting penicillin allergy.[238] This procedure should eliminate the need to carry out such testing when the child is ill and in need of penicillin therapy. Using this approach, the risk of resensitization is about 1%. Conversely, penicillin skin testing is risky and probably superfluous among patients with a strong history of penicillin allergy because physicians may be hesitant to give the drug even in patients with negative skin tests.[239] Overall, however, the data support the use of penicillin skin tests in managing patients with histories of penicillin allergy, regardless of the severity of the previous reaction. Penicillin skin testing is rapid, and the risk of a serious reaction is minimal when performed by trained personnel, using recommended drug concentrations, and completing skin prick tests before attempting intradermal skin tests. Testing should be completed shortly before administration of the drug, and possibly repeated before subsequent courses of β-lactam antibiotic treatment.[216,228] In one small study, 16% of adults receiving intravenous penicillin therapy had positive skin tests 1 to 12 months after completion of treatment.[240]

Table 17-13 summarizes the reagents used for β-lactam antibiotic skin tests and the recommended starting concentrations of these reagents, which are adequately sensitive but have a low risk for provoking a systemic or nonspecific irritant reaction. In patients with histories of life-threatening reactions to penicillin, it is advisable to dilute the skin test reagents 100-fold for initial testing. Prick testing is accomplished by pricking through a drop of the reagent placed on the volar surface of the forearm and observing for 15 to 20 minutes. A significant reaction is a wheal 3 mm or larger than the control with surrounding erythema. If negative, intradermal skin tests should follow. Using a tuberculin or allergy syringe, 0.02 mL of the reagent is injected, sufficient to raise a 2- to 3-mm bleb on the volar surface of the forearm. After 15 to 20 minutes, a positive test produces a wheal of 5 mm or larger with surrounding erythema. If the results are equivocal or difficult to interpret, the tests should be repeated. Some investigators disagree about what constitutes an acceptable positive skin test.[236]

Because penicillin MDM is not commercially available and skin testing with other β-lactam antibiotics has not been standardized or the results validated, test dosing is recommended in patients with histories of penicillin allergy and negative skin tests to PPL and penicillin G potassium.[2] How the physician approaches this procedure depends on the severity of the previous reaction and the experience of the managing physician. After documenting the need for the drug, obtaining informed consent, and preparing to treat anaphylaxis, and with a physician in constant attendance, 0.001 mg (1 U) of the therapeutic β-lactam antibiotic is administered by the desired (oral, intravenous) route. The patient is observed for signs of pruritus, flushing, urticaria, dyspnea, and hypotension. In their absence, at 15-minute intervals, subsequent doses are given as outlined in Table 17-14. If a reaction occurs during this procedure,

TABLE 17-13. *β-Lactam antibiotic skin tests*

Skin test reagents	Route	Drug test concentration	Skin test volume	Dose
Benzylpenicilloyl-polylysine* (Pre-Pen; 6×10^{-5} M)	Prick Intradermal	Full strength Full strength	1 drop 0.02 mL	
Penicillin G potassium* (freshly prepared)	Prick Intradermal (Serial 10-fold dilutions optional)§	10,000 U/mL 10,000 U/mL	1 drop 0.02 mL	200 U
Penicillin minor determinant mixture† (10^{-2} M)	Prick Intradermal (Serial 10-fold dilutions optional)§	Full strength Full strength	1 drop 0.02 mL	
Cephalosporins and other penicillins‡	Prick Intradermal (Serial 10-fold dilutions optional)§	3 mg/mL 3 mg/mL	1 drop 0.02 mL	60 μg
Aztreonam‡	Prick Intradermal (Serial 10-fold dilutions optional)§	3 mg/mL 3 mg/mL	1 drop 0.02 mL	60 μg
Imipenem‡	Prick Intradermal (Serial 10-fold dilutions optional)§	1 mg/mL 1 mg/mL	1 drop 0.02 mL	20 μg
Histamine (Histatrol; positive control)	Prick Intradermal	1 mg/mL 0.1 mg/mL	1 drop 0.02 mL	
Saline or diluent (negative control)	Prick Intradermal	NA NA	1 drop 0.02 mL	

*Testing validated.
†Testing validated; reagents not available (except at some medical centers).
‡Testing not validated. Negative tests do not rule out possibility of a reaction.
§Serial skin tests may be prudent when previous reaction was anaphylactic in nature.

it is treated with epinephrine and antihistamines, and the need for the drug should be reevaluated and desensitization considered if this agent is essential. This is a conservative test dosing schedule and may even be useful in situations in which skin testing with PPL and penicillin G potassium has not been successfully completed. More experienced physicians may elect to shorten this procedure, and one suggestion has been to test dose with $^1/_{100}$ of the therapeutic dose ($^1/_{1000}$ of the therapeutic dose if the previous reaction was severe), and then move quickly to the full therapeutic dose if there is no reaction.[213]

Because there is a small risk associated with skin testing and test dosing, in vitro tests have obvious appeal. Solid-phase immunoassays, such as the RAST and the enzyme-linked immunosorbent assay, have been developed to detect serum IgE antibodies against the major penicilloyl determinant. The RAST assay generally correlates with skin testing to PPL but is more time-consuming and less sensitive. A RAST assay for MDM-specific IgE antibodies is unavailable,[241] a serious deficiency when evaluating a patient with possible anaphylactic sensitivity to a β-lactam antibiotic. RAST assays for cephalosporins and other antimicrobial drugs have been reported but are only available for research. Thus, RAST and other in vitro analogues have limited clinical usefulness.

TABLE 17-14. *Suggested test dosing schedule for β-lactam antibiotics*

Dose (mg)*	Dose (U)*
0.001	1
0.005	10
0.01	20
0.05	100
0.10	200
0.50	800
1	1600
10	16,000
50	80,000
100	160,000
200	320,000

Full dose may be administered.

*400,000 U penicillin G potassium is roughly equivalent to 250 mg of other β-lactam antibiotics.

Management of Patients With Histories of Penicillin Allergy

Optimal management of patients with histories of penicillin or other β-lactam antibiotic allergy is the use of an equally effective, non–cross-reacting antibiotic. In most situations, adequate substitutes are usually available,[242] and consultation with infectious disease experts are valuable. Aztreonam, a monocyclic β-lactam antibiotic, has little cross-reactivity with penicillins or cephalosporins but should be used cautiously in patients with prior anaphylactic reactions to these agents.[231] Unfortunately, this antibiotic's activity is limited to aerobic gram-negative bacilli, including *Pseudomonas aeruginosa*.

If alternative drugs fail, induce unacceptable side effects, or are less effective, skin testing and, if necessary, test dosing with the β-lactam antibiotic of choice should be completed. If skin tests are positive, the patient reacts to test doses, or such testing is not done, administration of the β-lactam antibiotic, using a desensitization protocol, is advised.

Infections in which this becomes a more frequent consideration include enterococcal endocarditis, brain abscess, bacterial meningitis, overwhelming sepsis with staphylococcal or pseudomonal organisms, listerial infections, neurosyphilis, and syphilis in pregnant women. In fact, penicillin desensitization is medically indicated among pregnant women with syphilis who demonstrate immediate hypersensitivity to that drug.[243] Also, data do not support the use of alternatives to penicillin for treatment of neurosyphilis and all stages of syphilis among HIV-infected patients.[242]

The usual scenario is a patient who presents with a reasonable history of penicillin allergy and, if available and performed, negative skin tests to PPL and penicillin G potassium. Because important minor determinants are unavailable for skin testing, test dosing as previously outlined is recommended. If a reaction occurs at any test dose, the need for the drug should be reevaluated. If essential, a desensitization protocol should be considered. A more unusual scenario is a patient with a positive history and positive skin tests to available penicillin reagents. These patients are at significant risk for anaphylaxis, particularly if their skin test reactivity was to minor determinants of penicillin. Desensitization protocols significantly reduce the risk of anaphylaxis in patients with positive skin tests.

Acute β-lactam antibiotic desensitization would generally be performed in an intensive care setting. A signed consent form is essential. It may be advisable to point out that alternatives to desensitization may even be more risky. β-adrenergic–blocking drugs, including ophthalmic drops, should be discontinued. Asthmatic patients should be under optimal control. Premedication with antihistamines and corticosteroids is not recommended because these drugs have not been proved effective in suppressing anaphylaxis and could mask mild allergic manifestations that may have resulted in a modification of the desensitization protocol.[216]

Before initiation of desensitization, an intravenous line is established, baseline vital signs are recorded, and the clinical state of the patient is noted. A baseline electrocardiogram and spirometry have been advocated by some as well as continuous electrocardiographic monitoring. During desensitization, vital signs and the clinical state of the patient are noted before each dose and at 5- to 10-minute intervals after each dose. A physician must be in constant attendance during the entire procedure.

Desensitization has been successfully accomplished using either the oral or intravenous routes of administration.[244,245] Oral desensitization is favored by some, who believe that the risk of a serious reaction is less. The intravenous route is chosen by others, who prefer absolute control over the drug concentration used and its rate of administration. Unfortunately, there is no completely standardized regimen, and there have been no direct comparative studies between oral and intravenous desensitizing protocols.

Regardless of the method chosen for desensitization, the basic principles are similar. The initial dose is typically $1/10,000$ of the recommended dose. Oral desensitization may begin with the dose tolerated during oral test dosing. Intravenous desensitization should begin with $1/10$ or $1/100$ (if the previous reaction was severe) of the dose that produced a positive skin test or intravenous test dose response. The dose is then usually doubled at 15-minute intervals until full therapeutic doses are achieved, typically within 4 to 5 hours. Representative protocols for intravenous (Table 17-15) and oral (Table 17-16) desensitization follow.

Table 17-15 outlines an intravenous desensitization protocol for penicillin G potassium or any other β-lactam antibiotic.[3] The dose to be administered is placed in a small volume of 5% dextrose and water for piggyback delivery into the already established intravenous line. It is given slowly at first, then more rapidly if no warning signs, such as pruritus or flushing, appear. If symptoms develop during the procedure, the flow rate is slowed or stopped, and the patient is treated appropriately. After symptoms subside, the flow rate is slowly increased once again. Once the patient has received and tolerated 800,000 U of penicillin G or 800 mg of any other β-lactam antibiotic, the full therapeutic dose can be given and therapy continued without interruption.

Table 17-16 provides a protocol for oral desensitization with β-lactam antibiotics. If the patient is unable to take oral medication, it may be administered through a feeding tube. Mild reactions during desensitization, such as pruritus, fleeting urticaria, mild rhinitis, or wheezing, require the dose to be repeated until tolerated. If a more serious reaction occurs, such as hypotension, laryngeal edema, or severe asthma, the next dose should be decreased to at least one third of the provoking dose and withheld until the patient is stable. If an oral form of the desired β-lactam agent is unavailable, intravenous desensitization should be considered. Once desensitized, treatment must not lapse.

Regardless of the route selected for desensitization, mild reactions, usually pruritic rashes, may be expected in about 30% of patients during and after the procedure. These reactions usually subside with continued treatment, but symptomatic therapy may be necessary.

TABLE 17-15. *Protocol for intravenous desensitization with β-lactam antibiotics*

β-Lactam concentration (mg/mL)	Penicillin G concentration (U/mL)	Dose no.*	Amount given (mL)	Dose given (mg/U)
0.1	160	1	0.10	0.01/16
		2	0.20	0.02/32
		3	0.40	0.04/64
		4	0.80	0.08/128
1	1600	5	0.15	0.15/240
		6	0.30	0.30/480
		7	0.60	0.60/960
		8	1.00	1.0/1600
10	16,000	9	0.20	2.0/3200
		10	0.40	4.0/6400
		11	0.80	8.0/12,800
100	160,000	12	0.15	15.0/24,000
		13	0.30	30.0/48,000
		14	0.60	60.0/96,000
		15	1.00	100.0/160,000
1000	1,600,000	16	0.20	200.0/320,000
		17	0.40	400.0/640,000
		18	0.80	800.0/1,280,000

Observe patient for 30 minutes; administer full therapeutic dose intravenously.

*Dose approximately doubled every 15 minutes.
Sullivan TJ. Drug allergy. In: Middleton E, Reed CE, Ellis EF, Adkinson NF, Yunginger JW, eds. Allergy: Principles and practice. 4th ed. St Louis: CV Mosby, 1993: 1726.

After successful desensitization, some patients may have predictable needs for future exposures to β-lactam antibiotics. Patients with cystic fibrosis, chronic neutropenia, or occupational exposure to these agents may benefit from chronic twice-daily oral penicillin therapy to sustain a desensitized state between courses of high-dose parenteral therapy.[246,247] Some investigators are concerned about the ability to maintain 100% compliance among cystic fibrosis patients in an outpatient setting and therefore prefer to perform intravenous desensitization each time β-lactam antibiotic therapy is required.[248]

In summary, β-lactam antibiotics can usually be administered by desensitization with minimal difficulty among patients with histories of allergy to these drugs and a positive reaction to skin testing or test dosing. Once successfully desensitized, the need for uninterrupted therapy until treatment has been completed is essential to avoid the return of anaphylactic sensitivity. Any lapse in therapy greater than 12 hours may permit such sensitivity to return. Mild reactions during and after desensitization are not an indication to discontinue treatment. Many reactions resolve spontaneously; some require symptomatic therapy.

Among successfully desensitized patients with positive histories of β-lactam allergy and positive responses to skin testing or test dosing, this same approach may be repeated before future courses of therapy. Also, because there appears to be some risk of resensitization after a course of therapy among patients with positive histories and negative skin tests or test dosing,[238,240] these procedures may be repeated before readministration of these agents.

Non–β-Lactam Antimicrobial Agents

Allergic reactions to non–β-lactam antimicrobial drugs, most commonly cutaneous eruptions, are common causes of morbidity and rare causes of mortality. Anaphylaxis to these agents is a rare event. The estimated overall incidence of a hypersensitivity-type reaction to these drugs is about 1% to 3%. Some antimicrobial agents, however, such as TMP-SMX, produce reactions more commonly; whereas others, such as tetracycline, are much less likely to do so.

Unlike the β-lactam antimicrobials, these drugs have been less well studied and also include a wide variety of chemical agents. Research has been hampered by the lack of information regarding the immunochemistry of most of these drugs and, therefore, the unavailability of proven immunodiagnostic tests to assist the physician. Although skin testing with the free drug and some in vitro tests have been described for sulfonamides, aminoglycosides, and vancomycin, no large series have validated their clinical usefulness.

Despite these shortcomings, when such agents, notably TMP-SMX, are medically necessary, protocols have been developed to administer these drugs. With the exception of sulfonamides and occasionally other non–β-lactam drugs, urgent administration is usually not required. Slow, cautious test dosing is generally a safe and effective method to determine whether the drug is now tolerated. An example is to begin with 0.1 mg orally and then, at 30- to 60-minute intervals, to administer 1 mg, 10 mg, and 50 mg. If there is no reaction, on the following day, 100 mg and 200 mg may be given. On occasion, particularly in life threatening *Pneumocystis* or *Toxoplasma* sp infections in AIDS patients, a rapid test dosing schedule

TABLE 17-16. *Protocol for oral desensitization with β-lactam antibiotics*

β-Lactam concentration (mg/mL)*	Dose no.[†]	Amount given (mL)[‡]	Dose given (mg)
0.5	1	0.10	0.05
	2	0.20	0.10
	3	0.40	0.20
	4	0.80	0.40
	5	1.60	0.80
	6	3.20	1.60
	7	6.40	3.20
5	8	1.20	6
	9	2.40	12
	10	4.80	24
50	11	1	50
	12	2	100
	13	4	200
	14	8	400

Observe patient for 30 minutes; give full therapeutic dose by route of choice.

*Dilutions prepared from antibiotic syrup, 250 mg/5 mL.
[†]Dose approximately doubled every 15 minutes.
[‡]Drug amount given in 30 mL water or flavored beverage.
Sullivan TJ. Drug allergy. In: Middleton E, Reed CE, Ellis EF, Adkinson NF, Yunginger JW, eds. Allergy: principles and practice. 4th ed. St Louis: CV Mosby, 1993: 1726.

may be required. Because most reactions to non–β-lactam antimicrobial agents are nonana-phylactic (IgE independent), desensitization is rarely indicated and may be dangerous. A discussion of some of these agents follows.

Sulfonamides

Background

The stimulus for increasing attention to sulfonamide hypersensitivity is due not only to the resurgence of the clinical use of these agents after the introduction of TMP-SMX for treatment of a wide variety of gram-positive and gram-negative bacterial infections, but also to their importance in the treatment of infectious complications in patients with AIDS. In patients infected with HIV, TMP-SMX is effective as prophylaxis and primary therapy for PCP, as prophylaxis for *Toxoplasma gondii* infections, and as treatment for *Isospora belli* gastroenteritis. The combination of sulfadiazine and pyrimethamine is most effective to treat chorioretinitis and encephalitis due to toxoplasmosis in HIV-positive patients. Another sulfonamide, sulfasalazine, is still an important drug in the management of inflammatory bowel disease.

The most common reaction ascribed to sulfonamide hypersensitivity is a generalized rash, usually maculopapular in nature, that develops 7 to 12 days after initiation of treatment. Fever may be associated with the rash. Urticaria is occasionally present, but anaphylaxis is a rare event. In addition, severe cutaneous reactions, such as Stevens-Johnson syndrome and TEN, may occur. Hematologic reactions, notably thrombocytopenia and neutropenia, serum sickness–like reactions, and hepatic and renal complications occasionally occur.

Diagnostic Testing

No in vivo or in vitro tests are available to evaluate the presence of sulfonamide allergy. There is some evidence, however, that some of these reactions are mediated by an IgE antibody directed against its immunogenic metabolite, N^4-sulfonamidoyl.[29] Further, studies using multiple N^4-sulfonamidoyl residues attached to polytyrosine carrier as a skin test reagent have been reported,[249] but additional studies are necessary to evaluate its clinical usefulness. Also, it appears that most sulfonamide reactions are IgE independent. Most adverse reactions are probably due to hydroxylamine metabolites, which induce in vitro cytotoxic reactions in peripheral blood lymphocytes of patients with sulfonamide hypersensitivity.[250–252]

Clinical confirmation of sulfonamide reaction is accomplished by test dosing. This is of concern particularly when treating HIV-positive patients with TMP-SMX, and also with the use of sulfasalazine in the management of inflammatory bowel disease.

Management of Sulfonamide Reactions in Patients With Acquired Immunodeficiency Syndrome

Patients infected with HIV appear to have an increased risk of hypersensitivity reactions to certain drugs.[49] The best-known example of a drug that produces hypersensitivity reactions in such patients is TMP-SMX. Cutaneous eruptions from TMP-SMX occur in 3.4% of medical inpatients[253] and in 29% to 65% of patients with AIDS treated for PCP with this drug.[254] A retrospective study comparing PCP in patients with AIDS to PCP in patients with other underlying immunosuppressive disorders reported adverse reactions to TMP-SMX in 65% of AIDS patients compared with 12% of patients with other immunosuppressive diseases, suggesting that the abnormality may result from the HIV infection rather than from PCP.[255] Such reactions are less frequent among HIV-infected African-American patients.[256] The exact pathogenesis of these reactions is unknown. It is generally accepted that the sulfamethoxazole moiety is responsible for these reactions. Trimethoprim may be a potentiating factor, however.

With a reasonable or definite history of a previous reaction, the preferred approach is to use alternative drugs with similar efficacy. However, TMP-SMX is the drug of choice for treatment of PCP in AIDS patients. Pentamidine is a reasonable alternative to TMP-SMX but is also associated with serious adverse reactions.[257] Cautious readministration of these agents becomes an important consideration. This can be risky, however, because reactions may be severe or delayed in appearance, the disease may progress during the attempt, and the reaction may not be completely reversible. Conversely, these may be insignificant concerns when compared with expected fatal outcome from untreated PCP.

The literature does not provide a standardized protocol for cautious administration of these drugs. A recommended test dosing schedule (sometimes referred to as desensitization) for TMP-SMX begins with administration of 1% of the full dose on day 1, 10% on day 2, 30% on day 3, and the full dose on day 4.[2] By taking several days to complete, delayed reactions may become evident. When more urgent administration is necessary, TMP-SMX has been given intravenously in doses of 0.8, 7.2, 40, 80, 400, and 680 mg (based on the SMX component) at 20-minute intervals.[258] More prolonged courses of oral test dosing, such as 10 and 26 days, have been described.[259,260] Delayed reactions may be treated with 80 mg/day of prednisone and antihistamines to permit completion of the course of therapy for PCP.

Test dosing with intravenous pentamidine has been carried out in the face of a previous reaction to this agent. A stock solution containing 200 mg pentamidine in 250 mL dextrose in water (0.8 mg/mL) is prepared. Starting with a 1:10,000 dilution of this solution, 2 mL is given intravenously over 2 minutes. At 15-minute intervals, 2 mL of 1:1000, 2 mL of 1:100, and 2 mL of 1:10 dilution are administered. After this, 250 mL full-strength solution is given over 2 hours. Successful treatment with aerosolized pentamidine in patients with adverse reactions to systemic pentamidine has been reported using a rapid test dosing schedule.[261]

Rare reports have been made of anaphylactic-like reactions in patients with previous TMP-SMX cutaneous reactions.[262] Several investigators have reported an association between the progression of HIV disease and serum IgE levels.[263] Oral desensitization with TMP-SMX in one such patient has been described, beginning with 0.00001 mg (SMX component) and progressing to full dose treatment in 7 hours.[264] This procedure is rarely indicated and is dangerous.

Prophylaxis against PCP has been suggested for AIDS patients with CD4 cell counts below 200 cells/mm³, for patients with unexplained persistent fever (more than 37.8°C or 100°F) for 2 weeks, for oropharyngeal candidiasis regardless of CD4 cell count, and for patients who have recovered from an episode of PCP.[265] TMP-SMX is the drug of choice. If there has been a previous reaction to this agent, oral test dosing followed by daily administration has been effective.[266] If this is not tolerated, aerosolized pentamidine given by nebulizer once a month has been recommended. For patients who are unable to tolerate both drugs, dapsone may be a reasonable alternative. It appears that TMP-SMX is more effective than aerosolized pentamidine and dapsone.[267]

Sulfadiazine, together with pyrimethamine, is the treatment of choice for toxoplasmosis in HIV-infected patients. Among patients who react to sulfadiazine, clindamycin and pyrimethamine are effective alternatives for treatment of *T gondii* encephalitis. If this fails, rapid test dosing with sulfadiazine can be accomplished by using 1 mg, 10 mg, 100 mg, 500 mg, 1000 mg, and 1500 mg at 4-hour intervals.[268] Delayed cutaneous reactions can be treated with prednisone in an effort to complete the recommended course of therapy.

As noted previously, there are no standard protocols for cautious administration of sulfonamides. In addition to those cited, others have appeared in the literature, and more will probably follow.[259,260,264,269–271] All share the same principles, with the doses recommended, method of delivery, increment in doses, and interval between dosing based on the severity and type of the previous reaction and the urgency for treatment. Such strategies have generally been successful and could be applied to other drugs, for example, antituberculous regimens, which appear to result in an increased incidence of hypersensitivity reactions in patients with AIDS.

Management of Sulfasalazine Reactions in Patients With Inflammatory Bowel Disease

The active therapeutic component in sulfasalazine is 5-aminosalicylic acid, which is linked by an azobond to sulfapyridine. After oral ingestion, sulfasalazine is delivered intact to the colon, where bacteria split the azobond to release 5-aminosalicylic acid, which acts topically on inflamed colonic mucosa. The sulfapyridine component is largely absorbed systemically and accounts for most of the adverse effects attributed to sulfasalazine. The drug is used for mildly or moderately active ulcerative colitis and for maintaining remission of inactive ulcerative colitis. Its role in the management of Crohn's disease is less clear.

An estimated 2% of patients develop what is assumed to be a hypersensitivity reaction, usually a maculopapular rash, fever, or both. Oral 5-aminosalicylic acid preparations (e.g., olsalazine, mesalamine) are often preferred as first-line agents owing to their superior side-effect profile and equivalent therapeutic efficacy compared with sulfasalazine.[272]

For the occasional patient with possible drug allergy who requires sulfasalazine, test dosing has been recommended. One approach starts with a dilute suspension of the drug (liquid sulfasalazine suspension diluted with simple syrup), and the dose is slowly advanced[273] (Table 17-17). If a rash or fever develops, the dose may be reduced, and then advanced more slowly. This approach is ineffective for nonallergic toxicity (headache, nausea, vomiting, abdominal pain) and should not be considered for patients who have had severe reactions, such as Stevens-Johnson syndrome, TEN, agranulocytosis, or fibrosing alveolitis. Most patients were able to achieve therapeutic doses, although some patients required several trials.

With the new aminosalicylate preparations, newer corticosteroid enemas, and the use of other immunosuppressive drugs, the medical management of inflammatory bowel disease continues to improve, and the need for sulfasalazine should decrease.

Other Antimicrobial Agents

Aminoglycosides

Despite the introduction of newer, less toxic antimicrobial agents, the aminoglycosides continue to be useful in the treatment of serious enterococcal and aerobic gram-negative bacillary infections. These agents have considerable intrinsic toxicity, namely nephrotoxicity and ototoxicity.

Hypersensitivity-type reactions to aminoglycosides are infrequent and minor, usually taking the form of benign skin rashes or drug-induced fever. Anaphylactic reactions are rare but have been reported after tobramycin and streptomycin administration. Successful desensitization to tobramycin[274] and streptomycin[275] has been accomplished.

TABLE 17-17. *Test dosing with sulfasalazine*

Day	Dose (mg)
1	1
2	2
3	4
4	8
5–11	10
12	20
13	40
14	80
15–21	100
22	200
23	400
24	800
25–31	1000
32 on	2000

Purdy BH, Philips DM, Summers RW. Desensitization for sulfasalazine rash. Ann Intern Med 1984;100:512.

Vancomycin

Vancomycin is often an alternative treatment for serious staphylococcal and streptococcal infections in patients with severe hypersensitivity reactions to β lactam antibiotics.

Except for the "red man" or "red neck" syndrome, adverse reactions to vancomycin are exceedingly rare. Red man syndrome is characterized by pruritus and erythema or flushing involving the face, neck, and upper torso, occasionally accompanied by hypotension. This has been attributed to the nonimmunologic release of histamine.[276] This complication may be minimized by administering vancomycin over at least a 1- to 2-hour period. Pretreatment with antihistamines (e.g., hydroxyzine) may be protective. Vasopressors may be required if severe hypotension occurs.

Vancomycin has been reported to cause anaphylaxis. Successful desensitization to vancomycin has been reported in a patient with a positive intradermal skin test to the free drug.[208]

Fluoroquinolones

Fluoroquinolones are antimicrobial agents that have a broad range of activity against both gram-negative and gram-positive organisms. Skin rashes or pruritus has been reported in less than 1% of patients receiving these drugs. Anaphylactoid reactions, after the initial dose of ciprofloxacin, have been described.[58]

Tetracyclines

Tetracyclines are bacteriostatic agents with broad-spectrum antimicrobial activity. Hypersensitivity-type reactions, including morbilliform rashes, urticaria, and anaphylaxis, are rarely seen with tetracycline drugs. Doxycycline and demeclocycline may produce a mild to severe photo-toxic dermatitis; minocycline does not. Photosensitivity may occur with all tetracycline drugs.

Chloramphenicol

With the availability of numerous alternative agents and the concern about toxicity, chloramphenicol is used infrequently. In patients with bacterial meningitis and a history of severe β-lactam hypersensitivity, chloramphenicol is a reasonable choice. For treatment of rickettsial infections in young children or pregnant women, in whom tetracycline is contraindicated, this agent is useful.

Bone marrow aplasia is the most serious toxic effect. It is believed to be idiosyncratic and occurs in 1 in 40,000 cases of therapy. It tends to occur in patients who undergo prolonged treatment, particularly if the drug has been administered on multiple occasions. This might suggest an immunologic mechanism, but this has not been established.

Skin rash, fever, and eosinophilia are rarely observed. Anaphylaxis has been rarely reported.[277]

Macrolides

Erythromycin is one of the safest antibiotics. Hypersensitivity-type reactions are uncommon, usually benign skin rashes, fever, and eosinophilia. Cholestatic hepatitis occurs infrequently, most often in association with erythromycin estolate. Recovery is expected on withdrawal of the drug, although it may require a month to resolve.

The newer macrolides, azithromycin and Clarithromycin, are even better tolerated and less toxic. Cholestatic hepatitis has been reported with Clarithromycin.[278]

Clindamycin

Clindamycin is active against most anaerobes, most gram-positive cocci, and certain protozoa. The main concern with clindamycin use is *C difficile* pseudomembranous colitis.

A generalized morbilliform skin rash has been reported in up to 10% of patients in some series. Urticaria, drug fever, eosinophilia, and EM have occasionally been reported.

Metronidazole

Metronidazole is useful against most anaerobes, certain protozoa, and *Helicobacter pylori*. The most common adverse reactions are gastrointestinal. Hypersensitivity reactions, including urticaria, pruritus, and erythematous rash, have been reported. There is a case report of successful oral desensitization in a patient after what appeared to be an anaphylactic event.[279]

Antifungal Agents

Allergic reactions to amphotericin B are rare. A recent report described a patient with amphotericin B–induced anaphylaxis.[280] The patient was successfully challenged intravenously with amphotericin, using a desensitization-type protocol.

Hypersensitivity-type reactions, notably rash and pruritus, occur in 4% to 10% of patients receiving ketoconazole. Itraconazole has occasionally been associated with a generalized maculopapular rash. There is a report of successful oral desensitization in a patient with localized coccidioidomycosis with itraconazole.[281]

Antiviral Agents

Hypersensitivity reactions to antimicrobial and antiretroviral agents are common among HIV-infected patients. A patient was successfully desensitized to zidovudine using a protocol requiring 37 days.[282] Because limited drugs are available to treat people with HIV, such protocols may become increasingly necessary to provide treatment when alternatives are unavailable.

Antituberculous Agents

Many manifestations of hypersensitivity resulting from antituberculous drugs usually appear within 3 to 7 weeks after initiation of treatment. The most common signs are fever and rash, and the fever may be present alone for a week or more before other manifestations develop. The skin rash is usually morbilliform but may be urticarial, purpuric, or rarely exfoliative. Less common manifestations include a lupus-like syndrome (especially with isoniazid). Anaphylaxis rarely has been associated with streptomycin and ethambutol.

A common approach is to discontinue all drugs (usually isoniazid, rifampin, pyrazinamide) and to allow the reaction (usually a rash) to subside. Subsequently, each drug is reintroduced by test dosing to identify the responsible agent. Another drug then may be substituted for the causative agent. Another approach has been to suppress the reaction with an initial dose of 40 to 80 mg/day of prednisone while antituberculous therapy is maintained. This has resulted in prompt clearing of the hypersensitivity reaction. With adequate chemotherapy, steroids do not appear to affect the course of tuberculosis unfavorably. After taking prednisone for several months, the corticosteroid preparation may be discontinued, and the reaction may not reappear.

Multiple Antibiotic Sensitivity Syndrome

Patients who have reacted to any antimicrobial drug in the past have about a 10-fold increased risk of an allergic reaction to another antimicrobial agent.[43] The physician should be aware of this possibility and be prepared to institute treatment promptly.

Aspirin and Other Nonsteroidal Antiinflammatory Drugs

Background

Aspirin and NSAIDs rank second or third to the β-lactam antibiotics in producing allergic-type drug reactions. Unpredictable sensitivity reactions to these agents include (1) bronchospasm in certain patients with nasal polyps and asthma, and (2) an exacerbation of urticaria in many patients with ongoing urticaria or angioedema. The occurrence of both asthma and urticaria triggered by ASA administration in the same patient is rare.[283] In addition, among otherwise normal patients, anaphylactoid and urticarial reactions have occurred within minutes after the ingestion of ASA or a specific NSAID. Although ASA has been recommended to treat systemic mast cell disease, a subset of patients with this disorder experience anaphylactoid reactions after the ingestion of ASA and NSAIDs.[284]

The prevalence of *ASA-induced respiratory reactions* based on the patient's history alone is less than 10% among asthmatic patients older than 10 years of age[285]; based on oral challenge, it is 10% to 20%.[286] In the subpopulation of asthmatic patients with associated rhinosinusitis or nasal polyps, even without a history of ASA-induced respiratory reactions, the prevalence by oral challenge increases to 30% to 40%.[287] Among adult asthmatic patients with histories of ASA sensitivity, the prevalence of ASA-induced respiratory reactions after oral ASA challenges is confirmed in 66% to 97% of cases.[288] Among asthmatic children younger than 10 years of age, the prevalence of ASA sensitivity appears to be less but increases in frequency to that reported in adults during the teenage years. If adequate doses of certain other NSAIDs are used, they induce reactions in a significant number of patients reacting to ASA.

The typical patient is an adult with chronic nonallergic rhinosinusitis, often with nasal polyps, and nonallergic asthma. The asthma is often severe, requiring corticosteroids for optimal control. Most commonly, patients have had established respiratory manifestations for months or years before the first clear episode of an ASA-induced respiratory reaction. Such reactions usually occur within 2 hours after the ingestion of ASA or NSAIDs, may be severe and rarely are fatal. The reaction is often associated with profound nasal congestion, rhinorrhea, and ocular injection.[287]

One of the more attractive hypotheses to explain these ASA- and NSAID-induced respiratory reactions stems from the observation that these drugs share the property of inhibiting the generation of cyclooxygenase products, thereby permitting the synthesis of lipoxygenase products, most notably the leukotrienes, which are capable of inducing bronchospasm. To support this assertion, the 5-lipoxygenase inhibitor, zileuton, has been shown to block the decline in FEV_1 after ASA ingestion among ASA-sensitive asthmatic patients.[289]

A subpopulation of patients with *chronic urticaria* or *angioedema* experience an exacerbation of urticaria after ingesting ASA or NSAIDs.[290] Using appropriate challenge techniques, the prevalence is between 21% and 30%. A reaction is much more likely to occur when the urticaria is active at the time of challenge.[291] Avoidance of these agents eliminates acute exacerbations of urticaria after their ingestion but appears to have little effect on the ongoing chronic urticaria.

The prevalence of *anaphylactoid reactions* after the ingestion of ASA or specific NSAIDs is unknown. Characteristically, these patients appear to be normal and react to only one NSAID or to ASA. Cross-reactivity within the entire class of cyclooxygenase inhibitors is rare. Further, such reactions occur after two or more exposures to the same NSAID. These features suggest the possibility of an IgE-mediated response, but specific IgE against ASA or any NSAID has not been demonstrated. On occasion, urticaria or angioedema alone may occur after the ingestion of ASA or a specific NSAID in patients without ongoing chronic urticaria.

Diagnostic Testing

The diagnosis can usually be established by history and does not require confirmation. In some circumstances, the diagnosis is unclear or a specific diagnosis is required. Skin tests are of no value in the diagnosis of ASA or NSAID sensitivity. Also, no reliable in vitro tests are available for the detection of ASA sensitivity. The only definitive diagnostic test is oral test dosing.[290]

Among asthmatic patients, test dosing with ASA or NSAIDs can provoke a severe bronchospastic reaction and should be attempted only by experienced physicians capable of managing acute, severe asthma in an appropriate medical setting. The asthma should be under optimal control before test dosing is begun. The high risk of this procedure must be considered in relation to its potential benefit. A detailed description of a 3-day test dosing protocol may be found elsewhere.[290,292] A typical starting dose of ASA is 3 mg, progressing to 30 mg, 60 mg, 100 mg, 150 mg, 325 mg, and 650 mg at 3-hour intervals if there is no reaction. If a reaction occurs, subsequent ASA challenges are suspended, and the reaction is treated vigorously with bronchodilators. After an ASA-induced respiratory reaction, there is a 2- to 5-day refractory period during which the patient may tolerate ASA and all other NSAIDs.[293] Although not available in the United States, ASA-lysine has been used for inhalation challenge to verify ASA-sensitive asthmatic patients in Europe.[294] Considering the potential difficulties with test dosing and the fact that ASA and other NSAIDs can usually be avoided, such diagnostic challenges should be reserved for research purposes or for patients with suspected sensitivity to ASA or NSAIDs who require those agents for management of chronic conditions.

For patients with chronic urticaria, test dosing may be performed in an outpatient setting. For those with ongoing urticaria, treatment for the condition should be continued to avoid false-positive results.[291] If the urticaria is intermittent, test dosing can be accomplished during a remission. A typical ASA test dosing protocol is to give 100 mg and 200 mg twice in the morning at 2-hour intervals on day 1, and 325 mg and 650 mg on day 2.[292] Most patients react at doses of 325 mg or 650 mg, and the elapsed time before the reaction appears is 3 to 6 hours after ingestion of the drug. This protocol may be modified by including placebo capsules between ASA dosing.

Test dosing for anaphylactoid reactions is seldom indicated, and some would argue that it should never be attempted because of the risk of fatal anaphylaxis. As previously noted, however, anaphylactoid reactions are usually limited to either ASA or a single NSAID. Therefore, test dosing with another NSAID may demonstrate its safety for use in treating a medical condition. Unfortunately, if ASA sensitivity is the culprit, other NSAIDs are unacceptable alternatives as platelet inhibitors. For this reason, an oral ASA test protocol in an intensive care unit to reach a final dose of 80 mg has been reported.[295]

Management of ASA- and NSAID-Sensitive Patients

Once ASA and other NSAID sensitivity develops, it is present for life. Therefore, strict avoidance of these drugs is critical. Patients should be attentive to the variety of commonly available nonprescription preparations that contain ASA or NSAIDs, such as cold, headache, and analgesic remedies. All NSAIDs that inhibit cyclooxygenase pathways cross-react to varying degrees with ASA in causing respiratory reactions among ASA-sensitive asthmatic patients and in triggering urticarial reactions among patients with chronic urticaria who react to ASA. A list of NSAIDs that cross-react with ASA is provided in Table 17-18.

Among ASA-sensitive patients, acetaminophen is most commonly recommended as an alternative. In one study, however, high doses of acetaminophen, such as 1000 mg, were reported to provoke bronchospasm in about one third of ASA-sensitive asthmatic patients.[296] In general, acetaminophen-induced respiratory reactions are milder and of shorter duration than those induced by ASA. When asthma is stable, test dosing with acetaminophen may be attempted starting with 325 mg. If there is no reaction after 2 to 3 hours, 650 mg is given. After 3 more hours, if there has been no adverse reaction, 1000 mg of acetaminophen may be

TABLE 17-18. *Nonsteroidal antiinflammatory drugs that cross-react with aspirin*

Strong Inhibitors of Cyclooxygenase

Indomethacin (Indocin)

Sulindac (Clinoril)

Tolmetin (Tolectin)

Piroxicam (Feldene)

Diclofenac (Voltaren)

Ibuprofen (Motrin, Advil, Nuprin, Haltran, Medipren)

Naproxen (Naprosyn, Anaprox, Aleve)

Fenoprofen

Ketoprofen (Orudis, Oruvail)

Flurbiprofen (Ansaid)

Ketorolac (Toradol)

Meclofenamate (Meclomen)

Mefenamic acid (Ponstel)

Diflunisal (Dolobid)

Etodolac (Lodine)

Nabumetone (Relafen)

Oxaprozin (Daypro)

Weak Inhibitors of Cyclooxygenase

Acetaminophen (Tylenol, Datril, Excedrin, Midol, Percogesic)

Salsalate (Disalcid)

Phenylbutazone (Butazolidin)

Noninhibitors of Cyclooxygenase

Dextropropoxyphene (Darvon)

Choline magnesium trisalicylate (Trilisate)

Dipyridamole (Persantine)

Hydroxychloroquine (Plaquenil)

given.[297] Salsalate is also a weak cyclooxygenase inhibitor that has provoked asthma in 20% of ASA-sensitive asthmatic patients when given 2000 mg.[298] Dextropropoxyphene and choline magnesium trisalicylate have no effect on cyclooxygenase in vitro and do not appear to cross-react in ASA-sensitive asthmatic patients. Although there have been occasional reports of bronchospastic reactions to hydrocortisone sodium succinate (Solu-Cortef) among ASA-sensitive asthmatic patients, a report did not support this assertion.[299] Also, tartrazine (FD&C yellow dye) does not appear to cross-react with ASA in ASA-sensitive patients.[300]

A practical problem is what advice to give to historically non–ASA-sensitive asthmatic patients regarding the use of ASA and other NSAIDs. One approach is to caution such patients about the potential for such a reaction, particularly if they have nasal polyps and are steroid dependent.[301] Another suggestion is that asthmatic patients with normal sinus radiographs or computed tomographic scans of the sinuses and those with clear evidence of IgE-mediated inhalant respiratory disease have a low incidence of ASA-sensitivity.[302] Treatment with ASA or other NSAIDs may be medically necessary in some patients with ASA-sensitive asthma, such as in the management of a rheumatologic condition or to inhibit platelet aggregation for coronary artery disease prophylaxis. The term desensitization has been applied to this procedure, although many would prefer that this term be reserved for IgE-mediated reactions. The process is identical to oral test dosing with ASA for diagnostic purposes, except that the challenge continues after a positive respiratory reaction.[293] The dose of ASA that caused the reaction is reintroduced after the patient has recovered. If no further reaction occurs, at 3-hour intervals, the dose is gradually increased until either another reaction occurs or the patient can tolerate 650 mg of ASA without a reaction. Once successfully desensitized, cross-desensitization between ASA and all other NSAIDs is complete. This state can be maintained indefinitely if the patient takes at least one dose of ASA daily; if ASA is stopped, it persists for only 2 to 5 days.

ASA desensitization followed by long-term ASA treatment has been advocated for treatment of ASA-sensitive respiratory disease.[303] Such treatment has resulted in improvement in rhinosinusitis with prevention of nasal polyp reformation and improved sense of smell as well as a significant reduction in the need for systemic and inhaled corticosteroids.

Unlike ASA-sensitive asthma, ASA-sensitive urticaria or angioedema does not appear to respond to ASA desensitization.[304] Also, the indications for such among patients with ASA-induced anaphylactoid reactions are limited.[292] ASA desensitization has been employed to prevent synthesis of mast cell–derived PGD_2, a cyclooxygenase product thought to be largely responsible for systemic reactions among patients with systemic mast cell disease who also experienced anaphylactoid reactions after the ingestion of ASA or NSAIDs.[284]

Radiographic Contrast Media

Background

Nonfatal immediate generalized reactions (most commonly urticaria) occur in 2% to 3% of patients receiving conventional ionic hyperosmolar RCM and in less than 0.5% of patients receiving the newer lower osmolar agents. A large prospective study reported severe life-threatening (often anaphylactoid) reactions in 0.22% of those receiving the hyperosmolar media compared with only 0.04% of those receiving lower osmolar preparations.[305] It is clear that the lower osmolar RCM causes significantly fewer adverse reactions,[306] but severe reactions may occur.[307] In fact, the risk of a fatal reaction is the same with either class of RCM and is estimated to be 0.9 cases per 100,000 infusions.[308]

The overall prevalence of reactions to the noniodinated, gadolinium-based contrast agents for magnetic resonance imaging is about 1% to 2%. Severe systemic anaphylactoid reactions to these agents occur rarely, on the order of 1:350,000 injections.[309]

Some patients are at increased risk for an immediate generalized reaction to RCM. The most obvious and important risk factor is a history of a previous reaction to these agents. The exact reaction rate is unknown, but with ionic hyperosmolar RCM, it ranges between 17% and 60%.[310] The administration of nonionic lower osmolar agents to such patients reduces the risk to 5%.[311] Severe coronary artery disease, unstable angina, advanced age, female sex, and receipt of large volumes of contrast media are also risk factors.[307] Atopic and asthmatic patients appear to be more susceptible to anaphylactoid reactions to RCM.[305,312] There is some disagreement about the risk of an immediate generalized reaction to RCM among patients receiving β-adrenergic–blocking agents.[313, 314] The risk is probably not significantly increased; however, reactions may be more severe and less responsive to treatment. Among such patients, the use of lower osmolar RCM and possibly pretreatment with antihistamines and corticosteroids (see later) may be advisable. There is no evidence that patients who have reacted to topical iodine cleansing solutions, iodides, and shellfish are at increased risk for RCM reactions.

Typically, most reactions begin within 1 to 3 minutes after intravascular RCM administration, rarely after 20 minutes. Nausea, emesis, and flushing are most common and may be due to vagal stimulation. Such reactions are to be distinguished from immediate generalized reactions, which include pruritus, urticaria, angioedema, bronchospasm, hypotension, and syncope. Urticaria is the most common reaction. Most of these reactions are self-limiting and respond promptly to the administration of epinephrine and antihistamines. The potential for a fatal outcome must not be ignored, however, and trained personnel must be available to treat hypotension and cardiac or respiratory arrest.

The mechanism of RCM-induced immediate generalized reactions is not fully understood. These reactions are not IgE-mediated but probably involve mast cell activation with release of histamine and other mediators.

Diagnostic Testing

No in vivo or in vitro tests are available to identify potential reactors to RCM. Severe and fatal reactions have occurred after an intravenous test dose of 1 to 2 mL. Also, severe reactions have followed a negative test dose. Graded test dosing has been abandoned.

As noted earlier, a history of a previous reaction to RCM is the most essential information necessary to reduce the likelihood of a repeat reaction.

Management of Patients at Increased Risk for a Repeat RCM Reaction

Among patients with previous reactions to RCM, the incidence and severity of subsequent reactions has been reduced using pretreatment regimens of corticosteroids, antihistamines, and adrenergic agents. Using ionic, hyperosmolar RCM, pretreatment with prednisone and diphenhydramine reduced the prevalence of repeat reactions to about 10%, while the addition of ephedrine to this protocol reduced it further to 5%.[315] The addition of low osmolar, nonionic RCM to the prednisone-diphenhydramine regimen decreased the incidence of repeat reactions even further to 0.5%.[310,316] Most repeated reactions tended to be mild. Unfortunately, the high cost of these newer nonionic agents has limited their use.

The following summarizes a useful approach that can be recommended when patients with histories of a RCM-associated immediate generalized reaction require a repeated study[2]:

1. Document in the medical record the need for the procedure and that alternative procedures are unsatisfactory.
2. Document in the record that the patient or responsible person understands the need for the test, and that the pretreatment regimen may not prevent all adverse reactions.
3. Recommend the use of nonionic, lower osmolar RCM if available.
4. Pretreatment medications:
   A. Prednisone, 50 mg orally 13 hours, 7 hours, and 1 hour before the RCM procedure

B. Diphenhydramine, 50 mg intramuscularly or orally, 1 hour before the RCM procedure
C. Albuterol, 4 mg orally, 1 hour before the RCM procedure (withhold if the patient has unstable angina, cardiac arrhythmia, or other cardiac risks)
5. Proceed with the RCM study and have emergency therapy available.

In some situations, high-risk patients require an emergency RCM study. The following emergency protocol is recommended[2]:

1. Administer hydrocortisone, 200 mg intravenously, immediately and every 4 hours until the study is completed.
2. Administer diphenhydramine, 50 mg intramuscularly, immediately before or 1 hour before the procedure.
3. Administer albuterol, 4 mg orally, immediately before or 1 hour before the procedure.
4. Recommend the use of nonionic, lower osmolar RCM if available.

Because several hours are required for corticosteroids to be effective, it is best to avoid the emergency administration of RCM unless absolutely necessary. The medical record should note that there has not been time for conventional pretreatment and that there is limited experience with such abbreviated programs.

Also, anaphylactoid reactions to RCM may occur when these agents are administered by nonvascular routes, such as by retrograde pyelograms, hysterosalpingograms, myelograms, and arthrograms. Patients with previous reactions who undergo these procedures should receive pretreatment as described earlier.

Finally, the pretreatment protocols are only useful for the prevention of anaphylactoid reactions, but not for other types of life-threatening reactions, such as the adult respiratory tract distress syndrome or noncardiogenic pulmonary edema [317]

Local Anesthetics

Background

Patients who experience adverse reactions of virtually any type after the injection of a local anesthetic are often advised by their dentist or physician that they are allergic to these agents and should never receive "caines" in the future. Such patients are often denied the benefit of local anesthesia and may be subjected to the increased risk of general anesthesia.

Most commonly, these adverse effects appear to be the result of vasovagal reactions, toxic reactions, hysterical reactions, or epinephrine side effects. Contact dermatitis is the most common immunologic reaction to local anesthetics. On occasion, clinical manifestations suggestive of immediate-type reactions are described, but most reported series have shown that such reactions occur rarely, if ever.[318–320]

As shown in Table 17-19, local anesthetics may be classified as benzoic acid esters (group I) or others (group II). On the basis of local anesthetic contact dermatitis and patch testing studies, it appears that the benzoic acid esters often cross-react with each other but do not cross-react with agents in group II. Also, it appears that drugs in group II do no cross-react with each other and are less sensitizing.

Sulfites and parabens, which are used as preservatives in local anesthetics, may be responsible for allergic-like reactions. Such reactions are rare.[321] When confronted with this remote possibility, the pragmatic approach is to avoid preparations containing them. On the other hand, latex-containing products, such as gloves and rubber dams, are often used in dental and

TABLE 17-19. *Classification of local anesthetics*

Benzoic Acid Esters (group I)

Benzocaine*

Butamben picrate (Butesin)*

Chloroprocaine (Nesacaine)

Cocaine*

Procaine (Novocain)

Proparacaine*

Tetracaine (Pontocaine)

Amide or Miscellaneous Structures (group II)

Bupivacaine (Marcaine)†

Etidoocaine (Duranest)†

Lidocaine (Xylocaine)†

Mepivacaine (Carbocaine)†

Prilocaine (Citanest)†

Dibucaine (Nupercaine)†

Paramoxine (Tronothane)*

Dyclonine (Dyclone)*

Antihistamines

*Primarily topical agents.
†Contain amide structure.

surgical practices. Local or systemic reactions can occur in a latex-sensitive patient, and this possibility should be considered in the differential diagnosis of adverse reactions attributed to local anesthetic agents.

Diagnostic Testing

Skin testing as a part of a test dosing protocol is the preferred approach. Prick tests are usually negative. Positive intradermal skin tests are often found in otherwise healthy controls and do not correlate with the outcome of test dosing.[318,320] In vitro testing is not applicable.

Management of Patients With Histories of Reactions to Local Anesthetics

If the local anesthetic agent causing the previous reaction is known, a different local anesthetic agent should be selected for administration for reassurance. For example, if the drug is an ester, an amide could be chosen. If the drug was an amide, another amide could be used.

Another option is the use of an injectable antihistamine, such as diphenhydramine, as a local anesthetic.[322] Although this may provide reasonable anesthesia required for suturing, it is inadequate for dental anesthesia.

Unfortunately, the local anesthetic agent is often unknown, and the clinical details of the previous reaction are often vague, unavailable, or of uncertain significance. For this reason, the following protocol has been effective in identifying a local anesthetic agent that the patient will tolerate[2]:

1. Obtain informed consent.
2. Determine the local anesthetic agent to be used by the dentist or physician. It must not contain epinephrine. These are usually available as ampules.
3. At 15-minute intervals:
   Administer skin test using a prick test of the undiluted local anesthetic.
   If negative, inject 0.1 mL of a 1:100 dilution subcutaneously in an extremity.
   If no local reaction, inject 0.1 mL of a 1:10 dilution of local anesthetic subcutaneously.
   If no local reaction, inject 0.1 mL of undiluted local anesthetic agent.
   If no local reaction, inject 1 mL and then 2 mL of the undiluted local anesthetic agent.
4. After this procedure, give a letter to the patient indicating that the patient has received 3 mL of the respective local anesthetic with no reaction and is at no greater risk for a subsequent allergic reaction than the general population.
5. Such test dosing should be undertaken by physicians with training and experience in such tests and in the treatment of anaphylactic reactions.

This regimen should be completed shortly before the anticipated procedure, not weeks or months in advance. It should not be done simply to satisfy the curiosity of the patient or the referring dentist or physician. We are not aware of any patient with negative test dosing who reacted later when the local anesthetic agent was used for a procedure. The success of this approach is undoubtedly related to the rarity of true allergic reactions to local anesthetic agents. At the least, however, the protocol serves to allay the anxiety of patients and referring dentists and physicians and, at the most, it may permit one to identify safely that rare patient truly at risk for an allergic reaction to subsequent local anesthetic administration.

Insulin

Background

The exact incidence of insulin allergy is unknown, but it appears to be declining.[323] The increasing use of human recombinant DNA (rDNA) insulin may in part be responsible. However, human rDNA insulin has been associated with severe allergic reactions.[324] Alteration of the tertiary structure of the insulin molecule was the likely source of its immunogenicity. Patients with systemic allergy to animal source insulins have demonstrated cutaneous reactivity to human rDNA insulin.[325] In addition, IgE and IgG antibody directed against human rDNA insulin was detected in the sera of these patients.[326] In most patients, the antiinsulin antibody appears to be directed against a determinant present in all commercially available insulins.[327]

Most patients receiving insulin daily for several weeks, regardless of the preparation used, develop antibodies of all Ig classes to insulin. These antibodies may bind insulin, rendering it biologically inactive; however, the binding capacity is usually low, and insulin resistance does not occur.[328] About 40% of patients receiving animal (bovine, porcine) source insulin develop clinically insignificant immediate wheal-and-flare skin test reactivity to the insulin selected for treatment. The incidence of cutaneous reactivity in patients receiving human rDNA insulin is unknown. It has been suggested that the presence of antiinsulin IgG antibodies may serve as blocking antibodies and prevent allergic reactions in patients with antiinsulin IgE antibodies. Immunologic insulin resistance that is due to antiinsulin IgG antibodies may alternate or occur simultaneously with IgE-mediated insulin allergy.[329]

The most common, clinically important, immunologic reactions to insulin are local and systemic allergic reactions and insulin resistance.

Local allergic reactions are most common and usually appear within the first 1 to 4 weeks of treatment. They are usually mild and consist of erythema, induration, burning, and pruritus at the injection site. They may occur immediately (15 to 30 minutes) after the injection or may be delayed for 4 hours or more. Some patients have a biphasic IgE reaction in which the initial local reaction resolves within about an hour and is followed by a delayed indurated lesion 4 to 6 hours later that persists for 24 hours.[330] These local allergic reactions almost always disappear in 3 to 4 weeks with continued insulin administration. Occasionally, they may persist and may precede a systemic reaction. In fact, stopping treatment because of local reactions may increase the risk of a systemic allergic reaction when insulin therapy is resumed. Treatment of local reactions, if necessary at all, involves the administration of antihistamines for several weeks for symptomatic relief until the reaction disappears. On occasion, it may be necessary to switch to a different preparation.

Systemic allergic reactions to insulin are IgE mediated and are characterized by urticaria, angioedema, bronchospasm, and hypotension. Such reactions are rare. Most commonly, these patients have histories of interruption in insulin treatment. Systemic reactions occur most frequently within 12 days of resumption of insulin therapy and are often preceded by the development of progressively larger local reactions.

Immunologic insulin resistance is rare and is related to the development of antiinsulin IgG antibodies of sufficient titer and affinity to inactivate large amounts of exogenously administered insulin (in excess of 200 U/day). It occurs most commonly in patients older than 40 years of age, and usually appears during the first year of insulin treatment. When nonimmune causes of insulin resistance (obesity, endocrinopathies) have been excluded, treatment involves the use of corticosteroids, for example, 60 to 100 mg/day prednisone. This is effective in about 75% of patients, and improvement is expected during the first 2 weeks of treatment. The dose of prednisone is decreased gradually once a response has occurred, but many patients require small doses, such as 20 mg on alternate days, for up to 6 to 12 months.

Diagnostic Testing

About half of patients receiving insulin have positive skin tests to insulin. Therefore, such testing has limited value in the diagnostic evaluation. Skin testing is of value in selection of the least allergenic insulin (porcine, human) to be used for desensitization.

Management of Patients With Systemic Insulin Allergy

After a systemic allergic reaction to insulin, and presuming insulin treatment is necessary, insulin should not be discontinued if the last dose of insulin has been given within 24 hours. The next dose should be reduced to about one third of the dose that produced the reaction and then increased slowly by 2 to 5 U per injection until a therapeutic dose is achieved.[331]

When more than 24 hours has elapsed since the systemic allergic reaction to insulin, desensitization may be attempted cautiously if insulin is absolutely indicated. The least allergenic insulin may be selected by skin testing with commercially available insulins: porcine or human rDNA. Table 17-20 provides a representative insulin desensitization schedule.[2,332]

When no emergency exists, slow desensitization over several days is appropriate. The schedule may require modifications if large local or systemic reactions occur. In addition to

TABLE 17-20. *Insulin desensitization schedule*

Day	Time*	Insulin (U)	Route†
1	7:30 AM	0.00001‡	Intradermal
	12:00 noon	0.0001	Intradermal
	4:30 PM	0.001	Intradermal
2	7:30 AM	0.01	Intradermal
	12:00 noon	0.1	Intradermal
	4:30 PM	1	Intradermal
3	7:30 AM	2	Subcutaneous
	12:00 noon	4	Subcutaneous
	4:30 PM	8	Subcutaneous
4	7:30 AM	12	Subcutaneous
	12:00 noon	16	Subcutaneous
5	7:30 AM	20§	Subcutaneous
6	7:30 AM	25§	Subcutaneous

Increase by 5 U per day until therapeutic levels are achieved.

*In ketoacidosis, the doses may be given every 15 to 30 minutes.
Some physicians prefer to give all doses subcutaneously.
‡Day 1 through day 4: regular insulin.
§Day 5 and day 6: NPH or lente insulin.

being prepared to treat anaphylaxis, the physician must also be prepared to treat hypoglycemia, which may complicate the frequent doses of insulin required for desensitization.

More rapid desensitization may be required if ketoacidosis is present. The schedule suggested in Table 17-20 may be used, but the doses are administered at 15- to 30-minute intervals.

Desensitization is usually successful and is associated with a decline in specific IgE insulin-binding levels. Skin tests may actually become negative.[332] This is an example of true desensitization.

Streptokinase

Background

A nonenzymatic protein produced by group C β-hemolytic streptococci, streptokinase has been used increasingly for thrombolytic therapy but is associated with allergic reactions. The reported reaction rate ranges from 1.7% to 18%.[333] The descriptions of allergic reactions have not been well characterized but have included urticaria, serum sickness, bronchospasm, and hypotension. Both in vivo and in vitro evidence for an IgE-mediated mechanism has been reported.[334]

Diagnostic Testing

Because therapy must be instituted immediately, there is not sufficient time for an in vitro immunoassay. Intradermal skin tests with 100 IU of streptokinase are recommended.[335] Using this approach, patients who are at risk for anaphylaxis can be identified.

Management

If there is a negative skin test, streptokinase may be administered, but skin testing does not eliminate the possibility of a late reaction, such as serum sickness.[336]

If the skin test is positive, urokinase or recombinant tissue plasminogen activator may be used. Regimens of recombinant tissue plasminogen activator and streptokinase are equally effective in salvaging myocardium during an evolving infarction.[337]

Chymopapain

Background

Chymopapain is occasionally used for intradisk injection for chemonucleolysis of herniated lumbar intervertebral disks. It has been associated with anaphylaxis in 1% of patients, and there have been several fatalities.[338] Women are more likely than men to experience anaphylaxis.

Because anaphylaxis in patients treated with chymopapain has occurred on the initial injection, prior sensitization has been present. Chymopapain is obtained from a crude fraction called *papain* from the papaya tree and has enzymatic properties. Consequently, it is used for such purposes as tenderizing meat and clarifying beer or in solutions for use with soft contact lenses. It is likely that exposure to crude papain, a component of which is chymopapain, may sensitize patients to chymopapain.

Diagnostic Testing

Because anaphylaxis can occur after the first injection, it is desirable to have a method to identify patients at risk. Both in vivo skin tests and in vitro immunoassays have been used to detect antichymopapain IgE antibody.[339]

Skin testing with chymopapain has been useful in screening patients. Dilutions of chymopapain are made in saline with 0.1% human serum albumin as a stabilizer. If a histamine control is positive and a saline control is negative, prick tests are performed using 1 mg/mL and 10 µg/mL of chymopapain. If prick tests are negative, an intradermal skin test using 0.02 mL of 100 µg/mL chymopapain should follow. A positive reaction produces a wheal and erythema.

Management

If skin tests are negative, the intradisk injection can be done. If skin tests are positive, laminectomy should be considered.

The number of reactions to chymopapain is decreasing, largely owing to the decreased use of chemonucleolysis.

Drugs and Other Agents Used in the Perioperative Period

Immediate generalized reactions occurring during the perioperative period have received increasing attention. The estimated incidence is between 1 in 5000 and 1 in 15,000, with fatalities between 4% and 6%.[340] The evaluation and detection of such reactions is often complicated by the use of multiple medications and the fact that patients are unconscious and draped, which may mask the early signs and symptoms of such a reaction. During anesthesia, the only feature observed may be cardiovascular collapse or airway obstruction. Cyanosis with oxygen desaturation may be noted.

Neuromuscular-blocking agents (muscle relaxants) have been responsible for about half of these reactions,[341] but the possibility of latex allergy has become an increasingly important consideration. Other agents, such as intravenous induction agents (thiopental), opioid analgesics, blood transfusions, and plasma volume expanders, may also require some consideration. With the increased use of cardiopulmonary bypass surgery, the incidence of protamine-induced, immediate generalized reactions has risen. A discussion of some of these agents follows. A more comprehensive review of this subject can be found elsewhere.[342]

Neuromuscular-Blocking Agents (Muscle Relaxants)

Background

Neuromuscular-blocking agents are divided into two types: (1) depolarizing (e.g., succinylcholine), and (2) nondepolarizing or competitive (e.g., gallamine, pancuronium, tubocurarine, vecuronium). Immediate generalized reactions have occurred to both types, and sensitivity to both types has occurred in the same patient.

Initially, it was believed that clinical reactions with allergic features to these drugs were anaphylactoid. Although all of these agents are direct histamine releasers, with the exception of atracurium, mivacurium, and tubocurarine, intrinsic histamine-releasing activity of this group of agents is clinically insignificant.[343] Reactions that are more severe than simple flushing should be suspected of being IgE mediated.

These chemical agents contain quaternary or tertiary ammonium ions that, as small epitopes, may induce an IgE response.[344] Skin tests with appropriate dilutions of these agents have been positive in some patients but not in controls. Using in vitro tests for specific IgE antibodies against some of these agents has detected them in a high proportion of reactors.[345] There is significant cross-reactivity among the neuromuscular blockers as well as with other compounds that contain quaternary and tertiary ammonium ions. Those compounds occur widely in many drugs, foods, cosmetics, disinfectants, and other industrial materials. Patients may become sensitized through environmental contact with those materials. This could explain why some patients react to neuromuscular blockers without a history of exposure to them.[346]

Atopy does not appear to be a risk factor for the occurrence of anaphylactic reactions to those agents.[347] Most of these reactions occur in female patients, possibly owing to prior sensitization from exposure to ammonium ion epitopes found in cosmetics. It is unclear why these reactions are reported more frequently in Europe.

Diagnostic Testing

Patients who have had a suspected reaction to a neuromuscular blocker and who require further use of these agents should undergo intradermal skin testing with appropriate dilutions of the suspected agent and other blocking agents. Prick tests with undiluted stock solutions may eliminate agents to which the patient is highly sensitive. A protocol for skin testing with those agents is described elsewhere.[343] Using such, a negative skin test appears to be helpful in predicting that the drug may be safely given. In vitro tests are less sensitive.

Because sensitization can occur after environmental exposure to quaternary or tertiary ammonium ions, routine skin testing to these agents before surgery should be evaluated as a way to prevent such reactions during general anesthesia. However, this may not be cost-effective.

Management

Among patients who have experienced an immediate generalized reaction under general anesthesia, measures to prevent a second reaction should be considered. The physician should attempt to eliminate the possible role of other drugs or agents that may have contributed to the reaction, such as latex or antibiotics.

The use of volatile anesthetic agents or regional anesthesia may be a suitable alternative.

If a neuromuscular-blocking agent is essential, the role of skin testing appears to be gaining acceptance, but this may not be a practical consideration. If carried out according to a standardized protocol,[343] a positive test eliminates that agent from consideration, and a negative skin test appears reliable in predicting which agent can be safely given.

Without skin testing, a different muscle relaxant should be selected. Slow infusion of the agent is advised, and some have recommended a pretreatment protocol with antihistamines and corticosteroids, as described for the prevention of RCM reactions.[340] Although such a protocol is effective in preventing or modifying anaphylactoid reactions, it appears to have little or no effect in preventing IgE-mediated reactions.

Latex

Background

Latex is the natural milky rubber sap that is harvested from the rubber tree, *Hevea brasiliensis.* Latex allergy can cause contact dermatitis and IgE-mediated reactions during procedures involving latex exposure.

During the manufacturing process, various accelerators, antioxidants, and preservatives are added to ammoniated latex. Latex gloves are then formed by dipping porcelain molds into the compounded latex. The gloves are then oven heated, leached to remove water-soluble proteins and excess additives, cured by vulcanization, and finally powdered with cornstarch to decrease friction and provide comfort. Powder-free gloves are passed through a chlorination wash, which may also reduce the amount of water-soluble antigen.

The natural rubber latex allergens are proteins present in raw latex and are not a result of the manufacturing process.[348] These antigens can be leached from gloves by normal skin moisture and are adsorbed to the cornstarch powder. These cornstarch particles with absorbed latex allergen can become airborne and sensitize people by inhalation or produce symptoms in previously sensitized people.[349] Investigators have identified rubber elongation factor as a major rubber allergen.[350]

Contact dermatitis has been recognized for many years and is a type IV, cell-mediated reaction to low-molecular-weight accelerators and antioxidants contained in the rubber product.

In 1979, the first case of rubber-induced contact urticaria was reported.[351] Since then, many cases of IgE-mediated hypersensitivity reactions have been reported, including contact urticaria, rhinitis, asthma, and anaphylaxis.

Contact urticaria is the most common early manifestation of IgE-mediated rubber allergy, particularly in latex-sensitive health care workers who report contact urticaria involving their hands. These symptoms are often incorrectly attributed to the powder in the gloves or frequent hand washing.

Inhalation of latex-coated cornstarch particles from powdered gloves has evoked rhinitis and asthma in latex-sensitive people. Many of these patients are atopic, with histories of rhinitis due to pollens and of asthma due to dust mites and animal danders.[349] These reactions have been noted in health care workers and in people employed in a rubber glove factory.

Anaphylaxis is usually associated with parenteral or mucosal exposure. Reactions have occurred after contact with rubber bladder catheters or condoms and during surgery, childbirth, and dental procedures. Patients with latex-induced anaphylaxis during anesthesia often have a prior history of contact urticaria or angioedema from rubber products, such as gloves or balloons. Also, anaphylaxis has followed the blowing up of toy balloons. Fatal anaphylactic reactions have been reported only with rubber balloon catheters used for barium enemas.[352] These devices are no longer used in the United States.

In addition to health care workers, patients with spina bifida are at increased risk for latex sensitization as a result of repeated surgical procedures and repeated contact with bladder catheters and rubber gloves during removal of fecal impaction.[353]

The increased use of condoms and of rubber gloves by health care workers to prevent HIV infection is probably responsible for the increasing prevalence of sensitization. New glove manufacturing methods also may be contributing to the increased prevalence.

In addition to chronic latex exposure, other factors that appear to increase the likelihood of sensitization include possible cross-reactivity with bananas, avocados, passion fruit, and chestnuts.[354] Other plants, including poinsettias and *Ficus* plants, have proteins that may cross-react with latex and could increase the likelihood of sensitization among nursery or florist workers.[355]

Diagnostic Testing

The diagnosis of latex allergy is primarily based on the clinical history. Patients should be asked if they have ever noted erythema, pruritus, urticaria, or angioedema after contact with rubber products. Unexplained episodes of urticaria and anaphylaxis should be scrutinized. Also, the work history may uncover potential occupational exposure to latex.

In vivo and in vitro testing for the presence of latex-induced IgE antibodies has limited value. Skin prick tests using commercial latex reagents have been widely used in Europe and Canada. In the United States, there are no standardized, licensed latex extracts for diagnostic use. Some investigators have used their own extracts prepared from latex gloves. Latex gloves vary significantly in their allergen content,[356] however, and systemic reactions have occurred with these unstandardized preparations.[357] Intradermal skin testing for latex allergy is generally not recommended. Experienced allergists may prepare latex allergens for cautious prick and then intradermal tests beginning with low and than increasing concentrations.

"Use" tests have been advocated, wherein the patient's wet hands are exposed to latex gloves. Initially, one finger is exposed for 15 minutes and, if there is no reaction, the entire hand is exposed for an additional 15 minutes. In one series, 92% of patients with latex allergy had a positive provocative test.[358]

Latex-specific IgE antibodies have been demonstrated by immunoassay. RAST tests were positive in 50% to 90% of patients with positive skin tests. Modifications may improve sensitivity of the in vitro tests adequate for clinical use. In fact, the FDA has cleared a test system to aid in the diagnosis of patients suspected of having an allergic reaction to latex (Alastat Latex-Specific Allergen Test Kit, Diagnostic Products, Los Angeles).[359]

In summary, no reliable test for latex allergy is available. A standardized reagent for skin prick tests is the diagnostic method of choice, offering the best combination of speed and sensitivity. Unlike the delay in the availability of a standardized reagent for the detection of penicillin MDM sensitivity, a reliable skin test material for the diagnosis of latex allergy should soon be commercially available.

Management of Patients With Latex Allergy

Once the diagnosis of latex allergy is established, avoidance is the only effective therapy. Natural rubber latex is ubiquitous, and avoidance is often difficult. Extensive lists of medical and consumer natural rubber latex products are published elsewhere.[360,361] Compared with natural rubber latex, dry or crepe rubber products, such as automobile tires, have a low extractable protein content and therefore do not appear to be a problem in latex-allergic subjects. Also, "latex" in paints is not a problem in these patients.

Additional protective measures for patients with known latex allergy include wearing a Medic Alert bracelet, having autoinjectable epinephrine (Epipen) available, and keeping a supply of nonlatex gloves for emergencies. Because there has been association between latex allergy and certain foods, latex-sensitive patients should be asked about reactions to bananas, avocado, kiwi fruit, chestnuts, and passion fruit and advised to be cautious when ingesting them.

Preventing occupational exposure of health care workers requires the use of nonlatex, low-antigen-containing or powder-free gloves, and latex substitutes for nonglove products. Polyvinylchloride or polystyrene gloves are available, although their use may involve some sacrifice in barrier protection.

In operating rooms, the airborne latex allergen level can elicit respiratory symptoms in highly sensitive workers and patients. Latex-free operating rooms should be available, particularly during procedures in children with spina bifida.

For latex-sensitive patients undergoing surgery, in addition to the usual avoidance measures, premedication with corticosteroids and antihistamines has been recommended. Despite of these precautions, life-threatening intraoperative anaphylaxis has been reported.[362]

Until FDA standards are developed that ensure a low extractable protein content in natural rubber latex products, the incidence of latex sensitization will continue to be a significant public health care problem.

Protamine Sulfate

Background

Protamine is a small polycationic polypeptide (molecular weight, 4500) derived from salmon sperm. It is used to retard the absorption of certain insulins (NPH) and to reverse heparin anticoagulation. This latter application has increased significantly with the increased use of cardiopulmonary bypass procedures, cardiac catheterization, hemodialysis, and leukopheresis. Increased reports of life-threatening adverse reactions have coincided with increased use.

Acute reactions to intravenous protamine may be mild and consist of rash, urticaria, and transient elevations in pulmonary artery pressure. Other reactions are more severe and include bronchospasm, hypotension, cardiovascular collapse, and death.[363] The exact incidence of these reactions is unknown. A prospective study of patients undergoing cardiopulmonary bypass surgery revealed a reaction rate of 10.7%, although the severe reaction rate was 1.6%.[364]

Certain patient populations are at higher risk for developing adverse reactions to intravenous protamine. Diabetics treated with protamine-containing insulins have a 40-fold increased risk (2.9% versus 0.07%).[365] Initially, it was believed that men who have had vasectomies were at increased risk; however, the incidence of protamine reactions in this population is not significantly increased.[366] A history of fish allergy is not a significant risk factor.[365] Previous exposure to protamine intravenously may increase the risk of a reaction on subsequent administration.[363]

The exact mechanism by which protamine produces adverse reactions is not completely understood.[367] Some reactions appear to be IgE-mediated anaphylaxis, while others may be complement-mediated anaphylactoid reactions due to heparin–protamine complexes or protamine–antiprotamine complexes.

Diagnostic Testing

Although skin prick tests have been recommended using 1 mg/mL of protamine, in normal volunteers there was an unacceptable rate of false-positive reactions.[364] Using more dilute solutions did not appear to be predictive of an adverse reaction to protamine. Although serum antiprotamine IgE and IgG antibodies have been demonstrated in vitro, this has not been helpful in evaluating potential reactors.

Management

No widely accepted alternatives to the use of protamine to reverse heparin anticoagulation have been developed. Allowing heparin anticoagulation to reverse spontaneously has been advocated, but at the risk of significant hemorrhage. Pretreatment with corticosteroids and antihistamines may be considered, but there are no studies to support this approach. Hexadimethrine (Polybrene) was used in the past to reverse heparin anticoagulation, but the potential for renal toxicity has led to its removal. It may be available, however, as a compassionate-use drug for patients who previously had a life-threatening reaction to protamine. Test dosing may be valuable, but it is unproved. Emergency treatment for anaphylaxis should be immediately available.

Other Agents Used During the Perioperative Period

Intravenous induction agents, notably thiopental, have occasionally been associated with immediate generalized reactions during anesthesia. Positive intradermal skin tests to 0.25 mg/mL of thiopental have been reported in patients with such reactions.[368] A thiopental RAST test has been developed and is positive in many patients with positive skin tests.[369] Although neuromuscular-blocking agents are thought to be most often responsible for such reactions during anesthesia, one study found evidence of thiopental allergy in more than half of patients with histories of immediate generalized reactions during anesthesia.[370] The predictive value of skin tests and RAST tests to thiopental is uncertain.

Opioid analgesics induce mast cell mediator release by a direct effect rather than by an IgE-mediated mechanism. In vitro studies indicate that cutaneous mast cells are uniquely sensitive to opioids, whereas gastrointestinal and lung mast cells and circulating basophils are less likely to release histamine when exposed to these drugs.[371] Therefore, most opioid-induced reactions appear to be self-limiting cutaneous reactions restricted to pruritus, urticaria, and rarely, mild hypotension.

Skin testing with codeine, morphine, and meperidine produces a positive reaction in all humans due to direct mast cell activation. No in vitro tests are applicable.

If analgesia is essential, it is best to select an agent that differs from the one that caused the initial reaction. Pentazocine and fentanyl, although less potent, may be substitutes because they are less likely to result in mast cell activation.

Test dosing is the only method available to determine sensitivity.[2] The drug must be given *subcutaneously* to avoid contact with cutaneous mast cells and the resultant local reaction. The first dose of morphine should be 0.1 mg, and if there is no reaction, the doses can be increased to 0.5 mg, 1 mg, 2 mg, and 4 mg at 15-minute intervals. If a reaction occurs, the dose can be reduced and given more frequently, or test dosing with a different opioid may be considered. Nausea and vomiting are common side effects. The patient should be reassured that this does not represent an allergic reaction.

Antibiotics are commonly administered during the perioperative period and may be responsible for immediate generalized reactions. A discussion of allergic reactions to antibiotics was provided earlier.

Reports have been made of generalized reactions to bacitracin that is used to irrigate wounds at the end of a surgical procedure to reduce the rate of postoperative infection.[372]

Fluorescein sodium is used for angiograms to assess tissue perfusion and viability. Immediate generalized reactions and death have been reported infrequently.[373] These reactions appear to be anaphylactoid, and no immunologic studies have been reported.

Blood transfusions and plasma infusions may elicit immediate generalized reactions in 0.1% to 0.2% of these procedures. Anaphylactic shock occurs in 1 in 20,000 to 1 in 50,000 patients.[374] Patients with IgA deficiency should receive preparations from IgA-deficient donors because they may have preexisting serum IgE or IgG antibodies to IgA. Alternatively, thoroughly washed red blood cells may be administered. Pretreatment with corticosteroids and antihistamines may be helpful in some situations, but severe reactions can occur, and epinephrine must be readily available for treatment.

Plasma volume expanders may produce immediate generalized reactions in a small number of patients receiving these preparations.[375] Most of these reactions appear to be anaphylactoid and may be responsive to pretreatment with corticosteroids and antihistamines.

Ethylene oxide is used for gas sterilization of medical materials that do not tolerate heat sterilization. Anaphylaxis to ethylene oxide–sterilized devices has been described in patients receiving hemodialysis and undergoing plasmapheresis. Ethylene oxide can conjugate to human serum albumin to form an immunogen. RAST[376] and enzyme-linked immunosorbent assay[377] tests have detected IgE antibodies to ethylene oxide in most patients who have had generalized reactions during hemodialysis. Devices sterilized with ethylene oxide used during anesthesia, such as heart bypass pumps, can potentially cause anaphylaxis.

BIOLOGIC AGENTS: SERUM THERAPY AND IMMUNIZATIONS

Treatment and prevention of disease through manipulation of the immune system is a major achievement of modern medicine that has eliminated smallpox and has nearly eradicated polio, tetanus, diphtheria, pertussis, measles, mumps, and rubella in the United States. Extensive serum therapy began in the 1890s with the use of horse antisera to diphtheria and tetanus toxins. Until the use of antibiotics in the 1940s, treatment of infectious disease often involved the use of type-specific antisera to bacteria or their toxins. Today, active immunization to prevent infectious diseases has limited the use of passively transferred, immunologically active serum products; however, passive immunization with serum immunoglobulin concentrates still have an important role in well-defined clinical situations.

Immune Sera Therapy: Heterologous and Human

Background

The two major allergic reactions that may follow an injection of heterologous antisera are anaphylaxis and serum sickness. Anaphylaxis is less common and is more likely to occur among patients who are atopic and have IgE antibodies directed against the corresponding animal dander, most commonly horse. For this reason, these patients may react after the first injection of antisera. Serum sickness is more common and is dose related.

Modern immunization procedures and the availability of human immune serum globulin (ISG) and specific human ISG preparations have reduced the need for heterologous antisera. Equine antitoxins, however, may still be required in the management of snake bites (pit vipers and coral snake, black widow spider bite, diphtheria and botulism).[378] Antilymphocyte and antithymocyte globulins, prepared in horses and rabbits, have been used to provide immuno suppression and to treat autoimmune disease. Murine monoclonal antilymphocyte antibodies have also produced immediate generalized reactions, but such reactions do not appear to be IgE-dependent.[379]

When available and appropriate, human ISG preparations should be used in preference to animal antisera. Although infrequent, immediate generalized reactions have followed their administration. Intramuscular ISG preparations contain high-molecular-weight IgG aggregates that are biologically active and that may activate serum complement to produce anaphylactoid reactions. Anaphylaxis has also followed the administration of both intramuscular and intravenous human ISG among IgA-deficient patients who may produce IgE and IgG antibodies directed against IgA.[380] These patients are at risk of anaphylaxis on infusion of IgA-containing blood products. Only one preparation of intravenous ISG (Gammagard) is sufficiently IgA poor to be considered in the treatment of IgA-deficient patients.

Tests Before Heterologous Antisera Administration

Before administering heterologous antisera to any patient, regardless of history, skin testing *must* be performed on the volar surface of the forearm to demonstrate the presence of IgE antibodies and to predict the likelihood of anaphylaxis. Prick skin tests using antisera diluted 1:10 with normal saline and a saline control are performed. If negative after 15 minutes, intradermal skin tests using 0.02 mL of a 1:100 dilution of antisera and a saline control are completed. If the history suggests a previous reaction, or if the patient has atopic symptoms after exposure to the corresponding animal (usually horse), intradermal testing is begun using 0.02 mL of a 1:1000 dilution. A negative skin test virtually excludes significant anaphylactic sensitivity, but some recommend giving a test dose of 0.5 mL of undiluted antisera intravenously before proceeding with recommended doses. This approach does not exclude the possibility of a late reaction, notably serum sickness 8 to 12 days later.

Desensitization

When there is no alternative to the use of heterologous antisera, desensitization has been successful despite a positive skin test to this material. The procedure is dangerous and may be more difficult to accomplish in patients who are allergic to the corresponding animal dander.

Several protocols are recommended for desensitization. An intravenous infusion should be established in one or both arms. The package insert often recommends a schedule. A conservative schedule begins with the subcutaneous administration of 0.1 mL of a 1:100 dilution in an extremity, where a tourniquet may be placed proximally if required. The dose is doubled every 15 minutes. If a reaction occurs, it is treated, and desensitization is resumed using half the dose provoking the reaction. After reaching 1 mL of the undiluted antiserum, the remainder is given by slow intravenous infusion.

At times, more rapid delivery of the antisera may be required.[381] Here, intravenous infusions are established in both arms; one to administer the antisera and the other for treatment of complications. Premedication with 50 to 100 mg diphenhydramine intravenously is followed by slow infusion of the antisera through one of the intravenous lines. If there is no reaction after 15 minutes, the infusion rate may be increased. If a reaction occurs, the antisera infusion is stopped and the reaction treated with epinephrine. After the reaction has been controlled, the slow infusion is reestablished. Most patients can be given 80 to 100 mL over 4 hours. If there is no reaction, it is possible to give that amount in the first hour.

After successful desensitization, serum sickness usually develops in 8 to 12 days. When the dose of antisera is in excess of 100 mL, virtually all patients experience some degree of serum sickness. Treatment with corticosteroids is effective, the prognosis is excellent, and long-term complications are rare.

Tetanus Toxoid

Although minor reactions, such as local swelling, are common after tetanus toxoid or diphtheria–tetanus toxoid vaccinations, true IgE-mediated reactions are rare. Surveys estimate the risk of a systemic reaction to be 0.00001%.[382]

Because diphtheria toxoid is not available as a single agent, it is impossible to separate the true incidence of diphtheria-associated reactions from those due to tetanus toxoid.

When it appears necessary to administer tetanus toxoid to a patient with a history of a previous adverse reaction, a skin test–graded challenge may be performed.[383,384]

One recommended approach is to begin with a prick test using undiluted toxoid. If negative, at 15-minute intervals, 0.02 mL of successive dilutions of toxoid 1:1000 and 1:100 are injected intradermally. If the prick test was positive, the beginning dilution is 1:10,000. Subsequently, 0.02 mL and 0.20 mL of a 1:10 dilution are given subcutaneously. This may be followed by 0.05 mL, 0.10 mL, 0.15 mL, and 0.20 mL of full-strength toxoid given subcutaneously. Some prefer to wait for 24 hours after 0.10 mL is given to detect delayed reactivity. After that, the balance of full-strength material may be given for a final total dose of 0.50 mL.

Measles, Mumps, and Rubella Vaccine in Egg-Allergic Children

Background

Because the live attenuated virus used in the measles, mumps, and rubella (MMR) vaccine is grown in cultured chick embryo fibroblasts, concern has been raised regarding its administration to egg-allergic children. The fibroblast cultures used to produce MMR vaccine contain no or trivial amounts of egg allergen. For this reason, and also based on extensive clinical experience, it has been suggested that egg-allergic children be given MMR vaccine without preliminary skin testing with the vaccine.[385] Reactions to MMR vaccine have been described in children who tolerate eggs. This suggests that the reaction may be due to some other component, such as the gelatin included in the vaccine.[386]

The American Academy of Pediatrics recommends that egg-allergic children undergo skin testing with MMR vaccine before administration. If the skin test is positive, desensitization should be performed.

Until this controversy is fully resolved, the following approach appears reasonable for egg-allergic children.

Skin Testing

A prick test is performed with a 1:10 dilution of MMR vaccine in normal saline, and a normal saline control. Intradermal skin tests, after a negative prick skin test, are probably unnecessary and may be misleading. After a negative prick test, the vaccine may be administered in the routine fashion.

Desensitization

After a positive prick skin test to MMR vaccine, at 15-minute intervals, the following dilutions of vaccine are administered subcutaneously: 0.05 mL of a 1:100 dilution, 0.05 mL of a 1:10 dilution, and 0.05 mL of the undiluted vaccine. Subsequently, at 15-minute intervals, increasing amounts of the undiluted vaccine (0.10 mL, 0.15 mL, and 0.20 mL) are given until the total immunizing dose of 0.50 mL is received.[387] Using this protocol, systemic reactions have been reported; hence, a physician must be prepared to treat anaphylaxis. After completion of the procedure, it is advisable to keep the patient under observation for an additional 30 minutes.

Influenza and Yellow Fever Vaccine in Egg-Allergic Patients

Background

Allergic reactions to influenza vaccine are rare, and the vaccine may be given safely to people who are able to tolerate eggs by ingestion, even if they demonstrate a positive skin test to egg protein. Anaphylaxis has been reported at a rate of 0.024 in 100,000.[388] Among asthmatic patients, there was some concern about inducing bronchospasm after administration; however, there appears to be no evidence of asthmagenicity after influenza vaccine.[389] The patient with moderate or severe asthma is at risk from natural infection and benefits from influenza vaccination.

Although yellow fever vaccine is not required in the United States, travelers to endemic areas may require immunization. Of the egg-based vaccines, yellow fever vaccine contains the most egg protein. Two of 493 patients with a positive history of egg allergy had anaphylaxis after yellow fever immunization; both of these patents were positive by skin test to both egg and the vaccine.[390]

Tests

For patients with a clear history of egg allergy or when in doubt, skin testing with the appropriate vaccine is a reliable method to identify patients at risk.[391] A prick test is performed with a 1:10 dilution of the vaccine in normal saline, and a normal saline control. If negative or equivocal, an intradermal skin test using 0.02 mL of a 1:100 dilution of the vaccine is performed, and a saline control. If negative, the vaccine may be administered in a routine fashion.

Desensitization

After a positive skin test to the vaccine, if it is considered essential, 0.05 mL of a 1:100 dilution is administered intramuscularly; and at 15- to 20-minute intervals, 0.05 mL of a 1:10 dilution, then 0.05 mL of undiluted vaccine, is administered, followed by 0.10 mL, 0.15 mL, and 0.20 mL of undiluted vaccine for a total dose of 0.50 mL. Using this format, patients develop adequate protective antibody titers.[392]

Cancer Chemotherapeutic Agents

A brief discussion of hypersensitivity reactions to antitumor agents was presented earlier in the section describing immediate generalized reactions under the clinical classification of allergic drug reactions. With the exception of altretamine, the nitrosoureas, and dactinomycin, all other antitumor agents have been recognized to cause hypersensitivity reactions in at least a few cases.[59] All four types of Gell and Coombs reactions (see Table 17-4) have been associated with these agents, but most appear to be type I. L-Asparaginase, paclitaxel, cisplatin, and analogues have been more frequently associated with immediate generalized reactions. A few case reports of type I reactions have been described for most of these agents.

The mechanisms of hypersensitivity reactions to cancer chemotherapeutic agents have been investigated in only a few patients. Although some of these reactions appear to be IgE mediated, most are probably IgE independent.

Diagnostic Testing

No reliable in vivo or in vitro tests are available. Positive skin tests have been reported in patients who sustained an immediate generalized reaction to carboplatin and cisplatin.[60] In most situations, however, skin testing or test dosing does not appear to be worthwhile.[59]

Management

A patient who develops an immediate generalized reaction with hypotension should not be treated again with the inciting agent unless there are special circumstances. If a suitable analogue or another drug in the same chemical class is available, it should be substituted in the hope that clinically significant cross-reactivity will not occur. The development and use of pegaspargase as an alternative to L-asparaginase is an example of such.

If the previous reaction was not life-threatening, the reinstitution of therapy with the inciting drug may be possible after the prophylactic use of corticosteroids and antihistamines in the manner recommended for prevention of RCM reactions. In addition to pretreatment, slowing the rate of administration of the agent may be helpful. When paclitaxel was given over a 24-hour period, the incidence of reactions decreased significantly from about 10% to only sporadic cases.

As always, the potential for anaphylaxis must be considered, and the medical staff must be prepared to manage this emergency.

Anticonvulsant Hypersensitivity Syndrome

Background

The anticonvulsant hypersensitivity syndrome is a potentially fatal drug reaction with cutaneous and systemic reactions to arene oxide–producing anticonvulsants, namely phenytoin, carbamazepine, and phenobarbital.[393] The incidence is estimated to be between 1 in 1000 and 1 in 10,000 exposures.

Typically, there is fever, rash, and lymphadenopathy with multisystem abnormalities, most notably hepatitis, which is the most common cause of death. The rash is usually morbilliform and pruritic, but there is often periorbital and facial edema. Rarely, the eruption is Stevens-Johnson syndrome or TEN.

The syndrome is similar for all three drugs noted. The mechanism is unknown, but some features suggest an allergic reaction. There appears to be a high rate of cross-reactivity among these drugs.[394]

Management

Patients with anticonvulsant hypersensitivity syndrome probably should not be treated with a different arene oxide–producing anticonvulsant. No in vitro tests are available to discriminate among these three agents and to predict cross-reactivity.

A substitute anticonvulsant other than these three drugs should be selected if possible. A benzodiazepine may be substituted for seizure control. A new anticonvulsant, Gabapentin, may be useful because it does not contain the arene oxide structure.

Test dosing is an option but is extremely dangerous. It should not be attempted until the patient has completely recovered from the previous reaction, and it should have the endorsement of a neurologist. Using phenytoin as an example, slow and cautious test dosing may begin with 1 mg/day for 1 week, 5 mg/day for 1 week, 25 mg/day for 1 week, and 100 mg/day for 1 week.[2] Subsequently, the dose may be gradually increased by the neurologist.

At the first indication of any cutaneous reaction, the drug is stopped, and prednisone, 60 to 80 mg/day, is administered. Although the cutaneous reaction of anticonvulsant hypersensitivity syndrome appears to respond to corticosteroids, they may not reverse the noncutaneous manifestations.[395]

FINAL COMMENTS

Although pretreatment, test dosing, and desensitization are strategies that, in most situations, permit the administration of an essential drug to a patient with a history of a previous reaction to that agent, the physician must always be aware of and be prepared to treat a potential reaction. For those physicians inexperienced in managing allergic reactions, it is prudent to seek consultation with an experienced allergist who manages hypersensitivity reactions on a daily basis.

One cannot ignore the medicolegal implications under these circumstances. Informed consent, clear documentation of the necessity of the procedure, and appropriate consultation with specialists are to be noted in the medical record. This protects the patient, physician, and facility where such protocols are conducted.

REFERENCES

1. DeSwarte RD. Drug allergy. In: Patterson R, Grammer LC, Greenberger PA, Zeiss CR, eds. Allergic diseases: diagnosis and management. 4th ed. Philadelphia: JB Lippincott, 1993:395.
2. Patterson R, DeSwarte RD, Greenberger PA, Grammer LC, Brown JE, Choy AC. Drug allergy and protocols for management of drug allergies. Allergy Proc 1994;15:239.
3. Sullivan TJ. Drug allergy. In: Middleton E, Reed CE, Ellis EF, Adkinson NF, Yuninger JW, eds. Allergy: principles and practice. 4th ed. St Louis: CV Mosby, 1993:1726.
4. Anderson JA. Allergic reactions to drugs and biological agents. JAMA 1992;268:2845.
5. Classen DC, Pestotnik SL, Evans RS, Burke JP. Computerized surveillance of adverse drug events in hospitalized patients. JAMA 1991;266:2847.
6. Jick H. Adverse drug reactions: the magnitude of the problem. J Allergy Clin Immunol 1985;74:555.
7. Armstrong B, Dinan B, Jick H. Fatal drug reactions in patients admitted to surgical services. Am J Surg 1976;132:643.
8. Porter J, Jick H. Drug-related deaths among medical inpatients. JAMA 1977;237:879.
9. Jick H. Drugs: remarkably nontoxic. N Engl J Med 1974;291:284.
10. Spilker B. Guide to clinical trials. New York: Raven Press, 1991:565.
11. Scott HD, Rosenbaum SE, Waters WJ. Rhode Island physicians' recognition and reporting of adverse drug reactions. RI Med J 1987;70:311.
12. Kessler DA. Introducing MedWatch: a new approach to reporting and device adverse effects and product problems. JAMA 1993;269:2765.
13. Honig PK, Wortham DC, Zamani K, Conner DP, Mullin JC, Cantilena LR. Terfenadine-ketoconazole interaction: pharmacokinetic and electrocardiographic consequences. JAMA 1993;269:1513.
14. DeSwarte RD. Drug allergy: problems and strategies. J Allergy Clin Immunol 1984;74:209.
15. Schatz M, Patterson R, DeSwarte RD. Non-organic adverse reactions to aeroallergen immunotherapy. J Clin Allergy Immunol 1976;58:198.
16. Wolf S. The pharmacology of placebos. Pharmacol Rev 1959;11:689.
17. Penn I. Cancers following cyclosporine therapy. Transplantation 1987;43:32.
18. Kelly CP, Pothoulakis C, LaMont JT. Clostridium difficile colitis. N Engl J Med 1994;330:257.
19. Gelfand JA, Elin RJ, Berry FW, et al. Endotoxemia associated with the Jarisch-Herxheimer reactions. N Engl J Med 1976;295:211.
20. McInnes GT, Brodie MJ. Drug interactions that matter: a critical appraisal. Drugs 1988;36:83.
21. Affrime MB, Lorber R, Danzig M, Cuss F, Brannan MD. Three month evaluation of electrocardiographic effects of loratadine in humans. J Allergy Clin Immunol 1993;91:259.
22. Hansten PD, Horn JR. Drug interactions. 6th ed. Philadelphia and London: Lea & Febiger, 1989.
23. Beutler E. Glucose-6-phosphate dehydrogenase deficiency. N Engl J Med 1991;324:169.
24. Landu BM. Pharmacogenetics. Med Clin North Am 1969;53:839.
25. DeSwarte RD. Drug allergy: an overview. Clin Rev Allergy 1986;4:143.
26. Ring J. Pseudoallergic drug reactions. In: Korenblat PE, Wedner HJ, eds. Allergy: theory and practice. 2nd ed. Philadelphia: WB Saunders, 1992:243.
27. deWeck AL. Pharmacologic and immunochemical mechanisms of drug hypersensitivity. Immunol Allergy Clin North Am 1991;11:461.
28. Levine BB. Immunologic mechanisms of penicillin allergy: a haptenic model system for the study of allergic diseases in man. N Engl J Med 1966;275:1115.
29. Carrington DM, Earl HS, Sullivan TJ. Studies of human IgE to a sulfonamide determinant. J Allergy Clin Immunol 1987;79:442.
30. Sullivan TJ. Dehaptenation of albumin substituted with benzylpenicillin G determinants. J Allergy Clin Immunol 1988;81:222.
31. Didier A, Cador D, Bongrand P, et al. Role of quaternary ammonium ion determinants in allergy to muscle relaxants. J Allergy Clin Immunol 1987;79:578.
32. Coombs RRA, Gell PGH. Classification of allergic reactions responsible for clinical hypersensitivity and disease. In: Gell PGH, Coombs RRA, Lachman PJ, eds. Clinical aspects of immunology. 3rd ed. Oxford: Blackwell Scientific Publications, 1975:761.

33. VanArsdel PP Jr. Classification and risk factors for drug allergy. Immunol Allergy Clin North Am 1991;11:475.
34. Adkinson NF Jr. Risk factors for drug allergy. J Allergy Clin Immunol 1984;74:567.
35. Enright T, Chua-Lim A, Duda E. The role of a documented allergic profile as a risk factor for radiographic contrast media reactions. Ann Allergy 1989;62:302.
36. Perry HM, Tan EM, Carmody S, et al. Relationship of acetyltransferase activity to antinuclear antibodies and toxic symptoms in hypertensive patients treated with hydralazine. J Lab Clin Med 1970;76:114.
37. Woosley RL, Drayer DE, Reidenberg MM, et al. Effect of acetylator phenotype on the rate at which procainamide induces antinuclear antibodies and the lupus syndrome. N Engl J Med 1978;298:1157.
38. Reider MJ, Vetrecht J, Shear NH, Cannon M, Miller M, Stielberg SP. Diagnosis of sulfonamide hypersensitivity reactions by in vitro "rechallenge" with hydroxylamine metabolites. Ann Intern Med 1989;110:286.
39. Wooley PH, Griffin J, Panayi GS, et al. HLA-DR antigens and toxic reactions to sodium aurothiomalate and D-penicillamine in patients with rheumatoid arthritis. N Engl J Med 1980;303:300.
40. Roujeau JC, Huynh TN, Bracq C, et al. Genetic susceptibility to toxic epidermal necrolysis. Arch Dermatol 1987;123:171.
41. Attaway NJ, Jasin HM, Sullivan TJ. Familial drug allergy. J Allergy Clin Immunol 1991;87:227.
42. Sullivan TJ, Ong RC, Gilliam LK. Studies of the multiple drug allergy syndrome. J Allergy Clin Immunol 1989;83:270.
43. Moseley EK, Sullivan TJ. Allergic reactions to antimicrobial drugs in patients with a history of prior drug allergy. J Allergy Clin Immunol 1991;87:226.
44. Kamada MM, Twarog F, Leung DYM. Multiple antibiotic sensitivity in a pediatric population. Allergy Proc 1991;12:347.
45. Sullivan TJ. Management of patients allergic to antimicrobial drugs. Allergy Proc 1992;12:361.
46. Moss RB. Sensitization to aztreonam and cross-reactivity with other beta-lactam antibiotics in high-risk patients with cystic fibrosis. J Allergy Clin Immunol 1991;87:78.
47. Bierman CW, Pierson WE, Zeitz SJ, et al. Reactions associated with ampicillin therapy. JAMA 1972;220:1098.
48. Harb GE, Jacobson MA. Human immunodeficiency virus (HIV) infection: does it increase susceptibility to adverse drug reactions? Drug Safety 1993;9:1.
49. Bayard PJ, Berger TG, Jacobson MA. Drug hypersensitivity reactions and human immunodeficiency virus disease. J Acquir Immune Defic Syndr 1992;5:1237.
50. Kovacs JA, Hiemenz JW, Macher AM, et al. Pneumocystis carinii pneumonia: a comparison between patients with the acquired immunodeficiency syndrome and patients with other immunodeficiencies. Ann Intern Med 1984;100:663.
51. Toogood JH. Risk of anaphylaxis in patients receiving beta-blocker drugs. J Allergy Clin Immunol 1988;81:1.
52. Dukes MNG, ed. Meyler's side effects of drugs: an encyclopedia of adverse reactions and interactions. 12th ed. New York: Elsevier, 1992.
53. Dukes MNG, ed. Side effects of drugs, annual 19. New York: Elsevier, 1995.
54. Greenberger PA. Drug Allergies. In: Rich RR, Fleisher TA, Schwartz BD, Shearer WT, Strober W, eds. Clinical immunology: principles and practice. St Louis: Mosby Year-Book, 1996:988.
55. Porter J, Jick H. Boston Collaborative Drug Surveillance Programs: drug induced anaphylaxis, convulsions, deafness, and extrapyramidal symptoms. Lancet 1977;1:587.
56. Herrera AM, deShazo RD. Current concepts in anaphylaxis. Immunol Allergy Clin North Am 1992;12:517.
57. Weiss ME, Adkinson NF, Hirshman CA. Evaluation of allergic drug reactions in the perioperative period. Anesthesiology 1989;71:483.
58. Davis H, McGoodwin E, Reed TG. Anaphylactoid reactions reported after treatment with ciprofloxacin. Ann Intern Med 1989;111:1041.
59. Weiss RB. Hypersensitivity reactions. Semin Oncol 1992;19:458.
60. Windom HH, McGuire WP III, Hamilton RG, Adkinson NF. Anaphylaxis to carboplatin: a new platinum chemotherapeutic agent. J Allergy Clin Immunol 1992;90:681.
61. Weiss RB, Donehower RC, Wiernik PH, et al. Hypersensitivity reactions from Taxol. J Clin Oncol 1990;8:1263.
62. Weiss ME. Drug allergy. Med Clin North Am 1992;76:857.
63. Laxenaire MC, Monneret-Vautrin DA, Guaént JL. Drugs and other agents involved in anaphylactic shock occurring during anesthesia: a French multicenter epidemiological inquiry. Ann Fr Anesth Reanim 1993;12:91.
64. Weiler JM, Gellhaus AA, Carter JG, et al. A prospective study of the risk of an immediate adverse reaction to protamine sulfate during cardiopulmonary bypass surgery. J Allergy Clin Immunol 1990;85:713.
65. Grammer LC, Paterson BF, Roxe D, et al. IgE against ethylene oxide-altered human serum albumin in patients with anaphylactic reactions to dialysis. J Allergy Clin Immunol 1985;76:511.
66. Seggev JS, Ohta K, Tipton WR. IgE mediated anaphylaxis due to a psyllium-containing drug. Ann Allergy 1984;53:325.
67. Rohr AS, Pappano JE. Prophylaxis against fluorescein-induced anaphylactoid reactions. J Allergy Clin Immunol 1992;90:407.
68. Hamstra RD, Block MH, Schocket AL. Intravenous iron dextran in clinical medicine. JAMA 1980;243:1726.
69. Dykewicz MS, Rosen ST, O'Connell MM, et al. Plasma histamine but not anaphylatoxin levels correlate with generalized urticaria from infusions of antilymphocyte monoclonal antibodies. J Lab Clin Med 1992;120:290.
70. Dixon FJ, Vasquez JJ, Weigle WO, et al. Pathogenesis of serum sickness. Arch Pathol 1968;63:18.

71. Bielory L, Gascon P, Lawley TJ, et al. Human serum sickness: a prospective analysis of 35 patients treated with equine anti-thymocyte globulin for bone marrow failure. Medicine 1988;67:40.

72. Davidson JR, Bush RK, Grogan EW, et al. Immunology of a serum sickness/vasculitis reaction secondary to streptokinase used for acute myocardial infarction. Clin Exp Rheumatol 1988;6:381.

73. Erffmeyer JE. Serum sickness. Ann Allergy 1986;56:105.

74. Platt R, Dreis MW, Kennedy DL, et al. Serum sickness-like reactions to amoxicillin, cefaclor, cephalexin, and trimethoprim-sulfamethoxazole. J Infect Dis 1988;158:474.

75. Barnett EV, Stone G, Swisher SN, et al. Serum sickness and plasmacytosis: clinical, immunologic, and hematologic analysis. Am J Med 1963;35:113.

76. Lawley TJ, Bielory L, Gascon R, Yancey B, Young NS, Frank MM. A prospective clinical and immunologic analysis of patients with serum sickness. N Engl J Med 1984;311:1407.

77. Gilliland BC. Drug-induced autoimmune and hematologic disorders. Immunol Allergy Clin North Am 1991;11:525.

78. Morrow JD, Schroeder HA, Perry Jr HM. Studies on the control of hypertension by hyphex. II. Toxic reactions and side effects. Circulation 1953;8:829.

79. Ladd AT. Procainamide-induced lupus erythematosus. N Engl J Med 1962;267:1357.

80. Pistiner M, Wallace DJ, Nessim S, et al. Lupus erythematosus in the 1980's: a survey of 570 patients. Semin Arthritis Rheum 1991;21:55.

81. Steinberg AD, Gourley MF, Klinman DM, Tsokos GC, Scott DE, Krieg AM. Systemic lupus erythematosus. Ann Intern Med 1991;115:548.

82. Lahita R, Kluger J, Drayer DE, et al. Antibodies to nuclear antigens in patients treated with procainamide or acetylprocainamide. N Engl J Med 1979;301:1382.

83. Stec GP, Lertora JJL, Atkinson Jr AJ, et al. Remission of procainamide-induced lupus erythematosus with N-acetylprocainamide therapy. Ann Intern Med 1979;90:799.

84. Blomgren SE, Condemi JJ, Bignall MC, et al. Antinuclear antibody induced by procainamide: a prospective study. N Engl J Med 1969;281:64.

85. Gleichmann E, Pals ST, Rolink AG, et al. Graft-versus-host reactions: clues to the etiopathology of a spectrum of immunological disease. Immunol Today 1984;5:324.

86. Fauci AS. Vasculitis. J Allergy Clin Immunol 1983;72:211.

87. Hunder GG, Arend WP, Bloch DA, et al. The American College of Rheumatology 1990 criteria for the classification of vasculitis: introduction. Arthritis Rheum 1990;33:1065.

88. Arellano F, Sacristán JA. Allopurinol hypersensitivity syndrome: a review. Ann Pharmacother 1993;27:337.

89. Bigby M, Jick S, Jick H, Arndt K. Drug-induced cutaneous reactions: a report from the Boston Collaborative Drug Surveillance Program on 15,438 consecutive inpatients, 1975 to 1983. JAMA 1986;256:3358.

90. Kauppinen K. Rational performance of drug challenge in cutaneous hypersensitivity. Semin Dermatol 1983;2:227.

91. Kauppinen K, Stubb S. Drug eruptions: causative agents and clinical types. A series of in-patients during a 10-year period. Acta Derm Venereol 1984;64:320.

92. Roujeau JC, Stern RS. Severe adverse cutaneous reactions to drugs. N Engl J Med 1994;331:1272.

93. Levenson DE, Arndt KA, Stern RS. Cutaneous manifestations of adverse drug reactions. Immunol Allergy Clin North Am 1991;11:493.

94. Alanko K, Stubb S, Kauppinen K. Cutaneous drug reactions: clinical types and causative agents. A five-year survey of in-patients (1982–1985). Acta Derm Venereol 1989;69:223.

95. Hedner T, Samuelsson O, Lunde H, Lindholm L, Andren L, Wiholm BE. Angio-oedema in relation to treatment with angiotensin converting enzyme inhibitors. Br Med J 1992;304:941.

96. Orfan N, Patterson R, Dykewicz MS. Severe angioedema related to ACE inhibitors in patients with a history of idiopathic angioedema. JAMA 1990;264:1287.

97. Chin HL, Buchan DA. Severe angioedema after long term use of an angiotensin-converting-enzyme inhibitor. Ann Intern Med 1990;112:312.

98. Anderson MW, deShazo RD. Studies of the mechanism of angiotensin-converting enzyme (ACE) inhibitor-associated angioedema: the effect of an ACE inhibitor on cutaneous responses to bradykinin, codeine, and histamine. J Allergy Clin Immunol 1990;85:856.

99. Angelini G, Vena GA, Meneghini CL. Allergic contact dermatitis to some medicaments. Contact Derm 1985;12:263.

100. Storrs FJ. Contact dermatitis caused by drugs. Immunol Allergy Clin North Am 1991;11:509.

101. Rudzki E, Zakrzewski Z, Rebandel P, et al. Cross reactions between aminoglycoside antibiotics. Contact Derm 1988;18:314.

102. Elias J, Levinson A. Hypersensitivity reactions to ethylenediamine in aminophylline. Am Rev Resp Dis 1981;123:550.

103. Storrs FJ, Rosenthal LE, Adams RM, et al. Prevalence and relevance of allergic reactions in patients patch tested in North America-1984 to 1985. J Am Acad Dermatol 1989;20:1038.

104. Rietschal RL, Adams RM. Reactions to thimerosal in hepatitis B vaccines. Dermatol Clin 1990;8:161.

105. Fisher AA. Contact dermatitis from topical medicaments. Semin Dermatol 1982;1:49.

106. Korkij W, Keyoumars S. Fixed drug eruption. Arch Dermatol 1984;120:520.

107. Huff JC, Weston WL, Tonnesen MG. Erythema multiforme: A critical review of characteristics, diagnostic criteria, and causes. J Am Acad Dermatol 1983;8:763.
108. Brice DL, Krzemien BS, Weston WL, Huff JC. Detection of herpes simplex virus DNA in cutaneous lesions of erythema multiforme. J Invest Dermatol 1989;93:183.
109. Finan MC, Schroeter AL. Cutaneous immunofluorescence study of erythema multiforme: correlation with light microscopic patterns and etiologic agents. J Am Acad Dermatol 1984;10:497.
110. Tonnesen MG, Harrist TJ, Wintroub BV, et al. Erythema multiforme: microvascular damage and infiltration of lymphocytes and basophils. J Invest Dermatol 1983;80:282.
111. Correia O, Delgado L, Ramos JP, Resende C, Torrinha JA. Cutaneous T-cell recruitment in toxic epidermal necrolysis: further evidence of CD8+ lymphocyte involvement. Arch Dermatol 1993;129:466.
112. Cheriyan S, Patterson R, Greenberger PA, Grammer LC, Latall J. The outcome of Stevens-Johnson Syndrome treated with corticosteroids. Allergy Proc 1995;16:151.
113. Adam JE. Exfoliative dermatitis. Can Med Assoc J 1968;99:661.
114. Nicolis GD, Helwig EB. Exfoliative dermatitis: a clinicopathologic study of 135 cases. Arch Dermatol 1973;109:682.
115. Bigby M, Stern RS, Arndt KA. Allergic cutaneous reactions to drugs. Primary Care 1989;16:713.
116. Epstein JH, Wintroub BV. Photosensitivity due to drugs. Drugs 1985;30:42.
117. Nalbandian RM, Mader IJ, Barret JL, Pearce JF, Rupp EC. Petechiae, ecchymoses, and necrosis of skin induced by coumarin congeners. JAMA 1965;192:603.
118. Bauer KA. Coumarin-induced skin necrosis. Arch Dermatol 1993;129:766.
119. Goldstein SM, Wintroub BW, Elias PM, Wuepper KD. Toxic epidermal necrolysis. Unmuddying the waters. Arch Dermatol 1987;123:1153.
120. Amon RB, Dimond RL. Toxic epidermal necrolysis: rapid differentiation between staphylococcal-induced disease and drug-induced disease. Arch Dermatol 1975;111:1433.
121. Bastuji-Garin S, Rzany B, Stern RS, Shear NH, Naldi L, Roujeau JC. Clinical classification of cases of toxic epidermal necrolysis, Stevens-Johnson syndrome, and erythema multiforme. Arch Dermatol 1993;129:92.
122. Heinbach DM, Engrav LH, Marvin JA, Harnar TJ, Grube BJ. Toxic epidermal necrolysis. A step forward in treatment. JAMA 1987;257:2171.
123. Guillaume J-C, Ronjeau J-C, Revuz J, Penso D, Touraine R. The culprit drugs in 87 cases of toxic epidermal necrolysis (Lyell's syndrome). Arch Dermatol 1987;123:1166.
124. Stern RS, Chan HL. Usefulness of case report literature in determining drugs responsible for toxic epidermal necrolysis. J Am Dermatol 1989;21:317.
125. Ronjeau JC, Huynh TN, Bracq C, Guillaume JC, Revuz J, Touraine R. Genetic susceptibility to toxic epidermal necrolysis. Arch Dermatol 1987;123:1171.
126. Twarog FG. Hypersensitivity to pancreatic extracts in parents of patients with cystic fibrosis. J Allergy Clin Immunol 1977;59:35.
127. Pozner LH, Mandarano C, Zitt MJ, Frieri M, Weiss NS. Recurrent bronchospasm in a nurse. Ann Allergy 1986;56:14.
128. Coutts II, Dally MB, Newman Taylor AJ, et al. Asthma in workers manufacturing cephalosporins. Br Med J 1981;283:95.
129. Hunt LW, Rosenow EC, III. Asthma-producing drugs. Ann Allergy 1992;68:453.
130. Mecker DP, Wiedemann HP. Drug-induced bronchospasm. Clin Chest Med 1990;11:163.
131. Fraley DS, Bruns FJ, Segel DP, Adler S. Propanolol-related bronchospasm in patients without a history of asthma. S Med J 1980;73:238.
132. Lunde H, Herdner T, Samuelsson O, et al. Dyspnea, asthma, and bronchoconstriction in relation to treatment with angiotensin converting enzyme inhibitors. Br Med Jour 1994;308:18.
133. Simon SR, Black HR, Moser M, et al. Cough and ACE inhibitors Arch Intern Med 1992;152.1698.
134. Lacourciere Y, Lefebvre J, Nakhle G, et al. Association between cough and angiotensin converting enzyme inhibitors versus angiotensin II antagonists: The design of a prospective, controlled study J Hypertens 1994;12:S49.
135. Israili ZH, Hall WD. Cough and angioneurotic edema associated with angiotensin-converting enzyme inhibitor therapy. A review of the literature and pathophysiology. Ann Intern Med 1992;117:234.
136. Bush RK, Taylor SL, Holden K, et al. Prevalence of sensitivity to sulfiting agents in asthmatic patients. Am J Med 1986;81:816.
137. Goldfarb G, Simon RA. Provocation of sulfite sensitive asthma. J Allergy Clin Immunol 1984;73:135.
138. Simon RA, Stevenson DD. Lack of cross sensitivity between aspirin and sulfite in sensitive asthmatics. J Allergy Clin Immunol 1987;79:257.
139. Pisani RJ, Rosenow EC, III. Drug-Induced Pulmonary Disease. In: Simmons DH, Tierney DF, eds. Current pulmonology. vol 13. St. Louis: Mosby Year-Book, 1992:311.
140. Holmberg L, Boman G, Bottiger IE, et al. Adverse reactions to nitrofurantoin. Analysis of 921 reports. Am J Med 1980;69:733.
141. Sostman HD, Matthay RA, Putman CE, et al. Methotrexate-induced pneumonitis. Medicine 1976;55:371.
142. Martin WJ II, Rosenow EC III. Amiodarone pulmonary toxicity. Part I. Chest 1988;93:1067.
143. Kennedy JI. Clinical aspects of amiodarone pulmonary toxicity. Clin Chest Med 1990;11:119.

144. Manicardi V, Bernini G, Bossini P, et al. Low-dose amiodarone-induced pneumonitis: evidence of an immunologic pathogenic mechanism. Am J Med 1989;86:134.
145. Kennedy JI, Myers JL, Plumb VJ, et al. Amiodarone pulmonary toxicity: clinical, radiologic, and pathologic correlations. Arch Intern Med 1987;147:50.
146. Evans RB, Ettensohn DB, Fawaz-Estrup F, et al. Gold lung: recent developments in pathogenesis, diagnosis, and therapy. Semin Arthritis Rheum 1987;16:196.
147. Cooper JAD Jr, White DA, Matthay RA. Drug-induced pulmonary disease. Part 1: Cytotoxic drugs. Am Rev Respir Dis 1986;133:321.
148. Holoye P, Luna M, Mackay B, et al. Bleomycin hypersensitivity pneumonitis. Ann Intern Med 1978;88:47.
149. Kavaru MS, Ahmad M, Amirthalingam KN. Hydrochlorothiazide-induced acute pulmonary edema. Cleve Clin J Med 1990;57:181.
150. Kline JN, Hirasuna JD. Pulmonary edema after freebase cocaine smoking—not due to an adulterant. Chest 1990;97:1009.
151. Brashear RE. Effects of heroin, morphine, methadone, and propoxyphene on the lung. Semin Respir Med 1980;2:59.
152. Heffner JE, Sahn SA. Salicylate-induced pulmonary edema: clinical features and prognosis. Ann Intern Med 1981;95:405.
153. Andersson BS, Luna MA, Yee C, et al. Fatal pulmonary failure complicating high-dose cytosine arabinoside therapy in acute leukemia. Cancer 1990;65:1079.
154. Spry CJF. Eosinophilia and allergic reactions to drugs. Clin Haematol 1980;9:521.
155. Davis P. Significance of eosinophilia during gold therapy. Arthritis Rheum 1974;17:964.
156. Stafford BT, Crosby WH. Late onset of gold-induced thrombocytopenia. JAMA 1978;239:50.
157. Shulman NR. A mechanism of cell destruction in individuals sensitized to foreign antigens and its implications in autoimmunity. Ann Intern Med 1964;60:506.
158. Stricker RB, Shuman MA. Quinidine purpura: evidence that glycoprotein V is a target platelet antigen. Blood 1986;67:1377.
159. Chong BH. Heparin-induced thrombocytopenia. Blood Rev 1988;2:108.
160. Chong BH, Fawaz I, Cade J, et al. Heparin-induced thrombocytopenia: studies with a new low molecular weight heparinoid, Org 10172. Blood 1989;73:1592.
161. Salama A, Mueller-Eckhardt C. On the mechanisms of sensitization and attachment of antibodies to RBC in drug-induced immune hemolytic anemia. Blood 1987;69:1006.
162. Swanson MA, Chanmougan D, Swartz RS. Immunohemolytic anemia due to antipenicillin antibodies. N Engl J Med 1966;274:178.
163. Worlledge SM, Carstairs KC, Dacie JV. Autoimmune hemolytic anemia associated with alpha-methyldopa therapy. Lancet 1966;2:135.
164. Vincent PC. Drug-induced aplastic anemia and agranulocytosis incidence and mechanisms. Drugs 1986;31:52.
165. Young GAR, Vincent PC. Drug-induced agranulocytosis. Clin Haematol 1980;3:483.
166. Willson RA. The liver: its role in drug biotransformation and as a target of immunologic injury. Immunol Allergy Clin North Am 1991;11:555.
167. Lewis JH, Zimmerman HJ. Drug-induced liver disease. Med Clin North Am 1989;73:775.
168. Black M. Acetaminophen hepatotoxicity. Ann Rev Med 1984;34:577.
169. Zimmerman HJ, Lewis JH. Drug-induced cholestasis. Med Toxicol 1987;2:112.
170. Mitchell JR, Zimmerman HJ, Ishak KG, et al. Isoniazid liver injury: Clinical spectrum, pathology and probable pathogenesis. Ann Intern Med 1976;84:181.
171. Kenna JG, Neuberger JM, Williams R. Evidence for expression in human liver of halothane induced neoantigens recognized by antibodies in sera from patients with halothane hepatitis. Hepatology 1988;8:1635.
172. Christ DD, Kenna JG, Satoh H, Pohl LR. Enflurane metabolism produces covalently bound liver adducts recognized by antibodies from patients with halothane hepatitis. Anesthesiology 1988;69:833.
173. Knobler H, Levij IS, Gavish D, Chajek-Shaul T. Quinidine-induced hepatitis. A common and reversible hypersensitivity reaction. Arch Intern Med 1986;146:526.
174. Zimmerman HJ. Drug-induced chronic hepatic disease. Med Clin North Am 1979;63:567.
175. Boulton-Jones M, Sissons JGP, Nash PF, et al. Self-induced glomerulonephritis. Br Med J 1974;3:387.
176. Treser G, Cherubin C, Longergan ET, et al. Renal lesions in narcotic addicts. Am J Med 1974;57:687.
177. Sternlieb I, Bennett B, Scheinberg H. D-penicillamine induced Goodpasture's syndrome in Wilson's disease. Ann Intern Med 1975;82:673.
178. Silverberg DS, Kidd EG, Shnilka TK, et al. Gold nephropathy. A clinical and pathological study. Arthritis Rheum 1970;13:812.
179. Case DB. Proteinuria during long-term captopril therapy. JAMA 1980;244:346.
180. Kleinknecht D, Vanhille P, Morel-Maroger L, et al. Acute interstitial nephritis due to drug hypersensitivity. An up-to-date review with a report of 19 cases. Adv Nephrol 1983;12:277.
181. Porile JL, Bakris GL, Garella S. Acute interstitial nephritis with glomerulopathy due to nonsteroidal antiinflammatory agents: A review of its clinical spectrum and effects of steroid therapy. J Clin Pharmacol 1990;30:468.
182. Galpin JE, Shinaberger JH, Stanley TM, et al. Acute interstitial nephritis due to methicillin. Am J Med 1978;65:755.

183. Charleswarth, EN. Phenytoin induced pseudolymphoma syndrome: an immunologic study. Arch Dermatol 1977;113:477.
184. McCarthy LJ, Aguilar JC, Ransberg R. Fatal benign phenytoin lymphadenopathy. Arch Intern Med 1979;139:367.
185. Tomecki KH, Catalano CJ. Dapsone hypersensitivity. Arch Dermatol 1981;117:38.
186. Fenoglio JJ Jr, McAllister HA Jr, Mullick FG. Drug related myocarditis. I. Hypersensitivity myocarditis. Hum Pathol 1981;12:900.
187. Taliercio CP, Olney BA, Lie JT. Myocarditis related to drug hypersensitivity. Mayo Clin Proc 1985;60:463.
188. Kounis NG, Zavras GM, Soufras GD, Kitrow MP. Hypersensitivity myocarditis. Ann Allergy 1989;62:71.
189. Ten RM, Klein JS, Frigas E. Allergy skin testing. Mayo Clin Proc 1995;70:783.
190. Adkinson NF Jr. Diagnosis of immunologic drug reactions. NER Allergy Proc 1984;5:104.
191. Calkin JM, Maibach HI. Delayed hypersensitivity drug reactions diagnosed by patch testing. Contact Dermatitis 1993;29:223.
192. Patterson R. Diagnosis and treatment of drug allergy. J Allergy Clin Immunol 1988;81:380.
193. Baldo BA, Harle DG. Drug allergenic determinants. Monogr Allergy 1990;28:11.
194. Weiss ME, Nyham D, Zhikang P, et al. Association of protamine IgE and IgG antibodies with life-threatening reactions to intravenous protamine. N Engl J Med 1989;320:886.
195. Dobozy A, Hunyadi J, Kenderessy ASZ, Simon N. Lymphocyte transformation test in the detection of drug hypersensitivity. Clin Exp Dermatol 1981;6:367.
196. Livini E, Halevy S, Stahl B, Joshua H. The appearance of macrophage migration–inhibition factor in drug reactions. J Allergy Clin Immunol 1987;80:843.
197. Kalish RS, LaPorte A, Wood JA, Johnson KL. Sulfonamide-reactive lymphocytes detected at very low frequency in the peripheral blood of patients with drug-induced eruptions. J Allergy Clin Immunol 1994;94:465.
198. Schwartz LB. Tryptase, a mediator of human mast cells. J Allergy Clin Immunol 1990;86:594.
199. Appel GB. A decade of penicillin related acute interstitial nephritis: More questions than answers. Clin Nephrol 1980;13:151.
200. Rosenthal A. Followup study of fatal penicillin reactions. JAMA 1959;167:118.
201. Singer JZ, Wallace SL. The allopurinol hypersensitivity syndrome: unnecessary morbidity and mortality. Arthritis Rheum 1986;29:82.
202. Lawson DH, Jick H. Drug prescribing in hospitals: an international comparison. Am J Public Health 1976;66:644.
203. Pau AK, Morgan JE, Terlingo A. Drug allergy documentation by physicians, nurses, and medical students. Am J Hosp Pharm 1989;46:570.
204. Kuehm SL, Doyle MJ. Medication errors: 1977–1988. Experience in medical malpractice claims. NJ Med 1990;87:27.
205. Hanaford PC. Adverse drug reaction cards carried by patients. Br Med J 1986;292:1109.
206. Altman LC, Petersen PE. Successful prevention of an anaphylactoid reaction to iron dextran. Ann Intern Med 1988;109:346.
207. Chandler MJ, Ong RC, Grammer LC, Sullivan TJ. Detection, characterization, and desensitization of IgE to streptomycin. J Allergy Clin Immunol 1992;89:178.
208. Anné S, Middleton E Jr, Reisman RE. Vancomycin anaphylaxis and successful desensitization. Ann Allergy 1994;73:402.
209. Webster E, Panush RS. Allopurinol hypersensitivity in a patient with severe, chronic tophaceous gout. Arthritis Rheum 1985;28:707.
210. Sullivan TJ, Wedner HJ. Drug allergy. In: Korenblat PE, Wedner HJ, eds. Allergy: theory and practice. 2nd ed. Philadelphia: WB Saunders, 1992:541.
211. Graff-Lonnevig V, Hedlin G, Lindfors A. Penicillin allergy: a rare paediatric condition? Arch Dis Child 1988;63:1342.
212. Sullivan TJ, Wedner HJ, Shatz GS, Yecies LD, Parker CW. Skin testing to detect penicillin allergy. J Allergy Clin Immunol 1981;68:171.
213. Shepherd GM. Allergy to B-lactam antibiotics. Immunol Allergy Clin North Am 1991;11:611.
214. Idsoe O, Guthe T, Willcox RR, et al. Nature and extent of penicillin side-reactions with particular reference to fatalities from anaphylactic shock. Bull WHO 1968;38:159.
215. Berkelman RL, Finton RJ, Elsea WR. Beta-adrenergic antagonists and fatal anaphylactic reactions to oral penicillin. Ann Intern Med 1986;104:134.
216. Weiss ME, Adkinson NF Jr. Immediate hypersensitivity reactions to penicillin and related antibiotics. Clin Allergy 1988;18:515.
217. Task Force on Asthma and the Other Allergic Diseases. NIAID Task Force Report. Bethesda, Md: Department of Health, Education, and Welfare, 1979. National Institutes of Health Publication 79-387/G.
218. Shapiro S, Stone D, Siskind D, et al. Drug rash with ampicillin and other penicillins. Lancet 1969;2:969.
219. Wintroub BV, Stern R. Cutaneous drug reactions: pathogenesis and clinical classification. J Am Acad Dermatol 1985;13:167.
220. Neu HD. The new beta-lactamase-stable cephalosporins. Ann Intern Med 1982;97:408.
221. Silviu-Dan F, McPhillips S, Warrington RJ. The frequency of skin test reactions to side-chain penicillin determinants. J Allergy Clin Immunol 1993;91:694.

222. Gonzalez J, Miranda A, Martin A, et al. Sensitivity to amoxycillin with good tolerance to penicillin. J Allergy Clin Immunol 1988;81:222. Abstract.
223. Erffmeyer JE. Reactions to antibiotics. Immunol Allergy Clin North Am 1992;12:633.
224. Grieco MH. Cross-allergenicity of the penicillins and the cephalosporins. Arch Intern Med 1967;119:141.
225. Petz L. Immunologic cross-reactivity between penicillins and cephalosporins: a review. J Infect Dis 1978;137:574.
226. Anné S, Reisman RE. Risk of administering cephalosporin antibiotics to patients with histories of penicillin allergy. Ann Allergy Asthma Immunol 1995;74:167.
227. Van Arsdel PP Jr. Allergy to cephalosporins. JAMA 1991;265:2254.
228. Saxon A, Beal GN, Rohr AS, Adelman DC. Immediate hypersensitivity reactions to B-lactam antibiotics. Ann Intern Med 1987;107:204.
229. Igea JM, Fraj J, Davila I, Cuevas M, Cuesta J, Hinojosa M. Allergy to cefazolin: study of in vivo cross reactivity with other beta lactams. Ann Allergy 1992;68:515.
230. Saxon A, Adelman DC, Patel A, Hajdu R, Calandra GB. Imipenem cross-reactivity with penicillin in humans. J Allergy Clin Immunol 1988;82:213.
231. Adkinson NF Jr. Immunogenicity and cross-allergenicity of aztreonam. Am J Med 1990;88:125.
232. Fernandez-Rivas M, Carral CP, Cuevas M, Marti C, Moral A, Senent CJ. Selective allergic reactions to clavu-lanic acid. J Allergy Clin Immunol 1995;95:748.
233. Hoffman DR, Hudson P, Carlyle SJ, Massello W III. Three cases of fatal anaphylaxis to antibiotics in patients with prior histories of allergy to the drug. Ann Allergy 1989;62:91.
234. Sogn D, Evans R III, Shepherd G, et al. Results of the NIAID collaborative clinical trial to test the predictive value of skin testing with major and minor penicillin derivatives in hospitalized adults. Arch Intern Med 1992;152:1025.
235. Warrington RJ, Simons FER, Ho HW, et al. Diagnosis of penicillin allergy by skin testing: the Manitoba experience. Can Med Assoc J 1978;118:787.
236. Lin R. A perspective on penicillin allergy. Arch Intern Med 1992;152:930.
237. Adkinson NF Jr. Side-chain specific beta-lactam allergy. Clin Exp Allergy 1990;20:445.
238. Mendelson LM, Ressler C, Rosen JP, Selcow JE. Routine elective penicillin allergy skin testing in children and adolescents: study of sensitization. J Allergy Clin Immunol 1984;73:76.
239. Redelmeier DA, Sox HC Jr. The role of skin testing in penicillin allergy. Arch Intern Med 1990;150:1939.
240. Parker PJ, Parrinello JT, Condemi JJ, Rosenfeld SI. Penicillin resensitization among hospitalized patients. J Allergy Clin Immunol 1991;88:213.
241. Adkinson NF Jr. Tests for immunological drug reactions. In: Rose NF, Friedman H, eds. Manual of clinical immunology. Washington, DC: American Society for Microbiology, 1986:692.
242. Segreti J, Trenholme GM, Levin S. Antibiotic therapy in the allergic patient. Med Clin North Am 1995;79:935.
243. Bochner BS, Lichtenstein LM. Anaphylaxis. N Engl J Med 1991;324:1785.
244. Sullivan T, Yecies L, Shatz G, Parker CW, Wedner HJ. Desensitization of patients allergic to penicillin using orally administered B-lactam antibiotics. J Allergy Clin Immunol 1982;69:275.
245. Borisk L, Tamir R, Rosenwasser L. Intravenous desensitization to beta-lactam antibiotics. J Allergy Clin Immunol 1987;80:314.
246. Stark BJ, Earl HS, Gross GN, Lumry WR, Goodman EL, Sullivan TJ. Acute and chronic desensitization of penicillin-allergic patients using oral penicillin. J Allergy Clin Immunol 1987;79:523.
247. Brown LA, Goldberg ND, Shearer WT. Long-term ticarcillin desensitization by the continuous oral adminis-tration of penicillin. J Allergy Clin Immunol 1982;69:51.
248. Moss RB. Drug allergy in cystic fibrosis. Clin Rev Allergy 1991;9:211.
249. Gruchalla RS, Sullivan TJ. Detection of human IgE to sulfamethoxazole by skin testing with sulfamethoxazoyl-poly-L-tyrosine. J Allergy Clin Immunol 1991;88:784.
250. Shear NH, Spielberg SP, Grant DM, Tang BK. Differences in metabolism of sulfonamides predisposing to idio-syncratic toxicity. Ann Intern Med 1986;105:179.
251. Rieder MJ, Vetrecht J, Shear NH, et al. Diagnosis of sulfonamide hypersensitivity reactions by *in vitro* "rechal-lenge" with hydroxylamine metabolites. Ann Intern Med 1989;110:286.
252. Carr A, Tindall B, Penny R, et al. *In vitro* cytotoxicity as a marker of hypersensitivity to sulphamethoxazole in patients with HIV. Clin Exp Immunol 1993;94:21.
253. Jick H. Adverse reactions to trimethoprim-sulfamethoxazole in hospitalized patients. Rev Infect Dis 1986;4:426.
254. Carr A, Cooper DA, Penny R. Allergic manifestations of human immunodeficiency virus infection. J Clin Immunol 1991;11:52.
255. Kovacs JA, Hiemenz JW, Macher AM, Stover D, et al. *Pneumocystis carinii* pneumonia: a comparison between patients with the acquired immunodeficiency syndrome and patients with other immunodeficiencies. Ann Intern Med 1984;100:663.
256. Colebunders R, Izaley L, Bila K, Kabumpangi K, Melameka N, Nyst M. Cutaneous reactions to trimethoprim-sulfamethoxazole in African patients with acquired immunodeficiency syndrome. Ann Intern Med 1987;107:599.
257. Sattler FR, Cowan R, Nielson DM, et al. Trimethoprim-sulfamethoxazole with pentamidine for treatment of *Pneumocystis carinii* pneumonia in the acquired immunodeficiency syndrome. Ann Intern Med 1988;109:280.
258. Greenberger PA, Patterson R. Management of drug allergy in patients with acquired immunodeficiency syn-drome. J Allergy Clin Immunol 1987;79:484.

259. Absar N, Daneshvar H, Beall G. Desensitization to trimethoprim/sulfamethoxazole in HIV-infected patients. J Allergy Clin Immunol 1994;93:1001.

260. White MV, Haddad ZH, Brunner E, Sainz C. Desensitization to trimethoprim-sulfamethoxazole in patients with acquired immunodeficiency syndrome and *Pneumocystis carinii* pneumonia. Ann Allergy 1989;62:177.

261. Baum CG, Sonnabend JA, O'Sullivan M. Prophylaxis of AIDS-related *Pneumocystis carinii* pneumonia with aerosolized pentamidine in a patient with hypersensitivity to systemic pentamidine. J Allergy Clin Immunol 1992;90:268.

262. Sher MR, Suchar C, Lockey RF. Anaphylactic shock induced by oral desensitization to trimethoprim/sulfamethoxazole (TMP/SMZ). J Allergy Clin Immunol 1986;77:133.

263. Wright DN, Nelson RP, Ledford DK, et al. Serum IgE and human immunodeficiency virus (HIV) infection. J Allergy Clin Immunol 1990;85:445.

264. Finegold I. Oral desensitization to trimethoprim-sulfamethoxazole in a patient with AIDS. J Allergy Clin Immunol 1985;75:137.

265. Guidelines for prophylaxis against *Pneumocystis carinii* pneumonia for persons infected with human immunodeficiency virus. MMWR 1989;38(Suppl 5-5):1.

266. Hughes WT. Successful intermittent chemoprophylaxis for *Pneumocystis carinii* pneumonitis. N Engl J Med 1987;316:1627.

267. Martin MA, Cox PH, Beck K, Styer C, Beall GN. A comparison of the effectiveness of three regimens in the prevention of *Pneumocystis carinii* pneumonia in human immunodeficiency virus-infected patients. Arch Intern Med 1992;152:523.

268. Boxer MB, Dykewicz MS, Patterson R, Greenberger PA, Kelly JF. The management of patients with sulfonamide allergy. NER Allergy Proc 1988;9:219.

269. Yango MC, Kim K, Evans R III. Oral desensitization to trimethoprim-sulfamethoxazole in pediatric patients. Immunol Allergy Prac 1992;14:56.

270. Caballer BH, Fernandez-Rivas M, Lazaro JF, et al. Management of sulfadiazine allergy in patients with acquired immunodeficiency syndrome. J Allergy Clin Immunol 1991;88:137.

271. Moreno JN, Poblete RB, Maggio C, Gagnon S, Fischl MA. Rapid oral desensitization for sulfonamides in patients with the acquired immunodeficiency syndrome. Ann Allergy Asthma Immunol 1995;74:140.

272. Meyers S, Sachar DB, Present DH, Janowitz HD. Olsalazine sodium in the treatment of ulcerative colitis among patients intolerant of sulfasalazine: a prospective, randomized, placebo-controlled, double-blind, dose-ranging clinical trial. Gastroenterology 1987;93:1255.

273. Purdy BH, Philips DM, Summers RW. Desensitization for sulfasalazine rash. Ann Intern Med 1984;100:512.

274. Earl HS, Sullivan TJ. Acute desensitization of a patient with cystic fibrosis allergic to both B-lactam and aminoglycoside antibiotics. J Allergy Clin Immunol 1987;79:477.

275. Chandler MJ, Ong RC, Grammer LC, et al. Detection, characterization, and desensitization of IgE to streptomycin. J Allergy Clin Immunol 1992;89:178.

276. Polk RE, Healy DP, Schwartz LB, Rock DT, Garson ML, Roller K. Vancomycin and the red man syndrome: pharmacodynamics of histamine release. J Infect Dis 1988;157:502.

277. Palchick BA, Fink EA, McEntire JE, et al. Anaphylaxis due to chloramphenicol. Am J Med Sci 1984;288:43.

278. Yeu WW, Chau CH, Lee J, et al. Cholestatic hepatitis in a patient who received Clarithromycin therapy for a *M. chelonae* lung infection. Clin Infect Dis 1994;18:1025.

279. Kurohara ML, Kwong FK, Lebherz TB, Klaustermeyer WD. Metronidazole hypersensitivity and oral desensitization. J Allergy Clin Immunol 1991;88:279.

280. Kemp SF, Lockey RF. Amphotericin B: emergency challenge in a neutropenic, asthmatic patient with fungal sepsis. J Allergy Clin Immunol 1995;96:425.

281. Bittleman DB, Stapleton J, Casale TB. Report of successful desensitization to itraconazole. J Allergy Clin Immunol 1994;94:270.

282. Carr A, Penny R, Cooper DA. Allergy and desensitization to zidovudine in patients with acquired immunodeficiency syndrome (AIDS). J Allergy Clin Immunol 1993;91:683.

283. Lumry WR, Curd JG, Zeiger RS, et al. Aspirin sensitive rhinosinusitis: the clinical syndrome and effects of aspirin administration. J Allergy Clin Immunol 1983;71:588.

284. Butterfield JH, Kao PC, Klee GG, Yocum MW. Aspirin idiosyncrasy in systemic mast cell disease: a new look at mediator release during aspirin desensitization. Mayo Clin Proc 1995;70:481.

285. Giraldo B, Blumenthal MN, Spink WW. Aspirin intolerance and asthma: a clinical and immunological study. Ann Intern Med 1969;71:479.

286. Spector SL, Wangaard CH, Farr RS. Aspirin and concomitant idiosyncrasies in adult asthmatic patients. J Allergy Clin Immunol 1979;64:500.

287. Weber RW, Hoffman M, Raine, et al. Incidence of bronchoconstriction due to aspirin, azo dyes, non-azo-dyes and preservatives in a population of perennial asthmatics. J Allergy Clin Immunol 1979;64:32.

288. Pleskow WW, Stevenson DD, Mathison DA, et al. Aspirin-sensitive rhinosinusitis/asthma: spectrum of adverse reactions to aspirin. J Allergy Clin Immunol 1983;71:574.

289. Israel E, Fischer AR, Rosenberg MA, et al. The pivotal role of 5-lipoxygenase products in the reaction of aspirin-sensitive asthmatics to aspirin. Am Rev Respir Dis 1993;148:1447.

290. Stevenson DD. Diagnosis, prevention, and treatment of adverse reactions to aspirin and nonsteroidal anti-inflammatory drugs. J Allergy Clin Immunol 1984;74:617.

291. Mathison DA, Lumry WR, Stevenson DD, et al. Aspirin in chronic urticaria and/or angioedema: studies of sensitivity and desensitization. J Allergy Clin Immunol 1982;69:135.
292. Stevenson DD, Simon RA. Sensitivity to aspirin and nonsteroidal anti-inflammatory drugs. In: Middleton E Jr, Reed CE, Ellis EF, Adkinson NF Jr, Yunginger JW, eds. Allergy: principles and practice. 4th ed. St Louis: CV Mosby, 1993;1747.
293. Pleskow WW, Stevenson DD, Mathison DA, et al. Aspirin desensitization in aspirin-sensitive asthmatic patients: clinical manifestations and characterization of the refractory period. J Allergy Clin Immunol 1982;69:11.
294. Phillips GD, Foord R, Holgate ST. Inhaled lysine-aspirin as a bronchoprovocation procedure in aspirin-sensitive asthma: its repeatability, absence of late-phase reaction, and the role of histamine. J Allergy Clin Immunol 1989;84:232.
295. Stevenson DD. Aspirin and nonsteroidal anti-inflammatory drugs. Immunol Allergy Clin North Am 1995;15:529.
296. Settipane RA, Schrank PJ, Simon RA, Mathison DA, Christiansen SC, Stevenson DD. Prevalence of cross-reactivity with acetaminophen in aspirin-sensitive asthmatic subjects. J Allergy Clin Immunol 1995;96:480.
297. Fischer AR, Israel E. Identifying and treating aspirin-induced asthma. J Respir Dis 1995;16:304.
298. Stevenson DD, Hougham AJ, Schrank PJ, et al. Salsalate cross-sensitivity in aspirin-sensitive asthmatic patients. J Allergy Clin Immunol 1990;86:749.
299. Feigenbaum BA, Stevenson DD, Simon RA. Hydrocortisone sodium succinate does not cross-react with aspirin in aspirin-sensitive patients with asthma. J Allergy Clin Immunol 1995;96:545.
300. Stevenson DD, Simon RA, Lumry WR, et al. Adverse reactions to tartrazine. J Allergy Clin Immunol 1986;78:182.
301. Settipane GA. Aspirin and allergic diseases: a review. Am J Med 1983;74:102.
302. Stevenson DD, Mathison DA. Aspirin sensitivity in asthmatics: when may this drug be safe? Postgrad Med 1985;78:111.
303. Sweet JM, Stevenson DD, Mathison DA, et al. Long term effects of aspirin desensitization treatment for ASA sensitive patients with asthma. J Allergy Clin Immunol 1990;85:59.
304. Mathison DA, Lumry WR, Stevenson DD, et al. Aspirin in chronic urticaria and/or angioedema: studies of sensitivity and desensitization. J Allergy Clin Immunol 1982;69:135.
305. Katayma H, Yamaguchi K, Kozuka T, et al. Adverse reactions to ionic and nonionic contrast media: a report from the Japanese Committee on the safety of contrast media. Radiology 1990;175:621.
306. Wolf GL, Arenson RL, Cross AP. A prospective trial of ionic vs. nonionic contrast agents in routine clinical practice: comparison of adverse effects. Am J Radiol 1989;152:939.
307. Steinberg EP, Moore RD, Powe NR, et al. Safety and cost effectiveness of high-osmolality as compared with low-osmolality contrast material in patients undergoing cardiac angiography. N Engl J Med 1992;326:425.
308. Caro JJ, Trindale E, McGregor M. The risk of death and of severe nonfatal reactions with high-versus low-osmolality contrast media: a meta-analysis. AJR 1991;156:825.
309. Shellock FG, Hahn HP, Mink JH, Itskovich E. Adverse reaction to intravenous gadoteridol. Radiology 1993;189:151.
310. Greenberger PA, Patterson R. The prevention of immediate generalized reactions to radiocontrast media in high-risk patients. J Allergy Clin Immunol 1991;87:867.
311. Siegle RL, Halvosen R, Dillon J, et al. The use of iohexal in patients with previous reactions to ionic contrast material. Invest Radiol 1991;26:411.
312. Enright T, Chua-Lim A, Duda E, et al. The role of a documented allergic profile as a risk factor for radiographic contrast media reactions. Ann Allergy 1989;62:302.
313. Greenberger PA, Meyers SN, Kramer BL, Kramer BL. Effects of beta-adrenergic and calcium antagonists on the development of anaphylactoid reactions from radiographic contrast media during cardiac angiography. J Allergy Clin Immunol 1987;80:698.
314. Lang DM, Alpern MB, Visintainer PF, Smith ST. Increased risk for anaphylactoid reaction from contrast media in patients on B-adrenergic blockers or with asthma. Ann Intern Med 1991;115:270.
315. Greenberger PA, Patterson R, Tapio CM. Prophylaxis against repeated radiocontrast media reactions in 857 cases. Arch Intern Med 1985;145:2197.
316. Lasser EC, Berry CC, Mishkin MM, et al. Pretreatment with corticosteroids to prevent adverse reactions to nonionic contrast media. AJR 1994;162:523.
317. Ramesh S, Reisman RE. Noncardiogenic pulmonary edema due to radiocontrast media. Ann Allergy Asthma Immunol 1995;75:308.
318. Chandler MJ, Grammer LC, Patterson R. Provocative challenge with local anesthetics in patients with a prior history of reaction. J Allergy Clin Immunol 1987;79:883.
319. deShazo RD, Nelson HS. An approach to the patient with a history of local anesthetic hypersensitivity: experience with 90 patients. J Allergy Clin Immunol 1979;63:387.
320. Incaudo G, Schatz M, Patterson R, et al. Administration of local anesthetics to patients with a history of a prior reaction. J Allergy Clin Immunol 1978;61:329.
321. Schwartz HJ, Sher TH. Bisulfite sensitivity manifesting as allergy to local dental anesthesia. J Allergy Clin Immunol 1985;75:525.
322. Pollack CV, Swindle GM. Use of diphenhydramine for local anesthesia in "caine"-sensitive patients. J Emerg Med 1989;7:611.

323. Patterson R, Roberts M, Grammer LC. Insulin allergy: reevaluation after two decades. Ann Allergy 1990;64:459.
324. Fineberg SE, Galloway JA, Fineberg NS, Rathbun MJ, Hufferd S. Immunogenicity of recombinant DNA human insulin. Diabetologia 1983;25:465.
325. Grammer LC, Metzger B, Patterson R. Cutaneous allergy to human (recombinant DNA) insulin. JAMA 1984;251:1459.
326. Grammer LC, Roberts M, Patterson R. IgE and IgG antibody against human (recombinant DNA) insulin in patients with systemic insulin allergy. J Lab Clin Med 1985;105:108.
327. Grammer LC, Roberts M, Buchannan TA, Fitzsimons R, Metzger B, Patterson R. Specificity of IgE and IgG against human (recombinant DNA) insulin in human (or DNA) insulin allergy and resistance. J Lab Clin Med 1987;109:141.
328. Yallow RS, Berson SA. Immunologic aspects of insulin. Am J Med 1961;31:882.
329. Patterson R, Mellies CJ, Roberts M. Immunologic reactions against insulin. II. IgE anti-insulin and combined IgE and IgG immunologic insulin resistance. J Immunol 1973;110:1135.
330. deShazo R, Boehm T, Kumar D, Galloway J, Dvorak H. Dermal hypersensitivity reaction to insulin: correlations of three patterns to their histopathology. J Allergy Clin Immunol 1982;69:229.
331. Grammer LC, Chen PY, Patterson R. Evaluation and management of insulin allergy. J Allergy Clin Immunol 1983;71:250.
332. Mattson JR, Patterson R, Roberts M. Insulin therapy in patients with systemic insulin allergy. Arch Intern Med 1975;135:818.
333. McGrath KG, Patterson R. Anaphylactic reactivity to streptokinase. JAMA 1984;252:1314.
334. McGrath KG, Patterson R. Immunology of streptokinase in human subjects. Clin Exp Immunol 1985;62:421.
335. Dykewicz MS, McGrath KG, Davison R, Kaplan KJ, Patterson R. Identification of patients at risk for anaphylaxis due to streptokinase. Arch Intern Med 1986;146:305.
336. McGrath KG, Zeffren B, Alexander J, et al. Allergic reactions to streptokinase consistent with anaphylactic or antigen-antibody complex mediated damage. J Allergy Clin Immunol 1985;76:453.
337. Sherry S, Marder VJ. Streptokinase and recombinant tissue plasminogen activator (rt-PA) are equally effective in treating acute myocardial infarction. Ann Intern Med 1991;114:417.
338. Willis J, ed. Chymopapain approval. FDA Bull 1982;12:17.
339. Grammer LC, Patterson R. Proteins: chymopapain and insulin. J Allergy Clin Immunol 1984;74:635.
340. Moscicki RA, Sockin SM, Corsello BF, Ostro MG, Bloch KJ. Anaphylaxis during induction of general anesthesia: subsequent evaluation and management. J Allergy Clin Immunol 1990;86:325.
341. Didier A, Cador D, Bongrand P, et al. Role of quaternary ammonium ion determinants in allergy to muscle relaxants. J Allergy Clin Immunol 1987;79:578.
342. Keith PK, Dolovich J. Anaphylactic and anaphylactoid reactions in the perioperative period. Immunol Allergy Clin North Am 1992;12:671.
343. Smith DL, deShazo RD. Local anesthetics and neuromuscular blocking agents. Immunol Allergy Clin North Am 1995;15:613.
344. Vervloet D. Allergy to muscle relaxants and related compounds. Clin Allergy 1985;15:501.
345. Baldo BA, Fisher MM. Detection of serum IgE antibodies that react with alcuronium and tubocurarine after life-threatening reactions to muscle-relaxant drugs. Anesth Intens Care 1983;11:194.
346. Baldo BA, Fisher MM. Substituted ammonium ions as allergenic determinants in drug allergy. Nature 1983;306:262.
347. Charpin D, Benzarti M, Hémon Y, et al. Atopy and anaphylactic reactions to suxamethonium. J Allergy Clin Immunol 1988;82:356.
348. Slater JE. Allergic reactions to natural rubber. Ann Allergy 1992;68:203.
349. Bubak ME, Reed CE, Fransway AF, et al. Allergic reactions to latex among health-care workers. Mayo Clin Proc 1992;67:1075.
350. Czuppon AB, Chen Z, Rennert S, et al. The rubber elongation factor of rubber trees (*Hevea brasiliensia*) is the major allergen in latex. J Allergy Clin Immunol 1993;92:690.
351. Nutter AE. Contact urticaria due to rubber. Br J Dermatol 1979;101:597.
352. Gelfand DW. Barium enemas, latex balloons, and anaphylactic reactions. AJR 1991;156:1.
353. Meeropol E, Kelleher R, Bell S, et al. Allergic reactions to rubber in patients with myelodysplasia. N Engl J Med 1990;323:1072.
354. Ahlroth M, Alenius H, Turjanmaa K, Makinen-Kiljunen S, Reunala T, Palosuo T. Cross-reacting allergens in natural rubber latex and avocado. J Allergy Clin Immunol 1995;96:167.
355. Carey AB, Cornish K, Schrank P, Ward B, Simon R. Cross-reactivity of alternate plant sources of latex in subjects with systemic IgE-mediated sensitivity to *Hevea brasiliensis* latex. Ann Allergy Asthma Immunol 1995;74:317.
356. Yunginger JW, Jones RT, Fransway AF, et al. Extractable latex allergens and proteins in disposable medical gloves and other rubber products. J Allergy Clin Immunol 1994;93:836.
357. Kelly KJ, Kurup VP, Zacharisen M, et al. Skin and serological testing in the diagnosis of latex allergy. J Allergy Clin Immunol 1993;91:1140.
358. Turjanmaa K, Reunala T, Rasanen L. Comparison of diagnostic methods in latex surgical contact urticaria. Contact Dermatitis 1988;19:241.

359. Parish ES, Kimbrough C, eds. Latex sensitivity test. FDA Bull 1995;25:2.
360. Hamann CP. Natural rubber latex protein sensitivity in review. Am J Contact Dermatitis 1993;4:4.
361. Kelly KJ. Management of the latex-allergic patient. Immunol Allergy Clin North Am 1995;15:139.
362. Setlock MA, Cotter TP, Rosner D. Latex allergy: failure of prophylaxis to prevent severe reaction. Anesth Analg 1993;76:650.
363. Sharath MD, Metzger WJ, Richerson HB, et al. Protamine-induced fatal anaphylaxis. J Thorac Cardiovasc Surg 1985;90:86.
364. Weiler JM, Gellhaus MA, Carter JG, Meng RL, Benson PM, Hottel RA. A prospective study of the risk of an immediate adverse reaction to protamine sulfate during cardiopulmonary bypass surgery. J Allergy Clin Immunol 1990;85:713.
365. Gottschlich GM, Graulee GP, Georgitis JW. Adverse reactions to protamine sulfate during cardiac surgery in diabetic and non-diabetic patients. Ann Allergy 1988;61:277.
366. Levy JH, Schwieger IM, Zaidan JR, Faraj BA, Weintraub WS. Evaluation of patients at risk for protamine reactions. J Thorac Cardiovasc Surg 1989;98:200.
367. Weiss ME, Adkinson NF Jr. Allergy to protamine. Clin Rev Allergy 1991;9:339.
368. Cheema A, Sussman GL, Janeclewicz Z, et al. Pentothal anaphylaxis. J Allergy Clin Immunol 1988;81:220.
369. Harle DG, Baldo BA, Smal MA, et al. Detection of thiopentone-reactive IgE antibodies following anaphylactoid reactions during anesthesia. Clin Allergy 1986;16:493.
370. Binkley K, Cheema A, Sussman G, et al. Generalized allergic reactions during anaesthesia. J Allergy Clin Immunol 1992;89:768.
371. Ebertz JM, Hermens JM, McMillan JC, et al. Functional differences between human cutaneous mast cells and basophils: a comparison of morphine-induced histamine release. Agent Actions 1986;18:455.
372. Sprung J, Schedewie HK, Kampine JP. Intraoperative anaphylactic shock after bacitracin irrigation. Anesth Analg 1990;71:430.
373. Heffner JE. Reactions to fluorescein. JAMA 1980;243:2029.
374. Greenberger PA. Plasma anaphylaxis and immediate type reactions. In: Rossi EC, Simon TL, Moss GS, eds. Principles of transfusion medicine. Baltimore: Williams & Wilkins, 1991:635.
375. Isbister JP, Fisher MMcD. Adverse effects of plasma volume expanders. Anesth Intens Care 1980;8:145.
376. Marshall CP, Pearson FC, Sagona MA, et al. Reactions during hemodialysis caused by allergy to ethylene oxide gas sterilization. J Allergy Clin Immunol 1985;75:563.
377. Grammer LC, Patterson R. IgE against ethylene oxide altered human serum albumin (ETO-HSA) as an etiologic agent in allergic reactions of hemodialysis patients. Artif Organs 1987;11:97.
378. Gifford J. Serum therapy and immunoprophylaxis. In: Altman LC, ed. Clinical allergy and immunology. Boston: GK Hall, 1984:359.
379. Dykewicz MS, Rosen ST, O'Connell MM, et al. Plasma histamine but not anaphylatoxin levels correlate with generalized urticaria from infusions of antilymphocyte monoclonal antibodies. J Lab Clin Med 1992;120:290.
380. Burks AW, Sampson HA, Buckley RH. Anaphylactic reactions after gamma globulin administration in patients with hypogammaglobulinemia: detection of IgE antibodies to IgA. N Engl J Med 1986;314:560.
381. Wingert WA, Wainschel J. Diagnosis and management of envenomation by poisonous snakes. South Med J 1975;68:1045.
382. Kobayashi RH. Vaccinations. Immunol Allergy Clin North Am 1995;15:553.
383. Jacobs RL, Lowe RS, Lanier BQ. Adverse reactions to tetanus toxoid. JAMA 1982;247:40.
384. Carey AB, Meltzer EO. Diagnosis and "desensitization" in tetanus vaccine hypersensitivity. Ann Allergy 1992;69:336.
385. James JM, Burks AW, Roberson PK, Sampson HA. Safe administration of the measles vaccine to children allergic to eggs. N Engl J Med 1995;332:1262.
386. Sakaguchi M, Ogura H, Inouye S. IgE antibody to gelatin in children with immediate-type reactions to measles and mumps vaccines. J Allergy Clin Immunol 1995;96:563.
387. Trotter AC, Stone BD, Laszlo DJ, Georgitis JW. Measles, mumps, rubella vaccine administration in egg-sensitive children: systemic reactions during vaccine desensitization. Ann Allergy 1994;72:25.
388. Retaillian HF, Curtis AC, Storr G, et al. Illness after influenza vaccination reported through a nation-wide surveillance system: 1976–1977. Am J Epidemiol 1980;111:270.
389. Campbell BG, Edwards RL. Safety of influenza vaccination in adults with asthma. Med J Aust 1984;140:773.
390. Harvey RE, Posey WC, Jacobs RL. The predictive value of egg skin tests and yellow fever vaccine skin tests in egg-sensitive individuals. J Allergy Clin Immunol 1975;63:196.
391. Miller JR, Orgel A, Meltzer EO. The safety of egg-containing vaccines for egg-allergic patients. J Allergy Clin Immunol 1983;71:568.
392. Kletz MR, Holland CL, Mendelson JS, Bielary L. Administration of egg-derived vaccines in patients with history of egg sensitivity. Ann Allergy 1990;64:527.
393. Vittorio CC, Muglia JJ. Anticonvulsant hypersensitivity syndrome. Arch Intern Med 1995;27:2285.
394. Reents SB, Linginbahl WE, Davis SM. Phenytoin-carbamazepine cross-sensitivity. Ann Pharmacother 1989;23:235.
395. Silverman AK, Fairley J, Wong RC. Cutaneous and immunologic reactions to phenytoin. J Am Acad Dermatol 1988;18:721.

Allergic Diseases, 5th Edition,
edited by Roy Patterson, Leslie Carroll Grammer, and
Paul A. Greenberger. Lippincott–Raven Publishers, Philadelphia, © 1997.

18

Contact Dermatitis

Raymond G. Slavin

*R.G. Slavin: Division of Allergy and Immunology,
St. Louis University Health Sciences Center, St. Louis, MO 63104.*

Pearls for Practitioners
Roy Patterson

- Dermatitis around the eyes and on the cheeks can result from nail polish. Test for it on the forearm.
- You may have to clear the skin with topical steroids before patch testing.
- Dyshydrotic eczema often is labeled as an allergic reaction by patients.
- Contact dermatitis may have unusual sources. I have seen contact dermatitis from poison ivy in a man who skinned a rabbit; the rabbit had been nesting in poison ivy. Dogs' coats can transmit the poison ivy oleoresin to humans in the same manner.

Allergic contact dermatitis is a skin condition seen by all physicians and with new chemical sensitizers being introduced into the environment constantly, undoubtedly physicians will be seeing more instances of it. Contact dermatitis is the most common occupational disease and as such is important to both the individual and to society. Diagnosing allergic contact dermatitis and eliciting the cause requires all of the physician's patience, thoroughness, and acumen.

The patient with allergic contact dermatitis may be uncomfortable and at times may be disabled. The chronicity of the disease may be depressing to the patient. An inability to pursue employment or recreation are common.

IMMUNOLOGIC BASIS

Allergic contact dermatitis seems indistinguishable in its immunologic mechanism from other classic forms of the delayed, or cellular, type of hypersensitivity. Most clinical allergic problems are related to diseases associated with the immediate type of hypersensitivity, which depends on humoral antibody. In contrast, delayed or cellular hypersensitivity depends on sensitized lymphocytes.

Sensitization

The inductive or afferent limb of contact sensitivity begins with the topical application to the skin of a chemically reactive substance called a hapten. The hapten may be organic or inorganic and is generally of low molecular weight. Its ability to sensitize depends on its penetrating the skin and forming covalent bonds with proteins. The degree of sensitization is directly proportional to the stability of the hapten–protein coupling. In the case of the commonly used skin sensitizer, dinitrochlorobenzene, the union of the chemical hapten and the tissue protein occurs in the Malpighian layer of the epidermis, with the amino acid sites of lysine and cysteine being most reactive.[1] Skin lipids might exert an adjuvant effect comparable to the myoside of *Mycobacterium tuberculosis*.

Langerhans cells are of crucial importance in the induction of contact sensitivity.[2] These dendritic cells in the epidermis cannot be seen on routine histologic sections of the skin by light microscopic examination, but they can be identified easily by special stains. They possess Ia antigens and receptors for the Fc portion of IgG and complement, much like macrophages. The role of Langerhans cells in contact sensitivity reactions is predicted on the following observations. First, in contact hypersensitivity reactions, an apposition of lymphocyte-like cells and Langerhans cells can be seen microscopically. Second, the Langerhans cell has been shown to bind antigen in the skin and carry it by means of dermal lymphatics to the draining lymph nodes. Third, the Langerhans cell develops morphologic characteristics of secretion and increased enzymatic activity at the site of contact hypersensitivity reactions. Contact sensitivity may begin in more than one site.[3]

After the allergen is applied epicutaneously, it is ingested by the Langerhans cell by pinocytosis and is partially degraded; the resultant peptide is then brought to the cell surface, where it binds to the Ia antigen. The Langerhans cell then presents the processed antigen to T-helper cells either in the skin or in the draining lymph node. For the allergic response to proceed, the antigen-bearing Langerhans cell must contact CD4-positive T cells (T-helper cells) that have, on their surface, specific receptors for the contact allergen and class II antigen (Ia or HLA-DR).[4]

The specificity of the contact sensitivity response resembles that of delayed hypersensitivity (cellular) rather than immediate hypersensitivity (humoral). When a hapten–protein complex induces an immune response, circulating antibody produced is directed toward, or is specific for, the hapten. The delayed hypersensitivity usually is directed toward the protein carrier as well. This *carrier specificity* is clearly evident in contact sensitivity.[5]

Elicitation

The interaction of Langerhans-containing antigen cells and T-helper cells results in release of interleukin-1 (IL-1) by the Langerhans cell. IL-1 in turn activates T cells to release interleukin-2 (IL-2) and interferon gamma (IFN-γ). IL-1 also may increase antigen-presenting cell function and upregulates Ia expression on the Langerhans cells themselves. IL-2 stimulates T cells to secrete IFN-γ or immune interferon, which activates cytotoxic T cells, natural killer cells, and macrophages. These changes culminate in the epidermal spongiosis (intercellular edema) and dermal infiltrate that are characteristic of allergic contact dermatitis. The specifically sensitized CD4 helper T cells localize the response to the site of challenge by producing IL-2 and IFN-γ. They also provide the immunologic memory that accounts for the more rapid and intense response that occurs after reexposure to the contact allergen.[4]

Histopathology

The histologic picture in allergic contact dermatitis reveals that the dermis is invaded by mononuclear inflammatory cells, especially about blood vessels and sweat glands. The epidermis is hyperplastic with mononuclear cell invasion. Frequently, intraepidermal vesicles form, which may coalesce to form large blisters. The vesicles are filled with serous fluid containing granulocytes and mononuclear cells. In experimental contact sensitivity, in addition to mononuclear phagocyte and lymphocyte accumulation, basophils are seen. This is an important distinction from hypersensitivity reactions of the tuberculin type, in which basophils are completely absent.

The existence of an IgE-mediated delayed contact hypersensitivity response after epicutaneous challenge with a reactive hapten has been demonstrated.[6] In mice that have been passively sensitized with IgE anti-dinitrophenol antibody, epicutaneous antigen challenge results in an early and delayed contact hypersensitivity response. This suggests that some cases of allergic contact dermatitis in humans may be mediated at least partially by IgE antibodies.

Transfer

The delayed type of hypersensitivity can be transferred with sensitized lymphocytes. In humans, a cell-free dialyzable fraction obtained from sensitized lymphocytes can transfer delayed hypersensitivity.[7] In this respect, allergic contact dermatitis again resembles delayed hypersensitivity. Successful transfer of contact sensitivity can be accomplished with viable lymphoid cells both in experimental animals[8] and in humans,[9] although not as easily as with tuberculin or other types of bacterial sensitivity. Peripheral blood lymphocytes, exudative cells from the vesicles of contact dermatitis, and cell-free blister fluid all have successful transferred contact sensitivity in humans.

Control Mechanisms of Contact Sensitivity

In experimental contact sensitivity, both the duration and the magnitude of the contact sensitivity are regulated.[3] In the mouse, contact sensitivity wanes concomitantly with the production of antiidiotypic antibodies. Contact sensitivity also depends on the dose of the antigen. Supraoptimal doses of the contactant induce suppressor cells, with a resultant reduction in the response.

Tolerance or unresponsiveness to a contact allergen may be produced by exposure to the antigen before to sensitization. The route of presentation is also crucial in determining whether tolerance or sensitization results. The epicutaneous or subcutaneous routes favor sensitization, whereas the intravenous or oral routes favor tolerance.

CLINICAL FEATURES

History

Allergic contact dermatitis occurs most frequently in middle-aged and elderly persons, although it may appear at any age. In contrast to the classic atopic diseases, contact dermatitis is as common in the population at large as in the atopic population, and a history of concomitant or family allergy is of no help. No familial tendency in humans toward the development of allergic contact dermatitis has been demonstrated.

The interval between exposure to the responsible agent and the occurrence of clinical manifestations in a sensitized subject is usually 12 to 48 hours, although it may be as early as 4 hours and as late as 72 hours. The incubation or sensitization period between initial exposure and the development of skin sensitivity may be as short as 2 to 3 days in the case of a strong sensitizer such as poison ivy, or several years for a weak sensitizer such as chromate. A situation analogous to serum sickness may seen both experimentally and clinically. If sufficient allergen from the sensitizing exposure remains to react with the sensitized skin after the incubation period has elapsed, a spontaneous exacerbation may occur at the site of the sensitizing exposure. In addition, a flare-up may occur at a previously involved site weeks to years after exposure to the allergen or a closely related allergen at a distant site. Once the sensitivity is established, it generally persists for many years; however, there are instances in which the sensitivity has been lost after several years.

The patient usually notices the development of erythema, followed by papules, and then vesicles. Pruritus follows the appearance of the dermatitis and is uniformly present in allergic contact dermatitis.

Physical Examination

The appearance of allergic contact dermatitis depends on the stage at which the patient presents. In the acute stage, erythema, papules, and vesicles predominate, with edema and occasionally bullae (Fig. 18-1). The boundaries of the dermatitis generally are sharply marginated.

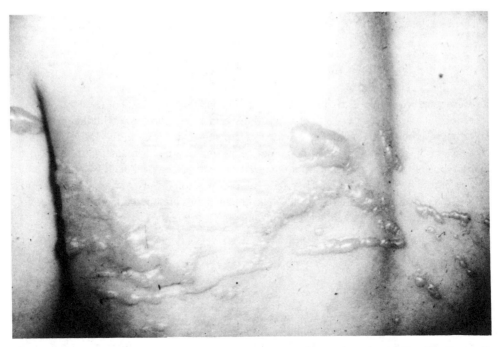

FIG. 18-1. The acute phase of contact dermatitis caused by poison ivy. Notice the linear distribution of vesicles. (Courtesy of Dr. Gary Vicik, St. Louis University School of Medicine, St. Louis, MO.)

Edema may be profound in areas of loose tissue such as the eyelids and genitalia. Acute allergic contact dermatitis of the face may result in a marked degree of periorbital swelling that resembles angioedema. The presence of the associated dermatitis should help the physician to make the distinction easily.

In the subacute phase, vesicles are less pronounced, and crusting, scaling, and the beginning of lichenification may be present. In the chronic stage, few papulovesicular lesions are evident, and thickening, lichenification, and scaliness predominate.

Different areas of the skin vary in their ease of sensitization. Pressure, friction, and perspiration are factors that seem to enhance sensitization. The eyelids, neck, and genitalia are among the most readily sensitized areas, whereas the palms, soles, and scalp are more resistant. Tissue that is irritated, inflamed, or infected is more susceptible to allergic contact dermatitis. A clinical example is the common occurrence of contact dermatitis in an area of stasis dermatitis that has been topically treated.

Differential Diagnosis

The skin conditions most frequently confused with allergic contact dermatitis are seborrheic dermatitis, atopic dermatitis, and primary irritant dermatitis.

In seborrheic dermatitis, there is a general tendency to oiliness of the skin and a predilection to lesions of the scalp and the nasal labial folds. Pruritus is not a prominent feature, and the lesions are irregular and covered with a greasy coating.

Atopic dermatitis (see Chap. 15) generally has its onset in infancy or early childhood. The skin is dry, and although pruritus is a prominent feature, it appears before the lesions and not after them, as in the case of allergic contact dermatitis. The areas most frequently involved are the flexural surfaces. The margins of the dermatitis are indefinite, and the progression from erythema to papules to vesicles is not seen.

The dermatitis caused by a primary irritant is a simple chemical or physical insult to the skin—for example, what is commonly called "dishpan hands" is a dermatitis caused by household detergents. A prior sensitizing exposure to the primary irritant is not necessary, and the dermatitis develops in many normal persons. This dermatitis begins shortly after exposure to the irritant, in contrast to the 12 to 48 hours after exposure in allergic contact dermatitis. The eruption begins with mild dryness, redness, and scaling. On continued exposure, fissuring, crusting, and lichenification may result. Primary irritant dermatitis usually is confined to the hands, and may be indistinguishable in its physical appearance from allergic contact dermatitis.

Skin conditions may coexist. It is not unusual to see allergic contact dermatitis caused by topical ointment applied for the treatment of atopic dermatitis and other dermatoses.

Another contact skin condition is photocontact dermatitis. This is an eruption caused by the interaction between a chemical and ultraviolet (UV) light.[10] The diagnosis is based on finding the eruption only on the parts of the body exposed to UV irradiation. The sensitizer usually is an ingested drug such as tetracycline, griseofulvin, or sulfa compounds or a topically applied substance such as a cold tar extract. In one form, termed the *phototoxic reaction*, cell damage can occur on the first exposure to sunlight. No sensitizing period is required, and the mechanism is nonimmunologic. The clinical appearance is that of an exaggerated sunburn reaction. The second form of photoreaction is a true contact photoallergic dermatitis. Contact is made with a photosensitizing substance, and then a delayed hypersensitivity reaction is induced by UV light of an appropriate wave length. Because an incubation period is necessary, no reaction occurs on first exposure. In this form of reaction, the sensitizing allergen undergoes a chemical alteration on exposure to the UV component of sunlight. The clinical appearance is a scaly eczematous eruption. Some drugs may cause both phototoxic and photoallergic reactions.

A variant of allergic contact dermatitis is *contact urticaria*.[11] This is an immediate wheal-and-flare response generated by a wide variety of contactants. There are three categories of contact urticaria, based on the mechanism of action. The first is nonimmunologic. It affects most individuals and occurs as a result of the direct release of mediators from mast cells. Urticariogenic agents causing this reaction include arthropod bodies, hairs, and nettles. The second category is allergic, and probably represents a type 1 hypersensitivity reaction with demonstration of antigen-specific IgE. Causes include foods (such as fish and egg), medications (such as penicillin G), silk, and animal saliva. The reaction may range from localized urticaria to urticaria and anaphylaxis. The third category appears to combine features of both the allergic and nonallergic types, and the mechanism is unknown. Ammonium persulfate, an oxidizing agent in hair bleach, is a common cause. Some patients with contact urticaria present with an immediate localized wheal-and-erythema response. Most appear with a relapsing dermatitis or generalized urticaria. Some patients complain only of itching, burning, and tingling of the skin. The specific diagnosis is made with an open patch test. The substance in question is spread on the forearm and observed for 30 minutes for the appearance of a macular erythematous reaction that evolves into a wheal. If the result of the open test is negative, then a closed patch test may be applied. In the allergic type of contact urticaria, the clinician should be careful of a systemic reaction to the patch test.

IDENTIFYING THE OFFENDING AGENT

History and Physical Examination

Once the diagnosis of allergic contact dermatitis is made, vigorous efforts should be directed toward determining the cause. A careful, thorough history is mandatory. The period from exposure to clinical manifestations must be kept in mind and an exhaustive search made for exposure to a sensitizing allergen in the patient's occupational, home, or recreational environment. The location of the dermatitis most often relates closely to direct contact with a particular allergen. At times this is straightforward, such as dermatitis of the feet because of contact sensitivity to shoe materials, or dermatitis of the wrist, the ear lobes, or the neck due to contact with jewelry. At other times, the relation of the dermatitis to the direct contact allergen may not be as obvious, and being able to associate certain areas of involvement with particular types of exposure is helpful. For example, contact dermatitis of the face often results from cosmetics directly applied to the area. Other possibilities must be kept in mind, however, such as hair dye, shampoo, and hairstyling preparations. Contact dermatitis of the eyelid, although often caused by eye shadow, mascara, and eye liner, also may be caused by nail polish. Involvement of the thighs may be caused by keys or coins in pants pockets. Therefore, the physician must be familiar with various distribution patterns of contact dermatitis that may occur in association with particular allergens.

Frequently, the distribution of the skin lesions may suggest several possible sensitizing agents, and patch testing (described later) is of special value. Certain allergens may be airborne, and exposure may occur by this route. Dermatitis caused by ragweed oil sensitivity occasionally is seen among farmers. Smoke from burning the poison ivy plant may contain the oleoresin as particulate matter, thus exposing the sensitive individual. Another route of acquiring poison ivy contact dermatitis without touching the plant is by indirect contact with clothing or animal fur containing the oleoresin. Also remember that systemic administration of a drug or a related drug that has been previously used topically and to which the patient has been sensitized can elicit a generalized eruption. An example is sensitivity to ethylenediamine. A patient may develop localized contact dermatitis to topically applied ethylenediamine hydrochloride used as a stabilizer in such compounds as triamcinolone acetonide (Mycolog) cream; a generalized eruption may occur when aminophylline is administered orally.[12]

The oral mucosa also may be the site of a localized allergic contact reaction, resulting in contact stomatitis or stomatitis venenata.[13] The relatively low incidence of contact stomatitis compared with contact dermatitis is attributed to the brief duration of surface contact, the diluting and buffering action of saliva, and the rapid dispersal and absorption because of extensive vascularity. Although distinctly uncommon, well-documented cases of contact stomatitis exist. Agents capable of producing contact stomatitis include dentifrices, mouthwashes, dental materials such as acrylic and epoxy resins, and foods. The clinical response may include gingivitis or stomatitis with erosive or ulcerative lesions.

Patch Testing

Principle

Patch testing or epicutaneous testing is the diagnostic technique of applying a specific substance to the skin with the intention of producing a small area of allergic contact dermatitis. It can be thought of as reproducing the disease in miniature. The patch generally is kept in place for 48 to 96 hours (although reactions may appear after 24 hours in markedly sensitive patients), with the patch site then observed for the gross appearance of a localized dermatitis resembling the primary lesion. The same principles of proper interpretation of a positive patch test result apply as in the case of the immediate wheal-and-erythema skin test reaction (see Chap. 2). A positive patch test reaction is not absolute proof that the test substance is the actual cause of dermatitis. It may reflect a previous episode of dermatitis, or it may not have any clinical relevance. The positive patch test result must correlate with the patient's history and physical examination.

Testing With the Appropriate Substance

The patient is exposed to myriad chemical and plant substances in everyday life, many of which have the potential to cause allergic contact dermatitis. Frequently, the history and physical examination disclose the cause of the dermatitis, and the patch test only corroborates the evidence. On other occasions, the history and location of the dermatitis suggest a particular category of exposure; patch testing appropriate to the particular category should then be performed. Categories include the patient's occupation, hobbies, household articles, clothing, cosmetics, plant exposure, and topical medications. Several interviews and exhaustive questioning may be necessary before a clue to the particular exposure is found. In some instances, there may be little or no suggestion of the offending agent; then, application of a standard group of substances known to be common causes of allergic contact dermatitis is indicated. Table 18-1 lists the components of a standard screening tray.[14] Substances for the standard series can be obtained from Hermal Pharmaceutical Laboratories (163 Delaware Avenue, Delmar, NY 12054).

The physician should become familiar with the potent sensitizers and with the various modes of exposure. Keep in mind the possibility of cross-reactivity to other allergens because of chemical similarities. Sensitivity to paraphenylenediamine, for example, also may indicate

TABLE 18-1. *Standard screening tray*

Benzocaine, 5%	Formaldehyde (contains methanol), 1%
Mercaptobenzothaizole, 1%	Ethylenediamine dihydrochloride, 1%
Colophony, 20%	Epoxy resin, 1%
p-Phenylenediamine, 1%	Quarternium 15, 2%
Imidazolidinyl urea (Germall 115), 2%	p-tert-Butylphenol formaldehyde resin, 1%
Cinnamic aldehyde, 1%	Mercapto mix, 1%
Lanolin alcohol (wool wax alcohols), 30%	Black rubber p-phenylenediamine mix (PPD), 0.6%
Carba mix, 3%	Potassium dichromate, 0.25%
Neomycin sulfate, 20%	Balsam of Peru, 25%
Thiuram mix, 1%	Nickel sulfate (anhydrous), 2.5%

Slavin RG, Ducomb DF. Allergic contact dermatitis. Hosp Pract 1989;24:39.

sensitivity to para-aminobenzoic acid and other chemicals containing a benzene ring with an amino group in the *para* position.

The five most common causes of allergic contact dermatitis in the United States are *Toxicodendron* (poison ivy, poison oak, poison sumac), paraphenylenediamine, nickel, rubber compounds, and ethylenediamine hydrochloride. Latex-induced contact dermatitis affects health care workers, patients with spina bifida, and manufacturing employees who prepare latex-based products.

Table 18-2 lists some of the most potent sensitizers and their most frequently presenting forms. It is not complete and is not intended as a general survey. More detailed information on other sensitizers, environmental exposures, and preparation of testing material can be found in several standard texts.[15–17]

Techniques

Because contact dermatitis is a systemic sensitivity, it should be possible to use any areas of the skin for patch testing. In rare instances of small, isolated areas of dermatitis, patch testing at a far distant site may give negative results. Generally, the back is used for patch testing. After washing the skin with alcohol or acetone, the skin is allowed to dry. The test materials are applied in rows directly on the skin, or covered with a small gauze flat, or placed on the gauze portion of an adhesive bandage. Recently, North American and international contact dermatitis research groups have adopted the A1-test as the standardized method for epicutaneous testing. This device is a cellulose disc attached to a polyethylene-coated aluminum backing. An alternative method is the Finn chamber, which consists of a round aluminum chamber. Its major advantages are that more patches can be applied and the reaction sites are smaller than in the A1-test.

The thin-layer rapid-use epicutaneous test is a standardized, ready-to-apply patch test system made of polyester covered with a film of allergens incorporated into a hydrophilic polymer. The patches are mounted on nonwoven cellulose tape with acrylic adhesive, covered with siliconized plastic, and packed in an airtight and light-impermeable envelope. When the test strip is affixed to the skin, perspiration hydrates the film and transforms it to a gel, releasing the allergen.

TABLE 18-2. *Potent sensitizers and their presenting forms*

Contactant	Exposure
Ethylenediamine hydrochloride	Mycolog cream (not ointment), aminophylline, hydroxyzine, antihistamines
Paraphenylenediamine	Hair dye; fur dye; black, blue, and brown clothing
Mercury	Topical ointments, disinfectants, insecticides
Nickel	Coins, jewelry, buckles, clasps, door handles
Formalin (formaldehyde)	Cosmetics, insecticides, wearing apparel (drip-dry, wrinkle-resistant, water-repellent)
Potassium dichromate	Leather (chrome tanning), yellow paints
Copper	Coins, alloys, insecticides, fungicides
Paraben	Cosmetics, pharmaceuticals
Epoxy resin	Adhesives
Sodium hypochlorite	Bleach, cleansing agents
Carba mix	Rubber, lawn and garden fungicides
Imidazolidinyl urea	Preservative in cosmetics
Latex	Rubber gloves, toys, condoms
Thiouram	Rubber (accelerator), fungicides, wood preservatives
Mercaptobenzothiazole	Rubber compounds (accelerator), anticorrosion agent
Phenyl-beta-naphthylamine	Rubber compounds (antioxidant)
P-tert-butylphenol	Rubber, plastics, adhesives

Inert materials should be moistened with a drop of saline. The gauze is held in place by adhesive tape.

There may be indications for so-called open testing in which the test substance is not covered by gauze or tape. Such indications include testing with substances that are irritating if occluded, for example, hair sprays, perfumes, after-shave lotions, antiperspirants, and plant oleoresins. Open testing also should be used when testing with substances suspected of being photosensitizers.

After 48 hours, the patches are removed, and after waiting 20 to 30 minutes to allow nonspecific mechanical irritation to subside, the reactions are read. Generally, the site of a positive response to a patch test itches. As stated earlier, the disease is reproduced in miniature, and in a positive reaction, vesicles on an erythematous edematous base are present. A true allergic reaction persists for several days. Irritative skin reactions subside in a few hours; therefore, when there is doubt, the area should be examined the following day. Positive patch test reactions often show an increase in the next 24 hours. Therefore, all test sites should be reexamined routinely at 72 hours. Some positive reactions may not occur for 96 hours or even 1 week, as in the case of neomycin. The reading should be directed to the center of the patch, where the skin was not in contact with the tape. Arbitrary grading of patch test results is +, erythema; ++, erythema and papules; +++, erythema, papules, and vesicles; ++++, erythema, papules, vesicles, and severe edema.

Materials to be used in testing may be obtained from commercial allergy supply houses. Remember, however, that the patient is an excellent source and that the materials the patient brings from the home or workplace may be extremely valuable.

Precautions

Several precautions must be observed in patch testing. The application of the test material itself may sensitize the patient. Potent materials that may sensitize on the first application include plant oleoresins, paraphenylenediamine, and methylsalicylate. Patch testing and especially repeated patch testing should not be performed unnecessarily. In testing, the clinician has to avoid provoking nonspecific inflammation. The testing material must be dilute enough to avoid a primary irritant effect. This is especially important when testing with a contactant not included in the standard patch test materials. To be significant, a substance must elicit a reaction at a concentration that does not cause reactivity in a suitable number of normal controls. Patch testing should never be performed in the presence of an acute or widespread contact dermatitis. False-positive reactions may be obtained because of increased reactivity of the skin. In addition, a positive patch test reaction with the offending agent may cause a flare-up of the dermatitis. The patient should be carefully instructed at the time of patch test application to remove any patch that is causing severe irritation. If the patch is left on for the full 48 hours, such an area actually may slough. As mentioned earlier, an anaphylactoid reaction can occur when testing for contact urticaria.

Systemic corticosteroids in sufficient doses decrease or ablate a delayed skin test reaction. However, a clinically significant epicutaneous or patch test reaction is not affected by smaller doses of corticosteroids, such as 20 mg or less of prednisone daily. Patch testing can be performed even when steroids are given in sufficient doses to completely suppress the clinical eruption. Topical application of corticosteroids suppresses the patch test reaction to a greater degree than systemic treatment.

COMPLICATIONS

The most common complication of allergic contact dermatitis is secondary infection caused by the intense pruritus and subsequent scratching. An interesting but poorly understood complication is the occasional occurrence of the nephrotic syndrome and glomerulonephritis in severe generalized contact dermatitis caused by poison ivy or poison oak.[18]

MANAGEMENT

General management strategies are outlined in Table 18-3.[19]

SYMPTOMATIC TREATMENT

The inflammation and pruritus of allergic contact dermatitis require symptomatic therapy.

For limited, localized allergic contact dermatitis, cool tap water compresses and a topical corticosteroid are the preferred modalities. Hydrocortisone is the only corticosteroid that should be applied to the face. The compresses minimize oozing, are economical, and are easy for patients to make from a soft, smooth cotton cloth such as a diaper or tea towel. Further, the compresses facilitate the absorption of a topical steroid and enhance its antiinflammatory property. The steroid should be in the form of a cream, not an occlusive ointment.[17] When the dermatitis is particularly acute or widespread, systemic corticosteroids should be employed. In instances when further exposure can be avoided, such as poison ivy dermatitis, there

TABLE 18-3. *Management of the allergic contact dermatitis*

Limited, localized reaction
> Cool tap water compresses
> Topical corticosteroid cream

Extensive, acute reaction
> Oral prednisone: 40–60 mg/d initially (adult); slow taper over 2 wk

Prophylaxis
> Antigen avoidance
> Protective clothing
> Barrier cream

should be no hesitation in administering systemic corticosteroids. This is a classic example of a self-limited disease that responds to a course of oral corticosteroid therapy. The popular usage of a 4- to 5-day decreasing steroid regimen often results in a flare of the dermatitis several days after discontinuing the steroids. It is probably best to continue the treatment for 10 to 14 days. There seems to be no need for prolonged antihistamine therapy in such instances. The response to systemic corticosteroids generally is dramatic, with improvement apparent in only a few hours. Three rules to be applied to systemic corticosteroid therapy in acute contact dermatitis are (1) use the least expensive preparation (prednisone); (2) use enough; (3) avoid prolonged administration.

A large initial dosage of prednisone, 40 to 60 mg/day in divided doses for an adult, should be given with a slow taper over 2 weeks.

For secondary infection resulting from scratching because of the pruritus of allergic contact dermatitis, antibiotics may be needed. Because of the risk involved in sensitization from topical antibiotics, the oral or injectable forms are preferred.

PROPHYLAXIS

The physician has a responsibility to patients not only to treat disease but also to prevent it. For that reason, topical applications of medications that have a high index of sensitization should be avoided. Included in this group are benzocaine, nitrofurazone (Furacin), antihistamines, neomycin, penicillin, sulfonamides, and ammoniated mercury. Legislation may be necessary to eliminate medications that are sensitizers and irritants.

When the offending agent causing allergic contact dermatitis is discovered, careful instruction must be given to the patient so that it may be avoided in the future. The physician should discuss all of the possible sources of exposure, and when dealing with occupational dermatitis, should have knowledge about suitable jobs for patients. In the case of chemical sensitivity, this list of sources may be extensive. When dealing with a plant sensitizer, the patient should be instructed in the proper identification of the offending plant.

If sensitization has occurred, the amount of information about the allergen is correlated with the condition of the skin. It has been shown that if the patient is aware of the allergen and informed about the variety of substances that contain it, the skin condition is much more satisfactory than if the patient knows little about the allergen.[20]

Sometimes exposure cannot be avoided, either because of the patient's occupation or because of the ubiquitous nature of the allergen.

The use of protective clothing is beneficial, as is the use of newly available barrier creams such as Stokoguard outdoor cream (Stockhausen–Skin Protection Division, P.O. Box 16025, Greensboro, NC 27416).

REFERENCES

1. Eisen HN, Belman S. Studies of hypersensitivity to low molecular weight substances. II. Reactions of some allergic substituted dinitrobenzenes with cysteine or cysteine of skin proteins. J Exp Med 1953;98:533.
2. Silberberg-Sinakin I, Gigli I, Baer RL, et al. Langerhans cells: role in contact hypersensitivity and relationship to lymphoid dendritic cells and to macrophages. Immunol Rev 1980;53:203.
3. Claman HN, Miller SD, Conlon PJ, et al. Control of experimental contact sensitivity. Adv Immunol 1980;30:121.
4. Belsito DV. The pathophysiology of allergic contact dermatitis. Clin Rev Allergy 1989;7:347.
5. Gell PGH, Benacerraf B. Studies on hypersensitivity. IV. The relationship between contact and delayed sensitivity: a study on the specificity of cellular immune reactions. J Exp Med 1961;113:571.
6. Ray MC, Tharp MD, Sullivan TJ, et al. Contact hypersensitivity reactions to dinitrofluorobenzene mediated by monoclonal IgE anti-DNP antibodies. J Immunol 1983;131:1096.
7. Lawrence HS. The transfer in humans of delayed skin sensitivity to streptococcal M substance to tuberculin with disrupted leukocytes. J Clin Invest 1955;34:219.
8. Landsteiner K, Chase MW. Experiments on transfer of cutaneous sensitivity to simple compounds. Proc Soc Exp Biol Med 1942;49:688.
9. Epstein WL, Kligman AM. Transfer of allergic contact-type delayed sensitivity in man. J Invest Dermatol 1957;28:291.
10. Duvivier A. Atlas of clinical dermatology. Philadelphia: WB Saunders, 1986:215.
11. Von Kroch G, Maibach HI. The contact urticaria syndrome: an update review. J Am Acad Dermatol 1981;6:328.
12. Fisher AA. New advances in contact dermatitis. Int J Dermatol 1977;16:552.
13. Archard HO. Common stomatologic disorders. In: Fitzpatrick TB, Arndt KA, Clark WH, et al., eds. Dermatology in general medicine. New York: McGraw-Hill, 1971:760.
14. Slavin RG, Ducomb DF. Allergic contact dermatitis. Hosp Pract 1989;24:39.
15. Fisher AA. Contact dermatitis. 3rd ed. Philadelphia: Lea & Febiger, 1985.
16. Schwartz L, Tullipan L, Peck SM. Occupational diseases of the skin. 3rd ed. Philadelphia: Lea & Febiger, 1957.
17. Sheldon JM, Lovell RG, Matthews KP. A manual of clinical allergy. 2nd ed. Philadelphia: WB Saunders, 1967:268.
18. Rytand DA. Fatal anuria, the nephrotic syndrome and glomerular nephritis as sequels of the dermatitis of poison oak. Am J Med 1968;5:548.
19. Slavin RG. Allergic contact dermatitis. In: Fireman P, Slavin RG, eds. Atlas of allergies. 2nd ed. London: Mosby-Wolfe, 1996:219.
20. Breit R, Turk RBM. The medical and social fate of the dichromate allergic patient. Br J Dermatol 1976;94:349.

Allergic Diseases, 5th Edition,
edited by Roy Patterson, Leslie Carroll Grammer, and
Paul A. Greenberger. Lippincott–Raven Publishers, Philadelphia, © 1997.

19

Nasal Polyposis, Sinusitis, and Nonallergic Rhinitis

David I. Bernstein

*D.I. Bernstein: Division of Immunology, ML563,
University of Cincinnati College of Medicine, Cincinnati, OH 45267-0563.*

Pearls for Practitioners
Roy Patterson

- In most cases, polyps can be controlled with topical steroids and occasional short courses of prednisone.
- There comes a time, however, when surgical polypectomy is necessary. The polyps are likely to come back, so be prepared to control them and try to keep them small.
- Recurrent sinusitis requires vigorous therapy and possible surgical intervention. Don't wait too long.
- Anosmia in a patient with nonallergic rhinitis is a problem. It may be temporarily reversible, but recovery is not likely.
- Nasal neurosis, with intense fixation on the nose, normal findings on examination, and failure to respond to good topical corticosteroid therapy is rare, but frustrating for the physician. Psychological help is rarely accepted
- Annual influenza immunization is a "must" for patients with asthma, the geriatric population, and health care workers. Patients with recurrent sinusitis should be immunized, as should workers in frequent close contact with the public such as barbers and beauticians.

NASAL POLYPS

Nasal polyps have been recognized and treated since ancient times.[1] The "aspirin triad" or occurrence of nasal polyps in association with asthma and aspirin sensitivity was first identified in 1911.[2] Nasal polyps usually arise from mucosa of the ethmoid, maxillary, or sphenoid sinuses, and result from inflammation and edema of mucosal tissue that prolapses through the sinus ostia. Histologic sections of nasal polyp tissue exhibit infiltration with eosinophils, plasma cells, lymphocytes, and mast cells.[3] Polypoid tissue is rich in ground substance containing acid mucopolysaccharide.[4,5]

The overall incidence or prevalence of nasal polyposis is unknown. Nasal polyps are diagnosed more frequently in men and during the third and fourth decades of life. Most clinical data indicate that there is no greater prevalence of nasal polyps among atopic compared with normal populations.[2,6,7] Nasal polyps are much less common in children than in adults. If nasal polyps are recognized in a child, the clinician must exclude cystic fibrosis, where the prevalence of nasal polyps ranges between 6.7% and 26%.[8,9] Of 211 polyp patients reported by Settipane and associates,[10] 71% also had asthma. Approximately 14% of the latter patients with nasal polyps reported aspirin intolerance. The prevalence could be underestimated in that 8% of nasal polyp patients without histories of salicylate sensitivity exhibit aspirin intolerance when challenged with aspirin.[10,11]

Clinical Presentation

Perennial nasal congestion, rhinorrhea, and anosmia (or hyposmia) are common presenting symptoms. Nasal and osteomeatal obstruction may result in purulent nasal discharge and sinusitis. Enlargement of nasal polyps may lead to broadening of the nasal bridge,[12] and rarely, nasal polyps can encroach into the orbit, causing compression of ocular structures and resulting in unilateral proptosis, which falsely suggests the presence of an orbital malignancy.[13]

A thorough examination with a nasal speculum is necessary for identification of nasal polyps. More complete visualization of nasal polyps can be accomplished by flexible rhinoscopy. Nasal polyps appear as bulbous translucent to opaque growths, and are best visualized extending from the middle and inferior nasal turbinates, causing partial or complete obstruction of the nasal canals. Frontal, ethmoidal, and maxillary tenderness with purulent nasal discharge indicate concurrent acute or chronic paranasal sinusitis. Sinus radiographic studies are rarely necessary for identification of nasal polyps. Common radiographic changes observed in patients with chronic nasal polyposis include the following: widening of the ethmoid labyrinths; mucoceles or pyoceles within the paranasal sinuses; and generalized loss of translucence in the maxillary, ethmoid, and frontal sinuses.[12]

Causes

The pathogenesis of nasal polyposis has not been defined. Allergic mechanisms have been investigated, but no consistent association has been established between atopy and nasal polyposis. Mast cells and their mediators could play a role in that mast cells as well as eosinophils are found in abundance in nasal polyp tissue. Bunstead and colleagues[14] detected measurable amounts of histamine, a mast cell and basophil mediator, in nasal polyp fluid. Allergen-induced release of histamine and proinflammatory mediators (e.g., leukotrienes) has been demonstrated after passive sensitization of nasal polyp tissue with allergic serum.[15] Growth factors have been isolated from polypoid tissue that stimulate in vitro proliferation of basophils, mast cells, and eosinophils, which could amplify and sustain tissue inflammation.[16,17] Increased numbers of CD8+ T cells are found in nasal polyps,[18] and immunoglobulin (IgG, IgM, IgA, and IgE) levels are elevated in polyp fluid.[19]

A variety of other factors may contribute to the pathogenesis of nasal polyps. In culture, nasal polyp tissue readily supports the growth of influenza A virus, although this does not establish a causative role for viral infection.[20] Autonomic imbalance, endocrine abnormalities, and abnormal vasomotor responses may contribute to the formation of nasal polyps. Although nasal polyposis seems to be an acquired condition, a higher than expected prevalence of nasal polyps, asthma, and aspirin intolerance have been reported in certain families.[21] For many years, it was hypothesized that aspirin sensitivity associated with asthma and nasal polyps were linked by an abnormality in arachidonic acid metabolism, resulting in enhanced leukotriene synthesis using the lipoxygenase pathway. This hypothesis has been supported by demonstration of increased levels of leukotrienes in nasal secretions of nasal polyp patients after oral aspirin challenge.[11] In summary, it is postulated but not proven that allergic, infectious, environmental irritant, genetic, or metabolic factors may alone or in combination result in formation of nasal polyps.

Treatment

The surgical treatment of nasal polyposis often is unsatisfactory. Simple nasal polypectomy results in temporary relief of nasal obstructive symptoms but is often followed by recurrence. Medical treatment with topical intranasal glucocorticoids has been demonstrated to be more effective than surgical polypectomy.[22] In contrast to topical glucocorticoids, antihistamines and decongestants are unsatisfactory for decreasing the size of nasal polyps. A daily dose of 400 µg of intranasal beclomethasone dipropionate (Vancenase, Beconase) was shown to reduce nasal congestion, rhinorrhea, and sneezing symptoms in patients with nasal polyps.[23] Intranasal topical glucocorticoids reduce the size of polyps, thereby reducing the necessity for nasal polypectomy.[24] Although the initial recommended dosage of intranasal beclomethasone is two sprays (42 µg per actuation) in each nostril two times a day, the dose may be doubled if required. A double blind placebo-controlled 4-month study of budesonide (Rhinocort), a potent topical glucocorticoid, has demonstrated the drug to be effective in treating nasal polyps. The antiinflammatory effect of budesonide was demonstrated by decreased numbers of eosinophils in nasal biopsy specimens of treated patients.[25] Long-term treatment with daily intranasal glucocorticoids is safe and does not lead to atrophic changes in nasal mucosa.[26] If polyps fail to respond to intranasal glucocorticoids, a brief 5- to 7-day course of oral prednisone (30 to 35 mg/day) may be effective. The long-term use of oral glucocorticoids should be avoided. Once nasal polyps have been reduced in size with prednisone, maintenance dosages of intranasal glucocorticoids should be resumed to prevent recurrence. Coexistent sinus infection may render individuals refractory to intranasal glucocorticoids and therefore should be treated with appropriate courses of antibiotics.

If all attempts at medical management have failed, surgical intervention should be recommended, particularly in the presence of chronic sinusitis that has been refractory to antibiotics. Simple polypectomy may be indicated for complete nasal obstruction, which causes extreme discomfort. If nasal polyps are associated with persistent ethmoid sinusitis with obstruction of the osteomeatal complex, a more extensive surgical procedure is required. Sphenoethmoidectomy with complete marsupialization of the ethmoid sinus and resection of the middle turbinate is a definitive procedure that has been reported to effectively prevent recurrence of nasal polyps in approximately 85% of treated patients.[27]

Asthmatic patients undergoing nasal polypectomy or sinus surgery had previously been regarded to be at risk for postoperative bronchospasm, but this rarely occurs. Nonspecific airway responsiveness determined by methacholine challenge does not increase significantly in asthmatics after nasal polypectomy.[28] After recovery from polypectomy or sphenoethmoidectomy, maintenance intranasal glucocorticoids should be instituted to prevent recurrence of nasal polyps.[53]

SINUSITIS

Sinusitis is an inflammatory disorder of the mucosal lining of the paranasal sinuses that may be initiated by either infectious or noninfectious factors. Regardless of initiating events, the four physiologic derangements that contribute to the evolution of infectious sinusitis are as follows: (1) decreased patency of the sinus ostia; (2) a fall in the partial pressure of oxygen within the sinus cavities caused by impairment of ventilatory exchange; (3) diminished mucociliary transport; and (4) compromise of mucosal blood flow. Edematous obstruction of the sinus ostia is a consistent finding in both acute and chronic sinusitis; this condition causes a low-oxygen environment within the sinus cavity, which results in decreased mucociliary transport[29] and favors the growth of common bacterial pathogens, including *Streptococcus pneumoniae, Hemophilus influenza,* and anaerobic bacteria.

Viral upper respiratory infections often precede acute bacterial sinus infections. Sinusitis may follow environmental exposure to fumes or chemical vapors. Bacterial sinusitis has long been considered a complication of seasonal or perennial allergic rhinitis, although no good data support this assumption. Cigarette smokers and individuals with vasomotor rhinitis are more susceptible to recurrent or chronic sinusitis.

The microbial pathogens implicated in acute maxillary sinusitis have been studied extensively. Accurate identification of bacterial pathogens have been achieved by culturing antral aspirates by needle puncture of the maxillary sinus. Cultures of nasopharyngeal specimens are useless because they do not reflect bacterial isolates in the sinuses. The most frequent bacteria isolated from maxillary sinuses of adult patients are *S pneumoniae, H influenzae,* and assorted anaerobes.[30] Viruses are cultured from 8% of aspirates, whereas 15% to 40% of antral aspirates are sterile. Common isolates include rhinovirus, influenza type A, and parainfluenza viruses.[31]

In children with acute maxillary sinusitis, *S pneumoniae, H influenzae,* and *Moraxella catarrhalis* have been identified as the predominant pathogens.[32] Viruses were isolated from 4% of pediatric patients, and 20% of cultured aspirates were sterile. Anaerobic bacteria have been cultured from 88% of antral aspirates of adult patients with chronic sinusitis but are seldom identified in children.[33,34]

Mucormycotic sinusitis is caused by fungus of the genus *Mucor,* a zygomycete.[35] This organism is saprophytic, is abundant in the natural environment, and may be isolated easily from the throat and stools of normal individuals. *Mucor* can become an invasive pathogen in diabetic, leukemic, or otherwise immunosuppressed patients. Similarly, invasive aspergillosis may involve the paranasal sinuses in the immunocompromised host.[36] Allergic *Aspergillus* sinusitis is a recently recognized syndrome occurring in nonimmunocompromised patients, which results from a local hypersensitivity response to *Aspergillus fumigatus* colonizing the sinus cavities.[37] Rarely, tuberculosis or syphilis have been reported to cause infectious sinusitis. Atypical mycobacteria can cause sinusitis in patients with AIDS.[38]

Clinical Presentation

Episodes of acute sinusitis are preceded by symptoms suggestive of viral upper respiratory infections or other environmental stimuli, which can cause mucosal inflammation, hypertrophy, and obstruction of the sinus ostia. Common presenting symptoms include frontal or maxillary head pain, fever, and mucopurulent or bloody nasal discharge. Other clinical features include general malaise, cough, hyposmia, mastication pain, and changes in the resonance of speech. Pain cited as coming from the upper molars may be an early symptom of acute maxillary sinusitis. Children with acute maxillary sinusitis present most often with cough, nasal discharge, and fetid breath, whereas fever is less common.[32]

Symptoms associated with chronic sinusitis are less fulminant; facial pain, headache, and postnasal discharge are common symptoms. The clinician should be aware that chronic maxillary sinusitis may result from primary dental infections (i.e., apical granuloma of the molar teeth, periodontitis).[31] Pain associated with temporomandibular dysfunction may be incorrectly diagnosed as chronic sinusitis. Individuals with sinusitis may experience severe facial pain associated with rapid changes in position (e.g., lying supine or bending forward) or with rapid changes in atmospheric pressure that occur during air travel.

Episodes of acute or chronic sinusitis may be manifestations of other underlying problems. Local obstruction by a deviated nasal septum, nasal polyps, or occult benign or malignant neoplasm may explain recurrent sinus infections. Patients presenting with frequent sinus infections that respond poorly to antibiotics should be examined for primary or acquired immunodeficiency states. Common variable hypogammaglobulinemia and selective IgA deficiency combined with IgG2 and IgG4 subclass deficiencies are humoral immunodeficiencies that should be considered.[39] Disorders of ciliary dysmotility usually occur in male patients. Kartagener's syndrome is characterized by recurrent sinusitis, nasal polyps, situs inversus, infertility, and bronchiectasis.[40] Incomplete forms of ciliary dysmotility may occur without associated pulmonary or cardiac involvement. Nasal mucosal biopsy and electron microscopic examination can identify abnormalities in ciliary structure. Wegener's granulomatosis is a necrotizing vasculitis that presents with epistaxis, refractory sinusitis, serous otitis, nodular pulmonary infiltrates, and focal necrotizing glomerulonephritis.[41] Notice that chronic sinusitis or otitis media can precede pulmonary and renal manifestations for years before the disease becomes fulminant. Thus, early diagnosis and treatment of this condition before development of renal disease can be life-saving.

Diagnosis

Palpable tenderness, erythema, and warmth may be appreciated over inflamed frontal, ethmoid, or maxillary sinuses. Clinical history and physical examination can reliably identify purulent sinusitis in more than 80% of cases.[42,43] Sinus radiographs should be reserved for difficult diagnostic problems or for patients with sinusitis unresponsive to an initial course of antibiotics. Radiologic changes of sinus mucosal thickening of 8 mm or greater is a sensitive diagnostic marker of bacterial sinusitis. Minimal radiologic changes are common in many cases of sterile sinusitis as well as in asymptomatic individuals. Computed tomography (CT) of the sinuses is a valuable method for defining pathologic changes in the paranasal sinuses.[44] CT is particularly useful for defining abnormalities in the anterior ethmoid and middle meatal areas (osteomeatal unit), which cannot be visualized well on sinus roentgenograms. The CT coronal views (Fig. 19-1) are much less costly than a complete sinus CT and are adequate for determining the patency of the osteomeatal complex, which includes the ethmoid and maxillary ostia and infundibulum. Such information is essential for assessing the need for surgical intervention in the treatment of chronic sinusitis.

Complications

In the age of antibiotics, severe life-threatening complications of acute sinusitis are relatively uncommon. However, the clinician must be able to recognize clinical manifestations of potentially fatal complications of sinusitis so that prompt medical and surgical treatments can be initiated in a timely fashion.

Symptoms commonly associated with acute frontal sinusitis include frontal pain, local erythema and swelling, fever, and purulent nasal discharge. Serious complications of frontal

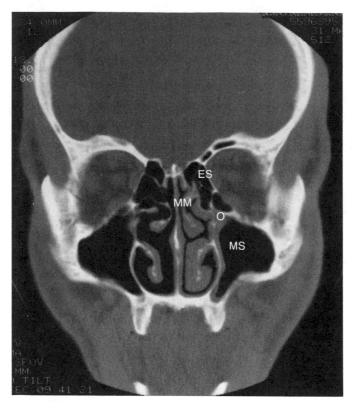

FIG. 19-1. Computed tomographic image of the paranasal sinuses. A coronal section exhibits significant sinus disease on the left with a relatively normal appearance on the right. The left middle meatus (MM) and maxillary ostium (O) are obstructed by inflamed tissue, causing significant obstruction of the left ethmoid (ES) and maxillary (MS) sinuses.

sinusitis may be attributed to the proximity of the frontal sinus to the roof of the orbit and anterior cranial fossa. Osteomyelitis can result from acute frontal sinusitis and may present as a localized subperiosteal abscess (Pott's puffy tumor). Sinus radiographs exhibit sclerotic changes in the bone contiguous to the frontal sinus. Intracranial complications of frontal sinusitis include extradural, subdural, and brain abscesses as well as meningitis and cavernous sinus thrombosis.[45] Acute ethmoiditis is encountered most commonly in children. Extension of inflammation into the orbit can result in unilateral orbital and periorbital swelling with cellulitis. This presentation can be distinguished from cavernous sinus thrombosis by the lack of focal cranial neurologic deficits, absence of retroorbital pain, and no meningeal signs. Affected patients usually respond to antibiotics, and surgical drainage is rarely necessary.

Cavernous sinus thrombosis is a complication of acute or chronic sinusitis, which demands immediate diagnosis and treatment.[45] The cavernous sinuses communicate with the venous channels draining the middle one third of the face. Cavernous sinus thrombosis often arises from a primary infection in the face or paranasal sinuses. Vital structures that course through the cavernous sinus include the internal carotid artery and the third, fourth, fifth, and sixth cranial nerves. Symptoms of venous outflow obstruction caused by cavernous sinus thrombosis include retinal engorgement, retrobulbar pain, and visual loss. Impingement of cranial nerves in the cavernous sinus can result in extraocular muscle paralysis and trigeminal sensory loss. If not treated promptly with high doses of parenteral antibiotics, septicemia and central nervous system involvement lead to a fatal outcome.

Acute sphenoid sinusitis is difficult to diagnose.[43,45] Affected patients report occipital and retroorbital pain, or the pain distribution may be nonspecific. Because of the posterior location of the sphenoid sinus, diagnosis of sphenoiditis may be delayed until serious complications are recognized. Extension of infections to contiguous structures may result in ocular palsies, orbital cellulitis, subdural abscess, meningitis, or hypopituitarism. Sinus radiographs often are unsatisfactory for evaluating sphenoiditis; sinus CT is a more effective diagnostic tool.

It has long been recognized that chronic or recurrent sinusitis may exacerbate asthma. Successful prevention and treatment of chronic sinusitis can be effective in controlling patients with difficult or refractory asthma. Slavin[46] described a group of steroid-dependent asthmatics with sinusitis in whom sinus surgery (i.e., the Caldwell-Luc procedure or sphenoidectomy) was performed. Asthma symptoms, steroid requirements, and nonspecific airway reactivity were reduced after surgery.

Treatment

Medical treatment of acute sinusitis should be initiated promptly. Oral decongestants alone or combined with antihistamines may diminish nasal mucosal edema and enhance sinus drainage. A 12-hour sustained-release oral preparation containing pseudoephedrine or phenyl-propanolamine is recommended in combination with a course of antibiotics. Topical nasal vasoconstrictors (e.g., oxymetazoline) used judiciously over the initial 2 to 3 days of treatment of acute sinusitis can facilitate drainage. Nasal lavage with saline can be effective for improvement of sinus drainage. Intranasal glucocorticoids may be a useful adjunctive treatment for decreasing mucosal inflammation and edema. For treating acute sinusitis, amoxicillin (250 to 500 mg three times daily) is the antibiotic of choice, which provides bactericidal activity against *H influenza, S pneumoniae*, and anaerobic bacteria. Amoxicillin is active against 60% to 80% of bacterial pathogens encountered in chronic sinusitis and should be administered for a duration of 21 to 28 days; briefer courses are associated with a greater probability of recurrence. In the penicillin-allergic patient, the alternative antibiotic of choice is trimethoprim-sulfamethoxazole.[34] Infection with penicillinase-producing organisms accounts for 25% of pediatric cases and 44% of adult patients with chronic sinusitis, and should be suspected in those patients who fail 14- to 21-day courses of amoxicillin.[33,47] In this situation, amoxicillin-clavulanic acid or an appropriate cephalosporin (e.g. cefuroxime), both of which are active against penicillinase-producing bacteria, should be substituted. Newer modified macrolide antibiotics (e.g. chlorithromycin, azithromycin), which have a broad spectrum of activity against pathogens implicated in sinusitis, can be used either in the penicillin- and sulfonamide-allergic patient or for treating patients who are unresponsive to amoxicillin.[48]

Intensive medical therapy may be unsuccessful in treating acute sinusitis. When fever, facial pain, and sinus radiographic changes persist in such patients, surgical drainage of infected sinuses may be indicated. Direct puncture and aspiration of affected sinuses should be performed by an otolaryngologist under local anesthesia. Parenteral antibiotics should be instituted if local extension of infection (i.e., cellulitis or osteomyelitis) occurs, or if the infection is suspected to have spread to vital central nervous system structures. For patients with maxillary sinusitis who do not respond to conservative drainage measures and aggressive antibiotic therapy, resection of diseased tissue within the sinuses is recommended.[46] Similar principles apply to the treatment of frontal, ethmoid, or sphenoid sinusitis. Adequate open drainage of frontal sinuses can be achieved by trephination through the roof of the orbit. If acute ethmoiditis is refractory to antibiotics, intranasal or external ethmoidectomy may be required. Sphenoid sinusitis, which often occurs with ethmoid sinusitis, may require a surgical aspiration and drainage procedure.

Patients with asthma who undergo sinus surgery should receive a thorough evaluation. Asthma must be under optimal control before the operation. In steroid-dependent patients, a brief course of oral steroids should be administered before surgery.

Intracranial complications of sinusitis (e.g., subdural emphysema or brain abscess) must be treated by prompt open surgical drainage and with parenteral antibiotics. Diffuse extension of osteomyelitis requires high-dose antibiotic treatment. Surgical debridement of localized osteomyelitis is recommended if a bony sequestrum of infection exists.

The treatment approach to chronic sinusitis and recurrent sinusitis should begin with identifying contributing factors such as underlying conditions (i.e., chronic allergic rhinitis, deviated nasal septum, rhinitis medicamentosa) and environmental factors (e.g., active or passive exposure to tobacco smoke, exposure to toxic irritants at work). In many cases, recurrent infections can be prevented by daily maintenance therapy with an oral 12-hour sustained release decongestant (i.e., pseudoephedrine or phenylpropanolamine). Oral phenylpropanolamine increases ostial and nasal patency, facilitating mucus drainage and thereby preventing infection.[49] Chronic use of topical glucocorticoids in combination with topical decongestants reduces nasal airway resistance and ameliorates radiographic changes in patients with chronic sinusitis.[50] Based on these reports, concurrent administration of nasal topical glucocorticoids and a 12-hour slow-release oral sympathomimetic (pseudoephedrine or phenylpropanolamine) is a rational strategy for prevention of recurrent sinusitis.

When all attempts at pharmacologic management have failed, surgery may be required for chronic or recurrent sinusitis. Functional endoscopic sinus surgery has supplanted older surgical procedures such as maxillary antrostomy (Caldwell-Luc). The basic principle of endoscopic techniques is to resect the inflamed tissues that obstruct the osteomeatal complex and the anterior ethmoids, and thus directly interfere with normal physiologic drainage. Inflammation or scarring of the latter structures obstructs drainage, resulting in spread of infection to the maxillary and frontal sinus cavities. As mentioned, sinus CT is essential in defining the specific disease in this area. Surgical resection of ethmoidal and osteomeatal structures is performed through the nose under guidance of a rigid endoscope. Diseased mucosa is resected, and narrow or stenotic areas, including the maxillary ostia, are widened.[51,52] This type of surgery is far more effective than the Caldwell-Luc procedure, which failed to restore normal physiologic drainage through the ostia. Because nasal endoscopic surgery is less invasive, postoperative morbidity has been markedly reduced in comparison with formerly used surgical techniques. A recent 4-year follow-up of 100 patients indicated general improvement in over 90% of patients. Recurrence of symptoms occurred as late as 3 years after surgery and primarily in patients who initially presented with nasal polyps, aspirin sensitivity, and reactive airways disease.[53]

NONALLERGIC RHINITIS

Symptoms of nonallergic rhinitis often are indistinguishable from those associated with perennial allergic rhinitis. Therefore, the evaluation and treatment of nonallergic rhinitis can be challenging. *Nonallergic rhinitis* is defined as inflammation of the nasal mucosa that is not caused by sensitization to inhalant aeroallergens. Lack of allergic causation must be proven by the absence of skin test reactivity to a panel of common aeroallergens.

Table 19-1 presents a classification for the nonallergic nasal disorders, which has been subdivided into inflammatory and noninflammatory disorders.[54]

Nonallergic vasomotor rhinitis is the most common of these disorders. This is an idiopathic condition characterized by perennial nasal congestion, rhinorrhea, and postnasal discharge. Ocular itching is noticeably absent. Typically, symptoms are increased early in the morning and aggravated by tobacco smoke, irritants, chemicals, perfumes, and various noxious odors. Symptoms are triggered by rapid changes in temperature. *Mixed perennial rhinitis* is diagnosed in allergic patients with prominent vasomotor symptoms.

Infectious rhinitis is suspected when purulent nasal discharge is present. Sinusoidal tenderness may indicate coexistent acute or chronic sinusitis. Atrophic rhinitis is a disorder of unknown origin, which often is seen in the elderly and is characterized by formation of thick, malodorous, dry crusts that obstruct the nasal cavity.[55] The nonallergic rhinitis with eosinophilia syndrome (NARES) is an inflammatory nasal disorder in which eosinophils are detectable in nasal secretions. The cause of this condition is unknown. Patients have negative skin test reactions to common inhalant aeroallergens.[56] The turbinates are pale with a purplish hue, edematous, or similar in appearance to what is observed in allergic rhinitis. NARES could represent a precursor to nasal polyposis. Nasal mastocytosis is another rare disorder than can be confirmed by the finding of increased mast cells in the nasal mucosa.

TABLE 19-1. *Classification scheme of nonallergic rhinitis*

Inflammatory
Infectious rhinitis
  Viral
  Bacterial
Atrophic rhinitis
Nonallergic rhinitis with eosinophilia (NARES)
Rhinitis associated with nasal polyposis
Nasal mastocytosis

Noninflammatory
Rhinitis medicamentosa caused by:
  Topical drugs
  Systemic drugs
Vasomotor rhinitis
Hormonal induced vasomotor instability
  Endocrine diseases—hypothyroidism
  Pregnancy
Rhinopathy associated with structural defects
  Deviated septum
  Head trauma resulting in CSF rhinorrhea
  Tumors
  Foreign bodies

Adapted from Middleton E. Chronic rhinitis in adults. J Allergy Clin Immunol 1988;81:971.

Nasal symptoms can result from the chronic use or abuse of topical and systemic medications, a syndrome referred to as *rhinitis medicamentosa*. A list of causative oral medications is shown in Table 19-2.[54] In addition to older antihypertensive agents, angiotensin-converting enzyme inhibitors have been reported to cause rhinorrhea and vasomotor symptoms in association with chronic cough, which resolve after withdrawal of the drug.[57] Excessive use of topical vasoconstrictor agents such as phenylephrine or oxymetazoline can result in epistaxis, "rebound" nasal congestion, and rarely cause nasal septal perforation.

Prominent nasal congestion is recognized in patients with hypothyroidism and myxedema. Approximately one third of pregnant women report nasal congestion and rhinorrhea during gestation.[58] This could be related to progesterone- or estrogen-induced nasal vasodilation and enhancement of mucus secretion. Other causes of nasal obstruction must be considered in the differential diagnosis. A grossly deviated nasal septum, nasal tumors, or a foreign body can be the source of unilateral nasal obstruction refractory to medical treatment. Cerebral spinal fluid (CSF) rhinorrhea is characterized by clear nasal discharge. It occurs in 5% of all basilar skull fractures but can be present in patients having no history of trauma. The use of glucose oxidase paper tests may result in an erroneous diagnosis. A glucose concentration of 40 mg/mL or greater in the CSF fluid confirms the diagnosis.

Evaluation begins with a careful history and examination with a nasal speculum. Nasal septal deviation is usually obvious. Pale, boggy nasal turbinates characteristic of allergic rhinitis may be seen in a patient with NARES or nasal polyps. The nasal mucosa appear beefy red or hemorrhagic in patients with rhinitis medicamentosa. Cytologic examination of a nasal mucus smear may reveal an abundance of neutrophils, which is suggestive of infectious rhinitis.[59] Nasal eosinophils are consistent with allergic rhinitis, NARES, or nasal polyposis. The absence of inflammatory cells on nasal smear should direct the physician to consider noninflammatory rhinopathies.

Treatment

The therapeutic approach to nonallergic nasal disorders is determined by findings derived from the diagnostic evaluation. Differentiation between inflammatory and noninflammatory nasal conditions is useful in selecting appropriate therapy.

TABLE 19-2. *Rhinitis medicamentosa: causative agents*

Antihypertensives	Psychotropic drugs
Reserpine	Thioridazine
Hydralazine	Chlordiazepoxide-amitryptiline
Guanethidine	
Methyldopa	**Ovarian hormonal agents**
Prazosin	Oral contraceptives
Beta-blockers	
Angiotensin-converting enzyme (ACE) inhibitors	

Treatment of Noninflammatory Rhinopathy

Patients with rhinitis medicamentosa should discontinue offending medications. Intranasal glucocorticoids may be of considerable benefit in these patients in decreasing mucosal edema. For vasomotor instability associated with endocrinologic changes during pregnancy, medications should be withheld if possible. If necessary, nasal topical steroids (e.g., beclomethasone) may be safe and effective for controlling chronic symptoms encountered during pregnancy. Nasal congestion associated with hypothyroidism and myxedema responds to thyroid hormone replacement. Nasal obstruction caused by a deviated septum requires septoplasty. Fifty percent of patients of CSF rhinorrhea recover spontaneously. When persistent, intravenous antibiotics should be started to prevent meningitis, and surgery often is required to repair a dural tear.

The treatment of vasomotor rhinopathy is problematic. Selection of therapy for vasomotor rhinitis is empiric, and there are variable responses to different regimens. Oral decongestants often are effective when given as 12-hour slow-release preparations (e.g., pseudoephedrine, phenylpropanolamine). Antihistamines alone or in combination with decongestants often are effective therapy for patients with concurrent allergic and vasomotor rhinitis. When the disease is refractory to oral decongestants, topical intranasal steroids should be added. Ipratropium, 80 µg four times daily, an anticholinergic agent, is proven to be effective in treating perennial nonallergic rhinitis.[60] The effect of anticholinergic agents has been attributed to inhibition of cholinergic nasal hyperresponsiveness, which is a feature of vasomotor rhinitis. In most patients, vasomotor symptoms can be successfully controlled with oral sympathomimetic agents combined with intranasal steroids or ipratropium. Environmental trigger factors or irritants such as cigarette smoke and fumes should be avoided.

Treatment of the Inflammatory Rhinitis

The syndrome of nonallergic rhinitis with eosinophilia responds best to intranasal glucocorticoids. Once initial control of daily symptoms has been achieved, doses can be reduced to the minimal levels required to prevent recurrence of symptoms. Infectious rhinitis and concurrent sinus infections should be treated with appropriate antibiotics. Viral-induced nasal symptoms can be treated symptomatically with antihistamine-decongestant preparations.

REFERENCES

1. Vancil ME. A historical survey of treatments for nasal polyposis. Laryngoscope 1969;79:435.
2. Moloney JR, Colins J. Nasal polyps and bronchial asthma. Br J Dis Chest 1977;71:1.
3. Cauna N, Hindover KII, Manzethi GW, et al. Fine structure of nasal polyps. Ann Otolaryngol 1972;81:41.
4. Weisskopf A, Burn HF. Histochemical studies of the pathogenesis of nasal polyps. Ann Otol Rhinol Laryngol 1959;68:509.
5. Taylor M. Histochemical studies on nasal polypi. J Laryngol Otol 1973;77:326.
6. Blumstein GI, Tuft L. Allergy treatment in recurrent nasal polyposis. Am J Med Sci 1957;234:269.
7. Settipane GA, Chaffee FH. Nasal polyp in asthma and rhinitis. J Allergy Clin Immunol 1977;59:17.
8. English GM. Nasal polyps and sinusitis. In: Middleton E, Reed CE, Ellis EF, eds. Allergy principles and practices. St Louis: CV Mosby, 1983:1215.
9. Cuyler JP, Monaghan AJ. Cystic fibrosis and sinusitis. J Otolaryngol 1989;18:173.
10. Settipane GA, Chaffee FH, Klein DE. A critical evaluation of aspirin challenge in patients with nasal polyps. J Allergy Clin Immunol 1982;69:148. Abstract.
11. Ferreri NR, Howland WC, Stevenson DD, Spiegelberg HL. Release of leukotrienes, prostaglandins, and histamine into nasal secretions of aspirin-sensitive asthmatics during reaction to aspirin. Am Rev Respir Dis 1988;137:847.

12. Lund VJ, Lloyd GAS. Radiological changes associated with benign nasal polyps. J Laryngol Otol 1983;97:503.
13. Rawlings EG, Olson RJ, Kaufman HE. Polypoid sinusitis mimicking orbital malignancy. Am J Ophthalmol 1979;87:694.
14. Bunstead RM, El-Ackad T, Smith JM, Brody MJ. Histamine, norepinephrine and serotonin content of nasal polyps. Laryngoscope 1979;89:832.
15. Kaliner M, Wasserman SI, Austen KF. Immunologic release of chemical mediators from human nasal polyps. N Engl J Med 1973;289:277.
16. Ohnishi M, Ruhno J, Bienenstock J, Dolovich J, Denburg JA. Hematopoietic growth factor production by cultured cells of human nasal polyp epithelial scraping: kinetics, cell source and relationship to clinical status. J Allergy Clin Immunol 1989;83:1091.
17. Sakaguchi K, Okuda M, Ushijima K, Sakaguchi Y, Tanigaito Y. Study of nasal surface basophilic cells in patients with nasal polyp. Acta Otolaryngol (Stockh) 1986;430(Suppl):28.
18. Stoop AE, Hameleers DMH, v Run Pe, Biewenga J, Van der Baan S. Lymphocyte and nonlymphoid cells in the nasal mucosa of patients with nasal polyps and of healthy subjects. J Allergy Clin Immunol 1989;84:734.
19. Chandra RK, Abol BM. Immunopathology of nasal polypi. J Laryngol Otol 1974;88:1019.
20. Ginzburg VP, Rosina EE, Sharova OK, Glendon YZ. The replication of influenza A viruses in organ cultures of human nasal polyps. Arch Virol 1982;74:293.
21. Falliers CJ. Familial coincidence of asthma, aspirin intolerance and nasal polyposis. Ann Allergy 1974;32:65.
22. Lildholdt T, Fogstrup J, Gammelguard N, et al. Surgical versus medical treatment of nasal polyps. Acta Otolaryngol 1988;105:140.
23. Mygind N, Pederson N, Prytz S, Sorensen H. Treatment of nasal polyps with intranasal beclamethasone diproprionate. Clin Allergy 1975;5:159.
24. Pederson CB, Mygind N, Prytz S, et al. Long term treatment of nasal polyps with beclamethasone diproprionate aerosol. Clin Otolaryngol 1976;82:252.
25. Holopainen E, Grahne B, Malmberg H, Makinen J, Lindqvist N. Budesonide in the treatment of nasal polyposis. Eur J Respir Dis 1982;122(Suppl):221.
26. Mygind N, Sorensen H, Pedersen CB. The nasal mucosa during long-term treatment with beclamethasone diproprionate aerosol. Acta Otolaryngol 1978;85:437.
27. Friedman WH, Katsantonis GP, Rosenblum BN, Cooper MH, Slavin R. Sphenoethmoidectomy: the case for ethmoid marsupialization. Laryngoscope 1986;96:473.
28. Miles-Lawrence R, Kaplan M, Chang K. Methacholine sensitivity in nasal polyposis and the effects of polypectomy. J Allergy Clin Immunol 1982;69:102.
29. Drettner B. Pathophysiology of paranasal sinuses with clinical implications. Clin Otolaryngol 1980;5:227.
30. Evans FD, Syndor JB, Moore WEC, et al. Sinusitis of the maxillary antrum. N Engl J Med 1975;293:735.
31. Gwaltney JM, Sydnor A, Sande MA. Etiology and antimicrobial treatment of acute sinusitis. Ann Otol Rhinol Laryngol 1981;90(3 Suppl 84):68.
32. Wald ER, Milmoe GJ, Bowen A, et al. Acute maxillary sinusitis in children. N Engl J Med 1981;304:749.
33. Brook I. Bacteriology of chronic maxillary sinusitis in adults. Am Otol Rhinol Laryng 1989;98:46.
34. Wald ER, Byers C, Guerra N, et al. Subacute sinusitis in children. J Pediatr 1989;115:29.
35. Lewis DR, Thompson DH, Fetter TW. Mucormycotic sphenoid sinusitis. Ear Nose Throat J 1981;60:32.
36. Stevens MH. Aspergillosis of the frontal sinus. Arch Otolaryngol 1978;104:153.
37. Katzenstein AL, Sale SR, Greenberger PA. Allergic *Aspergillus* sinusitis: a newly recognized form of sinusitis. J Allergy Clin Immunol 1983;79:89.
38. Naguib MT, Byers JM, Slater L. Paranasal sinus infection due to atypical mycobacteria in two patients with AIDS. Clin Infect Dis 1994;19:789.
39. Oxelius V, Laural A, Lindquist B, et al. IgG subclass in selective IgA deficiency. N Engl J Med 1981;304:1476.
40. Eliasson R, Mossberg B, Camner P, Afzelius BA. The immotile cilia syndrome. N Engl J Med 1977;291:1.
41. Abraham-Inpijn L. Wegener's granulomatosis, serous otitis media and sinusitis. J Laryngol Otol 1980;94:785.
42. Berg O, Berostedt H, Carenfelt C, Lind MG, Perols O. Discrimination of purulent from nonpurulent maxillary sinusitis. Ann Otolaryngol 1981;90:272.
43. Abramovich S, Smelt GJ. Acute sphenoiditis: alone and in concert. J Laryngol Otol 1982;96:751.
44. Forbes W, Fawcitt RA, Isherwood I, Webb R, Farrington T. Computed tomography in the diagnosis of diseases of the paranasal sinuses. Clin Radiol 1978;29:501.
45. Yarington CT. Sinusitis as an emergency. Otolaryngol Clin North Am 1979;12:447.
46. Slavin RG. Relationship of nasal disease and sinusitis to bronchial asthma. Ann Allergy 1982;49:76.
47. Goldenhersh MJ, Rachelefsky G, Dudley J, et al. The microbiology of chronic sinus disease in children with respiratory allergy. J Allergy Clin Immunol 1990;85:1030.
48. Casiano R. Azithromycin and amoxicillin in the treatment of acute maxillary sinusitis. Am J Med 1991;91(Suppl 3A):27.
49. Melen I, Friberg B, Andreasson L, Ivarsson A, Jannert M, Johansson C-J. Effects of phenylpropanolamine on ostial and nasal patency in patients treated for chronic maxillary sinusitis. Acta Otolaryngol (Stockh) 1986;101:494.
50. Sykes DA, Wilson R, Chan KL, Mackay IS, Cole PJ. Relative importance of antibiotic and improved clearance in topical treatment of chronic mucopurulent rhinosinusitis. Lancet 1986;Aug. 16:359.
51. Kennedy DW. Functional endoscopic sinus surgery. Arch Otolaryngol 1985;111:643.

52. Stammberger H. Endoscopic surgery for mycotic and chronic recurring sinusitis. Ann Otol Rhinol Laryngol 1985;94:1.
53. Schaitkin B, May M, Shapiro A, et al. Endoscopic sinus surgery: 4 year follow-up on the first 100 patients. Laryngoscope 1993;103:1117.
54. Middleton E. Chronic rhinitis in adults. J Allergy Clin Immunol 1988;81:971.
55. Goodman WS, de Souza FM. Otolaryngology. In: English GM, ed. Atrophic rhinitis. Philadelphia: JB Lippincott, 1990.
56. Mullarkey MF. Eosinophilic nonallergic rhinitis. J Allergy Clin Immunol 1988;82:941.
57. Berkin KE. Respiratory effects of angiotensin converting enzyme inhibitors. Eur Respir J 1989;2:198.
58. Schatz M, Hoffman CP, Zeiger RS, et al. Course and management of asthma. In: Middleton E, Reed C, et al, eds. Allergy: principles and practice. St Louis: CV Mosby, 1988:1093.
59. Meltzer E. Evaluating rhinitis: clinical, rhinomanometric and cytologic assessments. J Allergy Clin Immunol 1988;82:900.
60. Kirkegaard J, Mygind N, Melgaard F, et al. Ordinary and high dose ipratropium in perennial allergic rhinitis. J Allergy Clin Immunol 1987;79:588.

Allergic Diseases, 5th Edition,
edited by Roy Patterson, Leslie Carroll Grammer, and
Paul A. Greenberger. Lippincott–Raven Publishers, Philadelphia, © 1997.

20

Anaphylaxis

Kris G. McGrath

*K.G. McGrath: Section of Allergy and Immunology,
St. Joseph Hospital, Chicago, IL 60657–6274.*

Pearls for Practitioners
Roy Patterson

- After controlling acute anaphylaxis with epinephrine and H_1 blocking antihistamines, prednisone (60 mg for an adult) should be given to help prevent a late recurrence.
- *Idiopathic* anaphylaxis does not mean that the external cause has not been found, *but that there is no external cause*. Patients and their physicians have trouble accepting this.
- The emergency therapy for anaphylaxis, such as an Epipen, should be on the patient's person, not in the car or at home.
- Classification of anaphylaxis is as follows:
  1. *Allergic anaphylaxis:* This is immunologic, IgE antibody–mediated from an external allergy.
  2. *Pseudoallergic anaphylaxis:* This is caused by an external agent but is not IgE mediated and not immunologic. Reactions to radiographic contrast media are examples.
  3. *Idiopathic (nonallergic) anaphylaxis:* This is not caused by an unknown allergen. It occurs spontaneously.
- Munchausen's anaphylaxis is the result of purposeful self induction of true anaphylaxis. Diagnosis is difficult, and management, including psychiatric management, is difficult and often unsuccessful.

DEFINITION AND HISTORY

Anaphylaxis is the clinical manifestation of immediate hypersensitivity that occurs after the interaction between a specific antigen and a homocytotrophic antibody. This reaction occurs rapidly, often is dramatic, and is unanticipated. Death may occur through airway obstruction or irreversible vascular collapse. Anaphylaxis is the most severe form of an allergic reaction and should always be considered a medical emergency.

Such fatality was recognized as early as 2641 BC, when according to hieroglyphics, King Menses of Egypt was stung to death by a wasp or hornet. Portier and Richet[1] in 1902 noted that injection of a previously tolerated sea anemone antigen in a dog produced a fatal reaction as opposed to the anticipated prophylaxis. They termed this phenomenon anaphylaxis (Greek: *ana*—backward, *phylaxis*—protection).

Anaphylactoid (anaphylaxis-like) reactions are similar clinically to anaphylaxis. They are not mediated by antigen–antibody interaction but result from substances acting directly on mast cells and basophils, causing mediator release or acting on the tissues such as anaphyla-toxins of the complement cascade.

The most frequent cause of anaphylaxis in early reports was from horse serum used for diphtheria or tetanus antitoxins or as antiserum for infectious diseases.[2] Other causes of ana-phylaxis included diagnostic and therapeutic agents used in skin testing and allergen immuno-therapy and other foreign proteins.[3]

The development of modern drugs, therapeutic agents, and diagnostic agents has resulted in an increased incidence of anaphylaxis. These agents often are used by physicians in diag-nosis and treatment, requiring awareness of the problem and knowledge of preventive and therapeutic measures.

The following factors are associated with an increased incidence of anaphylaxis[4–9]:

- The nature of the antigen affects the risk of anaphylaxis. Certain antigens more often are the cause of anaphylaxis (e.g., penicillin among drugs, nuts, and shellfish among foods).
- Parenteral administration of a drug is more likely to result in anaphylaxis than is oral ingestion.
- An atopic history is associated with an increased incidence of anaphylaxis to latex, exer-cise, and radiographic contrast media (RCM). Idiopathic anaphylaxis patients have a higher prevalence of atopy. Atopic persons are not at increased risk of anaphylaxis from penicillin and Hymenoptera stings.
- Repeated interrupted courses of treatment with a specific substance and long durations between doses increase the risk of anaphylaxis.
- Immunotherapy extract injection to a symptomatic patient (especially undertreated asthma) during increased natural exposure to extract components may increase the risk of anaphylaxis.

EPIDEMIOLOGY

Occupation, sex, race, season of the year, and geographic location may provide the nature of the inciting agent, but evidence is lacking to substantiate these as predisposing factors.[5,10] Anaphylaxis has been estimated to occur in 1 of every 3000 patients and is responsible for more than 500 deaths a year.[5,11,12] Most studies conclude that an atopic person is at no greater risk than a nonatopic person for developing IgE-mediated anaphylaxis from penicillin or insect stings.[7,9] The most common causes of anaphylaxis are the antibiotics, especially peni-cillin. Penicillin has been reported to cause fatal anaphylaxis at a rate of 0.002%.[11,13] The most common cause of anaphylactoid reactions are from RCM. Life-threatening reactions after administration of RCM occur in approximately 0.1% of procedures. Fatal reactions occur in about 1:10,000 to 1:50,000 intravenous procedures. As many as 500 deaths per year occur after RCM administration.[14–17] Fatal reactions occur less frequently with lower osmolar RCM agents.[18] The next most common cause of anaphylaxis is Hymenoptera stings, with an incidence of 23 deaths per 150 million stings.[11,19–22] Fatalities from allergen immuno-therapy and skin testing are rare, with 6 fatalities from allergen skin testing and 24 fatali-ties from immunotherapy reported from 1959 to 1984.[23] In another study, 17 fatalities asso-ciated with immunotherapy occurred from 1985 to 1989.[24]

Not all persons who have had anaphylaxis have it again on reexposure to the same sub-stance. Those who do may react less severely than at the initial event. Factors suggested to explain this include the interval between exposures, the route of exposure, and the amount of the substance received.[11] The percentage of persons at risk for recurrent anaphylactic reac-tions has been estimated to be 10% to 20% percent for penicillins,[25] 20% to 40% for RCM,[26] and 40% to 60% for insect stings.[11,27]

Concern is growing regarding persons with recurrent unexplained anaphylaxis and idiopathic anaphylaxis; distinct subtypes are completely discussed in Chapter 21.

CLINICAL MANIFESTATIONS OF ANAPHYLAXIS

The manifestations of anaphylaxis vary with animal species. The guinea pig typically has acute respiratory obstruction; the rat, circulatory collapse with increased peristalsis; the rabbit, acute pulmonary hypertension; and the dog, circulatory collapse.

Humans vary greatly in the onset and course of anaphylaxis. The skin, conjunctivae, upper and lower airways, cardiovascular system, and the gastrointestinal tract may be affected solely or in combination. Neurologic involvement may also occur. Involvement of the respiratory and cardiovascular systems is of the most concern. In one series of anaphylactic deaths, 70% died of respiratory complications and 24% of cardiovascular failure.[28] Symptoms generally begin in seconds to minutes after exposure to the inciting agent. However, symptoms may be delayed for up to an hour. Initial signs and symptoms may include cutaneous erythema and pruritus, especially of the hands, feet, and groin. There can be a sense of oppression, impending doom, cramping abdominal pain, and a feeling of faintness or "light headedness." The skin findings may progress to urticaria and angioedema and usually last less than 24 hours. Respiratory symptoms may progress to include mild airway obstruction from laryngeal edema and, more severely, to asphyxia. Early laryngeal edema may manifest as hoarseness, dysphonia, or a "lump in the throat." Edema of the larynx, epiglottis, or surrounding tissues can result in stridor and suffocation. With lower airway obstruction and bronchospasm, the individual may complain of chest tightness or wheezing. Gastrointestinal manifestations include nausea, vomiting, abdominal pain, and intense diarrhea, which may be bloody. Of grave concern is when both airway obstruction and cardiovascular symptoms occur. This may include hypotension and vascular collapse (shock) followed by complications of asphyxia or cardiac arrhythmia. Myocardial infarction may be a complication of anaphylaxis.[29,30] Other frequent manifestations include nasal, ocular, and palatal pruritus; sneezing; diaphoresis; disorientation; and fecal or urinary urgency or incontinence. The initial manifestation of anaphylaxis even may be loss of consciousness. Dizziness, syncope, seizures, confusion, and loss of consciousness may occur as a result of cerebral hypoperfusion or as a direct toxic effect of mediator release.[11] Death may follow in minutes.[31] Late deaths may occur days to weeks after anaphylaxis but are often manifestations of organ damage experienced early in the course of anaphylaxis.[28] In general, the later the onset of anaphylaxis, the less severe the reaction.[32] In some patients, an early anaphylactic response may resolve only to be followed by a late or second (biphasic) episode of anaphylaxis.[33]

PATHOLOGIC FINDINGS

The anatomic and microscopic findings must be examined relative to the underlying illness from which the patient was being treated, the drugs administered, and the effect of secondary changes related to hypoxia, hypovolemia, and postanaphylaxis therapy.[5]

The prominent pathologic features of fatal anaphylaxis in humans are acute pulmonary hyperinflation, laryngeal edema, visceral congestion, pulmonary edema and intraalveolar hemorrhage, urticaria, and angioedema. In some patients, no specific pathologic findings are found.

Microscopic examination reveals noninflammatory fluid in the lamina propria of the areas just described, increased airway secretions, and eosinophilic infiltrates in bronchial walls.[31,34]

Sudden vascular collapse usually is attributed to vessel dilation or cardiac arrhythmia, but myocardial infarction may be sufficient to explain the clinical findings.[35] Myocardial damage may occur in up to 80% of fatal cases.[36] The most common electrocardiographic changes other than sinus tachycardia or infarction include T wave flattening and inversion, bundle branch block, supraventricular arrhythmia, and intraventricular conduction defects.[31,37]

The diagnosis of anaphylaxis is clinical, but the following laboratory findings help in unusual cases or in ongoing management. A complete blood count may show an elevated hematocrit secondary to hemoconcentration. Blood chemistries may reveal elevated creatine phosphokinase, aspartate aminotransferase, or lactate dehydrogenase if myocardial damage has occurred. Acute elevation of serum histamine, urine histamine, and serum tryptase have occurred, and complement abnormalities have been observed.[38] Plasma histamine has a short half-life and is not reliable for a postmortem diagnosis of anaphylaxis. Mast cell–derived tryptase (with a half-life of several hours), however, has been shown to be elevated for up to 24 hours after death from anaphylaxis and not from other causes of death. Serum tryptase may not be detected within the first 15 to 30 minutes of onset of anaphylaxis, and therefore persons with sudden fatal anaphylaxis may not have elevated tryptase in their postmortem sera.[39] The chest radiograph may show hyperinflation, atelectasis, or pulmonary edema, and ECG may reveal sinus tachycardia, atrial or ventricular arrhythmias, or myocardial infarction.

PATHOPHYSIOLOGY OF ANAPHYLAXIS

Anaphylactic reactions are initiated when a host interacts with a foreign material. This can be an IgE-mediated or a non–IgE-mediated process. Classic anaphylaxis occurs when an allergen combines with IgE antibody bound to the surface membranes of mast cells and circulating basophils. Mast cells are found in large numbers beneath mucosal and cutaneous surfaces in close association with blood vessels. The interaction between IgE and allergen activates a complex series of events, resulting in the release of many mediators of inflammation.[40] (Chemical mediators are discussed in detail in Chapter 4.) Histamine is a preformed vasoactive mediator in mast cell and basophil granules. Histamine acts on H_1 and H_2 receptors on target organs to increase vascular permeability, cause vasodilation, cause bronchial constriction, and enhance mucous secretion. Other important mediators include prostaglandins and leukotrienes that are synthesized de novo by activated mast cells (and other cell types). These mediators also cause bronchoconstriction, mucous secretion, and changes in vascular permeability. Platelet-activating factor (acetyl glyceryl ether phosphorylcholine) can alter pulmonary mechanics and lower blood pressure in animals.[41] In humans, it causes bronchoconstriction if inhaled and causes a wheal-and-flare reaction when injected into human skin. Its release has also been reported in cold urticaria, but whether platelet-activating factor participates in anaphylaxis remains speculative.[42]

A prominent accumulation of eosinophils occurs in anaphylactic reactions. This results from release of performed chemotactic factors and factors generated by IgE mast cell–basophil-dependent reactions such as leukotriene B_4. The eosinophil may act as an anti-inflammatory cell in the metabolism of vasoactive mediators or as an inflammatory leukocyte.[43] Mediators other than histamine are important, so attempts to block or treat anaphylaxis with antihistamines alone usually are inadequate. Also, these mediators do not explain all of the observed physiologic changes seen in anaphylaxis, suggesting other unidentified mechanisms and mediators involved.[11]

Non–IgE-induced bioactive mediator release from mast cells and basophils can be induced directly from the pharmacologic action of several substances and by complement components

(C3a, C5a). The latter occurs usually through activation of the complement system by antigen–antibody complexes. Non–IgE-mediated mast cell activation occurs with opiates, extracts of some foods, RCM, dextran, vancomycin, tubocurarine, and other muscle relaxants. Allergy skin tests based on IgE-mediated reactions are not useful in determining anaphylactoid reactions that depend on other mechanisms.

DIAGNOSIS AND DIFFERENTIAL DIAGNOSIS

Because of the profound and dramatic presentation, the diagnosis of anaphylaxis usually is readily apparent. When sudden collapse occurs in the absence of urticaria or angioedema, other diagnoses must be considered, although shock may be the only symptom of Hymenoptera anaphylaxis. These include cardiac arrhythmia, myocardial infarction, other types of shock (hemorrhagic, cardiogenic, endotoxic), severe cold urticaria, aspiration of food or foreign body, insulin reaction, pulmonary embolism, seizure disorder, vasovagal reaction, hyperventilation, globus hystericus, and factitious allergic emergencies. The most common is vasovagal collapse after an injection or painful situation. In a vasovagal collapse, pallor and diaphoresis are common features associated with presyncopal nausea. There is no pruritus or cyanosis. Respiratory difficulty does not occur, the pulse is slow, and the blood pressure can be supported without sympathomimetic agents. Symptoms are almost immediately reversed by recumbency and leg elevation. Hereditary angioedema must be considered when laryngeal edema is accompanied by abdominal pain. This disorder usually has a slower onset, lacks urticaria and hypotension, and often is accompanied by a family history of similar reactions. There is also a relative resistance to epinephrine, but epinephrine may have life-saving value in hereditary angioedema.

Idiopathic urticaria occurring with the acute onset of bronchospasm in an asthmatic patient may make it impossible to differentiate from anaphylaxis. Similarly, a patient experiencing a sudden respiratory arrest from asthma may be thought to be experiencing anaphylaxis because of severe dyspnea and facial fullness and erythema.

"Restaurant syndromes" may mimic anaphylaxis, such as scombroid fish poisoning and ingestion of monosodium glutamate or saurine, a histamine-like chemical also from spoiled fish.[44–47]

Many patients have flush reactions that mimic anaphylaxis. These include carcinoid flush, postmenopausal flush, chlorpropamide flush, flush caused by medullary carcinoma of the thyroid, flush related to autonomic epilepsy, and idiopathic flush.[44]

Excessive endogenous production of histamine may mimic anaphylaxis such as systemic mastocytosis, certain leukemias, and ruptured hydrated cysts.[44]

Other disorders include panic attacks, vocal cord dysfunction syndrome, Munchausen's stridor, and other factitious allergic diseases.[44,48,49]

Laboratory tests can help in differential diagnosis; for example, blood serotonin and urinary 5-hydroxy-indoleacetic acid level are elevated in carcinoid syndrome. Measuring plasma histamine levels may not be helpful because of its rapid release and short half-life. However, a 24-hour urine collection or spot sample for histamine or histamine metabolites can be helpful since urinary histamine levels are usually elevated for longer periods.[50] Measuring serum tryptase levels is useful if levels are found to be elevated, peaking 1 to 1½ hours after the onset of anaphylaxis with elevated levels persisting for 5 to 24 hours.[39,51]

A patient with Munchausen's stridor can be distracted from the vocal cord adduction by maneuvers such as coughing. Also, there are no cutaneous signs. In patients with vocal cord dysfunction, the involuntary vocal cord adduction can be confirmed by laryngoscopy during episodes, with an absence of cutaneous signs.[44,48,49]

A history of recent antigen or substance exposure and clinical suspicion are the most important diagnostic tools. IgE antibody can be demonstrated in vivo by prick skin testing. Skin prick testing can be useful in predicting anaphylactic sensitivity to many antigens. Caution must be exercised, beginning with dilute antigens. Anaphylaxis has followed skin testing with penicillin, insect sting extract, and foods. Passive transfer to human skin carries the risk of transmitting viral illnesses (i.e., hepatitis, HIV) and should not be done. The radioallergosorbent test (RAST) identifies nanogram quantities of specific antibody but is not as sensitive as skin testing. Other in vitro techniques include the release of histamine from leukocytes of sensitive individuals on antigen challenge, and the ability of a patient's serum to passively sensitize normal tissues such as leukocytes for the subsequent antigen-induced release of mediators.[5] Complement consumption has not been routinely used to define anaphylactic mechanisms. The only reliable test for sensitivity to agents that alter arachidonic acid metabolism, such as aspirin, other nonsteroidal antiinflammatory agents, and other suspected agents (i.e., tartrazine, benzoates), is carefully graded oral challenge with close clinical observation and measurement of pulmonary function, nasal patency, and blood pressure.

Substances capable of directly releasing histamine from mast cells and basophils may be identified in vitro using washed human leukocytes or by in vivo skin testing. These agents must release histamine in the absence of IgG or IgE antibody.[5]

FACTORS INCREASING THE SEVERITY OF ANAPHYLAXIS OR INTERFERING WITH TREATMENT

Many factors increase the severity of anaphylaxis or interfere with treatment, including the following:

- Presence of asthma
- Underlying cardiac disease
- Concomitant therapy with
  - β-Adrenergic blockers
  - Monoamine oxidase inhibitors
  - Angiotensin-converting enzyme (ACE) inhibitors.

Concomitant therapy with β-adrenergic blocking drugs or the presence of asthma exacerbate the responses of the airways in anaphylaxis and inhibit resuscitative efforts.[11,51–55] Furthermore, epinephrine use in patients on β-adrenergic blocking drugs may result in unopposed α-adrenergic effects, resulting in severe hypertension. However, case reports describe difficult-to-reverse anaphylactic shock. Rapid intravenous infusion of an allergen in a patient with a preexisting cardiac disorder may increase the risk of severe anaphylaxis.[11] β-Adrenergic blocking drugs should be used with caution, and preferably not at all in patients receiving immunotherapy and in idiopathic anaphylaxis. The difficulty in reversing anaphylaxis may occur in part from underlying cardiac disease for which β-adrenergic blockers have been given.

ACE inhibitors prevent the mobilization of angiotensin II, an endogenous compensatory mechanism, and can cause life-threatening tongue or pharyngeal edema themselves.[56] Monoamine oxidase inhibitors can increase the hazards of epinephrine by interfering with its degradation.[56]

Systemic reactions occur more frequently in patients with undertreated asthma who are receiving immunotherapy. It has been recommended that measurements of forced expiratory volume in 1 second (FEV_1) be performed before immunotherapy, with injections withheld if the FEV$_1$ is below 70% of the predicted volume.[23,57,58] However, this recommendation is not standard practice.

CAUSES OF ANAPHYLAXIS

Many substances have been reported to cause anaphylaxis in humans. These antigens are subdivided into proteins, polysaccharides, and haptens. A hapten is a low molecular weight organic compound that becomes antigenic when it or one of its metabolites form a stable bond with a host protein. With penicillin, both the parent hapten and nonenzymatic degradation products may form bonds with host proteins to form an antigen.[4]

The route of antigen exposure causing human anaphylaxis may be oral, parenteral, topical, or inhalational. An example of all four ways of entry is anaphylaxis associated with penicillin.

Table 20-1 lists common causes of anaphylaxis and anaphylactoid reactions in humans. This list is not all inclusive. The following discussion is a review of some important and interesting causes of anaphylaxis.

Penicillin

Penicillin is the most frequent cause of anaphylaxis in humans. Estimates of nonfatal anaphylactic reactions vary, ranging from 0.7% to 10%, and fatal reactions have been estimated at a frequency of 0.002%, or 1 fatality per 7.5 million injections.[4]

The most likely mode of administration to induce anaphylaxis is parenteral. Oral, inhalation, and diagnostic skin testing can cause anaphylaxis. Cross-reactivity exists between the various penicillins. If an individual is allergic to penicillin G, then other natural and synthetic penicillins must be considered to be allergenic in that person. Cross-reactivity also exists with cephalosporin antibiotics in some people with frequencies of 0% to 30%. Some have challenged this cross-reactivity.[59]

Penicillin haptens of importance are benzylpenicillin and semisynthetic penicillins. The benzylpenicilloyl group of benzylpenicillin quantitatively is the major haptenic determinant.[10,60] There is much cross-reactivity with α-aminobenzyl (ampicillin) penicilloyl hapten, but only minimal cross-reactivity with dimethoxyphenyl (methicillin) or oxacilleyl (oxacillin) penicilloyl haptens.[61] Penicillin therapy also induces the formation of antibodies for minor determinants derived from benzylpenicillin.[62] Cephalosporins induce the formation of a major determinant, the cephaloyl group, and minor determinants cross-reacting with those of benzylpenicillin.[61,63] Although reports vary, about 30% of patients with allergy to benzylpenicillin exhibit cross-reactivity to cephalosporins.[64] Clinical cross-reactivity between penicillin and a first- or second-generation cephalosporin ranges from about 5% to 16%. Aztreonam, a beta-lactam with a monobactam structure, can be used safely in patients with penicillin allergy.

Heterologous Antiserum

In the previously sensitized patient, horse serum can be a cause of anaphylaxis. The use of horse serum is less common since the advent of human tetanus antitoxin and rabies vaccine. Heterologous preparations were used at one time for numerous infections other than tetanus caused by pneumococci, meningococci, staphylococci, and the tubercle bacillus. Heterolo-

TABLE 20-1. *Causes of anaphylactic and anaphylactoid reactions in humans*

	Immunologic Mediator (IgE Antibody)		Immunologic Mediator (IgE Antibody)
Antibiotics	All	Orange	
Penicillins		Tangerine	
Cephalosporins		Sunflower seed	
Tetracyclines		Banana	
Sulfonamides		Mustard	
Nitrofurantoin	Possible	Pistachio, cashew	
Streptomycin		Tree nuts	
Vancomycin	No	**Allergy Extracts**	All
Chloramphenicol		Ragweed	
Ciprofloxacin		Grass	
Amphotericin B		Molds	
Miscellaneous Drugs/ Therapeutic Agents		Epidermals	
Acetylsalicylic acid	Possible	Hymenoptera	
Nonsteroidal antiinflammatory agents	Possible	**Hormones**	All
		Insulin	
Progesterone	Uncertain	Corticotropin	
Succinylcholine		Parathormone	
Thipental		ACTH	
D-Tubocurarine		Synthetic ACTH	
Mechlorethamine		Thymostimulin	
Opiates	No	**Enzymes**	All
Vaccines	Yes	Trypsin	
Antitoxins (horse)	Yes	Chymotrypsin	
Protamine sulfate	Varies	Penicillinase	
OKT3 monoclonal antibody	Yes	Asparaginase	
Foods	All	Chymopapain	
Nuts (peanut most common)		Streptokinase	
Shellfish		**Diagnostic Agents**	
Fish		Sodium dehydrocholate	No
Milk (raw)		Sulfobromophthalein	No
Buckwheat		Radiographic contrast media	No
Egg white		Benzylpenicilloly-polylysine (Pre-Pen)	Yes
Camomile tea (ragweed cross-reacts)			
Pinto bean		**Blood Products**	
Rice		Whole blood	Yes or some
Potato		Gamma globulin	

TABLE 20-1. *(Continued.)*

	Immunologic Mediator (IgE Antibody)		Immunologic Mediator (IgE Antibody)
Cryoprecipitate		Snake venom	
IgA		Fire ant	
Plasma		Triatoma	
Dialysis Exposure		**Polysaccharides/ Volume Expanders**	Uncertain
Ethylene oxide gas	Yes	Dextran	
AN69 membrane	No (bradykinin)	Acacia	
Venoms and Saliva	All		
Hymenoptera		**Seminal Plasma**	Yes
Deerfly		**Latex**	Yes

ACTH, corticotropin.

gous sera are used to treat snake bite, botulism, gangrene, diphtheria, spider bite, and organ transplant rejection. Skin testing should precede the use of such preparations to identify presence of IgE antibodies.[40]

Insect Stings

Systemic allergic reactions to insect stings occur in an estimated 3.3% of the population.[22,65,66] Approximately 40 deaths from insect stings occur annually in the United States. Serious nonfatal reactions occur in 1 to 10 per 100,000. The most common species are members of the order Hymenoptera, which includes hornets, wasps, honey bees, and yellow jackets. Fire ant stings also cause human anaphylaxis, particularly in the southern United States.

The patient may not accurately identify the specific insect, requiring confirmation of hypersensitivity by skin testing with purified venoms. A history of systemic reaction is associated with a 60% risk of similar or more severe reaction with future stings.[66] Severe reactions to insect stings with confirmed positive skin test results warrant the physician to advise the patient to undergo highly effective venom immunotherapy in addition to carrying epinephrine and practicing avoidance.[66] The efficacy of immunotherapy for fire ant hypersensitivity, which uses whole-body extract preparations, is not as established.[67] See Chapter 12 for a complete discussion of insect allergy.

Food

Foods are a common cause of anaphylaxis, and the sequence of events generally makes the diagnosis easy.[68] However, occasionally the physician and patient may not suspect the offending antigen. The most frequent causes of food anaphylaxis include crustaceans, legumes, fish, seeds, nuts, berries, egg whites, and dairy products. If the cause of food-induced anaphylaxis is not apparent from the patient's history, skin testing with food extracts may demonstrate IgE antibody and help determine the cause.[69] Skin testing with foods may cause anaphylaxis, requiring the use of diluted solutions, the prick test technique, physician presence, and the presence of emergency materials and equipment. Food antigenicity can be altered by cooking and processing, which may prevent a reaction such as occurs with potatoes. Food handling such as reported with kiwi fruit can cause anaphylaxis.[70] Cross-reactivity between foods exists such as with sunflower seeds and chamomile tea, which are in the ragweed family.[71,72] Food ingestion followed by exercise has been reported to cause anaphylaxis with celery, shrimp, squid, apple, wheat, hazelnut, abalone, and chicken.[73–76] These foods may be tolerated without exercise.

Food Additives

Papain in meat tenderizers has caused serious allergic reactions in some patients. Prick skin testing with papain and the meat tenderizer gave positive reactions. The reaction was confirmed by oral challenge and could be prevented with oral cromolyn sodium premedication.[77] Avoidance is preferred as a general rule.

Anaphylactic-type reactions have been reported to occur from metabisulfites. No IgE-mediated mechanism has been demonstrated,[78–80] and the relation to anaphylaxis is questionable. Sulfites have been used for centuries to preserve food and are cheaper and more effective than ascorbic acid. Sulfiting agents include sulfur dioxide and sodium or potassium sulfite, bisulfite, and metabisulfite. In addition to food preservation, these agents are used as sanitizers for containers, as antioxidants to prevent food discoloration, and as fresheners. They are found in foods such as beer, wine, shellfish, salad, fresh fruits and vegetables, potato, and avocado. The highest levels occur in restaurant foods with federal regulations restricting their use in foods served fresh.

Latex Anaphylaxis

The incidence of anaphylaxis to latex has not been determined or estimated. Between 1988 and 1992 the Food and Drug Administration received more than 1000 reports of latex anaphylaxis— 15 of these were fatal.[81] Children with spina bifida or severe urogenital defects, health care workers, and rubber industry workers seem to be at greater risk than the general population.[82] These reactions are mediated by IgE antibody to residual rubber tree proteins in latex gloves, condoms, and medical devices.[81,83] Exposure can be topical, inhalational, mucosal during condom use, from surgical and dental procedures, and intravenous. Any person at high risk should be tested.[82] Skin tests are more sensitive than serologic tests; however, no approved skin test reagent is available in the United States. Extracts have been made from raw latex and from finished rubber products. Systemic reactions to latex skin testing has been reported; thus, care must be exercised when skin testing with uncharacterized extracts.[82] In vitro testing is available by some commercial and university laboratories. High-risk individuals should be tested, and if found positive for latex-specific IgE or if a history of latex anaphylaxis exists, they should avoid latex. Injectable epinephrine should be carried in case of accidental exposure.

Drugs Used in General Anesthesia

The incidence of anaphylaxis in general anesthesia is approximately 1 in 5000 to 1 in 15,000 operations (one study estimated 1 in 980 to 1 in 22,000), with death varying in reports from 0.05% to 4% to 6%.[84–90] Induction agents and neuromuscular blocking drugs have caused reactions. These reactions have been anaphylactic (IgE mediated) and anaphylactoid. The induction agents include propanidid, alfathesin, thiopentone, methohexitone, propofol, and midazolam. Neuromuscular blocking drugs are predominantly implicated. These include D-tubocurarine, alcuronium, suxamethonium, gallamine, succinylcholine, pancuronium, vecuronium, and atracurium. Alcuronium is mostly used in Australia, and suxamethonium in France.[86] All of these drugs can induce histamine release. Nonspecific activation of the alternate pathway of complement may occur. The anaphylactic mechanism is the more frequent mechanism.[91,92] Preincubation with anti-IgE serum inhibits leukocyte histamine release. The presence of specific IgE against muscle relaxants also has been demonstrated. Cross-reactivity among these drugs exists, and variable results occur when intradermal and radioimmunoassay tests are done.[86,89]

The presence of skin manifestations may help to indicate an allergic reaction during general anesthesia, thus avoiding confusion with other causes of bronchospasm, hypotension, and cardiac arrhythmias. Some immediate-type reactions have occurred because of bolus injection of muscle relaxants rather than infusions over 1 minute, which are not associated with reactions.

Blood Components and Related Biologic Agents

Blood transfusions have induced anaphylactic reactions. A nonatopic recipient may be passively sensitized by transfusion of donor blood containing elevated titers of IgE.[93] Conversely, in rare cases, transfusion of an allergen or drug into an atopic recipient has caused plasma anaphylaxis. Most plasma reactions are not easily explained.

Anti-human IgA antibodies are present in about 40% of individuals with selective IgA deficiency. Some of the patients have allergic reactions varying from mild urticaria to fatal anaphylaxis, usually after numerous transfusions.[94] These antibodies usually are IgG but may be IgE mediated. These reactions can be prevented by using sufficiently washed red blood cells or by using blood from IgA-deficient donors.[95–98]

Serum protein aggregates (nonimmune complex) such as human albumin, human gamma globulin, and horse anti-human lymphocyte globulin can cause anaphylactoid reactions. These complexes apparently activates complement, resulting in release of bioactive mediators.[98,99]

Cryoprecipitate and factor VIII concentrate have been reported as causes of anaphylaxis. An IgE-mediated mechanism was demonstrated in one patient by leukocyte histamine release; positive skin test reactions to factor VIII, factor IX, and cryoprecipitate; and a positive RAST result to factor VIII. An attempt at pretreatment with corticosteroids and diphenhydramine and an attempt to desensitize did not prevent future reactions.[99,100]

Plasma expanders composed of modified fluid gelatins, plasma proteins, dextran, and hydroxyethyl starch have caused anaphylaxis. Skin testing and leukocyte histamine release may aid at predicting those at risk, but an immunologic mechanism is not clear.[101–103] Preinjection of 20 mL of dextran before infusion has been suggested as prophylaxis against dextran-induced anaphylaxis.[103]

Protamine sulfate derived from salmon testes caused an anaphylactic reaction in a patient allergic to fish, with such a risk suggested to be higher in infertile men or in one who has had a vasectomy.[104] However, fish hypersensitivity does not necessarily imply an increased risk of protamine reactions, which may not be IgE mediated, at least in a few cases. IgE antibodies to salmon obtained from patients who had experienced salmon anaphylaxis were not inhibited by protamine, suggesting lack of cross-reactivity.[105] There has been an increased use of protamine for medicinal purposes. These include the reversal of heparin anticoagulation during vascular surgery, cardiac catheterization, and the retardation of insulin absorption. Included are isophane, protamine zinc, and human insulins. Diabetic patients receiving daily subcutaneous injections of insulin containing protamine seem to have a 40- to 50-fold increased risk of life-threatening reactions when given protamine intravenously.[106,107] The mechanism seems to be caused by antibody-mediated mechanisms. In diabetic patients who had received protamine insulin injections, the presence of antiprotamine IgE antibody was a significant risk factor for acute protamine reactions, as was antiprotamine IgG. Patients having reactions to protamine without previous protamine insulin injections had no antiprotamine IgE antibodies. But in the group, antiprotamine IgG was a risk factor for protamine reactions.[108]

Streptokinase is a nonenzymatic protein produced by group C β-hemolytic streptococci. Streptokinase is used as a thrombolytic agent. Allergic reactions range in frequency from 1.7% to 18%. This includes anaphylaxis supported by in vitro and in vivo evidence. Intradermal skin testing with 100 IU of streptokinase is recommended before infusion. This dose causes an immediate reaction without a large delayed reaction in sensitive subjects. In patients with positive immediate cutaneous reactivity, an alternative thrombolytic agent should be used such as urokinase or recombinant rt-PA (Alteplase), which cost significantly more than streptokinase.[109–111]

An anaphylactoid reaction to recombinant rt-PA has been reported.[112] Antibodies to streptococcal antigens resulting from previous exposure are present in most persons, accounting for previous sensitization of affected patients.

Miscellaneous IgE-Mediated and Non–IgE-Mediated Anaphylaxis

The injection of chymopapain into herniated vertebral discs is called chemonucleolysis. This procedure has been associated with anaphylaxis in 1.2% of women and 0.4% of men with a death rate of 0.01%.[113] Chymopapain is obtained from papain, a crude fraction from the papaya, *Carcia papaya*.[114,115] It is used industrially as a meat tenderizing agent and to clarify beer and sterilize soft contact lenses. These exposures likely sensitize individuals who then receive and react to chymopapain injections. IgE-mediated allergy to papain has been reported in both occupational and nonoccupational settings.[77,115] Cutaneous skin testing by investigators has a 1% incidence rate of positive reactivity, approaching the historical incidence of anaphylaxis.[116,117] There were no instances of defined anaphylaxis caused by chymopapain in skin test–negative patients. Bernstein and colleagues[118] compared the incidence of positive skin test results with chymopapain and positive RAST results with chymopapain and found that RAST was less sensitive. This concurs with the concept that cutaneous testing is more sensitive than in vitro assays. Further, cutaneous testing provides immediate results. Therapeutic injection of chymopapain in patients who are skin test negative only can reduce the incidence rate of anaphylaxis below the historical rate of 1%.

Anaphylaxis has occurred after using ciprofloxicin,[119] cytarabine,[120] tetanus toxoid,[121] trichophytin,[122] ranitidine,[123] psyllium,[124] and cromolyn sodium.[125] Severe allergic reactions have been associated with ethylene oxide gas[126] used to sterilize supplies for chronic hemodialysis patients. IgE and IgG antibodies have been demonstrated against human serum albumin linked to ethylene oxide. Grammer and Patterson[127] demonstrated IgE antibodies against ethylene oxide–altered proteins as a likely explanation for some hemodialysis anaphylaxis. The ethylene oxide–human serum albumin (ETO-HSA) antigen was characterized by immunoelectrophoresis, gel filtration chromatography, and immunologic inhibition assays. Also, antibody to ETO-HSA has been detected in a peritoneal dialysis patient with allergic manifestations. In addition, during dialysis, anaphylactoid reactions (possibly mediated by bradykinin) have occurred because of AN69 membranes, especially in patients receiving ACE inhibitor drugs.[128,129]

Anaphylaxis after sexual intercourse has been reported in women.[130–132] One women's serum contained a heat-labile antibody that conferred anaphylactic sensitivity to human and monkey skin. The IgE antibody was directed against a glycoprotein in her husband's seminal fluid. In another woman, a defined antigen could not be determined, but a high level of serum IgE antibodies to partially purified seminal fraction IV has been demonstrated. Elevated levels of serum-specific IgE antibodies to human seminal plasma (HuSePl) also have been demonstrated. And, in one such patient, immunotherapy with HuSePl fractions prevented postcoital anaphylaxis.[132]

Allergic reactions to insulin are less common using human insulin produced by recombinant DNA methods, but reactions still occur.[133] This is possibly caused by tertiary structure differences between endogenous insulin and insulin obtained by recombinant DNA. Skin testing excludes insulin allergy when doubt exists and enables selection of the insulin preparation least likely to cause adversity. Desensitization protocols are available if no alternatives exist and if insulin must be given to the allergic patient.[134] The incidence of allergic reactions to insulins seems to be decreasing. In most cases, the patient experiences a local wheal and erythema at the site of insulin injection.

Life-threatening reactions after the administration of RCM occur in approximately 0.1% of procedures. Fatal reactions with RCM administration occur in about 1 in 10,000 to 1 in 50,000 intravenous procedures.[14–16] As many as 500 deaths per year may occur after RCM administration.[17] The immediate-type generalized reactions after RCM simulate anaphylaxis clinically but are not IgE mediated.

No method is available to identify individuals at risk of an initial reaction, but it is known that a person who had a previous reaction is at higher risk for a repeat reaction. Thus, individuals with previous adverse allergic reactions to RCM must be pretreated to reduce risk.[135] This should be done only if RCM administration is absolutely essential. A complete review of RCM allergy is found in Chapter 17. The introduction of lower osmolality RCM has not eliminated the problem of RCM reactions.

Idiopathic anaphylaxis is discussed in Chapter 21.

EXERCISE-INDUCED ANAPHYLAXIS

Exercise-induced anaphylaxis (EIA) occurs with vigorous exercise and may produce shock or loss of consciousness. Symptoms include urticaria, angioedema, nausea, vomiting, abdominal cramps, diarrhea, laryngeal edema, bronchospasm, and respiratory distress.[136,137] The reaction typically begins during exercise or after exercise is complete, and may occur only when exercise is performed shortly after a meal. Specific foods have been linked including celery, shrimp, apple, squid, abalone, wheat, hazelnut,[73–76] and chicken, but most cases are not associated with prior food ingestion.[73–76,138] These foods have been tolerated without exercise, and exercising without eating these foods does not cause anaphylaxis. It does not occur with each period of exercise, and the same amount of exercise on each occasion may not lead to anaphylaxis. About two thirds of patients with EIA have a family history of atopy, and about one half have a personal history of atopy.[137] One death has been reported from EIA.[139] Elevated concentrations of plasma histamine, serum lactate, and CPK have been demonstrated during episodes.[140] The exact mechanism is unknown, and it has been speculated that release of endogenous opioid peptides with vigorous exercise may release bioactive mediators in susceptible individuals.[40] There is evidence for mast cell activation from skin biopsy specimens.

Reproducibility in the laboratory using plastic occlusive suits does not always occur, which contrasts to raising core body temperature in patients with cholinergic urticaria.[136] Treatment is best provided by limiting exercise or stopping at the first sign of prodromal symptoms. Pretreatment with H_1 antihistamines is not always effective. The patient should employ self-discipline, use the "buddy system" of exercise, and keep injectable epinephrine available.

TREATMENT AND PREVENTION

The treatment of anaphylaxis should follow established principles for emergency resuscitation. Anaphylaxis has a highly variable presentation, and treatment must be individualized for a patient's particular symptoms and their severity. Treatment recommendations are based on clinical experience and an understanding of pathologic mechanisms and the known action of various drugs.[141] Rapid therapy is of utmost importance. The following approach is required to counteract the effects of mediator release, support vital functions, and prevent further release of mediators (Table 20-2).

At the first sign of anaphylaxis, the patient should be treated with epinephrine. Next, ask the patient if there is breathing difficulty, and then position recumbent for blood pressure determination. Assess airway patency and if the patient has had cardiopulmonary arrest. Basic cardiopulmonary resuscitation must be instituted immediately. If shock is present or impending, place the patient in a recumbent position and elevate the legs. Epinephrine is the most important single agent in treating anaphylaxis, and delaying it or failing to administer it is more problematic than its administration. Epinephrine in an aqueous solution of 1:1000 dilu-

TABLE 20-2. *Management of anaphylaxis*

1. Immediate: epinephrine 1:1000 0.3 mL IM (deltoid)

2. Record blood pressure and pulse

3. Depending on severity, degree of response, and the individual patient:

    a. IV benadryl 50 mg slowly

    b. Nasal oxygen

4. Repeat epinephrine every 15 min

5. Be prepared for intubation, hypotension

6. For severe bronchospasm:

    a. IV aminophylline

    b. Hydrocortisone sodium succinate (Solu-cortef) 200 mg IV push

7. For systolic blood pressure <90 mm Hg:

    a. 2 IV lines wide open

    b. Dopamine 400 mg (2 amp) in 500 mL D_5W; infuse until systolic blood pressure is 90 mm Hg, then titrate

    c. Norepinephrine (Levophed) 2 mg (1 amp) in 250 mL D_5W; titrate after reaching systolic of 90 mm Hg

8. For patients taking β-adrenergic blocking drugs:

    a. Glucagon 1–5 mg IV bolus, then titrate at 5–15 μg/min

    b. Atropine for bradycardia: 0.3–0.5 mg SQ every 10 min, maximum of 2 mg

IM, intramuscularly; IV, intravenous; D_5W, 5% dextrose in water; SQ, subcutaneously.

tion (0.30 to 0.50 mL; 0.01 mL/kg in children) is administered subcutaneously or intramuscularly in the upper extremity or thigh. If anaphylaxis resulted from an injection or sting, as long as the sting is not on the head, neck, hands or feet, a second injection of epinephrine may be given at the injection or sting site to reduce antigen absorption.[141]

Intravenous epinephrine should be used only in a terminal patient (dilute 1 mL of 1:1000 solution of epinephrine in 9 mL of saline solution; doses are .1 to .2 mL every 5 to 20 minutes). If the reaction is from an injection or sting, a tourniquet should be placed proximal to the site of the injection. The tourniquet should be released for 1 to 2 minutes every 10 minutes. Oxygen should be given in patients with cyanosis, dyspnea, or wheezing. The presence of preexisting chronic obstructive pulmonary disease must be determined.

Diphenhydramine can be administered intravenously (slowly over 20 seconds), intramuscularly, or orally (1 to 2 mg/kg), giving up to 50 mg in a single dose. Continue orally every 6 hours for 48 hours to reduce the risk of recurrence. Other rapidly absorbed antihistamines can be substituted.

If the patient does not respond to these measures and remains hypotensive or in persistent respiratory distress, hospitalization in an intensive care unit is essential. In these circumstances, begin intravenous fluids through the largest gauge line available at a rate necessary to maintain a systolic blood pressure above 100 mm Hg in adults and 50 mm Hg in children. If intravenous fluids are not effective, vasopressors such as levarterenol bitartrate (Levophed), dopamine (Intropin), or metaraminol (Aramine) may be tried. If bronchospasm persists, aminophylline can be cautiously administered intravenously, with serum theophylline monitoring.

Intubation and tracheostomy are necessary if upper airway obstruction is so severe that the patient cannot maintain adequate ventilation.

Corticosteroids are not helpful in the acute management of anaphylaxis. They should be used in moderate or severe reactions to prevent protracted or recurrent anaphylaxis. Aqueous hydrocortisone can be given in a dose of 5 mg/kg up to 200 mg (higher doses also are acceptable) immediately followed by 2 to 5 mg/kg every 4 to 6 hours. An equivalent dose of other corticosteroids preparations can be used intravenously, intramuscularly, or orally. Glucagon may be the drug of choice for patients taking β-adrenergic blockade medications because of its positive inotropic and chronotropic effects on the heart, which are independent of catechol receptors. The dose is an intravenous bolus of 1 to 5 mg followed by a 5- to 15-μg/minute titration. Atropine may be useful if the patient is bradycardic; the dose is 0.3 to 0.5 mg subcutaneously, repeated every 10 minutes to a maximum of 2 mg.[56]

After the patient's condition has been stabilized, maintain supportive therapy with fluids, drugs, and ventilation as long as it is needed to support vital signs and functions.

A careful history of previous adverse reactions to suspected antigens is mandatory before administering any medication. As in all allergic diseases, avoidance of a known antigen is the most effective prophylactic measure. Avoidance of a known food usually is easy, but accidental exposure still may occur from food mixtures. General measures can help avoid some stinging insect reactions. Drug avoidance is paramount based on a detailed history. Alternative drugs must be used. If the drug is absolutely essential, skin testing, test dosing, or desensitization may be attempted with great caution. Certain substances require pretreatment regimens such as RCM and protamine sulfate. Skin testing before drug use may be required such as with chymopapain, streptokinase, and local anesthetics. Oral food and substance challenge is discussed earlier in this chapter and in Chapter 14. Washed red blood cells, autotransfusion, and IgA-deficient blood are choices for IgA-deficient patients or IgG-deficient patients who have anti-IgA antibodies. Skin testing and RAST are discussed earlier in this chapter. General rules to reduce the risk of anaphylaxis are listed in Table 20-3.

TABLE 20-3. *Rules to reduce the risk of anaphylaxis*

1. Know the patient's allergy and medical history with medical record documentation

2. Know the patient's concurrent therapy

3. Administer drugs orally rather than parenterally if possible

4. Observe immunotherapy patients in the physician's office 30 min after the injection

5. Hold immunotherapy in the presence of undertreated asthma

6. Require the patient to carry, at all times, a statement of allergy in the form of a bracelet, necklace, or wallet card

7. Pretreat patients with a history of an anaphylactoid reaction (i.e., radiographic contrast media; see Chap. 17) if use of the agent is essential

8. Require patients with idiopathic anaphylaxis, or those at risk of accidental exposure to known anaphylactic agents, to carry an emergency treatment kit

EMERGENCY DRUGS AVAILABLE TO PATIENTS

Certain patients are at risk of unpredictable anaphylaxis. This includes stinging insect exposure, food allergy, latex allergy, and idiopathic anaphylaxis. These patients should carry with them at all times injectable epinephrine, an oral antihistamine, and a tourniquet (for bee stings). Examples of commercial kits are (1) Ana-kit (Bayer, West Haven, CT), a prefilled syringe that can deliver two doses of 0.3 mL 1:1000 aqueous epinephrine; and (2) an Epi-Pen (regular or junior, Center Labs, Port Washington, NY), a prefilled automatic injection device with 0.3 mL or 0.15 mL of 1:1000 aqueous epinephrine for idiopathic anaphylaxis, EIA, latex allergy, and food anaphylaxis. Patient education and instruction is required. After using these devices, the patient should go to the nearest medical facility and seek further definitive therapy.

REFERENCES

1. Portier P, Richet C. De l'action anaphylactique de certaines venins. Compt Rend Soc Biol 1902;54:170.
2. Lamson RW. Fatal anaphylaxis and sudden death associated with injection of foreign substances. JAMA 1924;82:1091.
3. Vaughn WT, Pipes DM. On the probable frequency of allergic shock. Am J Dig Dis 1936;3:558.
4. Weiszer I. Allergic emergencies. In: Patterson R, ed. Allergic diseases: diagnosis and management. Philadelphia: JB Lippincott, 1985:418.
5. Marquardt DL, Wasserman SI. Anaphylaxis. In: Middleton E Jr, Reed CE, Ellis EF, Adkinson NF Jr, Yunginger JW, Busse WW, eds. Allergy: principles and practice. St Louis: CV Mosby, 1993:1525.
6. Wiggins CA, Dykewicz MS, Patterson R. Idiopathic anaphylaxis: classification, evaluation, and treatment of 123 patients. J Allergy Clin Immunol 1988;82:849.
7. Horowitz L. Atopy as factor in penicillin reactions. N Engl J Med 1975;292:1243.
8. Van Metre TE, Adkinson NF Jr. Immunotherapy for aeroallergen disease. In: Middleton E Jr, Reed CE, Ellis EF, Adkinson NF Jr, Yunginger JW, Busse WW, eds. Allergy: principles and practice. St Louis: CV Mosby, 1993:1501.
9. Settipane GA, Klein DE, Boyd GK. Relationship of atopy and anaphylactic sensitization: a bee sting allergy model. Clin Allergy 1978;8:259.
10. Austen KF. The anaphylactic syndrome. In: Sampter M, Talmage DW, Frank MM, Austen KF, Claman HN, eds. Immunologic diseases. Boston: Little, Brown, 1988:1119.
11. Bochner BS, Lichtenstein LM. Anaphylaxis. N Engl J Med 1991;324:1785.
12. Boston Collaborative Drug Surveillance Program. Drug-induced anaphylaxis. JAMA 1973;224:613.
13. Idsoe O, Gruthe T, Wilcox RR, DeWeck AL. Nature and extent of penicillin side-reactions with particular references to fatality from anaphylactic shock. Bull WHO 1968;38:159.
14. Shehadi WH. Adverse reactions to intravascularly administered contrast media. Am J Roentgenol 1975;124:145.
15. Ansell G. Adverse reactions to contrast agents. Invest Radiol 1970;6:374.

16. Witten DW. Reaction to urographic contrast media. JAMA 1975;231:974.
17. Lasser EC, Lang J, Sovak M, et al. Steroids: theoretical and experimental basis for utilization in prevention of contrast media reactions. Radiology 1977;125:1.
18. Katayama H, Yamaguchi K, Kozuka T, et al. Adverse reactions to ionic and nonionic contrast media: a report from the Japanese Committee on the Safety of Contrast Media. Radiology 1990;175:621.
19. Parrish HM. Analysis of 460 fatalities from venomous animals in the United States. Am J Med Sci 1965;245:129.
20. Patterson R, Valentine M. Anaphylaxis and related allergic emergencies, including reactions due to insect stings. JAMA 1982;248:2632.
21. Golden DRK, Lichtenstein LM. Insect sting allergy. In: Kaplan AP, ed. Allergy. New York: Churchill Livingstone 1985:507.
22. Golden DBK. Epidemiology of allergy to insect venoms and stings. Allergy Proc 1989;10:103.
23. Lockey RF, Benedict IM, Turkeltauk PC, et al. Fatalities from immunotherapy (IT) and skin testing (ST). J Allergy Clin Immunol 1987;79:660.
24. Reid MJ, Lockey RF, Turkeltaub PC, et al. Survey of fatalities from skin testing and immunotherapy 1985–1989. J Allergy Clin Immunol 1993;92:6.
25. Weis ME, Adkinson NF. Immediate hypersensitivity reactions to penicillin and related antibiotics. Clin Allergy 1988;18:515.
26. Greenberger PA, Patterson R, Kelly J, et al. Administration of radiographic contrast media in high-risk patients. Invest Radiol 1980;15(Suppl 6):S40.
27. Hunt KJ, Valentine MD, Sobotka AK, et al. A controlled trial of immunotherapy in insect hypersensitivity. N Engl J Med 1978;299:157.
28. Barnard JH. Studies of 400 Hymenoptera sting deaths in the United States. J Allergy Clin Immunol 1973;52:525.
29. Levine HD. Acute myocardial infarction following wasp sting: report of two cases and critical survey of the literature. Am Heart J 1976;91:365.
30. Miline MD. Unusual case of coronary thrombosis. Br Med J 1949;1:1123.
31. James LP, Austen KF. Fatal systemic anaphylaxis in man. N Engl J Med 1967;270:597.
32. Siegel SC, Heimlich EM. Anaphylaxis. Pediatr Clin North Am 1962;9:29.
33. Stark BJ, Sullivan TJ. Biphasic and protracted anaphylaxis. J Allergy Clin Immunol 1986;78:76.
34. Delage C, Ivey WS. Anaphylactic deaths: a clinicopathic study of 43 cases. J Forensic Sci 1972;17:525.
35. Criep LH, Wochler TR. The heart in human anaphylaxis. Ann Allergy 1971;29:399.
36. Delange C, Mullick FG, Ivery NS. Myocardial lesions in anaphylaxis. Arch Pathol Lab Med 1973;95:185.
37. Booth BH, Patterson R. Electrocardiographic changes during human anaphylaxis. JAMA 1970;211:627.
38. Smith PL, Kagey-Sobotka A, Bleecker ER, et al. Physiologic manifestations of human anaphylaxis. J Clin Invest 1980;66:1072.
39. Yunginger JW, Nelson DR, Squillace DL, et al. Laboratory investigation of deaths due to anaphylaxis. J Forensic Sci 1991;36:857.
40. Bonner JR. Anaphylaxis. I. Etiology and pathogenesis. Ala J Med Sci 1988;25:283
41. McManus LM, Hanahan DJ, Demopoulos CA, Pinkard RN. Pathobiology of intravenous infusion of acetyl glyceryl ether phophorylcholine (AGEPC), a synthetic platelet activating factor (PAF) in the rabbit. J Immunol 1980;124:2919.
42. Grandel KE, Farr RS, Wanderer AA, et al. The association of platelet activating factor with primary acquired cold urticaria. N Engl J Med 1985;313:405.
43. Goetzl EJ, Wasserman SI, Ansten KF. Eosinophil polymorphonuclear leukocyte function in immediate hypersensitivity. Arch Pathol 1975;99:1.
44. Lieberman P. Distinguishing anaphylaxis from other serious disorders. J Respir Dis 1995;16:411.
45. Settipane GA. The restaurant syndromes. Arch Intern Med 1986;21:29.
46. Morrow SD, Margolies GR, Rowland BS, et al. Evidence that histamine is the causative totin of scombroid-fish poisoning. N Engl J Med 1976;295:117.
47. Hughes JM, Potter ME. Scombroid-fish poisoning. N Engl J Med 1991;324:766.
48. Patterson R, Schatz M. Factitious allergic emergencies: Anaphylaxis and laryngeal "edema." J Allergy Clin Immunol 1975;56:152.
49. McGrath KG, Greenberger PA, Zeiss CR. Factitious allergic disease: multiple factitious illness and familial Munchausen's stridor. Immunol Allergy Pract 1984;6:41.
50. Kaliner M, Dyer J, Merlins S, et al. Increased urinary histamine in contrast media reactions. Invest Radiol 1984;19:116.
51. LaRoche D, Vergnand M, Sillard B, et al. Biochemical markers of plasma histamine and tryptase. Anesthesiology 1991;75:945.
52. Newman RB, Schultz LK. Epinephrine-resistant anaphylaxis in a patient taking propranolol hydrochloride. Ann Allergy 1981;47:35.
53. Harmany PJ, Hopper GDK. Severe anaphylaxis and drug-induced beta blockade. N Engl J Med 1983;308:1536. Letter.
54. Jacobs RC, Rake GW, Fournier DC, et al. Potentiated anaphylaxis in patients with drug induced beta-adrenergic blockade. J Allergy Clin Immunol 1981;68:125.
55. Toogood JH. Risk of anaphylaxis in patients receiving beta-blocker drugs. J Allergy Clin Immunol 1988;81:1.

56. Lieberman P. Anaphylaxis: guidelines for prevention and management. J Respir Dis 1995;16:456.
57. Bousquet J, Hejjaeni A, Dhivert H, et al. Immunotherapy with a standardized *Dermatophagoides pteronyssinus* extract. III. Systemic reactions according to the immunotherapy schedule. J Allergy Clin Immunol 1990;85:473.
58. World Health Organization/International Union of Immunological Societies Working Group. Current status of allergen immunotherapy. Lancet 1989;i:259. Abstract.
59. Suresh A, Reisman RE. Risk of administering cephalosporin antibiotics to patients with histories of penicillin allergy. Ann Allergy Asthma Immunol 1995;74:167.
60. Parker CW. Allergic drug responses: mechanisms and unsolved problems. CRC Crit Rev Toxicol 1972;1:261.
61. Levine BB. Antigenicity and crossreactivity of penicillins and cephalosporins. J Infect Dis 1973;128:5364.
62. Levine BB, Redmond AP. Minor haptenic determinant-specific reagins of penicillin hypersensitivity in man. Int Arch Allergy Appl Immunol 1969;35:445.
63. Hamilton-Miller JMT, Newton GGP, Abraham EP. Products of aminolysis and enxymatic hydrolysis of the cephalosporins. Biochem J 1970;116:371.
64. Girard JP. Common antigenic determinants of penicillin G, ampicillin and the cephalosporins demonstrated in men. Int Arch Allergy Appl Immunol 1968;33:428.
65. Golden DBK, Valentine MD, Kagey-Sabotka A, et al. Prevalence of Hymenoptera venom allergy. J Allergy Clin Immunol 1982;69:124.
66. Hunt KH, Valentine MD, Sobotka AK, et al. A controlled trial of immunotherapy in insect hypersensitivity. N Engl J Med 1978;299:157.
67. Stablein JJ, Lockey RF. Adverse reactions to ant sting. Clin Rev Allergy 1987;5:161.
68. Golbert TM, Patterson R, Pruzansky JJ. Systemic allergic reactions to ingested antigens. J Allergy 1969;44:96.
69. Stricker WE, Anorve-Lopez E, Reed CE. Food skin testing in patients with idiopathic anaphylaxis. J Allergy Clin Immunol 1986;77:516.
70. Fine AA. Hypersensitivity reactions to kiwi fruit. J Allergy Clin Immunol 1981;68:235.
71. Noyes JH, Boyd GK, Settipane GA. Anaphylaxis to sunflower seed. J Allergy Clin Immunol 1979;63:242.
72. Bonner MH, Lee HJ. Anaphylactic reaction to chamomile tea. J Allergy Clin Immunol 1973;52:307.
73. Kidd J, Cohen S, Syssman A, Fink JN. Food-dependent exercise-induced anaphylaxis. J Allergy Clin Immunol 1982;69:103.
74. Tanaka S. An epidemiological survey on food dependent exercise-induced anaphylaxis in kindergartners, school children and junior high school students. Asia Pac J Public Health 1994;7:26.
75. Añibarro B, Dominguez C, Diaz JM, et al. Apple-dependent exercise-induced anaphylaxis. Allergy 1994;49:481.
76. Munoz MF, Lopez Cazana JM, Villas F, et al. Exercise-induced anaphylactic reaction to hazelnut. Allergy 1994;49:314.
77. Mansfield LE, Bowers CH. Systemic reaction to papain in a nonoccupational setting. J Allergy Clin Immunol 1983;71:301.
78. Prenner BM, Stevens JJ. Anaphylaxis after ingestion of sodium bisulfite. Ann Allergy 1976;37:180.
79. Schwartz HJ. Sensitivity to ingested metabisulfite: variations in clinical presentation. J Allergy Clin Immunol 1983;71:487.
80. Tarlo SM, Sussman GL. Asthma and anaphylactoid reactions to food additives. Can Fam Physician 1993;39:1119.
81. Sussman GL, Beezhold DH. Allergy to latex rubber. Ann Intern Med 1995;122:43.
82. Slater JE. Latex allergy: what do we know? J Allergy Clin Immunol 1992;90:279.
83. Oei HD, Tjiook SB, Chang KC. Anaphylaxis due to latex allergy. Allergy Proc 1992;13:121.
84. Fisher MM, Baldo BA. Anaphylactoid reactions during general anesthesia. Clin Anesthesiology 1984;2:677.
85. Vervloet D, Nizankowska E, Arnaud A, et al. Adverse reactions to suxamethonium and other muscle relaxants under general anesthesia. J Allergy Clin Immunol 1983;71:551.
86. Monevet-Vautrin DA, Guéant JL, Kamel L, Laxenaire MC, Kholty SEI, Nicolas JP. Anaphylaxis to muscle relaxants: cross-sensitivity studied by radioimmunoassays compared to intradermal tests in 34 cases. J Allergy Clin Immunol 1988;82:745.
87. Moscicki RA, Sockin SM, Corsello BF, Ostrow MG, Bloch KJ. Anaphylaxis during induction of general anesthesia: subsequent evaluation and management. J Allergy Clin Immunol 1990;86:325.
88. Laxenaire MC, Monevet-Vautrin DA, Vervloet D. The French experience of anaphylactoid rections. In: Sage DJ, ed. International anesthesiology clinics: anaphylactoid reactions in anesthesia. Boston: Little, Brown, 1985:145.
89. Fisher M, Baldo BA. Anaphylaxis during anesthesia: current aspects of diagnosis and prevention. Eur J Anaesth 1994;11:263.
90. Beard K, Jick H. Cardiac arrest and anaphylaxis with anesthetic agents. JAMA 1985;254:2742.
91. Vervloet D, Arnaud A, Senft M, et al. Leukocyte histamine release to suxamethonium in patients with adverse reactions to muscle relaxants. J Allergy Clin Immunol 1985;75:338.
92. Watkins J. Allergic and pseudoallergic mechanisms in anesthesia. In: Sage DJ, ed. International anesthesiology clinics: anaphylactoid reactions in anesthesia. Boston: Little, Brown, 1985:17.
93. Routledge RC, DeKretser DMH, Wadsworth LD. Severe anaphylaxis due to passive sensitization by donor blood. Br Med J 1976;1:434.
94. Wells JV, Buckley RH, Schanfield MS, et al. Anaphylactic reactions to plasma infusions in patients with hypogammaglobulinemia and anti-IgA antibodies. Clin Immunol Immunopathol 1977;8:265.

95. Vyas GN, Perkins HA, Yang YM, et al. Healthy blood donors with selective absence of immunoglobulin A: prevention of anaphylactic transfusion reactions caused by antibodies to IgA. J Lab Clin Med 1975;85:838.

96. Marrtinez-Sanz R, Marsal, Delaliana R, et al. Anaphylactic reaction associated with anti-IgA antibodies: description of one case successfully treated by means of extracorporeal circulation. J Cardiovasc Surg 1990;31:247.

97. Kumar ND, Sharma S, Sethi S, et al. Anaphylactoid transfusion reaction with anti-IgA antibodes in an IgA deficient patient: a case report. Indian J Pathol Microbiol 1993;36:282.

98. Ellis EF, Henny CS. Adverse reactions following administration of human gammaglobulin. J Allergy 1969;43:45.

99. Burman D, Hodson AK, Wood CBS, Brueton FW. Acute anaphylaxis, pulmonary edema and intravascular hemolysis due to cryoprecipitate. Arch Dis Child 1973;48:483.

100. Helmer RE, Alperin JR, Yunginger JW, et al. Anaphylactic reactions following infusion of factor VIII in a patient with classic hemophilia. Am J Med 1980;69:953.

101. Vervloet D, Senft M, Dygne P, et al. Anaphylaxis reactions to modified fluid gelatins. J Allergy Clin Immunol 1983;71:535.

102. Ring J. Anaphylactoid reactions to intravenous solutions used for volume substitution. Clin Rev Allergy 1991;9:397.

103. Renck H, Ljungström KG, Rosberg B, Dhunér KG, Dahl S. Prevention of dextran-induced anaphylactic reactions by hapten inhibition. Acta Chir Scand 1983;149:349.

104. Knape JTA, Schuller JC, Dehaas P, et al. An anaphylactic reaction to protamine in a patient allergic to fish. Anesthesiology 1981;55:324.

105. Greenberger PA, Patterson R, Tobin ML, Liotta JL, Roberts M. Lack of cross reactivity between IgE to salmon and protamine sulfate. Am J Med Sci 1989;296:104.

106. Stewart WS, McSweeney SM, Kellet MA, Faxon DP, Ryan TJ. Increased risk of severe protamine reactions in NPH insulin-dependent diabetics undergoing cardiac catheterization. Circulation 1984;70:788.

107. Goftschlich GM, Cravlee GP, Georgitis JW. Adverse reactions to protamine sulfate during cardiac surgery in diabetic and non-diabetic patients. Ann Allergy 1988;61:277.

108. Weiss ME, Nyhan D, Zhikang P, et al. Association of protamine IgE and IgG antibodies with life-threatening reactions to intravenous protamine. N Engl J Med 1989;320:886.

109. McGrath KG, Patterson R. Anaphylactic reactivity to streptokinase. JAMA 1984;252:1314.

110. McGrath KG, Zeffren B, Alexander J, et al. Allergic reactions to streptokinase consistent with anaphylactic or antigen-antibody complex mediated damage. J Allergy Clin Immunol 1985;76:453.

111. Dykewicz MS, McGrath KG, Davison R, Kaplan KJ, Patterson R. Identification of patients at risk for anaphylaxis from streptokinase. Arch Int Med 1986;146:305.

112. Massei D, Gill JB, Cairns JA. Anaphylactoid reaction during an infusion of recombinant tissue-type plasminogen activator for acute myocardial infarction. Can J Cardiol 1991;7:298.

113. Willis J, ed. Chymopapain approval. FDA Drug Bull 1982;12:17.

114. Drenth J, Jansonius JN, Koekoek R, et al. Structure of papain. Nature 1968;218:929.

115. Novey HS, Marchioli LE, Sokol WN, et al. Papain-induced asthma: physiological and immunologic features. J Allergy Clin Immunol 1979;63:98.

116. Grammer LC, Schafer M, Bernstein D, et al. Prevention of chymopapain anaphylaxis by screening chemonucleolysis candidates with cutaneous chymopapain testing. Clin Orthop 1988;234:15.

117. McCulloch JA, Canham WD, Dolovish J. Skin tests for chymopapain allergy. Ann Allergy 1985;55:609.

118. Bernstein DI, Gallagher JS, Ulmer A, Bernstein IL. Prospective evaluation of chymopapain sensitivity in patients undergoing chemonucleolysis. J Allergy Clin Immunol 1985;76:458.

119. Davis H, McGoodwin E, Reed TG. Anaphylactoid reactions after treatment with ciprolaxacin. Ann Int Med 1989;111:1041.

120. Rassiga AL, Schwartz HJ, Forman WB, et al. Cytarabine-induced anaphylaxis. Arch Intern Med 1980;140:425.

121. Zaloga GP, Chernow B. Life-threatening anaphylactic reations to tetnus toxoid. Ann Allergy 1982;49:107.

122. Klotz SD, Sweeny MJ, Dienst S, et al. Systemic anaphylaxis immediately after delayed hypersensitivity skin tests. Ann Allergy 1982;49:142.

123. Lazaro M, Compared JA, De la Hoz B, et al. Anaphylactic reaction to ranitidine. Allergy 1993;48:385.

124. Sussman GL, Dorian W. Psyllium anaphylaxis. Allergy Proc 1990;11:241.

125. Brown LA, Kaplan RA, Benjamin PA, et al. Immunoglobulin E–mediated anaphylaxis with inhaled cromolyn sodium. J Allergy Clin Immunol 1981;68:416.

126. Dolovich J, Bell B. Allergy to a product to ethylene oxide gas. J Allergy Clin Immunol 1978;762:30.

127. Grammer LC, Patterson R. IgE against ethylene oxide–altered human serum albumin (ETO-HSA) as an etiologic agent in allergic reactions of hemodialysis patients. Artif Organs 1987;11:97.

128. Schafer RM, Fink E, Schaefer L, et al. Role of bradykinin in anaphylactoid reactions during hemodialysis with AN 69 dialyzers. Am J Nephrol 1993;13:473.

129. Verresen L, Fink E, Lemke H, et al. Bradykinin is a mediator of anaphylactoid reactions during hemodialysis with AN 69 membranes. Kidney 1994;45:1497.

130. Frankland AW, Parish WE. Anaphylactic sensitivity to human seminal fluid. Clin Allergy 1979;4:249.

131. Kooistra JB, Yunginger JW, Santrach PJ, et al. In vitro studies of human seminal plasma allergy. J Allergy Clin Immunol 1980;66:148.

132. Mittman RJ, Bernstein DI, Adler TR, et al. Selective desensitization to seminal plasma protein fractions after immunotherapy for postcoital anaphylaxis. J Allergy Clin Immunol 1990;86:954.
133. Grammer LC, Metzger BE, Patterson R, et al. Cutaneous allergy to human (rDNA) insulin. JAMA 1984;251:1459.
134. Grammer LC. Insulin allergy. Clin Rev Allergy 1986;4:189.
135. Greenberger PA. Prophylaxis against repeat radiographic media reactions in 857 cases: adverse experience with cimetidine and safety of beta adrenergic antagonists. Arch Int Med;145:2197.
136. Sheffer AL, Soter NA, McFadden ER Jr, et al. Exercise-induced anaphylaxis: a distinct form of physical allergy. J Allergy Clin Immunol 1983;71:311.
137. Briner WW, Scheffer AL. Exercise-induced anaphylaxis. Med Sci Sports Exerc 1992;24:849.137.
138. Maulitz RM, Pratt DS, Schocket AL. Exercise induced anaphylactic reactions to shellfish. J Allergy Clin Immunol 1979;63:433.
139. Ausdermoore RW. Fatality in a teenager secondary to exercise-induced anaphylaxis. Pediatr Asthma Allergy Immunol 1991;5:21.
140. Tse KS, Yeung M, Ferrlera P. A study of exercise induced urticaria and angioedema. J Allergy Clin Immunol 1980;65:227. Abstract.
141. Bonner JR. Anaphylaxis. I. Etiology and pathogenesis. Ala J Med Sci 1988;25:283.

Allergic Diseases, 5th Edition,
edited by Roy Patterson, Leslie Carroll Grammer, and
Paul A. Greenberger. Lippincott–Raven Publishers, Philadelphia, © 1997.

21

Idiopathic Anaphylaxis

Roy Patterson and Kathleen E. Harris

*R. Patterson: Division of Allergy-Immunology, Department of Medicine,
Northwestern University Medical School, Chicago, IL 60611-3008.
K.E. Harris: Division of Allergy-Immunology, Department of Medicine
Northwestern University Medical School, Chicago, IL 60611-3008.*

Pearls for Practitioners
Roy Patterson

- These are about 30,000 cases of idiopathic anaphylaxis (IA) in the United States.
- Some physicians have difficulty accepting the diagnosis of IA even after seeing a case.
- The prognosis for IA is, in general, better than for severe, corticosteroid-dependent asthma.
- Even patients with malignant IA have a reasonably good prognosis.
- Undifferentiated somatiform IA has a poor prognosis for recovery. Acceptance of psychiatric care is not common.
- Increasing numbers of cases of pediatric IA are being identified. Some physicians have difficulty accepting this diagnosis also.
- The treatment regimens for IA of various classifications are, in general, successful.
- Corticosteroid-dependent IA does occur but is not common, and high doses of prednisone are rarely required.

Of the many unusual features of idiopathic anaphylaxis (IA), the following are some of the most striking. The disease was described about two decades ago,[1] and in the next 15 years IA was classified,[2] treatment regimens were established, and remission was induced in most cases. Fatalities have been described,[3] and the number of cases of IA in the United States has been estimated to be between 20,000 and 30,000.[4] Patients with frequent episodes have multiple emergency service visits and hospitalizations and usually are frightened. IA is not limited to the United States[5] and is likely to be distributed worldwide. When IA is identified and the treatment regimens instituted, the prognosis for control and remission is far better than for prednisone-dependent asthma in adults, since the latter problem generally persists for years with control but no remission.

The questions about IA thus become obvious. What were the explanations for recurrent IA before the disease was described? For such a costly, frightening, potentially fatal disease, why has there been so little interest on the part of the federal government and the major national allergy societies? Fortunately, the diagnostic methodology and treatment regimens are sufficiently successful that the alert physician who is aware of IA as the explanation for single or recurrent episodes of anaphylaxis with no apparent external cause can competently and successfully manage IA in pediatric or adult populations.

DESCRIPTIONS AND DEFINITIONS

Idiopathic anaphylaxis is an immediate-type life-threatening event with no external allergen triggering the onset through an IgE antibody–mediated reaction. Thus, foods, drugs, and venoms are not related to onset of episodes of IA but must be excluded during initial evaluation. The two major types of IA are (1) IA–angioedema (IA-A), in which airway obstruction occurs; and (2) IA–generalized (IA-G), in which the various systemic manifestations of anaphylaxis occur. The classification of IA relative to clinical manifestations and frequency is shown in Table 21-1.

TREATMENT REGIMENS

Treatment regimens evolved from experience in treating or preventing anaphylactic-type reactions such as those caused by radiographic contrast media.[6] As increasing numbers of patients were referred for management or opinions on management of IA, an algorithm was developed for guidance in management (Fig. 21-1).

TABLE 21-1. *Classification of idiopathic anaphylaxis*

Disease	Symptoms
Idiopathic anaphylaxis–generalized–infrequent (IA-G-I)	Urticaria or angioedema with bronchospasm, hypotension, syncope, or gastrointestinal symptoms with or without upper airway compromise with infrequent episodes (less than six episodes occurring per year).
Idiopathic anaphylaxis–generalized-frequent (IA-G-F)	Clinical manifestations as for IA-G-I but occurring more than 6 times per year.
Idiopathic anaphylaxis–angioedema–infrequent (IA-A-I)	Urticaria or angioedema with upper airway compromise such as laryngeal edema, severe pharyngeal edema, or massive tongue edema without other systemic manifestations with infrequent episodes (less than six episodes occurring per year).
Idiopathic anaphylaxis–angioedema–frequent (IA-A-F)	Clinical manifestations as for IA-A-I but occurring more than six times per year.
Idiopathic anaphylaxis–questionable (IA-Q)	Diagnosis is applied to a patient who is referred for management with a presumptive diagnosis of IA for which repeated attempts at documentation of objective findings are unsuccessful, response to appropriate doses of prednisone does not occur, and the diagnosis of IA becomes uncertain.
Idiopathic anaphylaxis–variant (IA-V)	Diagnosis is applied when symptoms and physical findings of IA vary from classic findings of IA. IA-V may subsequently be classified as IA-Q, IA-excluded, IA-A, or IA-G.
Undifferentiated somatoform IA	Symptoms mimic IA but no objective findings are seen and there is no response to the regimen for IA.

OUTCOME OF TREATMENT REGIMENS FOR IDIOPATHIC ANAPHYLAXIS

After initiation of the regimen for IA-G-frequent consisting of prednisone, hydroxyzine, and albuterol (see Fig. 21-1), the episodes of IA should cease while the patient is receiving daily prednisone. This may require 1 to 6 weeks of daily prednisone. If longer daily prednisone is required, the diagnosis of IA becomes questionable and alternate diagnoses must be considered, including those in the differential diagnosis of IA (listed on the next page).

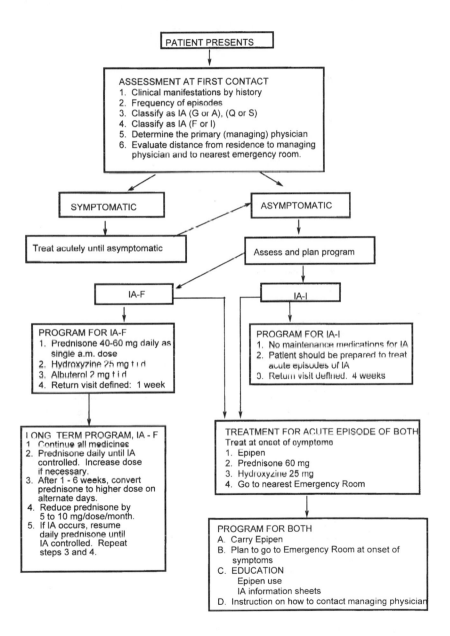

FIG. 21-1. The algorithm for initial assessment and management of idiopathic anaphylaxis (IA) of frequent (F) or infrequent (I) types at the patient's first visit. G, generalized; A, angioedema; Q, questionable; S, somatoform; a.m., morning; t.i.d., three times per day.

- Hereditary angioedema
- Systemic mastocytosis
- Hidden allergen (e.g., latex)
- Munchausen's anaphylaxis (purposeful self-exposure to antigen)
- Undifferentiated somatoform IA

If the patient's condition is not controlled by prednisone treatment (adult dosage, 60 mg daily for 6 weeks), the diagnosis likely is not IA, and undifferentiated somatoform IA[7] must be seriously considered.

After IA is controlled with daily prednisone, an alternate-day regimen of prednisone at a higher dose is initiated, and if the IA remains controlled, the dose of prednisone is cautiously reduced. If after a reduction of alternate-day prednisone an episode of IA occurs, daily prednisone must be resumed, followed by alternate-day prednisone at a higher dose and slower reduction.

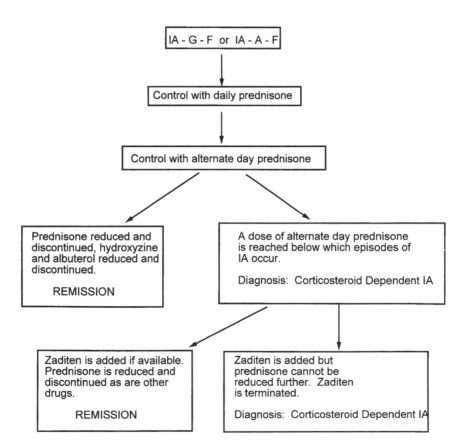

FIG. 21-2. The outcome and continued management of patients with idiopathic anaphylaxis (IA) at subsequent visits. For long-term management, patients should be seen initially at least every 4 weeks for reduction of prednisone dose. Clinical judgment is necessary to avoid excess prednisone or too rapid a reduction of prednisone dose. IA, idiopathic anaphylaxis; G, generalized; A, angioedema; F, frequent; I, infrequent.

The long-term result of this regimen is an induction of remission, and in most patients, the use of prednisone can be terminated (Fig. 21-2). If a dose of alternate-day prednisone is reached below which episodes of IA recur, the diagnosis of corticosteroid-dependent IA (CSD-IA) can be made. Patients with CSD-IA may respond to ketotifen (Zaditen; in countries where this drug is available), which allows further reduction and discontinuation of prednisone and possibly induces a remission. Alternatively, ketotifen may not alter the prednisone requirement, in which case ketotifen should be tapered and discontinued, with the diagnosis remaining CSD-IA.

IDIOPATHIC ANAPHYLAXIS–SINGLE EPISODE OR IDIOPATHIC ANAPHYLAXIS–INFREQUENT

A patient who has had even a single episode of IA should carry emergency therapy in the event of recurrence (see Fig. 21-1). When a single episode has been recent and sufficiently severe to suggest the likelihood of a fatality, the treatment course for IA-frequent (IA-F) (see Fig. 21-1) should be considered. Patients with IA-infrequent (IA-I) are managed with the availability of emergency therapy. However, these patients also may be considered for a course of prednisone, as is used for IA-F, to attempt to induce a remission of the IA syndrome.

PATIENT EDUCATION

A major goal in management of IA is the education of the patient, family, and sometimes the referring physician about IA. This includes teaching the patient the following. First, that there is *not* an external agent, and attention must be given to pharmacologic induction of a remission. Second, the patient should understand the risks of prednisone but that, in the method of management, prednisone treatment most likely will be terminated without residual side effects. Third, patients often demand explanations for IA, which include the theories of an autoimmune (anti-IgE) factor or the inappropriate release of cytokines such as histamine releasing factors, which are modified by prednisone therapy.[8]

UNDIFFERENTIATED SOMATOFORM IDIOPATHIC ANAPHYLAXIS

Undifferentiated somatoform idiopathic anaphylaxis is the term applied when patients who have no organic disease describe symptoms consistent with IA. The differentiation of organic from hysterical IA should be relatively simple, but the opposite is observed. In two series of cases,[7,9] the following general characteristics have been observed in a total of 19 cases: (1) the referring physician generally does not recognize the nonorganic nature of the problem; (2) the medical costs of hospitalizations, emergency service visits, and laboratory tests is extremely high; and (3) these patients may be treated excessively with unnecessary corticosteroids. An algorithm for the diagnosis of undifferentiated somatoform IA is shown in Figure 21-3. When the managing physician arrives at this diagnosis, further management may become difficult. Approaching the basis of the problem as psychological in origin with referral to a psychiatrist is the logical approach. This may be accepted by the patient. Alternatively, the patient may reject the concept of a psychological disorder as the explanation, often with hostility. Some of these patients can be treated by the allergist and generalist with safe, low doses of antihistamines and supportive ambulatory visits at increasing intervals. Other patients may continue to be admitted to hospital emergency services. They continue playing their role of a patient in anaphylaxis with unimaginable skill.

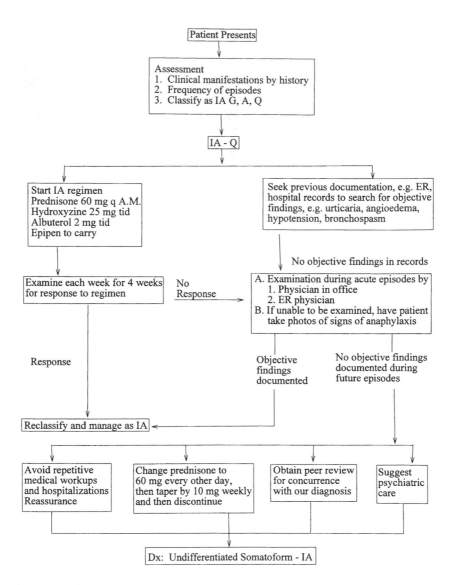

FIG. 21-3. An algorithm for diagnosis of undifferentiated somatoform idiopathic anaphylaxis. A.M., morning; G, generalized; A, angioedema; Q, questionable; ER, emergency room; Dx, diagnosis. (Reprinted with permission, Choy AC, Patterson R, Patterson DR, et al. Undifferentiated somatoform idiopathic anaphylaxis: nonorganic symptoms mimicking idiopathic anaphylaxis. J Allergy Clin Immunol 1995;96:893.)

PEDIATRIC IDIOPATHIC ANAPHYLAXIS

In our service, the ratio of pediatric IA to adult IA cases is about 1 pediatric IA case to 20 adult cases. For this reason, the diagnosis of IA in children may be delayed beyond the time seen for diagnosis in adults. In our series, however, the response to the regimen for IA (with dose adjustment for the pediatric population) appears to be equally successful and the prognosis is equally good as that for most adults.[10]

SUMMARY

Idiopathic anaphylaxis was identified about 20 years ago. It was classified and treatment regimens were adopted, tested, and proven effective. The prognosis for the individual patient is good, and reassuring a newly diagnosed patient of this is justified when the regimen described here is used. This is of particular value when patients and their families are extremely frightened. The series of cases of IA seen at the Northwestern Allergy-Immunology Service approximates 400 cases, with the last publication describing 335 patients.[11] One fatality has been documented.[12] Unfortunately, the prognosis for undifferentiated somatoform IA is not as good, but a diagnosis is important to prevent unnecessary hospitalizations.

REFERENCES

1. Bacal E, Patterson R, Zeiss CR. Evaluation of severe (anaphylactic) reactions. Clin Allergy 1978;8:295.
2. Wiggins CA, Dykewicz MS, Patterson R. Idiopathic anaphylaxis: classification, evaluation, and treatment of 123 patients. J Allergy Clin Immunol 1988;82:849.
3. Patterson R, Clayton DE, Booth BH, Greenberger PA, Grammer LC, Harris KE. Fatal and near fatal idiopathic anaphylaxis. Allergy Proc 1995;16:103.
4. Patterson R, Hogan MB, Yarnold P, Harris KE. Idiopathic anaphylaxis: an attempt to estimate the incidence in the United States. Arch Intern Med 1995;155:869.
5. Tejedor MA, Perez C, de la Hoz B, Jauregui I, Puras A, Alvarez-Cuesta E. Idiopathic anaphylaxis: clinical differences. J Allergy Clin Immunol 1992;89:349. Abstract.
6. Greenberger PA, Patterson R. The prevention of immediate generalized reactions to radiocontrast media in high-risk patients. J Allergy Clin Immunol 1991;87:867.
7. Choy AC, Patterson R, Patterson DR, et al. Undifferentiated somatoform idiopathic anaphylaxis: non-organic symptoms mimicking idiopathic anaphylaxis. J Allergy Clin Immunol 1995;96:893.
8. Patterson R, Harris KE. Idiopathic anaphylaxis: management and theories of pathogenesis. Clin Immunother 1995;4:265.
9. Patterson R, Greenberger PA, Orfan NA, Stoloff RS. Idiopathic anaphylaxis: diagnostic variants and the problem of nonorganic disease. Allergy Proc 1992;13:133.
10. Patterson R, Ditto A, Dykewicz MS, et al. Pediatric idiopathic anaphylaxis: additional cases and extended observations. Pediatr Asthma Allergy Immunol (in press).
11. Ditto AM, Harris KE, Krasnick J, Miller MA, Patterson R. Idiopathic anaphylaxis: a series of 335 cases. Ann Allergy Asthma Immunol 1996;77:285.
12. Krasnick J, Patterson R, Meyers GL. A fatality from idiopathic anaphylaxis. Ann Allergy Asthma Immunol 1996;76:376.
13. Patterson R, ed. Idiopathic anaphylaxis: Providence Oceanside Publications, Inc. (in press).

Allergic Diseases, 5th Edition,
edited by Roy Patterson, Leslie Carroll Grammer, and
Paul A. Greenberger. Lippincott–Raven Publishers, Philadelphia, © 1997.

22

Asthma

Paul A. Greenberger

*P.A. Greenberger: Division of Allergy-Immunology,
Northwestern University Medical School, Chicago, IL 60611-3008.*

Pearls for Practitioners
Roy Patterson

- If you treat a patient with asthma while that patient continues to smoke, you are helping that patient toward death.
- Cough equivalent asthma is asthma expressed as a cough. Diagnosis is made by excluding other causes of cough, giving a 2-week trial of prednisone at 30 mg daily, and having the cough disappear. Patients are subsequently managed by inhaled corticosteroids alone. If the cough doesn't disappear within 2 weeks of prednisone, the diagnosis is not cough equivalent asthma.
- Patients with corticosteroid-dependent asthma should be prepared for surgery with daily prednisone. Surgery includes dental work that is more than minimal, such as tooth extractions or root canal surgery.
- Patients should be instructed on the use of prednisone for travel, especially to foreign countries.
- Except for minimal asthma, inhaled corticosteroids are the first line of therapy.
- The primary cause of asthma is inflammation. Corticosteroids are antiinflammatory agents.
- Asthma triggered by pets, particularly cats, can be followed by respiratory infections and severe asthma requiring hospitalization. Paint fumes in the house can have the same result by nonspecific irritation.
- Patients whose asthma is controlled by an inhaled corticosteroid frequently reduce the dose, either forgetting to take it or because they think they don't need it.
- A patient hospitalized for asthma always should have an evaluation of the cause of the severe asthma, with measures taken to prevent readmission.
- Influenza vaccine should be given to every patient with asthma unless allergy to eggs exists.
- All patients with asthma can be managed so that they are not at risk of dying.
- Potentially fatal asthma is the diagnosis applied to patients who have had a near-fatal episode of asthma.
- Malignant potentially fatal asthma is the term applied to patients who do not comply with appropriate management principles.
- Munchausen's asthma is real asthma that patients induce by stopping medications.
- Factitious wheezing, like factitious stridor, is self-induced respiratory sounds. An experienced physician can learn to make the sounds.
- Death from asthma is preventable in every patient with asthma. Death from asthma cannot be prevented in every asthmatic.
- Asthma is asthma, not reactive airway disease.

continued

- Appropriate use of corticosteroids in asthma sometimes is followed by decreasing inflammation of the airways and decreased need for chronic corticosteroids.
- Teenagers often do not take the appropriate medications for asthma. The same is true for geriatric patients.
- Corticosteroidphobia in a patient with potentially fatal asthma is dangerous. Psychiatric care may be necessary but may not be accepted.
- Asthma is a disease of fluctuating severity. If a useless treatment is started just before spontaneous subsidence, the useless therapy may get the credit.
- Spontaneous subsidence of asthma often is seen during puberty but may occur later in life.
- The basic cause of asthma is not known. Nevertheless, effective therapy for all patients is available.

Asthma is a disease characterized by (1) hyperresponsiveness of bronchi to various stimuli, and (2) changes in airways resistance, lung volumes, and expiratory flow rates, with symptoms of cough, wheezing dyspnea, or shortness of breath. A joint committee of the American College of Chest Physicians and American Thoracic Society proposed the following definition: "A disease characterized by an increased responsiveness of the airways to various stimuli and manifested by slowing of forced expiration which changes in severity either spontaneously or as a result of therapy."[1] In 1991, a National Institutes of Health Expert Panel suggested that asthma was a disease characterized by (1) airway obstruction that is reversible—partially or completely, (2) airway inflammation, and (3) airway hyperresponsiveness.[2]

Asthma has been defined by a description of the response of the lung after a patient is exposed to various triggering factors. For example, terms such as allergic bronchitis, asthmatic bronchitis, allergic asthma, atopic asthma, nonallergic asthma, cough equivalent asthma,[3] and cardiac asthma[4,5] have been used to describe a particular type of asthma.[6] The central feature of asthma from a physiologic viewpoint is bronchial hyperresponsiveness to stimuli such as histamine or methacholine compared with patients without asthma. In population screening, such nonspecific hyperresponsiveness has been reported as sensitive but not specific.[6] Surprisingly, in a study of children aged 7 to 10 years, 48% of children with a diagnosis of asthma did not have bronchial hyperresponsiveness.[7] Asthma is characterized by wide variations of resistance to airflow on expiration (and inspiration), with remarkable transient increases in certain lung volumes such as residual volume, functional residual capacity (FRC), and total lung capacity (TLC).

Asthma is considered a reversible obstructive airways disease as compared with chronic obstructive pulmonary disease (COPD). Most patients with asthma experience symptom-free periods of days, weeks, months, or years between episodes, whereas chronic symptoms and fixed dyspnea characterize COPD. When daily symptoms of cough, wheezing, and dyspnea have been present for months in a patient with asthma, bronchodilator nonresponsiveness may be present. However, appropriate therapy reduces symptoms and improves the quality of life significantly along with improving pulmonary function status.

Whereas IgE-mediated bronchospasm can be demonstrated in many patients with asthma, not all patients with asthma are "allergic." Evidence does exist for IgE antibodies to respiratory syncytial virus[8] and parainfluenza virus,[9] however, so while the understanding of nonallergic asthma increases, perhaps the description of viral infection–triggered asthma will change. The sudden onset of wheezing dyspnea that occurs after ingestion of aspirin[10,11] or other nonsteroidal antiinflammatory drugs (NSAIDs)[12,13] is not an IgE-mediated reaction, but represents alterations of arachidonic acid metabolism such as blockage of the cyclooxygenase pathway with shunting of arachidonic acid into the lipoxygenase pathway. Potent lipoxygenase pathway products such as leukotriene D_4 (LTD_4) cause bronchospasm in aspirin- and NSAID-sensitive patients.[14,15] Most patients with asthma have symptoms precipitated by non-specific, non–IgE-mediated triggers such as cold air, air pollutants, exercise, crying or laughing, and changes in barometric pressure. Fortunately, pharmacologic therapy can minimize the effects of these nonspecific triggers.

GENETIC AND ENVIRONMENTAL FACTORS

Genetic and environmental factors are important in terms of development of asthma.[16] The approximate risk of an allergic-type disease in a child is 20%, but if one parent is allergic, this risk increases to 50%.[17–19] If both parents are allergic, there is a 66% chance of the child developing an allergic condition.[17–19] If allergy is defined as all IgE antibody–mediated diseases such as rhinitis, this does not necessarily apply to asthma.

In a prospective study of children evaluated during the first 6 years of life, the risk of a boy developing asthma was 14.3% versus 6.3% for girls.[20] These data support the notion of polygenic inheritance with greater prevalence in boys. In twin studies, the concordance for asthma in monozygotic twins reared together was similar to twins reared apart.[21] These data support a strong genetic effect on development of asthma. In a study of 6996 adult twin-pairs, the genetic components of asthma were found to be present but not as great.[22] Methacholine responsiveness, total serum IgE concentration, and immediate skin test reactivity have been found to be more concordant in monozygotic twins than in dizygotic twins,[23] which supports a genetic over environmental influence. Both factors should be considered as contributory, and production of specific antiallergen IgE seems to be affected by environmental and local allergic exposures in the genetically susceptible subject. The onset of early childhood asthma has not been associated with parental smoking[20]; however, once asthma begins, evidence exists for increased childhood respiratory symptoms from passive smoking from the mother but not the father.[24]

Environmental factors may be most important in the development of IgE. Frick and coworkers[25] demonstrated development of antiallergen IgE in association with increasing antiviral antibodies in a prospective study of high risk infants whose parents both had allergic diseases. Croup in early childhood has been associated with subsequent development of asthma.[26] Indoor allergen exposures from house dust mites[27] and cats[28] have been associated with the development of asthma, emphasizing that both viral infections[29] and allergens are involved in childhood wheezing.

COMPLEXITY OF ASTHMA

The cause of asthma remains unknown, although asthma is considered a complex inflammatory disease. Some important pathologic findings include a patchy loss of bronchial epithelium, usually associated with eosinophil infiltration,[30,31] contraction and hypertrophy of bronchial smooth muscles, bronchial mucosa edema, bronchial gland hyperplasia and hypersecretion of thick bronchial mucus, and basement membrane thickening.[32] There is subepithelial fibrosis that is composed of collagen types I, II, and V that contributes to the basement membrane thickening of asthma. Some physiologic characteristics of asthma include bronchial hyperresponsiveness to stimuli such as histamine,[33] methacholine,[34] or LTD_4,[35] at least a 12%

improvement in FEV_1 after inhalation of a β_2-adrenergic agonist unless the patient is experiencing status asthmaticus or has had severe, ineffectively treated airways obstruction and large changes in lung compliance, depending on severity of the disease. On a cellular level, during acute episodes of asthma, activated or hypodense eosinophils are present in increased numbers,[31,36] and eosinophil products such as major basic protein can be identified in sputum[37] and in areas where bronchial epithelium has been denuded.[38] Eosinophil cationic protein has been identified in areas of shed denuded bronchial epithelium. This cationic protein has been reported to be even more cytotoxic than major basic protein.[39] Mast cells in the bronchial lumen and submucosa are activated, and their many cell products are released, whether preformed or synthesized de novo. Macrophages and lymphocytes participate as well.

In addition, evidence supports the concept of neuroimmunologic abnormalities in asthma such as the lack of the bronchodilating nonadrenergic noncholinergic vasoactive intestinal peptide being present in lung sections from patients with asthma.[40] However, another study did not demonstrate absence of vasoactive intestinal polypeptide in tracheal or parenchymal lung tissues.[41] The bronchoconstricting neuropeptide substance P was identified in lower frequency in tracheas from patients with asthma compared with nonatopic controls, whereas substance P was present in equal amounts in parenchyma in sections from patients with asthma and from nonatopics. These findings do not support a deficiency of vasoactive intestinal polypeptide or an excess of substance P in tissue.[41] Substance P concentrations in induced sputum have been reported to be markedly elevated compared with control patients.[42]

These conflicting findings demonstrate the complexity of asthma, which, decades ago, was considered a psychological condition. Asthma is not a psychological disorder. Nevertheless, the burden of asthma as a chronic disease, especially when the patient has experienced repeated hospitalizations or emergency rooms visits, may result in psychological disturbances that coexist with asthma.[40–46]

INCIDENCE AND SIGNIFICANCE

Asthma affects over 10 million people in the United States.[47] Acute asthma is the most common childhood medical emergency.[48] The prevalence of asthma and asthma mortality rates are greater in urban rather than rural areas, in boys compared with girls, and in blacks compared with whites.[49] The prevalence of asthma in 6- to 11-year-old children has increased from 4.8% during 1971 to 1974, to 7.6% during 1976 to 1980,[50] to as high as 12.3% by 1992.[51] Such information was generated from questionnaire surveys in the United States. Apparent increased prevalence of asthma has been reported in the United Kingdom[52] and New Zealand[53] as well. The onset of asthma often occurs in the first two decades of life, especially during the first few years[54] or when the person is older than 40 years. However, intermittent respiratory symptoms may have existed for years before an actual diagnosis of asthma is made in patients older than 40 years of age.[54] The diagnosis of asthma is more likely to be given to women and nonsmokers, whereas men may be labeled as having chronic bronchitis, even when they do not have chronic sputum production for 3 months each year for 2 consecutive years. Asthma may have its onset in the geriatric population[55] and usually begins during or after an upper respiratory tract infection. The prevalence of asthma was found to be 6.5% of persons who were aged at least 70 years living in South Wales.[56]

Asthma morbidity can be enormous from a personal and family perspective as well as from the societal aspect. In 1988, there were about 15 million visits to physicians for asthma. The number of hospitalizations in the United States for asthma has increased almost 4 fold from 1965 to 1983 with absolute numbers growing from 127,000 to 459,000 per year.[57] The hospitalization rate for asthma increased from 48 to 166 per 100,000 children. In one study during 1988, 21% of children, with asthma had been hospitalized. The number of days of school missed from asthma is excessive as is work absenteeism. Asthma was thought to be occupationally related in 2% of the 6 million people with asthma in the United States in 1960. In contrast, in 1978, occupational causes were blamed for 15% of cases of asthma (United States total about 9 million) in a disability survey.[58,59] The high prevalence of occupational asthma as causes for respiratory symptoms in as many as 15% of newly diagnosed asthma[59] implies a major public health and economic issue in that some 250 different chemicals have been recognized as causes of asthma.[59]

Since 1960, the number of cases of asthma in the United States has increased from 6 million to over 10 million persons. Except for viral upper respiratory illnesses, asthma has been a major cause of school absenteeism. The number and percentage rate of fatalities from asthma has increased in the United States[47] and other countries including United Kingdom,[52] New Zealand,[53] Denmark,[60] France,[61] and Germany,[61] but not Canada.[62,63] The mortality rate in Germany still is double that of France, Denmark,[50] and the United States.[38] The extraordinarily high death rate in New Zealand of 7 per 100,000 of the population that occurred in the 1980s has been reduced to 4 per 100,000, which is similar to Australia.[62] The asthma death rates in the United States and Canada are about 2 per 100,000 of the population.[47,62] The exact number of persons dying from asthma is not known, but increases of death rates in patients aged 5 to 34 years have been noted.[47,49] This age range is used to minimize the number of confounding diagnoses such as COPD or chronic bronchitis. Some areas such as New York City and Chicago experienced high mortality rates, partly associated with lower socioeconomic conditions. In fact, 21.1% of all asthma deaths occurred in these two areas, despite having 6.8% of all 5- to 34-year-olds in the United States.[49] The fatality rate among nonwhites is much higher than whites.[47]

The costs of asthma include the direct costs of medications, hospitalizations, and physician charges in addition to indirect costs such as time lost from work with loss of worker productivity. The total cost in 1990 in the United States was estimated at $6.2 billion.[49] Emotional costs of asthma are great for the patient and the family if asthma is ineffectively managed or if the patient refuses to adhere to appropriate medical advice. The death of a family member from asthma is shocking since the person may be young and the fatal attack may not have been anticipated by others or even the patient. With current understanding and treatment of asthma, fatalities usually should be avoidable—asthma need not be a fatal disease. Over half of deaths from asthma occur outside of a hospital.[57] This finding has led some physicians to conclude that emergency medical services should be improved. One cannot dispute such an argument, but it is advisable for the physician managing the patient with asthma to have an emergency plan available for the patient or family so that optimally, asthma is not managed from a crisis orientation but rather on a preventive basis.

The number of prescriptions for asthma or COPD medications was estimated in 1985 to be 3% to 4% or 51 million of 1.5 billion prescriptions written in the United States for all medications.[64] From 1972 to 1985, the number of asthma and COPD prescriptions increased from 17 to 51 million.[64] Substantial increases in cromolyn by metered dose inhaler have occurred in recent years because of a simplified delivery system. The sales of inhaled corticosteroids have increased 12-fold from 1976 to 1991, whereas sales of β-adrenergic agonist inhalers increased threefold.[64] In summary, the prevalence of asthma has increased, although it is doubtful that any large changes have occurred. The hospitalization rates and fatality rates have increased, as have prescription medication prescriptions.

ANATOMY AND PHYSIOLOGY

The central function of the lungs is gas exchange with delivery into the blood stream of oxygen and removal of carbon dioxide. The lung is an immunologic organ and has endocrine and drug metabolizing properties too that affect respiration. The lung consists of an alveolar network with capillaries passing near and through alveolar walls and progressively larger intrapulmonary airways, including membranous bronchioles (1 mm or smaller noncartilaginous airways) and larger cartilaginous bronchi and upper airways. Inspired air must reach the gas exchange network of alveoli. The first 16 airway divisions of the lung are considered to be the conducting zone, whereas subsequent divisions from 17 to 23 are considered to be transitional and respiratory zones. The conducting zone consists of trachea, bronchi, bronchioles, and terminal bronchioles and produces what is measured as airways resistance. The terminal bronchioles as a rule have diameters as low as 0.5 mm. Respiratory bronchioles, alveolar ducts, and sacs comprise the transitional and respiratory zones[65] and are the sites of gas exchange.

The structure of bronchi and trachea is similar with cartilaginous rings surrounding the bronchi completely until the bronchi enter the lungs, at which time there are cartilage plates that surround the bronchi. When bronchioles are about 1 mm in diameter, the cartilage plates are not present. Smooth muscle surrounds bronchi and is present until the end of the respiratory bronchioles.

The lining mucous membrane of the trachea and bronchi is composed of pseudostratified ciliated columnar epithelium (Fig. 22-1). Goblet cells are mucin-secreting epithelial cells and are present in airways until their disappearance at the level of terminal bronchioles. In the ter-

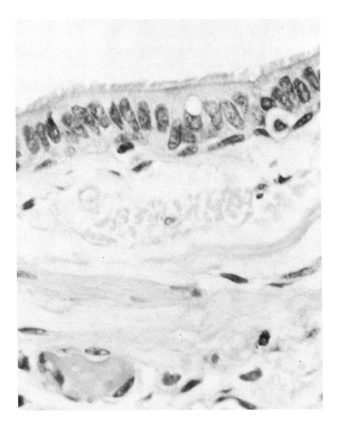

FIG. 22-1. Microphotograph of the wall of a normal bronchus. Notice the uniform ciliated epithelium and their bands of smooth muscle (Hematoxylin & eosin stain, ×250).

minal bronchioles, the epithelium becomes that of cuboidal cells with some cilia, clara (secretory) cells, and goblet cells until the level of respiratory bronchioles where the epithelium becomes alveolar in type. The cilia move in a watery lining layer proximally to help remove luminal material (debris, cells, mucus) by the ciliary "mucus escalator." Above the watery lining layer is a mucus layer. Other cells have been identified such as histamine-containing bronchial lumen cells,[66] alveolar macrophages, polymorphonuclear leukocytes, lymphocytes, eosinophils, and airway smooth muscle cells, which contribute to lung disease in different ways. The bronchial wall is characterized by mucosa, lamina propria, smooth muscle, submucosa, submucosal glands, and then cartilaginous plates. Submucosal glands produce either mucous or serous material, depending on their functional type. Mast cells can be identified in the bronchial lumen or between the basement membrane and epithelium. Mast cells have been recovered from bronchoalveolar lavage samples but their numbers are low in these samples.[67] Mast cell heterogeneity has been recognized based on contents and functional properties.[68] Briefly, mucosal mast cells are not recognized in a formalin-fixed specimen, but connective tissue mast cells are. Mucosal mast cells are present in the lung and contain tryptase, whereas connective tissue mast cells contain tryptase and chymotryptase.

Innervation

The nervous system and various muscle groups participate in respiration. Table 22-1 lists muscles, their innervation, and other respiratory responses such as by smooth muscle cells and bronchial glands and nonadrenergic, noncholinergic responses. Efferent parasympathetic

TABLE 22-1. *Innervation, muscles, and respiratory responses*

Efferents	Innervation
Muscles, cells or responses	
Sternocleidomastoid	C_2, C_3
Trapezius	C_3, C_4, spinal accessory nerve XI
Diaphragm	C_3–C_5
Scaleni	C_4–C_8
Intercostals	T_1–T_{11}
Smooth muscle cells	Vagus X
Bronchial glands	Vagus X, rare thoracic sympathetic
Epithelial sensory nerves (source of substance P, neurokinins, and vasoactive intestinal polypeptide)	Nonadrenergic, noncholinergic
Afferents	
Special function or site	
Irritant—cough (rapidly adapting) in trachea and main bronchi	Vagus X
Pulmonary stretch (slowly adapting) in trachea and main bronchi	Vagus X
C fibers in small airways or alveolar wall interstitium	Vagus X
Carotid body	Glossopharyngeal IX
CNS chemoreceptors	Medulla

(vagal) nerves innervate smooth muscle cells and bronchial glands. The vagus nerve also provides for afferent innervation of three types of sensory responses. The irritant (cough) reflex is rapidly adapting and originates in the trachea and main bronchi. Pulmonary stretch or slowly adapting afferents also are located in the trachea and main bronchi, whereas C fibers are located in small airways and alveolar walls. Afferent stimulation occurs through the carotid body (sensing oxygen tension) and nervous system chemoreceptors in the medulla (sensing hypercapnia).

Efferent respiratory responses include cervical and thoracic nervous system innervation of respiratory muscles such as listed in Table 22-1. Fortunately, not all respiratory muscles are essential for respiration should a spinal cord injury occur. In addition to efferent parasympathetic innervation of smooth muscle cells and bronchial glands, another source of efferent stimulation is through the nonadrenergic, noncholinergic epithelial sensory nerves. Stimulation of these nerves by epithelial cell destruction that occurs in asthma can trigger release of bronchospastic agonists such as substance P and neurokinins (A and B) through an antidromic axon reflex. The bronchodilating nonadrenergic noncholinergic neurotransmitter vasoactive intestinal polypeptide possibly opposes effects of other bronchospastic agonists such as substance P. An epithelial relaxing factor has been identified in preliminary studies that may not be present when bronchial epithelium has been shed.[69] The absence of vasoactive intestinal polypeptide or an epithelial relaxing factor could cause bronchoconstriction.

Smooth muscle cells participate in the Hering-Breuer inflation reflex in which inspiration leading to inflation of the lung causes bronchodilation. This reflex has been described in animals and humans. The clinical significance in human respiratory disease may be minimal. For example, often a patient with asthma who experiences some degree of bronchoconstriction when inhaling methacholine or histamine actually develops increased airways resistance during a deep inspiration. Patients without asthma and those with rhinitis demonstrate bronchodilation. During a bronchial challenge procedure in a patient with rhinitis, if the patient performs a forced vital capacity (FVC) maneuver by inhaling to TLC after inhaling the bronchospastic agonist in question, the resultant bronchodilation may mask any current airways obstruction. To obviate this possibility, the initial forced expiratory maneuver should be a partial flow volume effort, not a maximal one that requires maximal inspiration. Otherwise, the dose of agonist necessary to finally achieve a 20% decline in FEV_1, for example, will be higher than necessary.

PATHOPHYSIOLOGIC CHANGES IN ASTHMA

From a pathophysiologic perspective, the changes that occur in asthma are multiple, diverse, and complex. Further, some of the abnormalities such as bronchial hyperresponsiveness and mucus obstruction of bronchi can be present when patients are asymptomatic. The major physiologic abnormalities in asthma are (1) widespread smooth muscle contraction, (2) mucus hypersecretion, (3) mucosal and submucosal edema, (4) bronchial hyperresponsiveness, and (5) inflammation of airways. Obstruction to airflow during expiration and inspiration results with greater limitation during expiration. Hypertrophy and even hyperplasia of smooth muscle has been recognized in asthma. Smooth muscle contraction occurs in large or small bronchi. Challenge of patients with asthma by inhalation of histamine demonstrated two abnormal responses compared with patients without asthma.[70] First, the patients with asthma have increased sensitivity to histamine (or methacholine) since a smaller than normal dose of agonist usually is necessary to produce a 20% decline in FEV_1. Second, the maximal response to the agonist in asthma usually is increased over that which occurs in nonasthmatic nonrhinitis subjects. In fact, the maximal bronchospastic response (reduction of FEV_1) that occurs in the nonasthmatic nonrhinitis subject, if one occurs at all, reaches a plateau beyond which increases in agonist produce no further bronchoconstriction. In contrast, were it possible (and safe) to give a patient with asthma increasing amounts of an agonist such as histamine, increasing bronchoconstriction would occur. It is unclear why such different reactive responses occur in smooth muscle of patients with asthma.[71]

Hypersecretion of bronchial mucus may be limited or extensive in patients with asthma. Autopsy studies of patients who died from asthma after being symptomatic for days or weeks classically reveal extensive mucus plugging of airways. Large and small airways are filled with viscid mucus that is so thick, the plugs must be cut for examination.[72] Reid[72] has described this pattern as consistent with "endobronchial mucus suffocation." Other patients have mild amounts of mucus, suggesting that perhaps the fatal asthma episode occurred suddenly (over hours) and severe bronchial obstruction from smooth muscle contraction contributed to the patient's death. A virtual absence of mucus plugging, called "empty airways or sudden asphyxic asthma," has been reported.[72,73] Desquamation of bronchial epithelium can be identified on histologic examination[74] or when a patient coughs up clumps of desquamated epithelial cells (creola bodies). Bronchial mucus contains eosinophils that may be observed in expectorated spectrum. Charcot-Leyden crystals (lysophospholipase) are derived from eosinophils and appear as dipyramidal hexagons or needles in sputum. Viscid mucus plugs, when expectorated, can form a cast of the bronchi and are called Curschmann spirals.

Clinically, mucus hypersecretion is reduced or eliminated after treatment of acute asthma or inadequately controlled chronic asthma with systemic and then inhaled corticosteroids. Mucus from patients with asthma contains tightly bound glycoprotein and lipid as compared with mucus from patients with chronic bronchitis.[75] Macrophages have been shown to produce a mucus secretagogue as well as generate mediators and cytokines.[76]

The bronchial mucosa is edematous, as is the submucosa, and both are infiltrated with mast cells, activated eosinophils, and lymphocytes.[77] Venous dilation and plasma leakage occur along with the cellular infiltration. IgE has been identified in bronchial glands, epithelium, and basement membrane. Because plasma cell staining for IgE was not increased in number, it is thought that IgE is not produced locally, but since the lung is recognized as an immunologic organ, further work may show that IgE is produced in the lung.

The mechanism of bronchial hyperresponsiveness in asthma is unknown but is perhaps the central abnormality physiologically. Bronchial hyperresponsiveness occurs in patients with asthma to agonists such as histamine, methacholine, LTD_4, allergens, platelet-activating factor (PAF) and prostaglandin D_2 (short-lived response). Bronchial hyperresponsiveness is sensitive for asthma if a maximum dose of methacholine of 8 mg/mL is considered, which is necessary to cause a decline in FEV_1 of 20%. Patients with active symptomatic asthma often experience such a decline in FEV_1 when the dose of methacholine is 1 mg/mL or less. However, bronchial hyperresponsiveness is not specific for asthma since it occurs in other patients without asthma (Table 22-2).

Bronchial hyperresponsiveness is measured physiologically by reductions in expiratory flow rates (FEV_1) or decreases in specific conductance. Nevertheless, hyperresponsiveness consists of bronchoconstriction, hypersecretion, and hyperemia (mucosa edema). It has been easier to measure airway caliber by changes in FEV_1 than to measure changes in bronchial gland secretion, cellular infiltration, or blood vessels (dilation and increased permeability), which also contribute to hyperresponsiveness and cause airways obstruction. Indeed, there has yet to be an "inflammamometer" for asthma.

Often, on opening the thorax of a patient who has died from status asthmaticus, the lungs are hyperinflated and do not collapse (Fig. 22-2). Mucus plugging and obstruction of bronchi

TABLE 22-2. *Conditions of patients that may demonstrate bronchial hyperresponsiveness*

After a viral upper respiratory infection for 6 wk in nonasthma patients
In absence of changes in FEV$_1$ in patients with asthma
Chronic bronchitis
Left ventricular failure
Allergic rhinitis in absence of asthma
Apparently normal patients
Exposure to irritants
Smoking
In some normal infants
First-degree relatives of asthma patients
Sarcoidosis

FEV$_1$, forced expiratory volume in 1 second.

and bronchioles are present. In some cases, complicating factors such as atelectasis or acute pneumonia are identified. On histologic examination, there is a patchy loss of bronchial epithelium with desquamation and denudation of mucosal epithelium. Eosinophils are present in areas of absent epithelium, and immunologic staining has revealed evidence for eosinophil major basic protein at sites of bronchial epithelium desquamation. Activated (EG2 positive) eosinophils are present in the mucosa, submucosa, and connective tissue. Other histologic findings include hyperplasia of bronchial mucus glands, bronchial mucosal edema, smooth muscle hypertrophy, and basement membrane thickening (Fig. 22-3). The latter occurs from collagen deposition (types I, III, and V) and immunoglobulins as evidence of inflammation. The mucus plugs may contain eosinophils. Occasionally, bronchial epithelium is denuded, but histologic studies do not identify eosinophils. In some cases, neutrophils were present.[74] Other mechanisms of lung damage are present but not understood completely. Similarly, whereas many autopsy examinations reveal the classic pattern of mucus plugging (Fig. 22-4) of large and smaller bronchi and bronchioles leading to mucus suffocation or asphyxia as the terminal asthmatic event, some autopsies reveal empty bronchi.[72,73] Eosinophils have been identified in such cases in airways or in basement membranes but a gross mechanical explanation, analogous to mucus suffocation, is not present. A third morphologic pattern of patients dying from asthma is that of mild to moderate mucus plugging.[72]

Some patients dying from asthma have evidence for myocardial contraction band necrosis, which is different from myocardial necrosis associated with infarction. Contraction bands are present in necrotic myocardial smooth muscle cell bands in asthma, and, curiously, the cells are thought to die in tetanic contraction, whereas in cases of fatal myocardial infarction cells die in relaxation.

CONTROL OF AIRWAY TONE

The patency of bronchi and bronchioles is a function of many factors not fully understood.[78] Bronchomotor patency is affected by mediators secreted by mast cells, the autonomic nervous system, the nonadrenergic noncholinergic nervous system, circulating humoral substances, the respiratory epithelium, smooth muscle cells, and effects of cellular infiltration and glan-

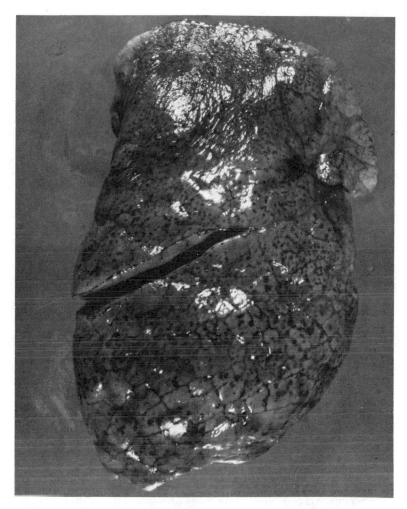

FIG. 22-2. Distended lung of patient who died in status asthmaticus.

dular secretions (Table 22-3). Even this list is oversimplified since asthma must be considered a complex condition in terms of pathophysiologic mechanisms.

Mediator release caused by mast cell activation results in acute and late bronchial smooth muscle contraction, cellular infiltration, and mucus production. Autonomic nervous stimulation contributes through vagal stimulation. The neurotransmitter for postganglionic parasympathetic nerves is acetylcholine, which causes smooth muscle contraction. Norepinephrine is the neurotransmitter for postganglionic sympathetic nerves. However, there appears to be little if any significant smooth muscle relaxation through stimulation of postganglionic sympathetic nerves. Exogenously administered epinephrine can produce smooth muscle relaxation. Circulating endogenous epinephrine apparently does not produce relaxation of smooth muscles. Sensory nerves in the respiratory epithelium are stimulated and lead to release of a host of neuropeptides that may be potent bronchoconstrictors or bronchodilators. Respiratory epithelium itself may contain bronchial relaxing factors that may become unavailable when epithelium is denuded. Tables 22-3 and 22-4 list some chemical mediators derived from mast cells and neuropeptides that may contribute to pathogenesis of asthma.

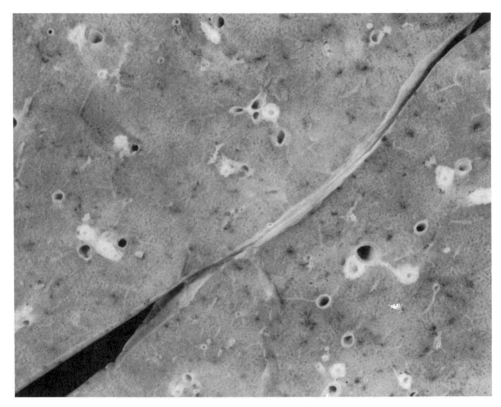

FIG. 22-3. Close-up of pulmonary parenchyma in a case of status asthmaticus. Bronchi are dilated and thickened.

Although much attention has been directed at understanding the contribution of IgE–mast cell activation in asthma, triggering or actual regulation of some of the inflammation of asthma may occur because of other cells in lungs of patients. Low-affinity IgE receptors are known to exist on macrophages, eosinophils, monocytes, lymphocytes, and platelets. These cells as well as mast cells in the bronchial mucosa or lumen can be activated in the absence of classic IgE-mediated asthma.

Bronchial biopsy specimens from patients with asthma demonstrate mucosal mast cells in various stages of activation in symptomatic and asymptomatic patients.[79,80] Mast cell hyperreleasibility may occur in asthma in that bronchoalveolar mast cells recovered during lavage contain and release greater quantities of histamine when stimulated by allergen or anti-IgE in vitro.[81,82]

Eosinophils are thought to contribute to proinflammatory effects by secretion of damaging cell products such as major basic protein, which can result in bronchial epithelial denudation, exposing sensory nerves, which leads to smooth muscle contraction. Eosinophils produce PAF, which is a potential bronchospastic agonist.[83] The PAF is proinflammatory in that it causes eosinophil and neutrophil chemotaxis, which produces positive feedback in terms of PAF production from attracted and newly activated eosinophils.[84] The latter can be demonstrated by their reduced density on centrifugation that occurs during acute episodes of asthma.

Increasing experimental data suggest a possible role of histamine releasing factors (HRFs) in asthma.[85–87] HRFs have been generated from mononuclear cells, neutrophils, pulmonary macrophages, and platelets. In vitro, for example, peripheral blood mononuclear cells from patients with asthma are stimulated with allergen and the supernatant is obtained. Subsequent

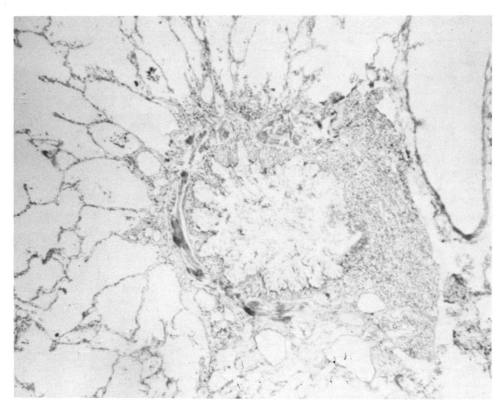

FIG. 22-4. Microphotograph of a dilated bronchus filled with a mucous plug. There is hypertrophy of the muscle layer, and the alveolar spaces are dilated.

incubation of supernatant with basophils results in histamine release. If basophils are representative of bronchial mast cells, then HRFs may affect airway tone by facilitating mast cell mediator release. On a cellular level, the control of airway tone is influenced by even more fundamental factors, including interleukin (IL)-1, IL-2, IL-3, IL-4, and interferon gamma, among others that influence lymphocyte development and proliferation as it relates to IgE production, for example, and IL-1, IL-3, and IL-5 as they relate to eosinophil development. IL-8, detected in bronchial epithelium, binds to secretory IgA and chemoattracts eosinophils, which generate PAF and leukotriene C_4 (LTC_4).

During an acute attack of asthma, there is an increase in inspiratory efforts, which applies greater radial traction to airways. Patients with asthma have great ability to generate increases in inspiratory pressures. Unfortunately, patients who have experienced nearly fatal attacks of asthma have blunted perception of dyspnea and impaired ventilatory responses to hypoxia.[88]

CLINICAL OVERVIEW

Clinical Manifestations

Asthma results in coughing, wheezing, dyspnea, sputum production, and shortness of breath. Symptoms vary from patient to patient and in the individual patient, depending on the activ-

TABLE 22-3. *Selected mast cell mediators and their proposed actions in asthma*

Mediator	Preformed	Newly synthesized	Actions
Histamine	+		Smooth muscle contraction (H_1 and via vagus); increased vascular permeability; vasodilator; mucus production (H_2)
Tryptase	+		Degrades vasoactive intestinal polypeptide; cleaves kininogen to form bradykinin, cleaves C_3
Eosinophil chemotactic factor	+		Eosinophil chemoattractant
Neutrophil chemotactic factor	+		Neutrophil chemoattractant
Peroxidase	+		Inactivates leukotrienes
Bradykinin		+	Smooth muscle contraction
Leukotriene D_4 (generated from leukotriene C_4)		+	Smooth muscle contraction; increases vascular permeability, mucus secretion
Prostaglandin D_2, $F_{2\alpha}$		+	Smooth muscle contraction; increases vascular permeability, mucus secretion
Platelet-activating factor		+	Smooth muscle contraction; increases vascular permeability, neutrophil and eosinophil chemoattractant; aggregates platelets; sensitizes airways to the agonists
Leukotriene B_4		+	Neutrophil and eosinophil chemoattractant

ity of asthma. Some patients experience mild nonproductive coughing after exercising or exposure to cold air as examples of transient mild bronchospasm. The combination of coughing and wheezing with dyspnea is a common finding in patients who have a sudden moderate to severe episode (such as might occur after aspirin ingestion in an aspirin-intolerant patient). Symptoms of asthma may be sporadic and often are present on a nocturnal basis. Some patients with asthma present with a persistent nonproductive cough as a main symptom of asthma. Typically, the cough has occurred on a daily basis and may awaken the patient at night. Repetitive spasms of cough are refractory to treatment with expectorants, antibiotics, and antitussives. The patient is likely to respond to antiasthma therapy such as inhaled β-adrenergic agonists or, if that is unsuccessful, inhaled corticosteroids. At times oral corticosteroids are necessary to stop the coughing and are useful as a diagnostic therapeutic trial. Pulmonary physiologic studies usually reveal large airway obstruction, as illustrated by reductions in FEV_1 with preservation of $FEF_{25\%-75\%}$ or small airways function.[89] The latter may be reduced in patients with this variant form of asthma. Conversely, some patients present with isolated dyspnea as a manifestation of asthma. Such patients have small airways obstruction with preservation of function of larger airways. The recognition of variant forms of asthma emphasizes that not all patients with asthma have detectable wheezing on auscultation. The medical history is invaluable, as is a diagnostic–therapeutic trial with antiasthma medications. Pulmonary physiologic abnormalities, such as reduced FEV_1, which responds to therapy, or bronchial hyperresponsiveness to methacholine can provide additional supportive data.

TABLE 22-4. *Selected neuropeptides and their proposed actions in asthma*

Neuropeptide	Actions
Vasoactive intestinal polypeptide	Smooth muscle relaxation Pulmonary vasodilator Stimulates adenylate cyclase Suppresses mucus secretion May be deficient in asthma
Substance P	Smooth muscle contraction Vasodilator Mucus secretion Increases capillary permeability
Neurokinin A	Smooth muscle contraction
Peptide histidine methionine	Inhibits vagal-induced bronchoconstriction Stimulates adenylate cyclase
Calcitonin gene-related peptide	Smooth muscle contraction

During an acute moderately severe episode of asthma or in longer term ineffectively controlled asthma, patients are likely to produce clear, yellow, or green sputum that can be viscid. The sputum contains eosinophils, which supports the diagnosis of asthma. In that either polymorphonuclear leukocytes or eosinophils can cause the sputum to be discolored, it is inappropriate to consider such sputum as evidence of a secondary bacterial infection. Patients with nonallergic asthma also produce eosinophil-laden sputum.

An occasional patient with asthma presents with cough syncope, a respiratory arrest that is perceived as anaphylaxis, chest pain, or pneumomediastinum or pneumothorax, or with symptoms of chronic bronchitis or bronchiectasis.

The physical examination may consist of no coughing or wheezing if the patient has stable chronic asthma or if there has not been a recent episode of sporadic asthma. Certainly, patients with variant asthma may not have wheezing or other supportive evidence for asthma. Usually, wheezing is present in other patients, which can be associated with reduced expiratory flow rates. Few patients always have wheezing on even tidal breathing, not just with a forced expiratory maneuver. Such patients may be asymptomatic and may have expiratory airflow obstruction when FVC or FEV_1 are measured. The physical examination must be interpreted in view of the patients' clinical symptoms and supplemental aids such as the chest roentgenogram or pulmonary function tests. There may be a surprising lack of correlation in some ambulatory patients between symptoms and objective evidence of asthma (physical findings and spirometric values).

An additional physical finding in patients with asthma is repetitive coughing on inspiration. Although not specific for asthma, it is frequently present in unstable patients. In normal patients, maximal inspiration to TLC results in reduced airways resistance whereas in patients with asthma, increased resistance occurs with a maximal inspiration. Coughing spasms can be precipitated in patients who otherwise may not be heard to wheeze. This finding is transient and, after effective therapy, does not occur. The patient with a severe episode of asthma may be found to have pulsus paradoxus and use of accessory muscles of respiration. Such findings correlate with an FEV_1 less than 1.0 L and air trapping, as manifested by hyperinflation of the FRC and residual volume.[90] The most critically ill patients have markedly reduced tidal volumes, and their maximal ventilatory efforts are no higher than their efforts during the acute event. The silent chest with absence or greatly reduced breath sounds indicates likely alveolar hypoventilation (normal or elevated arterial PCO_2) and hypoxemia. Such patients may require intubation or, in most cases, an admission to the intensive care unit. Great difficulty in speaking more than a half sentence before needing another inspiration is likely to be present in such patients.

Radiographic and Laboratory Studies

In about 90% of patients, the presentation chest roentgenogram is considered within normal limits.[91–93] The most frequently found abnormality is hyperinflation. The diaphragm is flattened, and there may be an increase in the anteroposterior diameter and retrosternal air space. The chest roentgenogram is indicated because it is necessary to exclude other conditions that mimic asthma or search for complications of asthma. Other conditions, including congestive heart failure, COPD, pneumonia, and neoplasms, are just some of the other common explanations for acute wheezing dyspnea that may mimic or coexist with asthma. Asthma complications include atelectasis as a result of mucus obstruction of bronchi, mucoid impaction of bronchi (often indicative of allergic bronchopulmonary aspergillosis), or pneumomediastinum or pneumothorax. Atelectasis often involves the middle lobe, which may collapse. The presence of pneumomediastinum or pneumothorax may have associated subcutaneous emphysema with crepitus on palpation of the neck, supraclavicular areas, or face (Figs. 22-5 and 22-6). Sharp pain in the neck or shoulders should be a clue to presence of a pneumomediastinum in status asthmaticus.

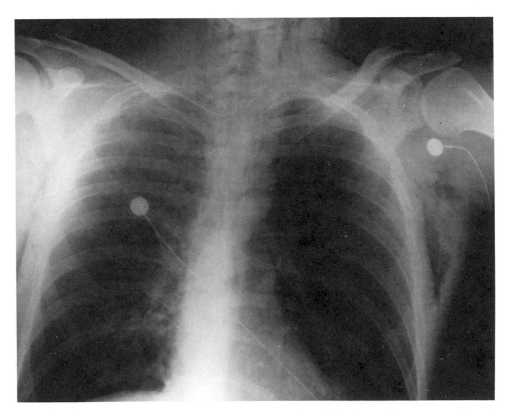

FIG. 22-5. Anteroposterior view of the chest of a 41-year-old woman demonstrates hyperinflation of both lungs, with pneumomediastinum and subcutaneous emphysema.

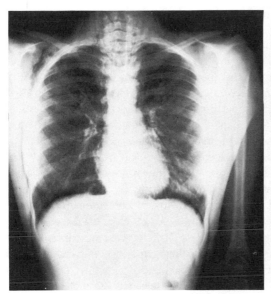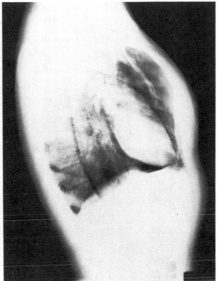

FIG. 22-6. (**A**) Posteroanterior and (**B**) lateral chest films of this 13-year-old asthmatic patient demonstrate hyperinflated lungs with bilateral perihilar infiltrates, pneumomediastinum, and subcutaneous emphysema in soft tissue of the chest and neck.

Depending on the patients examined, abnormal findings on sinus films may be frequent.[94] Taking such films is not indicated routinely but may identify unrecognized findings such as air–fluid levels, which may indicate infection or mucus membrane thickening (at least 4 mm, which is consistent with current or previous infection), and opacification of a sinus, or polyps. A computed tomography sinus examination may provide valuable additional information as to sinus disease, which is not appreciated fully by conventional sinus films.

Clinical research studies of acutely ill patients with asthma have been carried out with ventilation-perfusion (V/Q) scans. These procedures are not indicated in most cases, and in the markedly hypoxemic patient may be harmful since the technetium-labeled albumin macrospheres injected for the perfusion scan can lower arterial PO_2. Ventilation is extremely uneven.[95] Perfusion scans reveal abnormalities such that there may be matched V/Q inequalities. In some patients, the V/Q ratios in the superior portions of the lungs have declined from their relatively high values.[95] The explanation for such a finding is increased perfusion of upper lobes, presumably from reduced relative resistance relative to lower lobes that receive most of the pulmonary blood flow. Little evidence for shunting exists.[95] When a pulmonary embolus is suspected, the V/Q scan may be nondiagnostic in the patient with an exacerbation of asthma. In some patients with asthma and pulmonary embolus, areas of ventilation but not perfusion are identified so that the diagnosis may be made.

In the emergency room assessment of the patient with acute severe wheezing dyspnea, measuring arterial PO_2, PCO_2, and pH is invaluable. Whereas hypoxemia is a frequent and expected finding, the PCO_2 provides information as to the effectiveness of alveolar ventilation. This latter status is not assessed if just oxygen saturation is determined. The PCO_2 should be decreased initially during the hyperventilation stage of acute asthma. A normal or elevated PCO_2 is evidence of alveolar hypoventilation and may be associated with subsequent need for intubation to try to prevent a fatal outcome.

Pulmonary function measurements can be of assistance in helping to establish patient status. However, such measurements must be correlated with the physical examination. In the emergency room or ambulatory setting, many physicians determine spirometric values for expiratory flow rates with either peak expiratory flow rates (PEFRs) or FEV_1. These tests are effort-dependent, and acutely symptomatic patients may be unable to perform the maneuver satisfactorily. This could be from severe obstruction or patient inability or unwillingness to perform the maneuver appropriately. When properly performed, spirometric measurements can be of significant clinical use in assessing patient status. For example, patients presenting with spirometric determinations of 20% to 25% of predicted should receive immediate and intensive therapy and usually should be hospitalized. Frequent measurements of PEFR or FEV_1 in the ambulatory patient can establish a range of baseline values for day and night. Declines of over 20% from usual low recordings alert the patient to the need for more intensive pharmacologic therapy. Nevertheless, such measurements can be insensitive in some patients. Pulmonary physiologic values such as PEFR and FEV_1 have demonstrated value in clinical research studies, such as in documenting a 12% to 20% increase in expiratory flow rates after bronchodilator. Similarly, in testing for bronchial hyperresponsiveness, a 20% decline of FEV_1 is a goal during gradual administration of methacholine or histamine. Unfortunately, some patients are able to manipulate spirometric measurements to make a convincing case for occupational asthma. Thus, the physician must correlate pulmonary physiologic values with the clinical assessment. A complete set of pulmonary function tests should be obtained in other situations such as in assessing the degree of reversible versus nonreversible obstruction in patients with heavy smoking histories. The diffusing capacity for carbon monoxide is reduced in the COPD patient but is normal or elevated in the patient with asthma. Such tests should be obtained after 2 to 4 weeks of intensive therapy to determine what degree of reversibility exists. In the acutely ill patient with asthma, the diffusing capacity for carbon monoxide may be reduced. Thus, its usefulness in differentiating COPD from asthma is obscured if the wrong time to obtain this test is chosen.

The complete blood count should be obtained in the emergency setting. First, the hemoglobin and hematocrit provides status regarding anemia, which, if associated with hypoxemia, can compromise oxygen delivery to tissues. Conversely, an elevated hematocrit is consistent with hemoconcentration, such as occurs from dehydration or polycythemia. The latter does not occur in asthma in the absence of other conditions. The white blood cell count may be elevated from epinephrine (white blood cell demargination from vessel walls), systemic corticosteroids (demargination and release from bone marrow), or infection. In the absence of prior systemic corticosteroids, the acutely ill patient often has peripheral blood eosinophilia. For best accuracy, an absolute eosinophil count is required. However, in managing most patients with asthma—acutely symptomatic or long-term sufferers—eosinophil counts are not of value. The presence of eosinophilia in patients receiving long-term systemic corticosteroids suggests noncompliance or possibly rare conditions such as Churg-Strauss vasculitis, allergic bronchopulmonary aspergillosis, or eosinophilic pneumonia.[96] The percentage of eosinophilia usually does not exceed 10% to 20% of the differential. Higher values suggest an alternative diagnosis.

Sputum examination reveals eosinophils, eosinophils plus polymorphonuclear leukocytes (asthma and purulent bronchitis or bacterial pneumonia), or absence of eosinophils. In mild asthma, no sputum is produced. In the severely ill patient with asthma, sputum is thick, tenacious, and yellow or green. Major basic protein from eosinophils has been identified in such sputum.[37] Dipyramidal hexagons from eosinophil cytoplasm may be identified and are called Charcot-Leyden crystals. These crystals contain lysophospholipase. Curschmann spirals are expectorated yellow or clear mucus threads that are remnants or casts of small bronchi. Expectorated ciliated and nonciliated bronchial epithelial cells can also be identified, which emphasize the patchy loss of bronchial epithelium in asthma. On a related basis, high molecular weight neutrophil chemotactic activity has been identified in sera from patients with status asthmaticus.[97] This activity declined with effective therapy.

Serum electrolyte abnormalities may be present and should be anticipated in the patient presenting to the emergency department. Recent use of oral corticosteroids can lower the potassium concentration (as can β_2-adrenergic agonists) and cause a metabolic alkalosis. Oral corticosteroids may raise the blood glucose in some patients, as can systemic administration of β-adrenergic agonists. Elevations of atrial natriuretic peptide (antidiuretic hormone) can occur in acute asthma or COPD.[98,99] Clinically, few patients have large declines of serum sodium. Because intravenous fluids are administered, it is necessary to determine the current status of electrolytes and serum chemistry values. After prolonged high-dose corticosteroids, hypomagnesemia or hypophosphatemia may occur.

Rarely, a patient younger than 30 years may be thought to have asthma when the underlying condition is α_1-antitrypsin deficiency. More commonly, patients with wheezing dyspnea may have asthma and cystic fibrosis. The sweat chloride should be elevated markedly in such patients. A properly performed sweat chloride test is essential, as in the performance of other laboratory tests.

In the outpatient management of asthma, determining the presence or absence of antiallergen IgE is of value. For decades, skin testing for immediate cutaneous reactivity has been the most sensitive and specific method. Some physicians prefer in vitro tests instead. High-quality control for both skin testing and in vitro testing is essential. Both tests are subject to misinterpretation. Either method of demonstrating antiallergen IgE should be used as an adjunct to the narrative history of asthma, not as a substitution. More patients have immediate cutaneous reactivity or detectable in vitro IgE than have asthma that correlates with exposure to the specific allergen.

Complications of Asthma

Complications from asthma include death, adverse effects of hypoxemia or respiratory failure on other organ systems, growth retardation in children, pneumothorax or pneumomediastinum, rib fractures from severe coughing, cough syncope, and adverse effects of medications or therapeutic modalities used to treat asthma. Some patients develop psychological abnormalities because of the burden of a chronic illness such as asthma. Ineffectively treated asthma in children can result in chest wall abnormalities such as "pigeon chest" because of sustained hyperinflation of the chest in childhood.

In general, long-term asthma does not result in irreversible obstructive lung disease. However, an occasional patient with long-term asthma develops apparently irreversible disease in the absence of cigarette smoking or another obvious cause. Usually, such patients have asthma that has been oral corticosteroid dependent. Intensive therapy with oral corticosteroids does not result in expiratory flow rates of 80% of predicted. Patients do not become "respiratory cripples," as might occur from COPD, but pulmonary physiologic studies do not reveal return of parameters to the expected normal ranges. More studies are required. Such patients are not deficient in antiproteases that can be measured, and they do not have bullous abnormalities on chest roentgenogram. Computed tomography may demonstrate air trapping on expiration, however.

Pneumomediastinum or pneumothorax can occur in the patient presenting in status asthmaticus. Neck, shoulder, or chest pain is common, and crepitations can be detected in the neck or supraclavicular fossae. Rupture of distal alveoli results in dissection of air proximally by bronchovascular bundles. Then the air can travel superiorly in the mediastinum to the supraclavicular or cervical areas. At times, the air dissects to the face or into the subcutaneous areas over the thorax. Treating the patient's asthma with systemic corticosteroids is indicated to reduce the likelihood of hyperinflation and continued air leak. Unless the pneumothorax is large, conservative treatment is effective. Otherwise, thoracostomy with tube placement is necessary.

Fatalities from asthma are unnecessary since asthma is not an inexorably fatal disease. Fatalities do occur, and many factors have been suggested as explanations.[47,33,62,100–108] A few deaths from asthma unfortunately are unavoidable, despite appropriate medical care. A high percentage of deaths from asthma should be considered preventable. Survivors of major asthma events such as respiratory failure or arrest, pneumomediastinum or pneumothorax on two occasions, and repeated status asthmaticus despite oral corticosteroid treatment have potentially fatal asthma and are at higher risk of fatality compared with other patients with asthma.[44,106]

Uncontrolled asthma can lead to mucus plugging of airways and frank collapse of a lobe or whole lung segment. The middle lobe can collapse, especially in children. Repeated mucoid impactions should raise the possibility of allergic bronchopulmonary aspergillosis or cystic fibrosis.

Cough syncope or cough-associated cyanosis occurs in patients whose respiratory status has deteriorated and in whom status asthmaticus or need for emergency therapy has occurred. During severe airways obstruction from asthma during inspiration, intrathoracic pressure is negative since the patient must generate high negative pressures to apply radial traction on bronchi to maintain their patency. During expiration, the patient must overcome severe airways resistance and premature airways collapse. Increases in intrathoracic pressure during expiration with severe coughing as compared with intraabdominal pressure causes a decline in venous return to the right atrium. There also may be increased blood flow to the lung during a short inspiration, but that is accompanied by pooling in the pulmonary vasculature from the markedly elevated negative inspiratory pressure. There must be reduced blood flow to the left ventricle with temporary decreases in cardiac output and cerebral blood flow.

Pulsus paradoxus is present when there is a greater than 10 mm Hg decline in systolic blood pressure during inspiration. It is associated with severe airway obstruction and hyperinflation.[109] Electrocardiographic findings of acute asthma include sinus tachycardia as the most frequent finding, followed by right axis deviation, clockwise rotation, prominent R wave in lead V_1 and S wave in lead V_5, and tall peaked P waves consistent with cor pulmonale.[109]

Linear growth retardation can occur from ineffectively controlled asthma. Administration of oral corticosteroids is indicated to prevent repeated hospitalizations and frequent episodes of wheezing dyspnea. The child often responds with a growth spurt. Alternate-day prednisone does not result in growth retardation, especially when the dose is 30 mg or less on alternate days. Even high alternate-day doses in children can be tolerated reasonably well as long as status asthmaticus is prevented. Similarly, depot corticosteroids given every 2 to 3 weeks in high doses may result in growth retardation. Despite efficacy in asthma, such corticosteroid administration causes hypothalamic pituitary-adrenal suppression.[110] Their use should be considered only in the most recalcitrant children in terms of asthma management. Ineffective parental functioning or poor compliance usually accompanies such cases where reliable administration of prednisone and inhaled corticosteroids is impossible. The term *malignant potentially fatal asthma* has been suggested for such patients.[111]

Psychological Factors in Asthma

Asthma has evolved from a disorder considered to be psychological to one recognized as extremely complex and of unknown etiology. Psychological stress can cause modest reductions in expiratory flow rates such as occur when watching a terrifying movie.[112] Laughing and crying or frank emotional upheaval, such as an argument with a family member, can result in wheezing. Some patients require additional medication. Usually, if the patient has stable baseline respiratory status, severe asthma requiring emergency hospital care does not result. Nevertheless, some fatal episodes of asthma have been reported as associated with a high level of emotional stress. In an absence of how to quantitate stress and determine if there is a dose–response effect in asthma, such information must be considered as speculative. Specific personality patterns have not been identified in patients with asthma.

The patient with asthma may develop strategies to function with the burden of asthma as a chronic, disruptive, and potentially fatal disease. A variety of behavior patterns have been recognized such as the following: (1) disease denial with complacency, or outright denial of symptoms or of alerting the managing physician of a major change in respiratory symptoms or personally increasing mediations; (2) using asthma for obvious secondary gain, such as to avoid attending school or work, or to gain compensation; (3) developing compulsive or manipulative patterns of behavior that restrict the lifestyle of the patient and family members excessively; and (4) resorting to quackery. Some patients display hateful behavior toward physicians and their office staff personnel.[113,114] Psychiatric care can be of value in some cases, but often patients refuse appropriate psychiatric referrals. The use of peak expiratory flow monitoring devices can be misleading since patients can generate expected but truly inaccurate measurements. In contrast to theories implying that wheezing dyspnea in patients with asthma was primarily psychological, now the physician must decide how much of a patient's symptoms and signs are from asthma and how much might be psychological as a result of asthma. Indeed, a psychologist, psychiatrist, or social worker may help to identify what the patient might lose should asthma symptoms be suppressed to a greater degree than is present.

Major management problems occur when asthma patients also have schizophrenia, delusional behavior, neurosis, depression, or manic-depressive disorders.[115] Suicidal attempts are recognized from theophylline overdosing and unjustified cessation of prednisone. Repeated episodes of life-threatening status asthmaticus are difficult to avoid in the setting of untreated major psychiatric conditions.

The presence of factitious asthma indicates a significant psychiatric disturbance.[116] Initially, there must be trust established between the patient and physician. Abrupt referral of the patient to a psychiatrist can result in an unanticipated suicidal gesture or attempt. Psychiatric care can be valuable if the patient is willing to participate in therapy.

CLASSIFICATION OF ASTHMA

The following is a list of some types of asthma:

- Allergic asthma
- Nonallergic asthma
- Mixed asthma
- Potentially fatal asthma
  - Malignant potentially fatal asthma
- Aspirin-intolerant asthma
- Occupational asthma
- Exercise-induced asthma
- Variant asthma

• Factitious asthma
• Coexistent asthma and COPD.

It is helpful to categorize the type of asthma since treatment programs vary, depending on the type of asthma present. Some patients have more than one type of asthma.

Allergic Asthma

Allergic asthma refers to asthma caused by inhalation of allergen that interacts with IgE present in high-affinity receptors on bronchial mucosal mast cells. Allergic asthma often occurs from ages 4 to 40 years but has been recognized in the geriatric population[117] and in adult patients attending a pulmonary clinic for care.[118] Some physicians believe that many patients with asthma must have some type of allergic asthma because of elevated total serum IgE concentrations, antiallergen IgE,[119] and the frequent finding of peripheral blood or sputum eosinophilia. The use of the term allergic asthma implies that a temporal relation exists between respiratory symptoms and allergen exposure, and that the presence of antiallergen IgE antibodies can be demonstrated or suspected.

Respiratory symptoms may develop within minutes or in an hour after allergen exposure, or may not be obviously apparent when uninterrupted allergen exposure occurs. Common allergens associated with IgE-mediated asthma include pollens such as from trees, grasses, and weeds; fungal spores; dust mites; animal dander; and, in some settings, animal urine or cockroaches. IgE-mediated occupational asthma is considered under the category of occupational asthma. Allergen particle size must be less than 10 µm to penetrate into deeper parts of the lung because larger particles such as ragweed pollen (19 µm) impact in the oropharynx. Submicronic ragweed particles have been described that could reach smaller airways.[120] Particles smaller than 1 µm, however, may not be retained in the airways. Fungal spores such as *Aspergillus* species measure 2 to 3 µm, and the major cat allergen (*Fel* d I) has allergenic activity from 0.4 to 10 µm.[121] Another study demonstrated that 75% of *Fel* d I was present in particles of at least 5 µm, and 25% of *Fel* d I was present in particles less than 2.5 µm.[122]

The potential severity of allergic asthma should not be minimized since, experimentally, after an antigen-induced early bronchial response, bronchial hyperresponsiveness to an agonist such as methacholine or histamine can be demonstrated. This hyperresponsiveness precedes a late (3- to 11-hour) response.[123] In addition, fungal (mold)-related asthma may result in a need for intensive antiasthma pharmacotherapy, including inhaled corticosteroids and even alternate-day prednisone in some patients. Exposure to Alternaria alternata, a major fungal aeroallergen, was considered an important risk factor for respiratory arrests in 11 patients with asthma.[124] In children being evaluated long term for development of atopic conditions and having one parent with asthma or allergic rhinitis, asthma by 11 years of age was associated with exposure to high concentrations of *Dermatophagoides pteronyssinus*, a major mite allergen.[125] Similar results seem likely when children of atopic parents are exposed to animals in the house.

The diagnosis of allergic asthma should be suspected when symptoms and signs of asthma correlate closely with local patterns of pollenosis and fungal spore recoveries. For example, in the upper midwestern United States after a hard freeze in late November, which reduces (but does not eliminate entirely) fungal spore recoveries from outdoor air, patients who have "mold" asthma notice a reduction in symptoms and medication requirements. When perennial symptoms of asthma are present, potential causes of asthma include animal dander, dust mites, and, depending on the local conditions, fungal spores and pollens. Cockroach allergen (*Bla* g I) has been identified in numerous buildings and may be another cause of asthma. High indoor concentrations of mouse urine protein (*Mus* d I) have been identified with volumetric sampling, and monoclonal antibodies directed at specific proteins suggested additional indoor allergens. The physician should correlate symptoms with aeroallergen exposures, support the diagnosis by demonstration of antiallergen IgE antibodies, and institute measures where applicable to decrease allergen exposure. Some recommendations for environmental control have been made,[126] but may not be practical to implement for many patients and their families. Detection of cat allergen (*Fel* d I) in homes never known to have cat exposure is consistent with transport of *Fel* d I into such premises and the sensitivity of immunoassays for cat allergen. Nevertheless, recognizing that using sensitive immunoassays of airborne particulate matter reveals low concentrations of dust mites or cat dander, removing an animal from a home or covering a mattress and pillow properly is known to decrease the concentration of allergen to a level below which many patients have clinical asthma symptoms.

Although food ingestion can result in anaphylaxis, chronic asthma is not explained by food ingestion with IgE-mediated reactions. Food product inhalation such as occurs in bakers, egg handlers, flavoring producers, and in workers exposed to vegetable gums is known to produce occupational asthma mediated by IgE antibodies.

Nonallergic Asthma

Nonallergic asthma refers to many cases of asthma where IgE mediated airway reactions to common allergens are not present. Nonallergic asthma occurs at any age range as does allergic asthma, but as a generalization is more likely to occur in patients with asthma younger than 4 years of age and older than 40 years of age. Episodes of nonallergic asthma are triggered by upper respiratory tract infections or purulent rhinitis or sinusitis. In some cases, no infectious process can be identified. There is an absence of IgE-mediated asthma. Most patients have no evidence for IgE antibodies to common allergens. Occasionally, skin test reactions are positive, but despite presence of IgE antibodies, there is no temporal relation between exposure and symptoms. Often, but not exclusively, the onset of asthma occurs in the setting of a viral upper respiratory tract infection. Virus infections have been associated with mediator release and bronchial epithelial shedding, which could lead to ongoing inflammation and asthma symptoms.[127] Commonly recovered viruses that cause asthma are rhinoviruses, respiratory syncytial virus, parainfluenza viruses, influenza viruses, and adenovirus. Chronic sinusitis can be identified in some patients with asthma, as can nasal polyps with or without aspirin sensitivity.

Some experimental data exist linking the presence of antiviral IgE antibodies to asthma.[128] While the knowledge of mast cell activation grows, it may be recognized that antiviral IgE antibodies or other viral interactions with the lung and immune system trigger asthma that is considered to be nonallergic.

Allergen immunotherapy is not indicated and is not beneficial in patients with nonallergic asthma, despite the presence of antiallergen IgE.

Mixed Asthma

The term *mixed asthma* characterizes combined allergic and nonallergic triggers of asthma. Such patients experience both classic IgE-mediated asthma and chronic asthma that may not be explained by recent viral upper respiratory tract infections or episodes of purulent rhinitis or sinusitis. An example is a patient with grass- and ragweed-induced asthma, which, in the particular geographic area, is a recognized cause of asthma for 5 months of the year, whereas the patient has symptoms at other times for no obvious explanation.

Potentially Fatal Asthma

Potentially fatal asthma refers to the patient who is at high risk of an asthma fatality.[44,106] Patients have to fulfill one criterion from (1) respiratory acidosis or failure from asthma, (2) endotracheal intubation from asthma, (3) two or more episodes of status asthmaticus despite use of oral corticosteroids and other antiasthma medications, or (4) two or more episodes of pneumomediastinum or pneumothorax from asthma. Other factors have been associated with a potentially fatal outcome from asthma, and these criteria may not identify all high-risk patients. The physician managing the high-risk patient should anticipate a potential fatality in certain patients and try to prevent this outcome.[129] Asthma in the patient who is impossible to manage (because of noncompliance) is labeled malignant potentially fatal asthma.

Aspirin-Induced Asthma

Selected patients with asthma, often nonallergic, have unusual bronchial responses to aspirin and or NSAIDs.[130,131] The onset of acute bronchospastic symptoms after ingesting such agents can be within minutes (such as after chewing Aspergum) to within 3 hours. Some physicians accept a respiratory response that occurs within 8 to 12 hours after aspirin or NSAID ingestion; however, a shorter time interval seems more appropriate, such as up to 4 hours. In chronic asthma, variations in expiratory flow rates occur frequently so that confirming that aspirin produces a reaction at 8 hours requires carefully controlled studies. The most severe reactions occur within minutes to 2 hours after ingestion. With indomethacin, 1- or 5-mg oral challenges resulted in acute responses.[132] Cross-reaction exists so that certain NSIADs (indomethacin, flufenamic acid, and mefenamic acid) have a higher likelihood of inducing bronchospastic responses in aspirin-sensitive patients than phenylbutazone. Because fatalities have occurred in aspirin-sensitive patients with asthma, challenges should be carried out only with appropriate explanation to the patient, when an obvious need for the challenge (e.g., with rheumatoid arthritis) exists, and by experienced physicians. Interestingly, some aspirin-sensitive patients can be desensitized to aspirin after experiencing early bronchospastic responses.[132] Subsequent regular administration of aspirin does not cause acute bronchospastic responses.[132]

The aspirin triad refers to aspirin-sensitive patients with asthma who also have chronic nasal polyps.[10] The onset of asthma often precedes the recognition of aspirin sensitivity by years. Tartrazine (FDC yellow dye no. 5) was found to result in immediate bronchospastic reactions in 5% of patients with the aspirin triad.[10] Contrary results in double-blinded studies have been reported in that none of the patients responded to tartrazine.[133] The risks of inadvertent exposure to tartrazine by the aspirin-sensitive patient seem to be smaller than initially reported and range from nonexistent[133] to 2.3%.[134]

The drugs that produce such immediate respiratory responses have in common the ability to inhibit the enzyme cyclooxygenase, which is known to metabolize arachidonic acid into prostaglandin $F_{2\alpha}$ and thromboxanes. Structurally, these drugs are different. Data suggest that the blockade of cyclooxygenase diverts arachidonic acid into the lipoxygenase pathway with resultant production of LTC_4 and LTD_4.[14,15] The latter is a potent bronchospastic agonist. Aspirin-sensitive patients have higher resting prostaglandin $F_{2\alpha}$ concentrations and higher urinary leukotriene E_4 (LTE_4) concentrations[15] than aspirin-tolerant patients with asthma.

After ingesting aspirin, intolerant patients have an even greater rise in urinary LTE_4 than aspirin-tolerant subjects.[15]

Occupational Asthma

Occupational asthma has been estimated to occur in 2% to 15% of all patients with asthma.[59] Specific industry prevalence may be higher, such as 16% in snow crab processors in Canada.[135] Occupational asthma may be IgE mediated. When it is IgE mediated, accumulating longitudinal data support a time of sensitization followed by development of bronchial hyperresponsiveness and then bronchoconstriction.[59,135] After removal from the workplace exposure, the reverse sequence has been recorded. Malo and coworkers[135] documented that spirometry and bronchial hyperresponsiveness in ex–snow crab workers reached a plateau of improvement by 2 years after cessation of work exposure. The assessment of patients with possible occupational asthma is discussed in detail in Chapter 23. Some workers have early, late, dual, or irritant bronchial responses such as occurs to trimellitic anhydride, which is used in the plastics industry as a curing agent in the manufacture of epoxy resins.

The differential diagnosis of occupational asthma is complex and includes consideration of irritants, smoke, toxic gases, metal exposures, insecticides, organic chemicals and dusts, infectious agents, and occupational chemicals. In addition, true occupational asthma must be differentiated from coincidental adult-onset asthma that is not affected by workplace exposure. Some workers have chemical exposure and a compensation syndrome, but no objective asthma despite symptoms and usually a poor response to medications. The physician must exclude work-related neuroses with fixation on an employer as well as a syndrome of reactive airways dysfunction, which occurs after an accidental exposure to a chemical irritant or toxic gas.[136,137] Atopic status and smoking do not predict workers who will become ill to non–IgE-mediated chemicals. Atopic status and smoking are predictors of IgE-mediated occupational asthma.[59] Western red cedar workers display bronchial hyperresponsiveness during times of exposure with reductions in hyperresponsiveness during exposure-free periods. It is still uncertain if antiplicatic acid IgE is necessary for development of red cedar asthma because immediate skin test reactions are negative and bronchial responses are present. In vitro assay to detect IgE to plicatic acid–human serum albumin demonstrated elevated antibodies to this conjugate in workers.[138] The complexity of diagnosing occupational asthma cannot be underestimated in some workers. Respiratory symptoms may intensify when a worker returns from a vacation but may not be dramatic when deterioration occurs during successive days at work.

Avoidance measures and temporary pharmacologic therapy can suffice to confirm a diagnosis in some cases. Resuming exposure should produce objective bronchial obstruction and clinical changes. The physician must be aware that workers may return serial PEFR measurements that coincide with expected abnormal values during work or shortly thereafter. Such values should be assessed critically because they are effort-dependent and may be manipulated. Demonstration of IgE or IgG antibodies to the incriminated workplace allergen or to an occupational chemical bound to a carrier protein has been of value in supporting the diagnosis of occupational asthma and even in prospective use to identify workers who are at risk of developing occupational asthma.[139] Such assays are not commonly available but are of discriminatory value when properly performed.

If a bronchial provocation challenge is deemed necessary, it is preferable to have the employee perform a job-related task that exposes the employee to the usual concentration of occupational chemicals. Subsequent blinding may be necessary as well.

Exercise-Induced Asthma

Exercise-induced asthma refers to either an isolated disorder in patients with mild asthma or the inability to complete an exercise program in symptomatic patients with chronic asthma. Controlling the latter often permits successful participation in a reasonable degree of exercise. In patients with mild asthma whose only symptoms might be triggered by exercise, the pattern of bronchoconstriction is as follows: during exercise, the FEV_1 is slightly increased (about 5%), unchanged, or slightly reduced, but no symptoms occur, followed by declines of FEV_1 and onset of symptoms 5 to 15 minutes after cessation of exercise. The decline of FEV_1 is at least 20%. Airway hyperresponsiveness does not occur.[140] A subsequent decline of FEV_1 has been documented at 5 hours, which is consistent with a dual respiratory response. However, such declines also occurred on days in which no exercise challenge was conducted.[141] Clearly, even greater than 32% declines in FEV_1 5 hours after exercise in association with clinical symptoms are part of variations in pulmonary physiology of asthma and might result from loss of airway caliber from withdrawal of medications.[141]

Exercise-induced asthma resulting in a decline of FEV_1 of at least 20% is associated with inspiration of cold or dry air. In general, greater declines in spirometry and presence of respiratory symptoms are seen that are directly proportional to the level of hyperventilation and inversely proportional to inspired air temperature and extent of water saturation. The exact mechanism of bronchospasm remains controversial in that postexertional airway rewarming that causes increased bronchial mucosal blood flow has been suggested[142] and disputed[143] as possible mechanistic explanations. Clinically, it has been recognized that running outdoors while inhaling dry cold air is a far greater stimulus to bronchospasm than running indoors while breathing warmer humidified air or swimming.

Exercise-induced bronchospasm can occur in any form of asthma on a chronic basis but also can be prevented completely or to a great extent by pharmacologic treatment. In preventing isolated episodes of exercise-induced bronchospasm, medications such as inhaled β-adrenergic agonists inspired 10 to 15 minutes before exercise often prevent significant exercise-induced bronchospasm. Cromolyn by inhalation is effective, as are oral β-adrenergic agonists and theophylline, to a lesser extent. For patients with chronic asthma, overall improvement in their respiratory status by avoidance measures and regular pharmacotherapy minimizes exercise symptoms. Pretreatment with β-adrenergic agonists in addition to regular antiasthma therapy allows asthma patients to participate in exercise activities successfully.

Variant Asthma

Whereas most patients with asthma report symptoms of coughing, chest tightness, and dyspnea, and physicians are able to auscultate wheezing or rhonchi on examination, variant asthma refers to patients with asthma whose prime symptoms are paroxysmal and repetitive coughing or dyspnea in the absence of wheezing. The coughing often occurs after an upper respiratory infection, or exercise and after exposure to odors, fresh paint, or allergens. Sputum usually is not produced, and the cough occurs on a nocturnal basis. Antitussives, expectorants, antibiotics, and use of intranasal corticosteroids do not suppress the coughing. The chest examination reveals no wheezing or rhonchi. McFadden[89] documented increases in large airways resistance, moderate to severe reductions in FEV_1 (mean 53%), and bronchodilator responses. The mean residual volume was 152%, which is consistent with air trapping. In addition, patients with exertional dyspnea as the prime manifestation of asthma had

FEV_1 values still within normal limits but a residual volume of 236%,[89] but a not greatly increased airways resistance. Both types of patients had reduced small airways flow rates. Some patients can be heard to wheeze after exercise or after performing a FVC maneuver.

Pharmacologic therapy can be successful to suppress the coughing episodes or sensation of dyspnea, but often when inhaled β-adrenergic agonists have not been effective, the best way to suppress symptoms is with an inhaled corticosteroid. If using an inhaler produces coughing, a 5- to 7-day course of oral corticosteroids often stops the coughing.[144] At times, even longer courses of oral corticosteroids and antiasthma therapy are necessary.

Factitious Asthma

Factitious asthma presents diagnostic and management problems that often require multidisciplinary approaches to treatment.[116,145] The diagnosis may not be suspected initially because patient history, antecedent triggering symptoms, examination findings, and even abnormal pulmonary physiologic parameters may appear consistent with asthma. Nevertheless, there may be no response to appropriate treatment or worsening of asthma despite what would be considered effective care. Some patients are able to adduct their vocal cords during inspiration and on expiration make a rhonchorous sound, simulating asthma. Other patients have repetitive coughing paroxysms or "seal barking" coughing fits. A number of patients with factitious asthma are physicians, paramedical or nursing personnel, or have an unusual degree of medical knowledge. Psychiatric disease can be severe, yet patients seem appropriate in a given interview. Factitious asthma episodes do not occur during sleep, and the experienced physicians can distract the patient with factitious asthma and temporarily cause an absence of wheezing or coughing. Invasive procedures may be associated with conversion reactions or even respiratory "arrests" from breath-holding.

Coexistent Asthma and COPD

Usually, in the setting of long-term cigarette smoking with at least 40 pack years of smoking, asthma may coexist with COPD. Obviously, the patients with asthma or COPD should not smoke. Multiple medications may be administered in patients with asthma and COPD to minimize signs and symptoms. However, some dyspnea likely is fixed and not transient because of underlying COPD. The component of asthma can be significant, perhaps approximately 25% to 50% at first. However, with continued smoking, the reversible component—even using oral and inhaled corticosteroids, bronchodilators, theophylline, and anticholinergic agents—diminishes or becomes nonexistent. At that point, the lowest number of medications possible should be used. When there is no benefit from oral corticosteroids, it is advisable to taper and discontinue them.

Initially, such as after hospitalization for asthma, the patient with combined asthma and COPD may benefit from a 2- to 4-week course of oral corticosteroids. The effort to identify the maximal degree of reversibility should be made even when asthma is a modest component of COPD. The lack of bronchodilator responsiveness or peripheral blood eosinophilia does not preclude a response to a 2-week course of prednisone.

Long-term care of patients with coexistent asthma and COPD can be successful in improving quality of life and reducing or eliminating disabling wheezing. However, eventually, patients may die from end-stage COPD or coexisting cardiac failure.

NONANTIGENIC PRECIPITATING STIMULI IN ASTHMA

Hyperresponsiveness of bronchi in patients with asthma is manifested clinically by responses to various nonantigenic triggers. Examples include odors from cigarette smoke, fresh paint, cooking, cologne, perfumes, insecticides, and household cleaning agents.[146] In addition sulfur dioxide, combustion products, and air pollution—both indoor and outdoor—can trigger asthma signs and symptoms. Bronchospasm likely occurs on an irritant basis. Effective management of patients with asthma may permit patients to tolerate most inadvertent exposures with little troubling effects.

Gastroesophageal reflux has been a recognized trigger of asthma episodes.[147] Frank gastroesophageal reflux with aspiration into the bronchi has been associated with chronic cough, episodic wheezing, rhonchi, or even cyanosis if aspiration is severe. Reflux of gastric acid into the lower esophagus can precipitate symptoms of asthma without frank aspiration, perhaps by an esophagobronchial vagal reflex.[147] Medical therapy such as avoiding meals for 3 hours before sleeping, weight reduction, cessation of cigarette smoking, discontinuation of drugs that decrease gastroesophageal sphincter pressure (theophylline), diet manipulation, and raising the head of the bed 15 cm (6 inches) are among some interventions of value. Pharmacotherapy with H_2-histamine antagonists is advisable. Surgical intervention is indicated rarely but has been successful to varying degrees in about 60% of patients undergoing a Nissen transabdominal gastropexy.[148]

Congestive heart failure, when left sided, has been associated with exacerbations of asthma. Bronchial hyperresponsiveness has been recognized in nonasthmatic patients who developed left ventricular failure. When patients with asthma develop congestive heart failure, at times, sudden episodes of wheezing dyspnea can occur in the absence of neck vein distension or peripheral edema, which supports a diagnosis of left ventricular failure. Differentiating pulmonary edema from acute asthma may be difficult in brittle cardiac patients who have severe asthma or asthma, COPD, and left ventricular failure.

DIFFERENTIAL DIAGNOSIS OF WHEEZING

There are many causes of wheezing, dyspnea, and coughing, individually and collectively. A partial listing is presented.

I. Commonly encountered diseases or conditions
  A. Asthma
  B. Upper respiratory tract infections
    1. Bronchiolitis
    2. Croup
    3. Viruses (i.e., respiratory syncytial, rhinovirus, influenza, parainfluenza)
    4. Acute and chronic bronchitis
    5. Acute pneumonia
    6. Bronchiectasis
    7. Sinusitis
    8. Purulent rhinitis
  C. Congestive heart failure
    1. Left ventricular failure
    2. Mitral stenosis
    3. Congenital heart disease

    D. COPD

    E. Hyperventilation syndrome

    F. Pulmonary infarction or embolism

    G. Cystic fibrosis

    H. Laryngotracheomalacia

    I. Bronchopulmonary dysplasia

II. Less common conditions

    A. Tuberculosis

    B. Hypersensitivity pneumonitis

    C. Inhalation of irritant gases, odors, or dusts

    D. Physical obstruction of the upper airways

        1. Neoplasms (benign or malignant)

        2. Foreign bodies

        3. Acute laryngeal or pharyngeal angioedema

        4. Bronchial stenosis

            a. After intubation

            b. Granulomatous

            c. After burns

    E. Interstitial lung disease

    F. Pneumocystis carinii pneumonia

    G. Sarcoidosis

    H. Gastroesophageal reflux

III. Uncommon conditions

    A. Restrictive lung disease

    B. Churg-Strauss vasculitis

    C. Mediastinal enlargement

    D. Diphtheria

    E. Carcinoid tumor of main stem bronchi

    F. Thymoma

    G. Tracheoesophageal fistula

    H. Allergic bronchopulmonary aspergillosis

    I. α1-Antitrypsin deficiency

    J. Factitious coughing, wheezing, or stridor

    K. Vocal cord dysfunction

TREATMENT

The treatment of an asthmatic episode varies according to its clinical severity. Similarly, long-range treatment regimens depend on the type of asthma and its severity. The basic objective of treatment, as in other chronic illnesses, is to achieve significant control of symptoms to prevent physical and psychological impairment. In addition to clinical improvement, the practical goals of treatment are best measured by avoidance of hospitalizations and school or work absenteeism, and the ability of the patient to lead a normal, functional life with little or no impairment of exercise activities and sleep habits. The Expert Panel Report of the National Heart, Lung, and Blood Institute suggests specific management protocols for patients categorized with mild, moderate, and severe asthma.[2] The goals should maximize control of symptoms of asthma, permit as normal a lifestyle as possible, avoid nocturnal asthma, and achieve the best possible respiratory status.

Principles of Treatment

The treatment of asthma consists of therapeutic measures to control any inflammation, reverse bronchial mucosal edema, bronchospasm, hypersecretion of mucus, and V/Q imbalance. Depending on the severity of the attack, various degrees of hypocarbia or hypercarbia with its resultant acid–base changes also require specific therapy. Finally, other emergency measures may be necessary to prevent or reverse acute respiratory failure.

Preventive measures are important in the proper management of asthma. In exercise-induced asthma, appropriate premedication prevents symptoms. In allergic asthma, removing the offending allergen or allergens is of primary importance since it can reduce symptoms, the need for medication, and, eventually, bronchial hyperresponsiveness. If this is impossible, immunotherapy should be considered.[149–151] Protective measures also must be included to lessen the deleterious effects of certain aggravating factors. In addition, drugs that precipitate asthma must be avoided.

The best treatment of asthma consists of determining the clinical classification (see earlier), using necessary avoidance measures, drug therapy, allergen immunotherapy when indicated, and considering the effects of other conditions that may impact on the patient (Table 22-5).

Drug Therapy

Adrenergic Drugs

The peripheral effects of an adrenergic drug depend on its specific (alpha or beta) receptor-stimulating capacity, as well as the type and density of receptor present in the organ or tissue

TABLE 22-5. *Acute asthma tips*

In the Emergency Department

1. Establish severity of asthma

    Cannot speak in a sentence

    Accessory muscle use?

    Cyanotic?

    Heart rate 120/min or greater

    Cannot perform spirometry or peak flow is <200 L/min

    β_2-Adrenergic agonist overuse

    Marked nocturnal symptoms

2. Send the patient who clears after emergency therapy home with a short course of oral corticosteroid

3. Arrange follow-up care

In the Office

1. Does the patient need hospitalization or emergency therapy?

2. A combination of regular β_2-adrenergic agonist and inhaled corticosteroid may suffice; otherwise, add a short course of an oral corticosteroid

3. Check inhaler technique

4. Schedule follow-up care

5. Consider referral to an allergist-immunologist

TABLE 22-6. *Effects of adrenergic stimulation*

Alpha stimulation	β_1 stimulation	β_2 stimulation
Vasoconstriction	Cardiac stimulation	Bronchial relaxation
Intestinal relaxation	Chronotropic	Uterine relaxation
Contraction of uterus	Inotropic	Vascular smooth muscle relaxation
Contraction of ureter	Lipolysis	Stimulates skeletal muscle (tremor)
Contraction of dilator papillae		Stimulates liver and muscle glycogenolysis
Inhibition of insulin secretion		Stimulates skeletal muscle NaK ATPase (hypokalemia)

NaK, sodium potassium.

stimulated (Table 22-6). The bronchi contain predominantly β_2-adrenergic receptors, which promote bronchodilation. Beta receptors themselves may differ from organ to organ. Those in the heart are primarily β_1-adrenergic receptors, which increase cardiac contractibility and heart rate. Thus, adrenergic drugs possessing β_2-stimulating activity are most effective in treating asthma.

Biochemical mechanisms of action (Fig. 22-7) of the β-stimulating adrenergic drugs have not been completely clarified, but they are known to increase the rate of formation of 3'5'-cyclic adenosine monophosphate (cAMP) from adenosine triphosphate in the presence of adenylate cyclase. The increased cAMP in turn triggers other intermediate reactions, which ultimately result in both bronchodilation and inhibition of the mediator release in immediate hypersensitivity reactions. These effects reverse or inhibit some of the pathophysiologic events known to occur in asthma.

Continuing pharmacologic and biochemical research has resulted not only in a better understanding of the adrenergic receptor system, but also in the development of drugs with more specific stimulating or blocking action. The basic molecular structure of adrenergic drugs is the catechol nucleus, which consists of a benzene ring with hydroxyl groups at the 3 and 4 positions and a two carbon (alpha and beta) amide side chain at position 1 (Fig. 22-8). These drugs are quickly inactivated in vivo by cellular catechol-o-methyl transferase (COMT) and sulfatase (in the gut and liver). These enzymes alter the hydroxyl structure of the benzene ring, with the formation of a 3-methoxy radical in the case of COMT, and a sulfate with the action of sulfatase. These resultant compounds are devoid of bronchodilating properties. Monoamine oxidase (MAO) is another inactivating enzyme whose site of action is at the alpha carbon (amide-linked) of the side chain.

Various alterations of the molecular structure of the catecholamine nucleus have resulted in a variety of antiasthma drugs (see Fig. 22-8). Modification of the substitutents of the alpha carbon of the side chain (e.g., isoetharine, procaterol), as well as increasing the bulk of the substituent groups on the amide head (e.g., metaproterenol, terbutaline, albuterol) has resulted in greater and more specific β_2 stimulation. Alteration of the hydroxyl positions on the benzene ring from the 3,4 position (resorcinol structure) negates the effect of the COMT, thus giving these compounds a longer duration of action. A similar effect results from substitution of a saligenin in the 3-hydroxyl position (albuterol). Except for the substitution of a urea molecule at the 3-hydroxyl group, carbuterol is similar to albuterol. Compared with the older drugs (e.g., epinephrine, ephedrine, isoproterenol), the new adrenergic drugs possess more potent specific β_2 activity and a prolonged duration of action. Most are effective orally as well as by aerosol and parenteral administration. Salmeterol has a long side chain that binds effec-

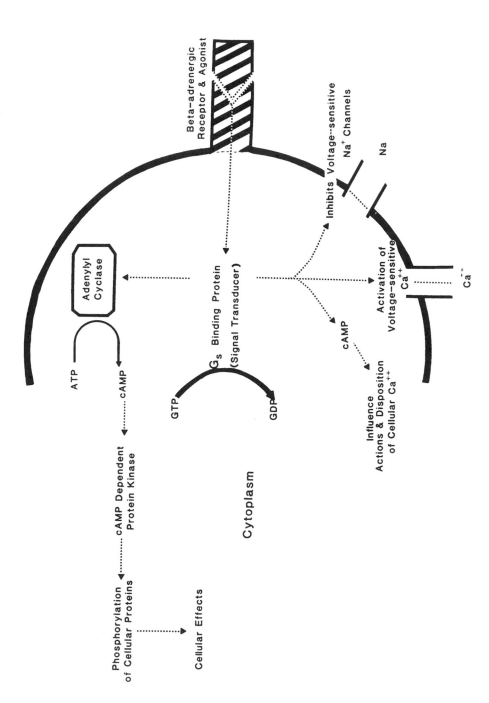

FIG. 22-7. A simplified schematic of beta-adrenergic receptor stimulation. Beta-adrenergic agonist stimulation of its receptor causes a conformational change in the guanine nucleotide-binding regulatory protein G_S. There is increased GTPase activity and then a transduced signal, resulting in activation of adenyl cyclase. This sequence raises the concentration of cAMP. The regulatory protein G_S couples beta-adrenergic receptors to adenyl cyclase and calcium channels. G_S interacts with the sodium channel, resulting in its inhibition.

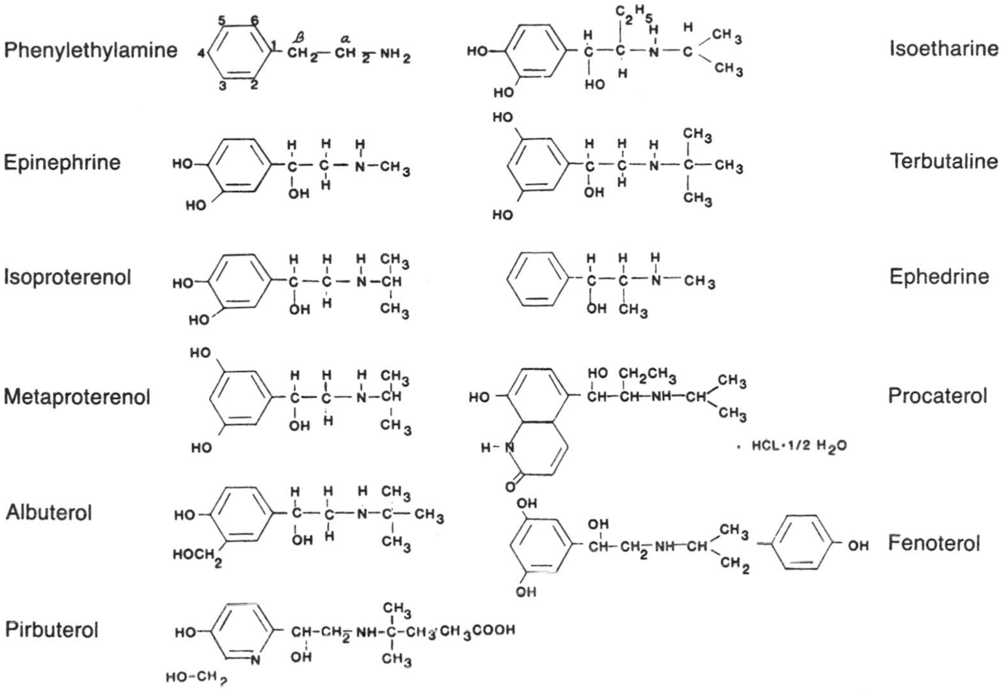

FIG. 22-8. The chemical structures of sympathomimetic drugs compared with phenylethylamine.

tively to the β_2-adrenergic receptor so that the drug can be administered every 12 hours. Salmeterol is eliminated (hydroxylated) by the liver.

The development of bronchial resistance or tolerance with continued use of adrenergics has been studied extensively. Some studies have shown evidence for the development of tolerance whereas other have not.[152,154] A 13-week double-blind study of inhaled isoproterenol and albuterol demonstrated statistically significant tachyphylaxis with albuterol but not with isoproterenol.[154] The tachyphylaxis of the duration of the bronchodilator (FEV$_1$) effect amounted to a decrease from 240 minutes to 168 minutes. Nevertheless, the peak bronchodilator response was preserved throughout the study. Most of the tachyphylaxis occurred by 4 weeks and did not increase substantially with continued use of albuterol. Interestingly, no tachyphylaxis was demonstrated with isoproterenol inhalations. After 13 weeks of inhaled bronchodilator therapy, however, the patients had statistically greater duration of bronchodilator effect with albuterol than with isoproterenol. This study demonstrated that either drug provides useful bronchodilating effects over a prolonged period, and that marked tachyphylaxis to albuterol inhalation must be rare. Excessive use of β-adrenergic inhalers has been associated with fatalities,[53,107,108] and it has been speculated that patients develop a false sense of security while continuing to be exposed to allergens.

Epinephrine

Epinephrine, because of its potent bronchodilating effect and rapid onset of action, is the drug of choice in acute asthma. It directly stimulates both α- and β-adrenergic receptors. The recommended adult dose is 0.30 mL of a 1:1000 solution administered subcutaneously. In infants and children, the dose is 0.01 mL/kg with a maximum of 0.25 mL. The dose may be repeated in 15 to 30 minutes if necessary. Nebulized epinephrine also is effective, but is less commonly used today.

Some side effects of epinephrine include agitation, tremulousness, tachycardia, and palpitation. Hypertension in the presence of acute asthma often resolves with epinephrine administration. This occurs because of a decrease in bronchospasm and from a decrease in peripheral vascular resistance by stimulation of β_2 receptors in smooth muscle of blood vessels in skeletal muscle. Epinephrine must be administered with caution in patients with cardiovascular disease and hypertension, but should not be considered contraindicated when bronchospasm is significant. Epinephrine is rapidly metabolized and, in the emergency setting, can be administered once and repeated once or twice more to determine if wheezing can be cleared. Otherwise, hospitalization is necessary. The maximum bronchodilator effect of epinephrine given subcutaneously is not less than that of inhaled β-adrenergic agonists and, occasionally, in the severely obstructed patient, exceeds what can be gained by aerosol therapy. Although epinephrine is an old drug, it is expedient, effective, and rapidly metabolized.

Ephedrine

Ephedrine, although less potent than isoproterenol and epinephrine, was used for decades because it was effective by oral administration and possessed a longer duration of action (3 to 6 hours). Its onset of action is approximately 1 hour, with a peak effect of 2 to 3 hours. This prolonged action results from the methyl substitution at the alpha carbon of the side chain, and the absence of 3,4-hydroxyl groups on the benzene ring, thus negating the effects of MAO and COMT (see Fig. 22-8). Ephedrine stimulates α- and β-adrenergic receptors directly and indirectly. Ephedrine is an integral component of some combination oral preparations available for treatment of asthma. The adult dose is 25 mg four times daily. For infants and children, the recommended dose is 0.5 mg to 1 mg/kg every 6 hours. Adverse effects of ephedrine are similar to those of epinephrine but are of lesser magnitude, except for central nervous system stimulation. Ephedrine currently is considered by many to be an outdated drug for antiasthma therapy because of the availability of β_2 agonists for inhalation or oral use. The 25-mg ephedrine capsule has been shown to have approximately the same efficacy as 2.5 mg of terbutaline. Ephedrine-theophylline-phenobarbital preparations are available without prescription. This combination is effective in management of asthma but is not preferred over β-adrenergic agonists delivered by metered dose inhalers combined with inhaled corticosteroids.

Pirbuterol

Pirbuterol (Maxair) is a selective β_2-adrenergic agonist that is structurally similar to albuterol. It is available as a metered dose inhaler with 300 actuations per canister. Each actuation releases 200 μg of pirbuterol. The maximal dosage is two inhalations every 4 to 6 hours. Pirbuterol is approved by the Food and Drug Administration (FDA) for children 12 years and older and adults. Pirbuterol also is available with an easy-to-use breath-activated unit (Maxair autohaler) with either 80 or 400 inhalations.

Metaproterenol

Metaproterenol (Alupent, Metaprel) is available for oral use (tablet and syrup), as well as for aerosol use by metered dose inhaler or nebulizer aerosol solution. The adult oral dose is 10 to 20 mg every 6 to 8 hours, and by aerosol one to three inhalations (650 μg per inhalation) every 6 hours. In children, the recommended oral dose is 10 mg every 6 to 8 hours for children ages 6 to 9 or those weighing 27 kg or less. For children weighing above 27 kg, 15 to 20 mg may be given every 6 hours. The concentration of the syrup is 10 mg/5 mL. The recommended aerosol dosage for children younger than 12 years of age is one to two inhalations every 6 hours.

Orally, the onset of action of metaproterenol is approximately 30 minutes, with a peak effect in 2 to 3 hours. By aerosol, its onset of action is within 2 to 10 minutes, and its duration of action is approximately 4 to 6 hours if asthma is not severe.

Metaproterenol is an effective bronchodilator with infrequent and minimal side effects. Tachycardia occurs in about 4% of the patients, and all other cardiovascular, CNS, and gastrointestinal side effects have a total incidence rate of less than 1%. The rate of side effects from oral administration may be less than seen with ephedrine, but still approximates 20%. The side effects from oral administration are tachycardia, nervousness, tremor, palpitations, nausea, and vomiting, which may limit its acceptance by patients.

Terbutaline

Terbutaline (Brethaire, Bricanyl) is effective subcutaneously, orally, and by metered dose inhalation. This drug is not approved by the FDA for use in children younger than 12 years of age. Subcutaneously, the adult dosage is 0.25 mL (0.25 mg), and it may be repeated in 15 to 30 minutes once with a maximum dose of 0.50 mg in 4 hours. In children aged 12 to 15 years, the dose is 0.01 mg/kg, with a maximum dose of dose of 0.25 mg. Given subcutaneously, it has not been found to differ significantly from epinephrine in onset or duration of action. Terbutaline and other beta agonists lose their "selectivity" when administered parenterally. Tachycardia may occur directly or on a reflex basis from stimulation of β_2 receptors in smooth muscle of peripheral vasculature, which causes vasodilation. Terbutaline was found to produce more tachycardia then epinephrine.[155] The adult oral dose is 5 mg three times daily, and for children aged 12 to 15 the recommended dose is 2.5 mg three times daily. Orally, the bronchodilating effect of terbutaline has its onset at about 30 minutes, peaks in 2 to 4 hours, and has a variable duration of from 3 to 7 hours. Side effects have a relatively high incidence, and include principally tremor, and also tachycardia and palpitation. With the 5 mg three times daily dosage in adults, tremor occurs in from 20% to 33% of patients; with the 2.5-mg three times daily dosage, tremor is significantly lessened. It is preferable to use the metered dose inhaler. There are 300 actuations with 200 μg terbutaline per actuation.

Saligenins

The characteristic feature of the saligenin compounds is the substitution of a methanol group for the hydroxyl group at the 3 position of the benzene ring (see Fig. 22-8). These compounds are not substrates for COMT so that they have longer action than isoproterenol.

Albuterol

Albuterol (Proventil, Ventolin) is effective orally, by aerosol, and subcutaneously. It is not approved for subcutaneous use in the United States. The FDA has not approved its use for children younger than 2 years of age. Tablets are 2 and 4 mg and can be administered every 6 to 8 hours. Longer lasting tablets (Proventil Repetabs, Volmax of 4 and 8 mg) can be administered every 12 hours. The elixir is 2 mg/5 mL at a dosage of 0.2 mg/kg up to 2 mg three times a day in children. The metered dose inhaler delivers 90 µg of albuterol per inhalation, and the maximum recommended frequency is two inhalations every 4 to 6 hours. Significant bronchodilation occurs within 15 minutes of inhalation, with maximum effect in 60 to 90 minutes. Useful bronchodilation lasts 3 to 6 hours. After oral ingestion, peak improvement in respiratory parameters occurs in 2 to 3 hours, with effects lasting 6 hours or longer. Side effects are similar to other β_2 agonists. By nebulizer administration, a 3-mL solution of 0.083% can be nebulized as a unit dose. Otherwise, the 0.5% solution is diluted (0.5 mL plus 2.5 mL saline). Alternatively, for chronic use, 0.5 mL of albuterol can be diluted with 2.0 mL cromolyn (Intal) nebulizer solution.

Continuously nebulized albuterol solution for treating acute episodes of asthma consists of preparing 7.7 mL of 0.5% albuterol in 100 mL saline. A pump infuses the solution at a rate of 14 to 21 mL/hour while the nebulizer supplies 100% oxygen. (However, initial studies have not demonstrated superior results compared with repeated nebulized albuterol administration).

Bitolterol

Bitolterol (Tornalate) is a prodrug (an ester) and must be deesterified in the lung. The active moiety is colterol. The recommended dosage is two to three inhalations every 6 hours. The dose released by the metered inhaler is 370 µg. Bitolterol is approved for use in children older than 12 years and in adults. The metered dose inhaler contains 300 actuations. The nebulizer solution should be 2 to 4 mL, but cromolyn should not be added to the nebulizer simultaneously.

Fenoterol

Fenoterol (Berotec) is structurally similar to metaproterenol and is a β_2-selective adrenergic agonist. Fenoterol is not approved for use in the United States. It is available as a metered dose inhaler, and the dosage is two inhalations every 6 hours. A 0.5% solution is available for nebulization. An excess number of fatalities has been reported in patients who used more than 1 canister per month,[108] so caution is advised.[53]

Procaterol

Procaterol (Pro-Air) is a potent β_2-adrenergic agonist not available in the United States. Procaterol is administered as a metered dose inhaler containing 10 µg per actuation with usual dosage of two inhalations every 6 to 8 hours. The inhaler contains 200 actuations. Procaterol has onset of action within 5 minutes.

Salmeterol

Salmeterol (Serevent) is a potent β_2-adrenergic agonist with a long half-life so that administration is one to two inhalations every 12 hours. It is 50 times more potent experimentally than albuterol, but provides similar peak bronchodilation as albuterol. Each metered dose inhaler provides the equivalent of 25 μg salmeterol per actuation. Units contain either 60 or 120 actuations. It is approved for use in children aged 12 years and older and for adults as a maintenance but not acute bronchodilator medication. A shorter acting β_2-adrenergic agonist may be added 4 to 6 hours after use of salmeterol. However, antiinflammatory (bronchoprotective) medications most likely should be administered concurrently.

Adverse Effects of Adrenergic Aerosols

Aerosols containing adrenergic drugs have been used in the treatment of asthma for 40 years. The immediate relief of this form of therapy has made it widely acceptable to both patients and physicians. Unfortunately, many patients assume an almost addictive relation with their inhalers, which results in overuse. The most common side effects are related to β_1 stimulation, resulting in cardiac symptoms, as listed earlier with epinephrine. Potential adverse effects from β_2-adrenergic agonists include overuse, systemic absorption across bronchial mucosa, delay in receiving antiinflammatory therapy, and fatalities.

Although subjective and objective improvement of airway obstruction is produced by inhaled beta agonists, the associated hypoxemia of asthma is not improved, and may be increased. This probably results from enhancing the already existing ventilation perfusion imbalance by either increasing aeration of those alveoli already overventilating in relation to their perfusion, or by reestablishing ventilation to nonperfused alveoli. Absorption of beta agonists from bronchial mucosa may result in systemic effects such as increased cardiac output.[156] Ventilation perfusion mismatching would occur by perfusion of underventilated alveoli. The resultant hypoxemia usually is clinically insignificant, unless the initial PO_2 is on the steep portion of the O_2–hemoglobin dissociation curves (less than 60 mm Hg). In moderately severe acute asthma, oxygen should be administered to correct the hypoxemia.

Of concern is the paradoxical response of increased bronchial obstruction seen in occasional patients using β-adrenergic agonists by inhalation. With an exacerbation of asthmatic symptoms, these patients may overuse inhalation therapy because of a decreasing response to proceeding inhalations. A cycle begins of increasing obstruction with increasing use of the aerosol. This may precede status asthmaticus. Patients who are identified as using β-adrenergic agonist inhalation or nebulizers excessively should have this therapy terminated. This can be accomplished by temporary use of prednisone to control underlying bronchospasm and airway inflammation. Before prescribing β-adrenergic agonists, the physician should warn patients about overuse. Overuse can be defined as more than manufacturer's recommendations or perhaps daily scheduled use even at manufacturer's recommendations. For short- to moderate-duration bronchodilators such as albuterol, pirbuterol, or terbutaline, I believe that the recommended scheduled use is not dangerous or unsafe in terms of controlling asthma. The ultimate safety of fenoterol and salmeterol needs to be established. I am concerned about the unanticipated fatalities in patients who received fenoterol or salmeterol and therefore believe that caution is indicated.

The essential consideration is that patients may delay seeking and obtaining proper therapy for asthma and instead attempt to decrease the symptoms with an inhaler or nebulizer. This delay allows underlying bronchoconstriction and hyperinflation of lung volumes to progress such that hypoxemia, hypercarbia, or respiratory failure may be present when the patient seeks acute medical care. The desire to increase the dosage of β-adrenergic agonists should be weighed against systemic effects as well as the failure to treat underlying mucus obstruction of bronchi and the many other inflammatory events in asthma.

Practical Considerations in the Use of Adrenergic Agents

For acute symptoms, aerosolized β-adrenergic agonists can be administered. Parenteral epinephrine is the drug of choice for acute asthma. Either may be repeated two to three times. If there is no response, the patient is in status asthmaticus, and hospitalization is required. If the patient does respond, bronchodilators should be given for sustained benefit, and corticosteroids are indicated to prevent a return of symptoms of asthma.

Subcutaneous terbutaline is favored by some physicians for acute treatment of asthma. Similar bronchodilation results with epinephrine or terbutaline[157,158] when equal doses are administered. Continuously nebulized albuterol has not been demonstrated to be superior to intermittently administered treatments.[159] Hypokalemia, tachycardia, or cardiac arrhythmias may occur.

Emergency room personnel should be instructed in administration of nebulized aerosols or metered dose inhalers with or without spacer devices. Some patients having severe attacks of asthma do not respond to nebulized β-adrenergic agonists but benefit from subcutaneous therapy. Ineffective delivery of $β_2$-adrenergic agonists can prevent adequate responses to therapy in severely ill patients. Conversely, some patients not responding to an initial subcutaneous injection of epinephrine or terbutaline may respond to inhaled therapy. Failure to respond to two treatments with nebulized β-adrenergic agonists usually indicates status asthmaticus. Further, continuously nebulized $β_2$-adrenergic agonists such as albuterol over 2 hours did not provide any additional benefit compared with two 5-mg boluses given hourly of aerosolized albuterol.[159] To some extent, the former is less labor intensive than nebulized treatments given at hourly intervals. The place of such an approach must be established.

For mild, intermittent asthma, inhaled or oral β-adrenergic agonists may be used as needed. As in many situations where multiple choices of drugs are available, the physician should become experienced with one or two preparations. When asthma is chronic, regular inhaled β-adrenergic agonists may be recommended, but alternatives include cromolyn or inhaled corticosteroids. An aerosolized beta agonist taken before exercise is an example of a useful method of pharmacotherapy for exercise-induced asthma.

For more significant chronic asthma, $β_2$-adrenergic agonists in combination with inhaled cromolyn, nedocromil, or corticosteroids are indicated. The combination of these agents may be additive, and the need for $β_2$-adrenergic agents reduced.

When β-adrenergic agonists are administered by inhalation, proper technique is essential. Patients may fail to expire fully to FRC before actuating their metered dose inhaler. Other patients may inhale too rapidly to TLC, take a submaximal inspiration, flex the neck during inspiration, forget to shake the canister before actuation, or fail to hold their breath for 8 to 10 seconds after a full inspiration. All of these variables may decrease drug delivery to the lung periphery and explain poor therapeutic responses. Rarely, the inhaler cap can be inhaled inadvertently or coins, paper clips, or capsules stored inside the metered dose inhaler are inhaled. When effective synchronization of inhalation with actuation of air inhaler cannot be corrected, improvement in patient care may be achieved by discontinuing the inhaler and using only oral medications.

Several devices are available which improve the dynamics of aerosol administration by a pressurized inhaler. Some of these include the tube spacer (10 × 3.2 cm), aerochamber, and collapsible reservoir aerosol system (11.5 cm long and 9 cm in diameter when inflated). These devices minimize aerosol deposition in the oropharynx and increase delivery to the airways. Further, by requiring a slower inspiration, more drug may be distributed to obstructed peripheral airways than with a rapid inspiration, which favors central airway deposition at the expense of the peripheral airways. Although increases in flow rates above that achieved with a metered dose inhaler have been documented in some patients, use of a space device does not improve the efficient use of a metered dose inhaler. For patients who have impaired inhaler technique, spacer devices are beneficial. Pirbuterol (Maxair autohaler) is an example of a breath-activated inhaler that simplifies inhaler technique.

Motor-driven nebulizers do not result in greater bronchodilation than that achieved with pressurized aerosol canisters.[160] Drug delivery by motor-driven nebulizers has been considered more efficacious because the patient inhales a relatively large concentration of drug from the nebulizer. For example, the dose of albuterol added to the nebulizer is 5 mg, which is 56 times the dose generated by the pressured canister (90 μg). However, perhaps 15% to 20% of the drug is actually nebulized during inspiration, and only 10% of the nebulized dose reaches the bronchi.[160] Thus, the dose delivered to the lung from the nebulizer may be similar to that given by a pressurized aerosol canister. The delivery system can cause nosocomial infections also. On the other hand, motor-driven nebulizers formalize the process of drug administration and do not require the patient to learn correct inhalation technique, as is needed for the metered dose inhalers.[160]

In summary, the physician should become familiar with a few bronchodilators and emphasize proper inhalation technique. In some patients, spacer devices or breath-activated units improve drug delivery. Physicians should recheck the patient's inhaler technique periodically because errors are made frequently that impede drug delivery and some patients use delivery devices improperly. The goal should be to have the patient use β_2-adrenergic agonists intermittently rather than on a scheduled basis.

As useful as the beta agonists are, even combined with cromolyn, inhaled corticosteroids, theophylline, and nedocromil, they are not capable of controlling severe asthma. This limitation must be kept in mind, and oral corticosteroids should be used when appropriate.

Corticosteroids

Overview

Corticosteroids are the most effective drugs in the treatment of asthma. Parenteral corticosteroids are indicated for the treatment of status asthmaticus, but objective evidence of improvement in flow rates and FEV_1 requires approximately 12 hours of therapy.[161] In some patients, beneficial effects occur by 6 hours.[162] Short-term outpatient administration decreases the incidence of return visits to emergency medical facilities.[163,164] Chronic administration prevents work and school absenteeism, disabling wheezing, and episodes of status asthmaticus or respiratory failure in severe asthmatics. A double-blind study in acutely ill children supports efficacy as well.[165] Because of their potentially serious side effects, their systemic use is advised only when other measures have not provided sufficient control of acute or chronic symptoms. Their indiscriminate employment in mild asthma is not indicated. Failure to use them when indicated, however, may result in unwarranted morbidity and mortality. In life-threatening asthma, corticosteroids are essential, but because of their delayed onset of action, they cannot replace other necessary emergency measures including β-adrenergic agonists, patent airway, and oxygen. Patients who are still wheezing after initial emergency treatment with beta agonists are in status asthmaticus and should receive systemic corticosteroids.

TABLE 22-7. *Antiinflammatory effects of corticosteroids in asthma*

Reduces symptoms (cough, wheezing, dyspnea) from asthma

Decreases mucus production

Improves oxygenation and time to discharge after status asthmaticus

Reduces recidivism to emergency departments after acute therapy

Can prevent deterioration leading to status asthmaticus

Reduces need for β_2-adrenergic agonists or theophylline

Improves morning expiratory flow rates and intraday variation

Prevents the late bronchoconstrictive response to aerosol allergen provocation

Modestly lessens nonspecific bronchial hypersensitivity

Reduces recovery of eosinophils and mast cells in bronchoalveolar lavage

Reduces eosinophilic infiltration in the respiratory epithelium and lamina propia

Reduces nos. of activated (CD25+ and HLA-DR+) lymphocytes in bronchoalveolar lavage

Reduces ex vivo bronchoalveolar (macrophage) cell synthesis of leukotriene B_4 and thromboxane B_2

Reduces bronchoalveolar lavage cells expressing mRNA for IL-4 and IL-5 with an increase in interferon gamma–positive cells

Increases the ratio of ciliated columnar cells to goblet cells in the bronchial epithelium

Increased nos. of intraepithelial nerves

Regenerates bronchial epithelium

IL, interleukin.

Patients who must be hospitalized for exacerbations of asthma should receive systemic corticosteroids immediately without attempting to determine if continued β-adrenergic agonists (or theophylline) will work without systemic corticosteroids.

Oral corticosteroids are of value in prevention of repeated emergency room visits or office visits in acutely ill patients who respond to β-adrenergic agonists and do not require hospitalization. A dosage regimen of 30 to 50 mg each morning of prednisone for 5 to 7 days often is effective in adults, and in children 1 to 2 mg/kg of prednisone is necessary, often the latter dosage for the first few days.

The exact mode of action of corticosteroids in asthma is not known, but it probably results from their many antiinflammatory effects (Table 22-7). Reduction of bronchial mucosal edema, mucus accumulation, suppression of the inflammatory response, and stabilization of membrane (vascular and lysosomal) permeability are some of their known effects that may relieve asthma. Corticosteroids stimulate lipomodulin, which inhibits the action of phospholipase A_2. This action of corticosteroids reduces the availability of arachidonic acid for production of its bioactive metabolites such as leukotrienes, prostaglandins, and thromboxanes. Mast cell release of lyso-PAF, which is also phospholipase A_2 dependent, is inhibited.[166] Corticosteroids restore β-adrenergic responses in bronchi and have been shown to decrease extraneuronal uptake of catecholamines. They also suppress IgE-dependent late-phase allergen reactions, and 1 week of oral corticosteroids can inhibit the early response to allergen. Corticosteroids potentiate the β-adrenergic–stimulated increases in activity of adenylate cyclase and subsequent increases in cAMP. Alone, they have not been shown conclusively to elevate cAMP levels. Corticosteroids inhibit the proliferation of mucosal-type mast cells but do not inhibit mast cell mediator release.[167]

In addition to their therapeutic importance, corticosteroids may be useful as a diagnostic tool. Often, it is helpful to document the extent of reversibility of a patient's signs and symptoms to establish whether the basic underlying process is asthma or irreversible obstructive airways disease. Therapeutic doses of corticosteroids for 7 to 14 days should significantly reverse the airway obstruction of asthma in most patients but results in little or no reversal in most patients with chronic bronchitis or emphysema. The initial therapeutic dose of prednisone in children is 2 mg/kg/day and in adults is from 40 to 80 mg/day.

Numerous analogues of cortisone and hydrocortisone are available. Varying their chemical configurations has conferred changes in duration of action, but more specifically, has resulted in a lessening of their mineralocorticoid effect. Unfortunately, the development of the newer synthetic analogues has not resulted in any preparation with only antiinflammatory properties without the concomitant undesirable effects on glucose and protein metabolism. Therefore, serious side effects can result from prolonged use of high doses of any of these preparations. The relative dose equivalents of available corticosteroids are shown in Table 22-8.

Despite the many possible side effects resulting from corticosteroids, absolute contraindications to their use, such as herpes simplex ophthalmicus, are rare. In the past, varicella infection constituted an absolute contraindication, but failure to maintain the current dose in a severe asthmatic patient who develops varicella may lead to worsening of asthma or to death.[168] Most of the serious side effects result from the prolonged use of large doses of corticosteroids. In most patients, chronic maintenance doses are relatively low, usually 2.5 to 15 mg of prednisone or its equivalent per day. Frequently, chronic patients with asthma who require corticosteroids may be managed adequately using an alternate-day prednisone schedule, which is clearly the therapy of choice. This schedule helps further reduce significant side effects. Long-term studies of steroid-dependent asthmatic patients accordingly have shown predominantly tolerable side effects, with few exceptions.

To minimize side effects, use these drugs for the shortest time necessary to achieve the clinical goal. A 3- to 5-day course of prednisone in therapeutic doses may be sufficient to reverse an occasional acute episode of asthma that has not responded adequately to the common modes of therapy. If oral corticosteroids are required for longer periods, abrupt discontinuation may be followed by the return of acute symptoms. Until significant clearing of signs and symptoms of asthma occur, prednisone or the equivalent should be administered at a steady dosage rate over the first 1 to 2 weeks. In a small group of patients who have abruptly

TABLE 22-8. *Relative dose equivalents of corticosteroids*

Corticosteroids	Equivalent antiinflammatory dose (mg)
Short-Acting	
Hydrocortisone	20
Prednisone	5
Prednisolone	5
Methylprednisolone	4
Intermediate-Acting	
Triamcinolone	4
Long-Acting	
Betamethasone	0.6
Dexamethasone	0.75

discontinued corticosteroids after prolonged use, a withdrawal syndrome may occur, consisting of malaise, emotional lability, myalgia, and low-grade fever.

In patients requiring maintenance oral therapy, the lowest possible dose compatible with adequate control of symptoms should be used, and there should be use of inhaled corticosteroids as well. The doses of prednisone usually needed to control asthma do not result in activation of peptic ulcers[169,170] or tuberculosis.[171] The incidence rate of peptic ulceration in users of oral corticosteroids is either the same as in nonusers (0.8%) or has a 1% greater frequency rate (1.8%).[169] The clinical importance of this doubling of the risk is uncertain. The incidence of peptic ulcers becoming manifest in corticosteroid-treated patients is so low as to call into question the importance of the association.[171] Thus, ulcer regimens or antituberculosis treatment are not indicated routinely. Notice that the chronic use of alternate-day or low-dose daily steroids has not been shown to be associated with an increased risk of infections, including tuberculosis.[171] In every patient requiring chronic oral corticosteroid therapy, however, follow-up surveillance is necessary for early detection and management of possible side effects.[172]

Annual ophthalmologic examinations to check for cataracts are recommended. In children, an accurate record of growth is indicated.

Supraphysiologic doses of systemic corticosteroids may be associated with loss of trabecular and cortical bone. The occurrence of osteopenia is not inevitable in all patients ingesting prednisone for prolonged periods.[173] In a group of patients with severe corticosteroid-dependent asthma who had been treated with prednisone an average of nearly 10 years, only 4 of 21 patients had cortical thickness below 2 standard deviations from normal, and only 1 patient had vertebral fractures. For those patients, aged 47 to 73 years, whose prednisone was administered as a single morning dose or on an alternate-day regimen, the incidence of vertebral fractures was not different from the age-matched population. In Caucasian or Asian patients with a family history of osteopenia or in selected other patients, the addition of therapy to increase calcium absorption has been recommended by some investigators. Long-term prospective studies with assessment of vertebral bone densities are needed so conclusions regarding therapy can be made.[174]

Because part of the corticosteroid-induced osteopenia may be attributable to decreased calcium absorption from the gastrointestinal tract, parathyroid hormone secretion may increase. To prevent the increased parathyroid hormone secretion, giving calcium or vitamin D or its active metabolites may be considered. Currently, data do not demonstrate the benefit of these measures in ambulatory corticosteroid-dependent asthmatic patients. Before initiating high-dose calcium or vitamin D supplementation, calcium levels in urine collected over a 24-hour period should be obtained. If urinary calcium is not elevated, calcium carbonate (40% calcium) can be administered as three 650-mg tablets per day such that 500 to 1000 mg of elemental calcium is available (1950 mg calcium carbonate $\times$ 0.4 = 780 mg calcium). Adequate calcium should be consumed in the diet, and calcium concentrations in urine should be obtained every 6 to 12 months thereafter to avoid calcium or vitamin D poisoning. Calcium supplementation (1 g daily) in patients receiving a median prednisone dosage of 15 mg daily reduced the urinary hydroxyproline–creatinine ratio, which is an indirect measure of bone resorption.[174] In that serum alkaline phosphatase and osteocalcin (bone gla protein)—indirect measures of bone formation—did not decrease, it was thought that bone mass could increase. Radiologic confirmation was not provided, however.[175]

Measures to correct abnormalities in mineral metabolism induced by oral corticosteroids require cooperative patients and physician expertise to avoid toxicity. Their use cannot be recommended for all patients receiving oral corticosteroids until data demonstrate utility in ambulatory asthmatic patients. Estrogen replacement therapy has proven of value in preventing bone loss in postmenopausal women and can be administered. Regular gynecologic examinations are necessary. Prevention of osteopenia is of paramount importance and should begin early since bone mass increases until about 45 years of age (or earlier) and then declines over years. Exercise, lack of sedentary lifestyles, avoidance of cigarette smoking, or overuse of thyroxine in euthyroid or possibly hypothyroid patients are some additional factors to address in terms of bone formation. In addition, adequate calcium intake of 1000 mg daily is advisable. Oral corticosteroids, if necessary long term, should be administered as alternate-day therapy with short-acting agents such as prednisone or methylprednisolone. Split daily doses should be avoided in stable ambulatory patients. Maximal dosage inhaled corticosteroids should be used. Patients with established osteoporotic fractures may require bisphonates, fluorides, estrogens, and calcium supplementation.

A potentially serious side effect from corticosteroids is suppression of the hypothalamic-pituitary–adrenal (HPA) axis. This results in an impaired ability to tolerate stress, and for this reason patients must receive increased doses of corticosteroids during stressful situations such as surgery, infectious illness, and even exacerbations of asthma. The extent of suppression, however, varies from patient to patient. The time required for a return to normal HPA activity after discontinuation of corticosteroids also varies and is unpredictable. In a rare patient, inability of the HPA axis to respond to stress may continue for up to 1 year after the cessation of therapy, and in other patients, normal HPA reactivity may persist despite their taking corticosteroids for as long as 10 years. Fortunately, surgery with modern anesthesia techniques rarely results in maximal adrenal output of about 300 mg cortisol.[176]

Maximal doses of inhaled corticosteroids on a daily basis should be used where indicated. To minimize the occurrence of adverse side effects from oral corticosteroids, the use of alternate-day prednisone therapy is recommended. The total daily dose of a short-acting corticosteroid preparation (prednisone, prednisolone) should be taken in the morning every 48 hours, as long as underlying airways obstruction is controlled adequately. Daily prednisone is indicated in the acutely ill patient. Often, a short course (5 to 7 days) of daily prednisone is required to control asthma. Alternate-day prednisone therapy should be considered for patients who still require corticosteroids after 2 weeks of daily medication of severe asthma. Most patients obtain adequate control of symptoms by this form of therapy with little deterioration in pulmonary function on the alternate day.[177]

Several studies confirm that alternate-day prednisone therapy has resulted in prevention or amelioration of some manifestations of Cushing's syndrome. The benefit is not caused simply by a reduction in the dose of prednisone. If patients who have been taking daily prednisone receive the identical or triple the dose every 48 hours, side effects are reduced. Specifically, amelioration of the following adverse effects of daily steroid administration has been reported when alternate-day prednisone is used: cushingoid facies and obesity, easy bruisability, poor wound healing, hypertension, glucose intolerance, inhibition of linear growth, and personality disturbances.[178] Delayed hypersensitivity is preserved with the alternate-day steroids, and the patient is not at increased risk of infection.[171] Antibody production is preserved on alternate-day and even on daily prednisone therapy. Suppression of the HPA axis is reduced greatly with the alternate-day prednisone schedule; however, although adrenal reserve is normal in most patients receiving even large doses of alternate-day prednisone, the metyrapone test may give abnormal results in some who are taking alternate-day steroids. Thus, in the presence of major stress (surgery, acute myocardial infarction), supplemental doses of corticosteroids should be administered immediately (100 mg hydrocortisone intravenously or intramuscularly immediately and every 8 hours). This dosage prevents complications from uncontrolled asthma but does not produce poor scar formation, decreased tensile strength, or wound infections.

Although major side effects are not observed usually in patients receiving less than 20 mg of prednisone daily (administered as a single morning dose), the physician should convert to an alternate-day regimen. One common mistake is to convert too rapidly. If a patient has been receiving split doses of prednisone on a daily basis, the first goal should be to establish control of the severe asthma with a single morning dose of prednisone. Once the patient is stable, tripling the daily dose on alternate days may be adequate for controlling the disease. Close patient supervision is essential during this critical changeover period. Some patients do not tolerate alternate-day steroid therapy, even with large doses of prednisone, and should be managed on daily steroids using a single morning prednisone dose. The half-life of prednisolone is about 200 minutes in patients requiring daily prednisone or alternate-day prednisone, and other pharmacokinetic parameters are similar.[179]

Parenteral Corticosteroids

Intravenous corticosteroids generally are employed for status asthmaticus. Hydrocortisone (Solu-Cortef), methylprednisolone (Solu-Medrol), prednisolone (Hydeltrasol), and dexamethasone (Decadron) are available.

Collins and coworkers[180] conducted a study to determine the fate of intravenously injected hydrocortisone hemisuccinate in acutely asthmatic and nonasthmatic subjects given varying loading doses. In both groups, peak plasma concentrations occurred at the same time, and the plasma half-life was identical. Peak plasma concentrations occurred within 60 minutes, and the half-life of a 4-mg/kg dose was 125 minutes. A dosage of 4 mg/kg every 4 to 6 hours is sufficient in status asthmaticus. When using large doses of hydrocortisone, replacing potassium is important. The serum glucose should be monitored.

Aerosol Corticosteroids

Topically active corticosteroids have been used by inhalation for the outpatient treatment of asthma, including beclomethasone dipropionate, dexamethasone, triamcinolone acetonide, flunisolide, budesonide, and fluticasone. Budesonide is not approved for use in the United States, but is an effective corticosteroid. Beclomethasone dipropionate has been used extensively in the United States since 1976, and has been employed worldwide since 1972. It is administered by metered aerosol (42 µg per inhalation). A beclomethasone dipropionate preparation available outside of the United States contains 250 µg per inhalation. The latter is given two to four times daily. The patient should understand completely how to inhale these drugs. Swallowing the equivalent amount of drug has been shown not to produce the desired results that are seen when the aerosol treatment is used correctly. The patient should expire to FRC, then breathe slowly up to TLC as the aerosol is delivered. The patient ideally should hold the breath for 8 to 10 seconds at the end of the deep inspiration. This is essential to ensure that the inhaled corticosteroid reaches the bronchi. Spacer devices can help as well.

When airway obstruction from asthma is severe, inhaled corticosteroids (or β-adrenergic agonists) may cause additional bronchial irritation, and asthma may become worse. In this situation, it is advisable to treat the patient with an adequate dose of oral corticosteroids. This may require doses of prednisone such as 40 mg daily for 1 week or more in adult patients. The recommended initial doses of beclomethasone dipropionate are three to four inhalations twice daily in children and up to ten inhalations bid in adults. Many adults are controlled with approximately one half this maximal dose. No suppression of the HPA axis as evaluated by diurnal cortisol levels, intravenous metyrapone tests, and intravenous corticotropin–cortisol responses was seen when children received no greater than 400 µg/day.[181] When a dose higher than this was used, however, the metyrapone test result was abnormal in some children.[182] Several children being managed with alternate-day prednisone with doses of 20 mg or less can be weaned successfully to inhaled corticosteroid alone. Long-term alternate-day corticosteroid therapy may be associated with some significant side effects in themselves (small chance of cataracts and adverse effects on bone mass), and topical inhaled rather than systemic steroids seem to be a superior alternative.

Beclomethasone dipropionate, when used in doses exceeding 800 µg/day in adults, has been associated with some abnormalities in the HPA axis. As evidence of its minimal systemic corticosteroid effect, several patients who are able to reduce the dose of oral corticosteroid for control of asthma by using beclomethasone dipropionate have experienced exacerbations of nasal polyps, allergic rhinitis, and atopic dermatitis. This same result occurs with other aerosol corticosteroids.

The original prednisone dosage and the duration of corticosteroid therapy do not affect the efficacy of beclomethasone dipropionate or other inhaled corticosteroids. Oropharyngeal candidiasis occurs with sufficient frequency that it should be suspected in all patients who develop a sore throat during steroid aerosol therapy. Miconazole troches or nystatin (Mycostatin) oral suspension are effective therapy in most cases. Rarely, hoarseness has occurred, which often resolves with temporary discontinuation of the inhaled corticosteroid. The prednisone dose should be increased if aerosol therapy is stopped in this situation to prevent status asthmaticus.

Bronchial mucosa atrophy has not been described in patients who have used topical corticosteroids in recommended doses even for long term. Because of the absence of serious side effects and with the impressive array of antiinflammatory effects (see Table 22-7), primary monotherapy of asthma with inhaled corticosteroids is recommended. The physician should individualize the therapeutic options and verify that IgE-mediated triggering allergens are avoided. In newly diagnosed patients with mild asthma, 600 µg twice daily of budesonide was considered superior compared with inhaled 375 µg of terbutaline twice daily,[183] Such patients were treated for 2 years with this moderately high dose of budesonide and then received budesonide 400 µg/day or placebo.[184] Not surprisingly, patients who received budesonide have better asthma control (FEV_1, peak flow, and bronchial responsiveness) than patients who received the placebo. Patients who initially had received terbutaline improved after therapy with 1200 µg/day of budesonide.[184]

Improvements in the degree of bronchial hyperresponsiveness have been reported after use of inhaled corticosteroids.[185,186] Clinically important improvements occur with administration of effective doses of inhaled corticosteroids.[187] Some patients benefit by use of spacer devices to improve delivery to the distal airways.[188] Increases in asthma may first be recognized by coughing during use of inhaled corticosteroids. Often, a short course of oral corticosteroids stops any progression of symptoms of asthma and permits effective use of inhaled medications. Increasing the number of inhalations of inhaled corticosteroids may result in effective treatment since bronchial obstruction from worsening asthma interferes with delivery of inhaled medications to the periphery.

Many patients can be managed effectively and safely with inhaled corticosteroids given twice daily. β_2-adrenergic agonists can be used supplementally but not necessarily on a scheduled regimen. Exacerbations of asthma are treated with a short course of prednisone or increase in inhaled corticosteroid depending on severity. A topical corticosteroid's efficacy in managing asthma should be considered as well as its potency. Usually, the more potent medication is chosen if efficacy (maximum achievable effect) is comparable (Fig. 22-9).

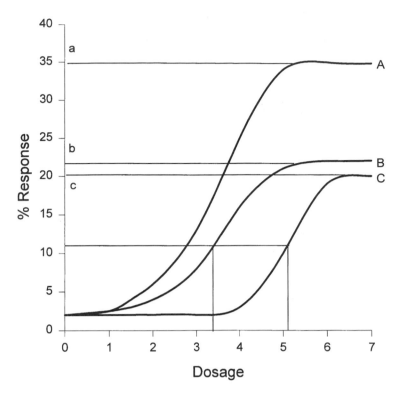

FIG. 22-9. Percent improvement from an inhaled corticosteroid is plotted on the y axis. Dosage is plotted on the x axis. The maximum achievable effect (efficacy) is greatest for drug A (35%) versus drugs B and C (about 20%, *points b* and *c*). Potency is illustrated by the fact that (on the x axis) a dose of 5.1 U of drug C is needed to achieve the same response as that produced by 3.4 U of drug B. Neither drug B nor C is as efficacious as drug A.

Depot Corticosteroids

Repository injectable preparations of corticosteroids are available but should be used only in rare cases, such as in malignant potentially fatal asthma where patients are almost unmanageable. They may be useful for better control of the patient with severe asthma who indiscriminately abuses inhaled or oral agents or for the noncompliant patient with life-threatening asthma. The preparations usually are associated with a profound and long-lasting HPA suppression.

Theophylline

Theophylline is not essential in managing asthma. The most important pharmacologic action of theophylline (1,3-dimethylxanthine) is bronchodilation. Other properties of the drug include central respiratory stimulation, inotropic and chronotropic cardiac effects, diuresis, relaxation of vascular smooth muscles, improvement in ciliary action, and reduction of diaphragmatic muscle fatigue.

Theophylline has been shown in vitro to increase cAMP concentrations by inhibiting phosphodiesterase, the enzyme that converts 3'5'-cAMP to 5'AMP. However, the inhibition of phosphodiesterase by theophylline was accomplished with concentrations that would be toxic in vivo; thus, theophylline's mechanism of action appears unclear but is unlikely to be attributable to phosphodiesterase inhibition. A possible explanation for bronchodilation from theophylline is adenosine antagonism.[189]

The 24-hour theophyllines (Uni-Phyl, Uni-DUR) offer greater convenience for patients. The apparent peak level occurred 13 hours after ingestion. Alternatively, Theo-Dur or Slo-Bid are reliable 12-hour preparations. Reductions in intestinal transit time by gastroenteritis or other diseases may prevent satisfactory absorption of theophylline. Conversely, food (fat) may increase absorption of some long-acting theophyllines.

Optimal bronchodilation from theophylline is a function of the serum concentration. Maximal bronchodilation usually is achieved with concentrations between 8 and 20 µg/mL. Some patients achieve adequate clinical improvement with serum theophylline levels at 5 µg/mL or even lower. The explanation for this phenomenon is that the bronchodilator effect of theophylline, as measured by percentage increase in FEV_1, is related to and fairly closely dependent on the logarithm of the serum concentration.[190] A dose-related improvement in pulmonary function was reported in six patients. The mean improvement in FEV_1 was 19.7% with theophylline concentration at 5 µg/mL, 30.9% at 10 µg/mL, and 42.2% at 20 µg/mL. Two graphical presentations of these data are shown in Figure 22-10. At these concentrations, improvement in pulmonary function occurs in linear fashion with the log of the theophylline concentration. However, using an arithmetic scale on the abscissa, improvement in pulmonary function occurs in a

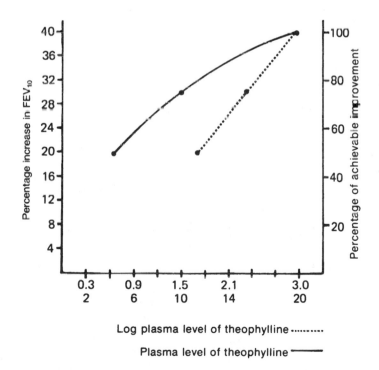

FIG. 22-10. Percentage of increase in forced expiratory volume in 1 second ($FEV_{1.0}$) is plotted against increasing concentration of theophylline. The log of the corresponding theophylline concentration is plotted on an arithmetic scale.

hyperbolic manner. Thus, although continued improvement occurs with increasing serum concentrations, the incremental increase with each larger dose decreases. Approximately 50% of the improvement in FEV_1 that is achievable with a theophylline concentration of 20 µg/mL is reached with concentration of 5 µg/mL and 75% of the improvement is reached with a concentration of 10 µg/mL.

Toxic effects of theophylline include nausea, vomiting, palpitation, agitation, seizures, and arrhythmias. In a retrospective study of 47 hospitalized adults, primarily older than 50 years of age, evidence of toxicity was less common in the range of 15 to 25 µg/mL than for over 25 µg/mL.[191] At a concentration of over 25 µg/mL, toxic reactions occurred in 11 of 14 patients. Life-threatening forms of theophylline toxicity, such as seizures, may occur without previous manifestations of toxicity such as nausea, tremulousness, or vomiting.[192] Seizures may take place with a theophylline level of 25 µg/mL.[192] High doses of theophylline cannot be maximally and safely used without determinations of serum concentration levels. A rare patient who is sensitized to the ethylenediamine base may show allergic reactions (urticaria or contact dermatitis) from aminophylline, and should be managed with 100% anhydrous theophylline preparations. Fortunately, this type of allergic reaction is rare.

Ninety percent of theophylline is metabolized through hepatic pathways (cytochromes P-450 and $P_1 450$), and 10% is excreted by the kidneys. Table 22-9 lists recommended initial doses of theophylline or aminophylline to be used during inpatient management. Table 22-10 lists some of the many factors that may alter the clearance of theophylline. Steady-state theophylline calculations have been published.[193]

Theophylline is valuable in treating mild to moderate asthma and may be well tolerated if peak concentrations are from 8 to 15 µg/mL. Compared with inhaled β-adrenergic agonists administered with inhaled corticosteroids, theophylline may add no apparent additional benefit.[194,195] Further, a metaanalysis of 13 studies on the treatment acute asthma did not reveal a benefit of aminophylline over adrenergic agonists.[196]

A greater measure of safety as determined by the therapeutic index may occur when other xanthines are used such as enprofylline[197] or bamiphylline.[198] However, these drugs are not available in the United States.

TABLE 22-9. *Recommended initial doses of aminophylline intravenously for status asthmaticus**

Patient population	Loading dose[†] (mg/kg over 20 min)	Maintenance (mg/kg/h)
Children 1–12 y	6	1.00
Adolescents 12–16 y	5.6	0.60
Adult (nonsmokers) <60 y	5.6	0.50
Congestive heart failure or COPD	5.6	0.25[‡]
Hepatic disease	5.6	0.25[‡]
Adults >60 y	5.6	0.25[‡]

COPD, chronic obstructive pulmonary disease.
*Calculated per ideal body weight, although use is controversial.
†Must be reduced or not given if previously ingested theophylline preparations still are being absorbed in gastrointestinal tract, resulting in detectable serum concentrations.
‡Clearance of theophylline may be so slow that avoidance of theophylline may be advisable.

TABLE 22-10. *Factors altering theophylline clearance*

Increased clearance	Decreased clearance
Active smoking (tobacco or marijuana)	Cor pulmonale
	Congestive heart failure
Passive smoking (tobacco)	Hepatic disease
High-protein, low-carbohydrate diet	Shock or critically ill state
	Pneumonia
Phenytoin*	Macrolide antibiotics (erythromycin,† troleandeomycin)
	Cimetidine
	Carbamazepine
	Ciprofloxacin
	Upper respiratory infections (viral)
	Age older than 60 y
	Fever
	Low-protein, high-carbohydrate diet

*Theophylline can inhibit phenytoin absorption.
†After 6 d of treatment.

Cromolyn

Cromolyn sodium (Intal) was shown to be effective in preventing bronchospasm from inhaled antigen in 1967.[199] It has been used in the United States since 1973 and has a high therapeutic index in contrast to theophylline. Cromolyn is a derivative of khellin, an active principle obtained from crude extracts of seeds from an eastern Mediterranean plant, *Ammi visnaga*. The drug is not well absorbed by the gastrointestinal tract, but when inhaled, approximately 8% is absorbed systemically. The unchanged drug is excreted in the urine and bile. It is available as a metered dose inhaler containing 112 or 200 actuations or by nebulized aerosol inhalation. Ampules contain 20 mg of cromolyn in 2 mL of diluent. Intal (Fisons) can be added to a nebulizer containing a β-adrenergic agonist for inhalation.

Cromolyn possesses no intrinsic bronchodilating or antihistaminic properties. In vitro studies have shown that cromolyn inhibits IgE mediated histamine release from mast cells and does not inhibit the antigen–antibody reaction on the mast cell. Cromolyn has been reported to increase cAMP levels by reducing calcium transport across mast cell membranes, which inhibit calcium-dependent antigen-induced mediator release.[200,201] In lymphocytes, cromolyn possibly inhibits phosphodiesterase activity, which could also indirectly increase levels of cAMP.[202] Concentrations of cromolyn were high, however. It has been shown experimentally that cromolyn inhibits the immediate and late reactions that follow bronchial provocation with antigen. Cromolyn inhibits the reduction in FEV_1 that occurs with exercise or cold air exposure during eucapnic hyperpnea. These experiments suggest that cromolyn may exert a protective effect on the bronchi on a nonimmunologic basis. Similarly, cromolyn inhalation abrogates sulfur dioxide–induced bronchospasm. Cromolyn has been demonstrated to decrease bronchial hyperreactivity to histamine and methacholine in children with asthma.

Cromolyn is considered an antiinflammatory agent for use in asthma because it blocks immediate and late bronchial reactions to inhaled allergens. The efficacy of cromolyn, however, is not apparent in all patients with asthma, and if improvement is not apparent after 2 months of use with concomitant clinical stabilization and reduced need for other medications, its use should be discontinued. Cromolyn is also effective in patients with exercise-induced asthma, and frequently but not exclusively benefits the atopic individual who must experience unavoidable animal exposure. When β_2-adrenergic agonists are not controlling asthma adequately, a trial of cromolyn may increase symptoms when bronchospasm is present. After improvement with prednisone, cromolyn is started; prednisone is tapered and terminated, and the efficacy of cromolyn is evaluated. It is important to recognize an adequate clinical response. Cromolyn is helpful in some cases of industrial asthma, primarily in the diagnosis of occupational asthma.

Serious, significant side effects from the use of cromolyn are nonexistent, but mild irritation of the tracheobronchial tree with slight bronchospasm may occur. The prior use of an inhaled sympathomimetic is helpful in relieving this minor side effect. Prolonged cromolyn use has reduced symptoms of asthma and the need for β-adrenergic agonists.[203] This does not occur in all patients.

Nedocromil

Nedocromil (Tilade) is a nonsteroid antiinflammatory drug that experimentally inhibits both early and late bronchial responses to allergen. Nedocromil inhibits afferent nerve transmission from respiratory nerves so that substance P may be limited in its effect as a bronchoconstrictor or trigger of cough. It also can decrease nonspecific bronchial hyperresponsiveness.[204] In vitro, nedocromil has been demonstrated to have antieosinophil activity as well as inhibiting activation of neutrophils, mast cells, macrophages, and platelets. Nedocromil is administered by metered dose inhaler with each actuation delivering 1.75 mg. The canister contains 112 inhalations, and the initial dosage for children ages 12 years and older and adults is two inhalations four times daily. The dosage may be reduced as improvement (cessation of coughing) occurs. Some adverse effects include unpleasant (bitter) taste and slight temporary yellowing of teeth from the inhaler contents.

Nedocromil is efficacious in patients with mild to moderate asthma[204,205] and in patients who require inhaled corticosteroids.[206]

Anticholinergics

Anticholinergic agents have been suggested for asthma to diminish cyclic guanosine monophosphate concentrations and to inhibit vagal efferent pathways. Bronchodilation then could occur in a multiplicative fashion when anticholinergics are administered with β-adrenergic agonists. Atropine and analogues such as ipratropium bromide have been shown to possess bronchodilating properties. Combination therapy of ipratropium bromide (Atrovent; 36 μg four times daily by aerosol) with theophylline and inhaled fenoterol, a β2-adrenergic agonist, resulted in statistically significant increases in flow rates compared with theophylline and fenoterol combined.[207] No increase in side effects occurred. Unfortunately, despite improved flow rates with the three-drug combination, there was no decrease in the number or severity of episodes of asthma during the study period. Some studies show no benefit from inhaled atropine (3.2 mg nebulized twice) compared with metaproterenol (15 mg nebulized twice) in acute asthma,[208] whereas another anticholinergic bronchodilator, glycopyrrolate, 2 mg, proved as beneficial as metaproterenol, 15 mg.[209] Monotherapy with anticholinergic bronchodilators is unlikely to replace sympathomimetic agents in acute asthma, in that the onset of action is slower than with β-adrenergic agonists. Why currently available anticholinergic bronchodilators are not especially successful in asthma management compared with that of COPD is not certain, aside from relative influence of cholinergic tone in bronchi in both conditions.

Smooth muscles have muscarinic (cholinergic) receptors of several types including M_1, M_2, and M_3. Smooth muscle contraction in large airways is primarily from M_3 stimulation, whereas in smaller airways M_1 and M_3 receptors are present. Vagal nerve–induced bronchoconstriction is mediated by M_1 receptors.[210]

Zileuton

Zileuton is a 5-lipoxygenase inhibitor that has been demonstrated to reduce asthma symptoms and increase baseline FEV_1 by 13.4%.[211] The drug is administered orally from 1.6 to 2.4 g/day. Zileuton is not approved for use in the United States but supports the notion that inhibiting the potent bronchoconstrictor LTD_4 is useful as a nonsteroidal antiinflammatory modality. Zileuton decreases urinary LTE_4 39% as a marker of suppressing the production of LTD_4.[211]

Nonspecific Measures

Protection From Meteorologic Factors

Increasing air pollution is a known worldwide health hazard. It is considered to be a major causative factor in certain conditions such as bronchitis, emphysema, and lung cancer. Urban surveys have shown adequately the deleterious effect of pollution on patients with chronic cardiopulmonary disease. The alarming morbidity and mortality rates resulting from thermal inversions in cities in the United States and elsewhere dramatize the seriousness of stagnating pollution. The patient with asthma, because of inherent bronchial hyperreactivity, may be more vulnerable to air pollution.

Industrial smog results from incomplete combustion of fossil fuels, and it consists of sulfuric acid, oxides of sulfur, nitrogen dioxide, carbon monoxide, and particulate material. Photochemical smog occurs from the action of ultraviolet radiation on nitrogen oxides or hydrocarbons from automobile exhaust. Ozone is the major constituent of photochemical smog.

Other meteorologic factors such as sudden changes in temperature, increases in relative humidity, and increasing or decreasing barometric pressure also may aggravate asthmatic symptoms in some patients. It is impossible to protect patients from these changes entirely. Why weather changes should aggravate asthma is not completely understood.

The breathing of cold, dry air is a potent stimulus that precipitates symptoms in many patients. The use of face masks may be beneficial in these patients.

Home Environment

Certain controls of the internal environment of the home (especially the bedroom) are beneficial. Extremes of humidity can adversely affect the patient with asthma; the optimal humidity should range from 40% to 50%. Low humidity dries the mucous membranes and becomes an irritative factor.

Most patients are benefited by air conditioning, but in a few patients, the cold air may increase symptoms. The reduction in spore counts in air-conditioned homes in part results from simply having the windows closed to reduce the influx of outdoor spores.[212]

Mechanical devices that purify circulating air may be helpful but are not essential. Conventional air filters such as those in a typical furnace vary in their effectiveness but in general remove only particles larger than 5 μm (e.g., pollens). Many inhalant particles, such as dust mites, fumes, smoke, some fungal spores, some rat urinary proteins, some cat allergen, bacteria, and viruses are smaller than 5 μm. Submicronic particles of ragweed have been identified that also would not be filtered.[213] Efficient air-cleaning devices include the electrostatic precipitator, which attracts particles of any size by high-voltage plates, nonelectronic precipitators useful for forced air heating systems, more efficient furnace filters, and air cleaners that use a high-efficiency particulate accumulator filtering system. The latter have helped reduce clinical symptoms, which is the primary requirement of any filtering system.[214] In general, an animal in the home environment produces too great a quantity of dander to be removed or reduced by air cleaners. Sensitive immunoassays have documented presence of urinary protein (*Mus* d I) from rodents in indoor environment air samples. Similar findings occur with cockroach fecal particles or saliva (*Bla* g 1). Control measures are difficult in such conditions but should be encouraged. It is not possible to reduce indoor concentrations of house dust mite (*Der* p 1) to a mite-free level. Clinical benefit to dust mite–sensitive patients, however, occurs if some avoidance measures are instituted. The mattress, box spring, and pillow should be covered with special zippered covers. For comfort, encasings with an outer layer of cotton or polyester material are recommended. Venetian blinds should be cleaned regularly or not installed, and attention to other dust collection sites should be given. The value of ascaricides or tannic acid (to denature mite antigen) needs to be established.[215]

The presence of moist basements and crawl spaces may provoke acute or chronic symptoms in certain patients allergic to fungal spores. Dehumidification and more effective drainage are advised.

Smoking

Cigarette smoking must be discouraged in all patients and their family members. Its deleterious effects probably result from bronchial irritation and impairment of antibacterial defense mechanisms. Cigarette smoke has been shown to impair mucociliary transport and to inhibit alveolar macrophage phagocytosis.

Bronchial lavage specimens from smokers demonstrated a twofold reduction in elastase inhibitory activity compared with nonsmokers. This is consistent with a functional antiprotease deficiency, and although not clearly relevant to the pathogenesis of asthma, suggests a mechanism for production of emphysema from smoking. Conversion to low-tar, low-nicotine cigarettes should not be advised because smokers may vary their smoking patterns to maintain their usual nicotine levels.[216] Although many modalities have been tried to achieve cessation of smoking, the failure rate remains high in most studies. In general, slowly decreasing the number of cigarettes smoked per day has not resulted in smoking cessation. Patients with asthma who continue to smoke often require progressive increments in medication. Keeping a patient with asthma controlled with medication while the patient continues to smoke is not good practice of medicine. When emphysema occurs, episodes of asthma may be tolerated poorly, and may result in frequent hospitalizations or in respiratory failure.

Passive smoking by nonasthmatic subjects has been associated with statistically significant reductions in flow rates. This finding raises the possibility that some asthmatic patients may experience increased symptoms in smoke-filled office rooms or homes.

Exercise

The subjective and psychological value of physical conditioning, especially in children with asthma, may be a helpful adjunct in treatment. A unique feature of asthma is the occurrence of bronchospasm with exertion. Many children or adults may be discouraged by their inability to participate in sports or to withstand other normal exertional activities. These feelings of inferiority promote additional physical and psychological incapacitation. An exercise program, once asthma has been stabilized with appropriate therapy, results in a noticeable increase in physical capacities. This, in turn, instills a sense of accomplishment and competition, so desperately needed to uplift a person's self-image. Inhaled β-adrenergic agonists or inhaled cromolyn taken 15 to 30 minutes before exercise decreases postexercise bronchospasm. It is advisable to inquire about the patient's current exercise tolerance and participation in sports, because this is a good guide to overall therapy.

Drugs to Use Cautiously or to Avoid

Antidepressants of the MAO inhibitor class are not recommended, because these substances may induce a hypertensive crisis when taken with sympathomimetic drugs that are commonly used in the medical treatment of asthma. The tricyclic group of antidepressants are much less likely to produce this complication and can be used with asthma medications.

Narcotics such as morphine and meperidine, because of their respiratory depressive properties, are contraindicated during exacerbations of asthma. Moreover, morphine can activate mast cells to release histamine. Even mild sedatives and tranquilizers should be avoided because they also induce varying amounts of respiratory depression. Small doses of these drugs may be used cautiously in the outpatient treatment of asthma patients with anxiety symptoms. Asthma should not be considered primarily as an expression of an underlying emotional disturbance, and its diagnosis alone is not an indication for the use of these drugs.

Excessive use of hypnotics for sleep also must be discouraged. Nocturnal reductions in PO_2 occur regularly in normal and in patients with asthma. Status asthmaticus is an absolute contraindication for the use of sedatives or tranquilizers. In this situation, even small doses of these drugs may cause respiratory depression.

Drugs possessing anticholinesterase properties may potentiate wheezing. This results from their parasympathomimetic enhancing effect caused by the inhibition of acetylcholine catabolism. These drugs represent the primary drug treatment of myasthenia gravis; if asthma coexists, a therapeutic problem arises. When anticholinesterases are necessary, maximal doses of beta agonists and inhaled corticosteroids may be necessary. The addition of oral corticosteroids may be indicated for more adequate control of asthma, but in some patients myasthenic symptoms may initially worsen with addition of corticosteroids.[217]

Propranolol and other β-adrenergic blocking drugs have gained wide clinical use in the treatment of cardiac arrhythmias, angina, hypertension, asymmetric septal hypertrophy, after myocardial infarction, for thyrotoxicosis, and for migraine. These drugs exert blocking properties on both cardiac and pulmonary beta receptors. As a result of the effect on the latter, it may enhance or trigger wheezing in overt and latent asthmatic patients. The adrenergic receptors of the lung are predominantly β_2 in type, and they subserve bronchodilation. When these receptors are blocked, bronchoconstriction may result. Should propranolol or other β-adrenergic antagonists be required in a patient with asthma, cautious increasing of doses with close supervision is recommended. Acute bronchospasm has been associated with conjunctival instillation of beta antagonists (timolol) for glaucoma.[218]

Bronchospasm has been described even for betaxolol, a β_1-adrenergic antagonist, which is less likely to cause declines in FEV_1 than timolol.[219] Occasionally, parasympathomimetic agents such as pilocarpine administered in the conjunctival sac can cause bronchospasm.[219] Make certain that the patient with chronic asthma first is stabilized, such as with inhaled β-adrenergic agonists and corticosteroids, so that any possible effects from necessary ophthalmic drugs are minimized.

Angiotensin-converting enzyme inhibitors, especially captopril, have been associated with cough and asthma, even on the first dose.[220,221] Discontinuation of the angiotensin-converting enzyme inhibitor is associated with rapid resolution of symptoms. This class of drugs is not contraindicated in patients with asthma, but awareness of this adverse drug reaction is necessary.

Specific Measures

Allergic Asthma

Specific allergy management must be included in the treatment regimen of allergic asthma. When one allergen is the primary cause (e.g., animal dander) and it can be removed from the environment, symptomatic relief is achieved. Most allergic patients, however, are sensitive to more than one allergen, and many allergens cannot be removed completely. In adults, inhalant allergens are the most frequent causative agents. Foods are rarely the cause of asthma, except occasionally in children and infants and often are incriminated erroneously.[222]

Patients may attribute their respiratory symptoms to aspartame or monosodium glutamate when such associations are not justified. Exposure to sulfur dioxide from sodium or potassium metabisulfite used as an antioxidant in foods can cause acute respiratory symptoms in patients with asthma. However, patients with stable asthma who are managed by antiinflammatory medications are not affected significantly by metabisulfite.

Certain basic environmental controls in the house are advisable. Dacron (or hypoallergenic) pillows are preferred and should be enclosed in special zippered covers. Box springs and mattresses should be enclosed similarly.

Other aspects may be considered with regard to the environmental control in the home. Basement apartments, because of increased moisture, are most likely to have higher levels of airborne fungi and mite antigens. For the highly dust-allergic patient, electrostatic furnace filters should be used and maintained properly. In patients with perennial symptoms, it is generally advisable that pets (e.g., cats, dogs, and birds) be removed from the house if there are symptoms from contact of if there is a positive skin test reaction.

When environmental control is either impossible or insufficient to control symptoms, allergen immunotherapy should be included as a form of immunomodulation. Efficacy in asthma has been documented for pollens, dust mite, and *Cladosporium*.[150] Other than modest effects, immunotherapy with cat dander extracts has not been impressive in reducing symptoms.

Johnstone and Dutton,[223] in a 14-year prospective study of allergen immunotherapy of asthmatic children, have shown that 72% of the treated group were free of symptoms at 16 years of age compared with only 22% of the placebo group. Of greater importance was a significantly increased improvement rate in those receiving the highest tolerable dose of antigen.

Nonallergic Asthma

Treatment of nonallergic asthma primarily involves the judicious use of drug therapy.

Convincing evidence is available that virus-induced upper respiratory infections initiate exacerbations of asthma. Important agents for children from age 1 to 5 years include respiratory syncytial virus, parainfluenza virus, and rhinovirus; for older children and adults, influenza virus, parainfluenza virus, and rhinovirus are important. Adenovirus infection rarely acts to initiate asthma attacks.

Annual influenza vaccination should be administered according to the recommendations by the Centers for Disease Control for children and adults. Prompt treatment of secondary bacterial infections such as purulent bronchitis, rhinitis, or sinusitis is desirable. Pneumococcal vaccine can be administered to patients with chronic asthma, although pneumococcal pneumonia is an infrequent occurrence.

Aspirin-Sensitive Asthma

Treatment for aspirin-sensitive asthma is similar to that for the nonallergic type, except for patients in whom there is clinical and skin test evidence of contributing inhalant allergy. It is important to avoid aspirin and NSAIDs, which may also produce adverse reactions. Patients must be informed that numerous proprietary mixtures contain aspirin, and they must be certain to take no proprietary medication that contains acetylsalicylic acid. Acetaminophen may be used as a safe substitute for aspirin, and other salicylates such as sodium salicylate, choline salicylate, or salicylate can be taken safely. The ingestion of aspirin or NSAIDs by patients commonly causes acute bronchoconstriction. Another group includes patients who have urticaria, angioedema, or a severe reaction resembling anaphylaxis. Some physicians include both groups of patients as aspirin reactors, but others consider that the group in whom aspirin causes asthma differs from the group in whom urticaria, angioedema, or the anaphylactic type of reaction occurs.

The exact mechanism by which these patients become intolerant to aspirin and the other substances is not known. The relation that this intolerance bears to rhinitis, nasal polyposis, and asthma is also unknown. A property common to all of these substances is their antiinflammatory effect. Aspirin and NSAIDs inhibit cyclooxygenase, which metabolizes arachidonic acid into prostaglandins and thromboxanes. Compared with patients with asthma, patients with aspirin-sensitive asthma have increased baseline urinary concentrations of LTE_4, a marker of 5-lipoxygenase products. After aspirin ingestion, there is even greater increase in urinary LTE_4 concentrations, consistent with synthesis of the potent agonist LTD_4.

In aspirin-sensitive asthma, potentially dangerous drugs must be avoided. In some situations, provocative dose testing with either aspirin or NSAIDs may be carried out to confirm the diagnosis. The physician should be in attendance at all times because of the explosiveness and severity of these reactions. Pulmonary function parameters and vital signs should be measured. Aspirin should be administered in serial doubling doses, beginning with 3 or 30 mg.[224] If 650 mg of aspirin has been given and there is not a 20% fall in FEV_1, it is unlikely that aspirin is significant in the patient's condition. When test-dosing with tartrazine, FDC yellow dye no. 5, begin with 1 mg, 5 mg, 15 mg, and 29 mg every hour.[225] Tartrazine sensitivity is not found in the absence of aspirin sensitivity. The aspirin (or NSAID) challenge, as described earlier, may be dangerous and should not be done without a clear indication. The physician should be experienced in this type of challenge, and the patient should be fully informed about potential risks and benefits.

Serial test dosing with aspirin in patients with aspirin-sensitive asthma has been reported as a possible specific therapeutic modality. Patients received increasing doses of aspirin as follows every 2 hours: 3 or 30 mg, 60 mg, 100 mg, 150 mg, 325 mg, and 650 mg. When a decrease in FEV_1 of 25% was achieved, the "provoking" dose was repeated every 3 to 24 hours until no bronchospastic response occurred. Patients then were treated for 3 months with aspirin and as a group experienced fewer nasal symptoms, but unfortunately only 50% of patients had a reduction in asthma symptoms.[226] The use of prednisone and other antiasthmatic medications was not different after aspirin "desensitization." Thus, although it is possible to administer aspirin cautiously to patients with proven bronchospastic responses to aspirin, the subsequent administration of aspirin for a 3-month period did not alter the severity of asthma, with only a few exceptions. The administration of aspirin or NSAIDs to aspirin-sensitive patients should be reserved for selected patients when it is necessary to confirm the diagnosis of aspirin hypersensitivity or to administer aspirin or related drugs for another disease (such as rheumatoid arthritis) for which suitable alternatives are not satisfactory.

Potentially Fatal Asthma

The diagnosis of potentially fatal asthma (defined earlier) is helpful because it identifies high-risk patients who are more likely to die of asthma.[44,129] Despite aggressive intervention such as early and intensive pharmacotherapy, allergen avoidance, and psychological evaluation, the death rate was found to be 7.1%, which is much greater than the asthma death rate overall of 0.0017%.[44] Patients with potentially fatal asthma do not have an inexorably fatal condition in that stabilization and clinical improvement can occur if patients are managed effectively and are compliant with office appointments and other factors. Some patient factors that complicate care of potentially fatal asthma and result in noncompliance include psychological or psychiatric conditions (schizophrenia, bipolar disorder, personality disorders), chaotic dysfunctional families, denial, anger, lack of insight, ignorance, and child abuse by proxy. In the latter situation, some parents refuse to permit essential medications such as prednisone to be administered to their children despite previous episodes of respiratory arrest or repeated status asthmaticus. Some physician factors that can contribute to ineffectively managed patients and potential fatalities include (1) lack of appreciation for limitations in effectiveness of β-adrenergic agonists, theophylline, and the combination in increasingly severe asthma; (2) prednisonephobia; (3) failure to increase the dosage of prednisone or to administer prednisone when asthma exacerbations occur, such as during an upper respiratory tract infection; (4) lack of availability to the patient; (5) prescribing excessively demanding regimens; and (6) limited understanding of importance of a quiet chest on auscultation in severely dyspneic patients.

In survivors of episodes of nearly fatal asthma, defined as acute respiratory arrest or presentation with PCO_2 of at least 50 mm Hg or impaired level of consciousness, blunted perceptions of dyspnea were identified when patients were hospitalized but normalized.[227] Similarly, the ventilatory response to inhalation of carbon dioxide was not different from that of other patients with less severe asthma or nonasthmatic subjects.[227] However, abnormal respiratory responses to decreases in inspired oxygen were identified.[88] This group of patients with potentially fatal asthma does not demonstrate persistent physiologic abnormalities that identify these high-risk patients as having intrinsically precarious asthma.

Potentially fatal asthma can be treated with inhaled corticosteroids, inhaled β-adrenergic agonists, and usually alternate-day or rarely daily prednisone in compliant patients. It is advisable to institute the nonspecific general areas of care discussed previously. In contrast, with malignant potentially fatal asthma patients, depot corticosteroids can be administered after appropriate documentation in the medical record and informing the patient. As for other types of asthma, preventing fatalities and status asthmaticus involves understanding asthma, knowing the patient, instituting stepwise but effective therapy, establishing a physician–patient relationship, and emphasizing early therapy for increasingly severe asthma.

Personal peak flow monitoring does not help the unreliable, noncompliant patient. A personal peak flow monitor will possibly improve asthma if it can formalize antiasthma therapy in the otherwise noncompliant patient.

CLINICAL MANAGEMENT

Treatment of the Acute Asthmatic Attack

In mild attacks, the use of inhaled or oral bronchodilators every 4 to 6 hours may suffice. Inhaled β-adrenergic agonists can be administered by metered dose inhaler with or without a spacer device, depending on patient technique, or by nebulizer. Patients must be advised about their proper use and warned against overuse. However, aqueous epinephrine, 1:1000, is the drug of choice and can be given subcutaneously, and the dose should be repeated every 15 to 20 minutes if necessary. More than three doses are not recommended. Once the acute attack has subsided, regular and continuous use of bronchodilators should follow for at least 3 to 5 days. If bronchodilators have not been effective acutely, intravenous aminophylline should be considered, although several studies have not demonstrated benefit for aminophylline and β-adrenergic agonists in acute asthma management.[196] Aminophylline must be administered over a period of at least 20 minutes to avoid acute toxicity. The recommended quantities are listed in Table 22-9. When signs and symptoms of asthma are refractory to two or three injections of epinephrine or inhaled β-adrenergic agonists with or without aminophylline, status asthmaticus exists, a medical emergency requiring corticosteroids. Its treatment is presented later.

There is no advantage in using terbutaline instead of epinephrine in the acute treatment of asthma. Subcutaneous injections of equal doses of terbutaline and epinephrine (0.25 mg) have been reported to elicit equal bronchodilation of similar duration in asthmatic adults.[157] In the same study, it was shown that greater bronchodilation was seen with 0.50 mg of both drugs. In children, similar bronchodilation was found between these two agents, measuring PEFR only. Furthermore, terbutaline has been associated with peripheral vasodilation because of vascular smooth muscle relaxation. A reflex tachycardia then may occur, which may be associated with ventricular arrhythmias. Thus, in the cardiac patient with acute asthma, epinephrine can be administered, but the dose lowered. Inhaled β-adrenergic agonists also may be used.

Because tachyphylaxis to β-adrenergic agonists has been demonstrated in vivo and in vitro in some studies, concern has been expressed that prior administration of beta agonists may abrogate clinical response from current emergency treatment of asthma. Failure of a patient to improve suggests increasingly severe asthma (bronchospasm, hyperinflation, mucus plugging of airways), not tachyphylaxis to beta agonists.

With the introduction of newer β₂-adrenergic agonists that are available by nebulized aerosol, some physicians choose to administer these drugs (albuterol, fenoterol) by inhalation. There has been no advantage, aside from perhaps the convenience of administering albuterol by continuous nebulization compared with every 2- to 4-hour treatments. Some patients, however, are unable to take a deep enough inspiration to deliver inhaled drug effectively, and subcutaneous therapy should be administered in such patients. As airway obstruction increases and the patient approaches status asthmaticus, little improvement in flow rates or clinical status would be expected after beta agonists (delivered by any route) with or without theophylline. Corticosteroids are indicated in this situation. If the patient receives two treatments with inhaled bronchodilators or two subcutaneous injections of epinephrine or terbutaline and is able to be released, a short effective course of prednisone will help prevent a return to the office or emergency room. Follow-up care should be planned (see Table 22-5).

Treatment of Chronic Asthma

The management of chronic asthma entails a continuous broad control that must be tailored to each patient. Features of general management (as discussed earlier) must be included in the treatment regimen. Significant allergic factors are treated by environmental control combined with appropriately administered allergen immunotherapy. In each patient, secondary contributing factors must be evaluated and controlled as best as possible. Some of these factors include cessation of smoking, compliance with medications, and treatment of concurrent medical diseases such as sinusitis, COPD, congestive heart failure, and medication intolerance.

Many patients with chronic asthma require some form of chronic bronchodilator therapy. In those with mild intermittent symptoms, inhaled or oral preparations taken only when symptoms occur may suffice. A patient who has asthma only with infection should be instructed to begin bronchodilators and possibly inhaled corticosteroids at the first sign of symptoms of coryza. Some children who wheeze only with upper respiratory infections may need to use bronchodilators or inhaled corticosteroids regularly because of the chronicity of pulmonary function abnormalities in asthma and frequent viral upper respiratory syndromes in children. This point needs to be explained clearly to the parents to obtain maximal benefit from antiasthma medications. Patients with persistent symptoms clearly require chronic daily medication. For routine outpatient care, in patients older than 5 years of age, there is no evidence that nebulizers are more effective than metered dose inhalers used properly (with or without a spacer device). Some plan for regular therapy is indicated.

If the patient is a corticosteroid-dependent asthmatic with nocturnal symptoms, effective control of these symptoms may be achieved either by increasing the morning prednisone dose or by increasing the use of inhaled corticosteroid. A patient being treated with chronic bronchodilator therapy using either beta agonists, theophylline, or a combination of these agents may have an exacerbation of asthma. In these cases, additional β-adrenergic agonists may result in side effects. Additional theophylline may result in toxicity. As illustrated in Figure 22-10, on average, a theophylline concentration of 10 µg/mL corresponds approximately to 75% of the bronchodilator response of a concentration of 20 µg/mL. In a study of nine stable asthmatic patients, statistically significant increases in FEV_1 were recorded when serum theophylline was increased from 6.4 to 12.8 µg/mL, but further increases were not observed when serum levels were 19.2 µg/mL.[228] Short-term corticosteroid therapy may be the most appropriate therapy. If longer use of corticosteroids or more frequent courses are required, inhaled corticosteroids and alternate-day prednisone should be considered once the patient has improved (Table 22-11).

When chronic use of sympathomimetics does not provide adequate control of asthma or cannot be tolerated, cromolyn, nedocromil, or inhaled corticosteroids should be tried. When cromolyn is used properly in chronic asthma, certain patients show definite improvement. If added to sympathomimetic agents, the additional benefit from cromolyn may or may not be seen. When additional treatment is required in patients using inhaled bronchodilators, however, a 2-month trial of cromolyn should be recommended. If unsuccessful, inhaled corticosteroid, inhaled nedocromil, and finally, alternate-day oral corticosteroids should be administered.

TABLE 22-11. *Chronic asthma tips*

1. Appreciate limitations of inhaled β_2-adrenergic agonists, theophylline, and cromolyn

2. Check and improve inhaler technique, even in patients using spacer devices

3. Reassess the patient after initial therapy and change management if satisfactory improvement has not occurred.

4. Emphasize antiinflammatory therapy as opposed to scheduled β_2-adrenergic agonists (and possibly theophylline).

5. Address allergic factors from the home, school, and workplace. Consider referral to an allergist-immunologist.

6. Exclude allergic bronchopulmonary aspergillosis.

7. Treat patients with inhaled corticosteroids and β_2-adrenergic agonists; many patients can be managed successfully with these.

8. Avoid excessively demanding medication regimens.

9. Arrange for emergencies or deteriorations in respiratory status by involving the patient or family, if possible.

10. Use oral corticosteroids early to decrease asthma symptoms in a patient who has deteriorated after an upper respiratory tract infection rather than as a "last resort."

11. Identify patients with potentially fatal asthma.

Because of their frequent recurrence, surgical removal of nasal polyps should be considered only after local corticosteroid aerosol; when coupled with good medical and allergy management, this has been effective in decreasing obstruction and infection. Sinus surgery also should be considered when more conservative treatment (medical and allergic) has resulted in little or no success in preventing recurrent sinusitis.

Anxiety or depression may aggravate asthma. When these conditions are present, antidepressants may be necessary. Psychological or psychiatric evaluation should be obtained. Occasionally, it has been assumed by the lay public and some members of the medical profession that asthma is primarily an expression of an underlying psychological disturbance. This attitude has inappropriately prevented proper medical and allergy management in some patients. In most patients, psychiatric factors are of little significance in the cause of the disease. Psychological factors may be a contributory aggravating factor in asthma, but this should not be construed as evidence that asthma is predominantly psychological. Asthma is a chronic disease that also may be associated with significant impairment of physical and social activity. These factors in themselves may lead to the development of psychoneurotic signs and symptoms. Often, when asthmatic symptoms are brought under control, concomitant improvement of the psyche occurs. When schizophrenia and corticosteroid-dependent asthma coexist, the physician may become frustrated because of the patient's prednisone phobia, noncompliance with medications or appointments, and abuse of emergency medical facilities.[45,115] Depot methylprednisolone (Depo-Medrol) may be beneficial or lifesaving in patients if they keep their medical appointments.

The decision to use a peak flow meter should be kept in perspective. If the patient is under effective control of asthma such that exercise tolerance is satisfactory, nocturnal wheezing is absent or infrequent, emergency room visits are avoided, and symptoms of asthma are uncommon or mild, little benefit from a peak flow meter would occur. If the peak flow meter can emphasize patient compliance with antiasthma measures and medication, then its addition to a regimen is valuable. Some patients submit peak flow diaries consistent with their expectations or perceptions of asthma. Other patients do not contact their physicians or intensify therapy for peak flow rates of 30% of predicted, nullifying any value to the patient or physician. There may be discrepancies between measurements of PEFR and FEV_1, resulting in over or underestimation of the FEV_1.[229]

Treatment of Intractable Asthma

Intractable asthma refers to persistent, incapacitating symptoms that have become unresponsive to the usual therapy, including moderate doses of corticosteroids. These cases fortunately are few, and most involve patients with the nonallergic or mixed type of asthma. Their constant medical and nonmedical requirements are heavy social and financial burdens on their families. For these reasons, institutions that care for the intractable asthmatic have been funded. Originally, it was believed that mere removal of the patient from the home would be beneficial, but with the accumulated years of experience it has become evident that the problem is more complex. Many patients, despite their long-term residence in these institutions, with optimal medical and psychological management, persist with disabling symptoms and corticosteroid dependence. Some investigators suggest that intractable asthma, because of its unique resistance to the commonly employed asthma therapy, may represent a variant of asthma with superimposed pathophysiologic mechanisms. An example of the latter would be α_1-antitrypsin deficiency, which may present early in its course as asthma. Most patients with intractable asthma, however, are not deficient in antiproteases. Their lung disease may represent an inflammatory process with bronchial mucosal edema, mucus plugging of airway, and decreased lung compliance instead of a primary bronchospastic state. In cases of intractable asthma, a home visit by the physician sometimes is beneficial for the patient and for the physician. For example, the finding that an animal resides in the home of an atopic "intractable" asthmatic may explain the apparent failure of corticosteroids to control severe asthma.

Most cases of intractable asthma are those with severe corticosteroid-dependent asthma in whom adequate doses of corticosteroids have not been used, either by physician or patient avoidance. After initiation of appropriate doses of prednisone and clearing of asthma, many patients can be controlled with alternate-day prednisone and inhaled corticosteroids. Others require moderate to even high doses of daily prednisone for functional control. Fortunately, this latter group is small. Occasionally, they are patients with severe lung damage secondary to allergic bronchopulmonary aspergillosis, or more frequently they have irreversible obstructive lung disease with a bronchospastic component. Alteration of the latter component can be achieved pharmacologically with bronchodilators and prednisone, but the irreversible obstructive component cannot be altered.

To reduce the prednisone dosage in patients with intractable asthma (severe corticosteroid-dependent asthma), some physicians recommend using methylprednisolone (Medrol) and a macrolide antibiotic troleandomycin to decrease the prednisone requirement. Although prednisone dosage can be reduced, the decreased clearance of methylprednisolone by the effect of troleandomycin on the liver still may result in cushingoid obesity or corticosteroid side effects, at times exceeding prednisone alone. Therefore, methylprednisolone and troleandomycin are reduced as the patient improves. This approach has little to offer.

High dosages of intramuscular triamcinolone have been recommended and are effective therapy, but were associated with expected adverse effects such as cushingoid facies, acne, hirsutism, and myalgia.[230] In adults, methotrexate (15 mg per week) was found to be steroid sparing in a group of patients whose daily prednisone dosage was reduced 36.5%.[231] A double-blind placebo-controlled trial over a shorter period, 13 weeks, did not disclose any benefit of methotrexate, in that both methotrexate and placebo-treated patients had prednisone reductions of about 40%.[232] Such a finding is consistent with the observation that entry into a study itself can have a beneficial effect. The use of methotrexate remains an experimental approach. Cyclosporin also has been disappointing.

In a study of the natural history of severe asthma in patients who required at least 1 year of prednisone in addition to other pharmacotherapy (β-adrenergic agonists, theophylline, and high-dose inhaled corticosteroids), avoidance measures, and possibly immunotherapy, prednisone-free intervals occurred that even lasted for several years.[233] It was uncommon to have greater prednisone requirements, although usually, in these severe cases of asthma, prednisone dosages were stable over time or reductions occurred. Adequate "wash-in" periods are needed in studies of such patients. Otherwise, credit may be given to a new therapy inappropriately.

The administration of gold therapy for asthma has been described but is associated with recognized toxicity.[234]

Uncontrolled studies with dapsone, hydroxychloroquine, and intravenous gamma globulin in the management of the difficult cases of asthma await further data.

Use of budesonide by inhalation may assist in management of difficult-to-control prednisone-dependent patients. The term *glucocorticoid resistant* asthmatic has been applied to patients who did not improve after 2 weeks of prednisone or prednisolone administration (40 mg daily for 1 week, 20 mg daily for week 2).[235,236] Experimentally, glucocorticoid receptor down-regulation on T-lymphocytes has been identified, suggesting that such patients may have impaired inhibition of activated T-lymphocytes in asthma. For example, dexamethasone in vitro did not inhibit T-lymphocyte proliferation to the mitogen phytohemagglutinin in the "glucocorticoid-resistant" subjects.[236]

STATUS ASTHMATICUS

Status asthmaticus is defined as severe asthma unresponsive to emergency therapy with β-adrenergic agonists. It is a medical emergency for which immediate recognition and treatment are necessary to avoid a fatal outcome. For practical purposes, status asthmaticus is present in the absence of meaningful response to epinephrine (two or three subcutaneous injections) or terbutaline (two subcutaneous injections) or two aerosol treatments with β-adrenergic agonists.

Several factors have been shown to be important in inducing status asthmaticus and contributing to the mortality of asthma. Approximately 50% of patients have an associated respiratory tract infection. Some have overused sympathomimetics before developing refractoriness. In the aspirin-sensitive asthmatic patient, ingestion of aspirin or related cyclooxygenase inhibitors may precipitate status asthmaticus. Exposure to animal dander (especially cat dander) in the highly atopic patient may contribute to development of status asthmaticus, particularly when this is associated with a respiratory infection. Withdrawal or too sudden of a reduction of corticosteroids may be associated with the development of status asthmaticus. In many situations, both the patient and physician are unaware of the severity of progression of symptoms, and often earlier and more aggressive medical management would have prevented status asthmaticus. The inappropriate use of sedatives and tranquilizers in the treatment of status asthmaticus has contributed to the development of respiratory failure. Overdose of theophylline has been cited as a cause of death or cardiac arrest in some patients.

Status asthmaticus requires immediate treatment with high-dose corticosteroids.

Patients with status asthmaticus must be hospitalized where close observation and ancillary treatment by experienced personnel are available. If respiratory failure occurs, optimal treatment often involves the combined efforts of the allergist, pulmonary disease critical care physician, and anesthesiologist.

TABLE 22-12. *Treatment of status asthmaticus*

1. Corticosteroid therapy (give immediately in the office or emergency department)

   Hydrocortisone (Solu-Cortef) 4 mg/kg intravenously every 4–6 h or methylprednisolone (Solu-Medrol) 0.5–1.0 mg/kg intravenously every 4–6 h or prednisone 1 mg/kg orally every 4–6 h

2. β-Adrenergic agonists

   Choice of approaches available:

   1. Epinephrine 0.01 mL/kg of 1:1000 solution, subcutaneously not to exceed 0.3–0.5 mL in adults; may repeat twice at 20-min intervals then at reduced frequency

   2. Terbutaline 0.25 mg subcutaneously; may be repeated in 30 min, then in 4 h

   3. Aerosolized therapy; albuterol, metaproterenol, terbutaline, or other agent; repeat in 30 min, then at reduced frequency

   4. If a patient does not respond to steps 1 or 2 (above), try step 3; if a patient does not respond to step 3, try step 1

3. Hospitalize

4. Laboratory studies

   WBC with differential

   Chest roentgenogram

   Pulse oximetry or arterial blood gas

   Serum electrolytes and chemistries

   Sputum Gram stain, culture, and sensitivities

   Bedside spirometer may be useful, but not essential

   Electrocardiogram

5. Oxygen therapy

6. Correct dehydration

   2–3 L/min nasal cannula (best guided by arterial blood gas determination)

7. Aminophylline therapy (controversial)

   Check theophylline concentration if chronic therapy; adjust therapy based on Tables 22-9 and 22-10; administration is optional because efficacy has been questioned during emergency use

8. Antibiotic therapy

   When indicated for purulent rhinitis, bronchitis, or sinusitis

9. Impending or acute respiratory failure

   Repeat β-adrenergic agonists

   Endotracheal intubation with assisted or controlled ventilation

WBC, white blood cell count.

Initial laboratory studies should include a complete blood count, Gram stain with culture and sensitivity of the sputum, chest x-ray, serum electrolytes, pulse oximetry, and perhaps arterial blood gas studies (Table 22-12). A bedside spirometer may be helpful in determining and following ventilatory parameters. However, there may be considerable improvement during treatment of status asthmaticus without improvement in FEV_1 or vital capacity. This apparent lack of spirometric improvement occurs although the hyperinflation of lung volumes is diminishing in association with a reduction in the elastic work of breathing. Of these laboratory aids, blood gas determinations are probably the most valuable. Not only are they important in guiding therapy, they are also important in providing a true assessment of sever-

TABLE 22-13. *Spirometry and blood gases in asthma as related to the stage or severity*

	FEV$_1$	Vital capacity	Po$_2$ (normal 90–100 mm Hg)	Pco$_2$ (normal 35–40 mm Hg)	pH (normal 7.35–7.43 mm Hg)
Stage I (respiratory alkalosis)	↓	Normal	Normal	↓	>7.43
Stage II (respiratory alkalosis)	↓↓	↓	↓	↓↓	>7.43
Stage III	↓↓↓	↓↓	↓↓	Normal	7.35–7.43 normal
Stage IV (respiratory acidosis)	↓↓↓↓	↓↓↓	↓↓↓	↑↑↑	<7.35

FEV$_1$, forced expiratory volume in 1 second; Po$_2$, partial pressure of oxygen; Pco$_2$, partial pressure of carbon dioxide.

ity. These determinations allow the classification of asthma into four stages of severity (Table 22-13). Stage I signifies the presence of airway obstruction only. Because of the associated hyperventilation, the PCO$_2$ is low, and the pH is therefore slightly alkalotic (respiratory alkalosis). The PO$_2$ in stage I is normal. Spirometric study shows only a decrease in FEV$_1$, with a normal vital capacity. As symptoms progress, obstruction of the airway increases, compliance decreases, and air trapping and hyperinflation develop. As a result of the latter changes, the FRC increases and the vital capacity is decreased. In stage II, V Q imbalance with hypoxemia occurs. These changes, however, are not enough to impair net alveolar ventilation; thus, although PO$_2$ is lowered, PCO$_2$ remains low, and an alkalotic pH persists. With progressive severity, net alveolar ventilation decreases and a transitional period exists (stage III), in which the PCO$_2$ increases and the pH decreases, so that both values appear to be normal. When the blood gas study shows hypoxemia in the presence of a normal PCO$_2$ and pH, close supervision with frequent determinations of pH and PCO$_2$ are essential to evaluate the adequacy of treatment and the possible progression to respiratory failure characterized by hypoxemia and elevated PCO$_2$ (stage IV). Clinical observation alone is inadequate in determining the seriousness of status asthmaticus.[237]

Treatment of Status Asthmaticus

Although many patients with status asthmaticus manifest signs of fright, restlessness, and anxiety, the use of sedatives and tranquilizers is contraindicated. Appropriate therapy for status asthmaticus eventually controls the anxiety as the asthma improves. Even small doses of sedatives and tranquilizers may suppress respiratory drive to an extent sufficient to induce respiratory failure.

Some patients in status asthmaticus are dehydrated. The hyperventilation and increased work of breathing cause water loss through the lungs and skin. Also, because of their respiratory distress, many patients have not maintained an adequate fluid intake.

Intravenous solutions of 5% dextrose, alternating with 5% dextrose in normal saline, meets basic sodium and chloride requirements. In patients with a compromised cardiovascular system, sodium and water overload must be avoided. Because a high dose of corticosteroids is used in these patients, adequate potassium supplementation must be included in the intravenous therapy. In some adults, 80 mEq of potassium chloride per 24 hours (not to exceed 20 mEq/hour) is indicated. Frequent serum electrolyte determinations provide the best guide for continued electrolyte therapy.

It is controversial whether aminophylline should be administered acutely. If it is used, aminophylline should be given intravenously using constant infusion according to Table 22-9.

Because all patients are hypoxemic, oxygen therapy is required. Ideally, blood gas determinations should guide proper therapy. Therapeutically, a PO_2 of 60 mm Hg or slightly higher is sufficient. This often can be accomplished with low flow rates of 2 to 3 L/minute by nasal cannula. Ventimasks calibrated to deliver 24%, 28%, and 35% oxygen also may be used. The necessity for higher concentration of oxygen to maintain a PO_2 of 60 mm Hg usually signifies the presence of thick tracheobronchial secretions and of V/Q mismatch. It is cautioned that, in patients with asthma complicated by COPD, chronic hypercapnia may be present, and hypoxemia remains as the only respiratory stimulus. Oxygen therapy during an acute respiratory insult in these patients may enhance progression to respiratory failure. Close clinical observation and frequent blood gas monitoring are important in preventing this complication. In infants and young children, fine mist tents in an oxygen-enriched atmosphere should be avoided because they obscure the patient from vision, may frighten the patient, and may not deliver adequate oxygen.

With evidence of infection (i.e., purulent sputum, fever, sinusitis, or roentgenographic evidence of pneumonitis), antibiotics should be administered. In some instances, infection may be present in the absence of these suggestive findings. For this reason and because of the seriousness of status asthmaticus, the early use of antibiotics is recommended in status asthmaticus. Drugs of choice include amoxicillin, erythromycin, and tetracycline. Results of sputum culture should dictate change in antibiotic therapy. If sinusitis is present, other antibiotics such as amoxicillin-clavulanate, cefaclor, trimethoprim-sulfamethoxazole, or in children, erythromycin-sulfisoxazole can be administered.

Large doses of corticosteroids are essential immediately in status asthmaticus. The exact dose of corticosteroids necessary for treatment of status asthmaticus is unknown but the doses must be high. Hydrocortisone, 4 mg/kg, may be given intravenously and repeated every 4 to 6 hours. Methylprednisolone, 0.5 to 1.0 mg/kg, may be given intravenously and repeated every 4 to 6 hours in situations where sodium retention would be detrimental. With improvement, oral doses of prednisone can be substituted at 60 to 80 mg/day in an adult and 2 mg/kg/day in children.

For acute dyspnea, subcutaneous epinephrine or terbutaline or aerosolized β-adrenergic agonists may be administered every 4 hours or more frequently; however, little or no effect may be seen in the first 24 hours. For most patients in status asthmaticus, postural drainage and chest percussion are not necessary as part of the treatment. Treatment of status asthmaticus is summarized in Table 22-12.

RESPIRATORY FAILURE

Most patients with status asthmaticus respond favorably to the management described previously. In those who continue to deteriorate, other aggressive measures must be included to prevent respiratory failure, which may be defined as a PCO_2 greater than 50 mm Hg or a PO_2 less than 50 mm Hg. The important features of treatment at this stage include measures to maintain adequate alveolar ventilation and to protect from the severe acid–base disturbances that may arise. At this point, the coordinated efforts of the anesthesiologist or critical care specialist chest physician and the allergist are important in providing proper and effective treatment.

Signs of impending respiratory failure result from the combined effects of hypercapnia, hypoxia, and acidosis. Clinically, because of fatigue, inability to talk, and exhaustion, thoracic excursion is decreased, and auscultation of the chest may show decreased respiratory sounds because of the decrease in air flow.[238] Because of accompanying stupor, the patient may appear to be struggling less to breathe. These two features may give a false impression of improvement. Signs and symptoms of hypoxia include restlessness, confusion or delirium, and central cyanosis, which is present when arterial saturation is less than 70% and arterial PO_2 is less than 40 mm Hg. Hypercapnia is associated with headache or dizziness, confusion, unconsciousness, asterixis, miosis, papilledema, hypertension, and diaphoresis. Other danger signs in the patient with status asthmaticus include the presence of pulsus paradoxus, marked inspiratory retractions, inability to speak in full sentences, and cardiac arrhythmias that may lead to cardiac arrest. Acute chest pain is consistent with myocardial ischemia or rib fractures, but when subcutaneous emphysema is present, chest pain suggests pneumomediastinum or pneumothorax. Acidosis and hypoxemia contribute to pulmonary vasoconstriction, with resultant pulmonary hypertension, strain of the right side of the heart, and eventual cardiac failure. The acidosis is primarily respiratory in origin, but with severe hypoxemia, aerobic metabolism is impaired, and there is an accumulation of pyruvic and lactic acid (end products of anaerobic metabolism). These result in a superimposed metabolic acidosis.

The presence of these signs and symptoms associated with development of acidosis and hypercapnia demand the institution of mechanical ventilation. Tracheal intubation is preferred to tracheostomy because of its ease, and also because the potential complications of the latter are prevented. Electrocardiographic monitoring is advised to facilitate the early detection and treatment of arrhythmias that may occur during or immediately after intubation. The monitoring should continue throughout the entire time of mechanical ventilation. Before intubation, mild sedation or light halothane anesthesia is suggested. Preoxygenation with humidified 100% oxygen is administered with the use of mask and bag. A muscle paralyzing drug (atracurium, vecuronium, or pancuronium) is administered to further facilitate intubation and ventilation.[237] A cuffed nasotracheal or orotracheal tube is inserted and attached to the ventilator. The orotracheal tube, because of its large diameter, allows for more efficient suctioning of secretions.

In status asthmaticus, high pulmonary pressures are present; volume-regulated ventilators are most efficient in overcoming these pressures and provide more efficient and smoother ventilation. Tidal volume settings can be 8 to 10 mL/kg.[237]

After instituting mechanical ventilation, many patients with only minimal sedation are able to trigger the machine themselves (assisted ventilation). For those who fight the machine, and despite mild sedation, are unable to accommodate to it, it is necessary to provide continuous muscle relaxation and have the machine completely take over their breathing (controlled ventilation). While the patient is being ventilated, obtain frequent blood gas determinations. Some hypercapnia can be accepted. Frequent gentle suctioning of tracheobronchial secretions is necessary. Ventilator-applied positive end-expiratory pressure should be limited or avoided to prevent pneumothorax.

Overtreatment with sodium bicarbonate must be avoided. With efficient mechanical ventilation, sudden removal of carbon dioxide may result in acute alkalosis, because the elevated levels of bicarbonate remain uncompensated. Hyperexcitability and convulsions then may occur. This complication is best treated by temporarily decreasing ventilation. Other factors such as depletion of potassium (from corticosteroids or diuretics) and chloride may occur in status asthmaticus, and also may contribute to alkalosis. Adequate replacement of these ions must be included in therapy.

The only possible contraindication to the use of mechanical ventilation is the presence of pneumothorax or pneumomediastinum. In view of the potential lethality of acute respiratory failure, these conditions are considered relative contraindications. Mechanical ventilation may be undertaken, provided that all other measures have been unsuccessful. Pneumothorax must be treated with a chest tube under water seal before ventilation is attempted.

In an extreme attempt to prevent mechanical ventilation when adequate time is available, intravenous isoproterenol may be administered in the intensive care setting in children. Isoproterenol infusions have been shown to be useful in the management of status asthmaticus in children. Using them in older patients may be valuable and may avoid the risks associated with intubation. Isoproterenol infusion in an 18-year-old patient, however, has been reported as a possible cause of myocardial necrosis.[239] Thus, the benefit–risk ratio of an isoproterenol infusion in adolescents and adults must be judged carefully. The maximal dose is determined by the heart rate (which should not exceed 200) or by the development of persistent arrhythmia. In 27 children who had a favorable response to intravenous isoproterenol, the PCO_2 was 66 mm Hg before and 35 mm Hg after treatment.[240] The maximal dose of isoproterenol was 0.44 µg/kg/minute, and the heart rate at that dose was 192. Some patients do not respond to this treatment, and for these patients intubation and mechanical ventilation must be instituted. Fortunately, intravenous isoproterenol should and can be avoided in most patients with respiratory failure.

COMPLICATIONS OF MECHANICAL VENTILATION

Mechanical ventilation, although lifesaving in acute respiratory failure, may be associated with specific complications.[237] Sudden occurrence of tachypnea, hypotension, tachycardia, and cyanosis usually indicates a serious complication such as kinking of the endotracheal tube with obstruction of a major bronchus, disconnection from the ventilator, a pneumothorax or pneumomediastinum, or obstruction of the endotracheal tube by secretions.

Oxygen toxicity from the chronic use of a high concentration of oxygen (50% to 100% for 48 hours or longer) is another complication that can occur with the use of mechanical ventilation. Frequent checks of the inspired oxygen concentration can prevent this from happening. The pulmonary changes found with oxygen toxicity are capillary congestion, interstitial edema, alveolar edema, fibrin deposition, hemorrhage, and atelectasis. These changes themselves may impair oxygen transport and contribute to hypoxemia. Later and irreversible changes of oxygen toxicity include capillary proliferation and fibrosis.

Abnormal fluid retention and weight gain also may occur with prolonged mechanical ventilation. The chest roentgenogram may assume the appearance of pulmonary edema. As expected, a decrease in vital capacity and compliance, with a tendency to hypoxemia, results. The cause of the water retention is not known, but subclinical heart failure or antidiuretic hormone release have been suggested as mechanisms. Water restriction and diuretic therapy constitute treatment for this complication.

Tracheal stenosis is a complication of cuffed endotracheal or tracheostomy tubes. This occurs as a result of the mucosal injury arising from cuff-induced pressure necrosis. Other factors such as local infection and hypotension may be contributory. The occurrence of stridor or loud wheezing, heard best at the mouth, suggest the possibility of this complication in a patient recently intubated. Modifications in tube design may lower the incidence of this complication. Fortunately, mechanical ventilation even for severe episodes of status asthmaticus is not required for more than 7 days, and thus this complication is less likely to occur.

A potentially fatal complication of mechanical ventilation is *Pseudomonas aeruginosa* pneumonitis or other nosocomial infection. The ventilators often are the source of infection, but the concomitant use of antibiotics and corticosteroids along with an impaired bronchopulmonary defense mechanism are important predisposing factors. The radiologic picture of this type of pneumonia is variable and may consist of bilateral or unilateral consolidation, nodular lesions, or abscess formation. The diagnosis is established by repeated cultures from tracheal and bronchial secretions, and specific antibiotic therapy is best determined by sensitivity studies.

Prolonged use of muscle relaxing agents can cause severe myopathy that requires rehabilitation measures.

PREPARING THE ASTHMATIC PATIENT FOR SURGERY

For elective surgery, the patient with asthma should be evaluated 1 week in advance as an ambulatory patient so that adequate treatment can be instituted to ensure optimal bronchopulmonary status. The patient should be treated with prednisone, whether or not the patient regularly requires corticosteroids. If the patient is a corticosteroid-dependent asthmatic patient currently on a maintenance dose, increase the dose of prednisone instead of relying on increased use of bronchodilators to ensure complete control of asthma. Meet with the patient on an ambulatory basis the day before surgery if necessary. If the patient is topical corticosteroid-dependent, a short course (4 to 5 days) of prednisone (25 to 40 mg/day) before surgery is recommended to maximize pulmonary function. Pulmonary function testing should be obtained, at least FVC and FEV_1. The main need for corticosteroids, however, is prevention of intraoperative or postoperative asthma.

Hydrocortisone, 100 mg intramuscularly or intravenously, should be started before surgery and continued every 8 hours until the patient can tolerate oral medications. Repeat doses of hydrocortisone are given after surgery so that a total of 300 mg of hydrocortisone is received on the day of surgery. If no postoperative asthma occurs, the hydrocortisone dose can be discontinued. The doses of prednisone and hydrocortisone needed to control asthma do not increase postoperative complications such as wound dehiscence.[241]

Preanesthetic sedation may be achieved with hydroxyzine, because it causes minimal respiratory depression. Regional anesthesia should be used when feasible, but if general anesthesia is required, halothane remains a valuable anesthetic. Desirable properties of halothane are smooth and rapid induction of anesthesia, and relaxation of bronchial smooth muscle, with a resultant increase in bronchial caliber and pulmonary compliance. It also has been shown that halothane possesses β-adrenergic stimulating activity.

In patients with asthma, inhalation induction and maintenance of anesthesia is preferred. Manipulation of the upper airway (e.g., suction, pharyngeal airways) may cause bronchospasm during light stages of anesthesia. Tracheal intubation is to be avoided when possible, but if deemed necessary it should be performed during deep levels of anesthesia. Some patients benefit from intrabronchial lidocaine.

After surgery, the patient must be examined carefully. Aerosol bronchodilators, deep breathing exercises, adequate hydration, and gentle coughing should be instituted to avoid accumulation of secretions and atelectasis.

COMPLICATIONS OF ASTHMA

Pneumothorax, pneumomediastinum, and subcutaneous emphysema can occur during an attack of severe asthma, although they are rare. These complications are thought to result from the rupture of overdistended peripheral alveoli. The escaping air then follows and dissects through bronchovascular sheaths of the lung parenchyma. Usually, the amount of air is minimal and no specific intervention is required. When severe tension symptoms occur, insertion of a chest tube under a water seal for pneumothorax may be needed. Tracheostomy may be required for severe tension complications of pneumomediastinum. A common feature of these conditions is chest pain; this is not expected with uncomplicated asthma, and when present should suggest the possibility of the extravasation of air. On auscultation of the heart, a crunching sound synchronous with the heartbeat may be present with pneumomediastinum (Hamman's sign).

Minimal areas of atelectasis may occur in asthma. Atelectasis of the middle lobe is a common complication of asthma in children. It is often reversible with bronchodilators and prednisone, given immediately to avoid the risk of bronchoscopy, or at least to prepare for this examination. It probably results from mucus plugging and edema of the middle lobe bronchus. When the atelectasis does not respond to the above treatment within a few days, bronchoscopy is indicated for both therapeutic and diagnostic reasons. Occasionally, children may develop atelectasis of other lobes or of an entire lung. Allergic bronchopulmonary aspergillosis (see Chap. 24) and cystic fibrosis must be excluded in these patients, as in any patient with asthma.

Rib fracture and costochondral strain may occur as a result of coughing with attacks of asthma. In a few patients, severe coughing from asthma may result in cough syncope.

Chronic bronchitis and emphysema are not complications of asthma. These conditions occur with irreversible destruction of lung tissue, whereas asthma is a reversible bronchospastic condition. In some patients, asthma and emphysema or chronic bronchitis may coexist. The identification of bronchiectasis in a patient with asthma should raise the possibility of allergic bronchopulmonary aspergillosis or undiagnosed cystic fibrosis. Hypoxemia from uncontrolled asthma has been associated with adverse effects on other organs, such as myocardial ischemia or infarction. A rare patient with long-term asthma seemingly develops "end-stage" asthma with severe airways obstruction and lung hyperinflation in the absence of smoking, occupational exposures, or other causes for lung damage.

MORTALITY

Death from asthma commonly occurs either as a result of status asthmaticus progressing to respiratory failure, or suddenly and unexpectedly from severe bronchospasm and hypoxia perhaps with a terminal cardiac arrhythmia. In England and Australia, an increase in deaths occurred in the mid-1950s that continued, peaking in the mid-1960s. This increase in mortality rate from asthma continues. The use of high concentrations of sympathomimetic aerosols had been suspected to be a contributing factor in some of these deaths, but is unlikely to be a satisfactory explanation. In the United States, the death rate from asthma had been declining in the last 25 years but has been increasing again. Fatality rates are lower in the United States and Canada than many countries such as New Zealand and Australia.

A 1980s surge in deaths in New Zealand and the availability of albuterol inhalers without prescription in that country has been considered possibly analogous to the earlier epidemics of the 1960s. Undue reliance on inhaled sympathomimetics by patients and physicians may contribute to fatalities in patients with severe exacerbations of asthma because essential corticosteroid therapy is not being administered. In addition, excessive deaths associated with the potent β_2-adrenergic agonist fenoterol have been reported.

The factors that have been implicated in contributing to asthma deaths include the use of sedation, the failure to use adequate doses of oral corticosteroids, theophylline toxicity, excessive use of adrenergic aerosols, noncompliance with physician instructions, and failure to initiate oral corticosteroids for exacerbations of asthma in patients weaned from oral steroids. The latter phenomenon may be exacerbated by the use of inhaled corticosteroids which do not substitute for oral corticosteroids acutely. High-risk chronic asthmatic patients include those who have had severe wheezing (often since the first year of life), frequent episodes of prolonged asthma requiring hospitalization or chronic corticosteroid use, chest deformities such as pigeon breast, wheezing between exacerbations of asthma, gross pulmonary function abnormalities when asymptomatic, or patients previously requiring mechanical ventilation during respiratory failure such as patients with potentially fatal asthma.[106] Patients with underlying restrictive lung disease tolerate status asthmaticus poorly as well. Some fatalities occur in the setting of no medical care or associated with substance abuse.[242]

THE FUTURE

Asthma management will be improved by continued research and stability of the family. Specific curative therapy can be realized only when basic pathologic mechanisms are understood. Then therapeutic modalities can be devised rationally to reverse the underlying pathogenetic processes. If indeed leukotrienes are major mediators of bronchospasm, the possibility exists that treating patients with a leukotriene antagonist[243] or lipoxygenase inhibitor[211] could reduce or eliminate the need for other medications. Although currently available calcium channel antagonists do not appear to have a place in the treatment of asthma, future research into membrane receptors may lead to improved pharmacotherapy. The advances already made provide for continued optimism for future treatment of asthma, as interactions of the lung, immune system, mast cell mediators and cell products, and adhesion molecules are understood in greater detail.

REFERENCES

1. American College of Chest Physicians, American Thoracic Society. Pulmonary terms and symbols. Chest 1975;67:583.
2. National Institutes of Health, National Heart, Lung, and Blood Institute, Expert Panel Report, National Asthma Education Program, Executive Summary: Guidelines for the diagnosis and management of asthma. Public Health Service, U.S. Department of Health and Human Services, NIH publication no. 91-3042A, 1991.
3. Carrao WM, Braman SS, Irwin RS. Chronic cough as the sole presenting manifestation of bronchial asthma. N Engl J Med 1979;30:633.
4. Quesenberry PJ. Cardiac asthma: a fresh look at an old wheeze. N Engl J Med 1989;320:1346.
5. Cabanes LR, Weber SN, Matran R, et al. Bronchial hyperresponsiveness to methacholine in patients with impaired left ventricular function. N Engl J Med 1989;320:1317.
6. Samet JM. Epidemiologic approaches for the identification of asthma. Chest 1987;91:74S.
7. Pattemore PK, Asher MI, Harrison AC, et al. The interrelationship among bronchial hyperresponsiveness, the diagnosis of asthma, and asthma symptoms. Am Rev Respir Dis 1990;142:549.
8. Welliver RC, Sun M, Rinaldo D, Orga PL. Predictive value of respiratory syncytial virus-specific IgE responses for recurrent wheezing following bronchiolitis. J Pediatr 1986;109:776.
9. Welliver RC, Duffy L. The relationship of RSV-specific immunoglobulin E antibody responses in infancy, recurrent wheezing, and pulmonary function at age 7–8 years. Pediatr Pulmonol 1993;15:19.
10. Samter M, Beers RF. Intolerance to aspirin: clinical studies and consideration to its pathogenesis. Ann Intern Med 1968;69:975.
11. Stevenson DD, Pleskow WW, Simon RA, et al. Treatment of aspirin sensitive asthma/rhinosinusitis with aspirin. J Allergy Clin Immunol 1983;71:272.
12. Vanselow NA, Smith JR. Bronchial asthma induced by indomethacin. Ann Intern Med 1967;66:568.
13. Santiago SM Jr, Klaustermeyer WR. Acute respiratory failure secondary to indomethacin in an aspirin-intolerant asthmatic patient. Ann Allergy 1976;37:138.

14. Israel E, Fischer AR, Rosenberg MA, et al. The pivotal role of 5-lipoxygenase products in the reaction of aspirin-sensitive asthmatic subjects to aspirin. Am Rev Respir Dis 1993;148:1447.
15. Shuaib Nasser SM, Patel M, Bell GS, et al. The effect of aspirin desensitization on urinary leukotriene E_4 concentrations in aspirin-sensitive asthma. Am J Respir Crit Care Med 1995;151:1326.
16. Ownby DR. Environmental factors versus genetic determinants of childhood inhalant allergies. J Allergy Clin Immunol 1990;86:279.
17. Luoma R, Koirvkko A, Viander M. Development of asthma, allergic rhinitis, and atopic dermatitis by the age of five years. Allergy 1983;38:339.
18. Ratner B, Silberman DE. Allergy: its distribution and hereditary concept. Ann Allergy 1952;9:1.
19. Wittig HJ, McLaughlin ET, Leifer KL, Belloit JD. Risk factors for the development of allergic disease: analysis of 2190 patient records. Ann Allergy 1978;41:84.
20. Horwood LJ, Fergusson DM, Hons BA, Shannon FT. Social and familial factors in the development of early childhood asthma. Pediatrics 1985;75:859.
21. Blumenthal MN, Yunis E, Mendell N, Elston RC. Preventive allergy: genetics of IgE-mediated diseases. J Allergy Clin Immunol 1986;78:962.
22. Lubs M-L E. Empiric risks for genetic counseling in familes with allergy. J Pediatr 1972;80:26.
23. Hopp RJ, Bewtra AK, Watt GD, Nair NM, Townley RG. Genetic analysis of allergic disease in twins. J Allergy Clin Immunol 1984;73:265.
24. Murray AB, Morrison BJ. Passive smoking by asthmatics: its greater effect on boys than on girls and on older than on young children. Pediatrics 1989;84:451.
25. Frick OL, German DF, Mills J. Development of allergy in children. I. Association with virus infections. J Allergy Clin Immunol 1979;63:228.
26. Weiss ST, Tager IB, Munoz A, et al. The relationship of respiratory illness in childhood to the occurrence of increased levels of bronchial responsivenness and atopy. Am Rev Respir Dis 1985;131:573.
27. Price JA, Pollock I, Little SA, et al. Measurement of airborne mite antigen in homes of asthmatic children. Lancet 1990;336:895.
28. Sporik R, Ingram JM, Price W, et al. Association of asthma with serum IgE and skin test reactivity to allergens among children living at high altitude: tickling the dragon's breath. Am J Respir Crit Care Med 1995;151:1388.
29. Martinez FD, Wright AL, Taussig LM, et al. Asthma and wheezing in the first six years of life. N Engl J Med 1995;332:133.
30. Gleich GJ, Motojima S, Frigas E, Kephart GM, Fujisawa T, Kravis LP. The eosinophilic leukocyte and the pathology of fatal bronchial asthma: evidence for pathologic heterogeneity. J Allergy Clin Immunol 1987;80:412.
31. Bousquet J, Chanej P, Lacoste JY, et al. Eosinophilic inflammation in asthma. N Engl J Med 1990;323:1033.
32. Kleinerman J, Adelson L. A study of asthma deaths in a coroner's population. J Allergy Clin Immunol 1987;80:406.
33. Salome CM, Peat JK, Britton WJ, Woolcock AJ. Bronchial hyperresponsiveness in two populations of Australian schoolchildren. I. Relation to respiratory symptoms and diagnosed asthma. Clinical Allergy 1987;17:271.
34. Cookson WOCM, Musk AW, Ryan G. Associations between asthma history, atopy and non-specific bronchial responsiveness in young adults. Clinical Allergy 1986;16:425.
35. Smith LJ, Greenberger PA, Patterson R, Krell RD, Bernstein PR. The effect of inhaled leukotriene D_4 in humans. Am Rev Respir Dis 1985;131:368.
36. Frick WE, Sedgwick JB, Busse WW. The appearance of hypodense eosinophils in antigen-dependent late phase asthma. Am Rev Respir Dis 1989;139:1401.
37. Frigas E, Loegering DA, Solley GO, Farrow GM, Gleich GJ. Elevated levels of eosinophil granule major basic protein in the sputum of patients with bronchial asthma. Mayo Clin Proc 1981;56:345.
38. Filley WV, Holley KE, Kephart GM, Gleich GJ. Identification by immunofluorescence of eosinophil granule major basic protein in lung tissues of patients with bronchial asthma. Lancet 1982;ii:11.
39. Fredens K, Dahl P, Venge P. Eosinophils and cellular injury: the Gordon phenomenon as a model. Allergy Proc 1985;6:346.
40. Ollerenshaw S, Jarvis D, Woolcock A, Sullivan C, Scheibner T. Absence of immunoreactive vasoactive intestinal polypeptide in tissue from the lungs of patients with asthma. N Engl J Med 1989;320:1244.
41. Lilly CM, Bai TR, Shore SA, et al. Neuropeptide content of lungs from asthmatic and nonasthmatic patients. Am J Respir Crit Care Med 1995;151:548.
42. Tomaki M, Ichinose N, Miura M, et al. Elevated substance P content in induced sputum from patients with asthma and patients with chronic bronchitis. Am J Respir Crit Care Med 1995;151:613.
43. Miller BD. Depression and asthma: a potentially lethal mixture. J Allergy Clin Immunol 1987;80:481.
44. Walker CL, Greenberger PA, Patterson R. Potentially fatal asthma. Ann Allergy 1990;64:487.
45. Sonin L, Patterson R. Corticosteroid dependent asthma and schizophrenia. Arch Intern Med 1984;144:554.
46. Yellowless PM, Ruffin RE. Psychological defenses and coping styles in patients following a life-threatening attack of asthma. Chest 1989;95:1298.
47. Current trends: asthma—United States, 1982–1992. MMWR 1995;43:952.
48. Kerem E, Tibshirani R, Canny G, et al. Predicting the need for hospitalization in children with acute asthma. Chest 1990;98:1355.

49. Weiss KB, Wagener DK. Changing patterns of asthma mortality: identifying target populations at high risk. JAMA 1990;264:1683.

50. Evans R III, Mullally DI, Wilson RW, et al. Prevalence, hospitalization and death from asthma over two decades: 1965–1984. Chest 1987;91:65.

51. Clark D, Gollub R, Green WF, et al. Asthma in Jemez Pueblo schoolchildren. Am J Respir Crit Care Med 1995;151:1625.

52. Burney PGJ. Asthma mortality: England and Wales. J Allergy Clin Immunol 1987;80:379.

53. Sears MR. Changing patterns in asthma morbidity and mortality. J Invest Allergol Clin Immunol 1995;5:66.

54. Burrows B. The natural history of asthma. J Allergy Clin Immunol 1987;80:373.

55. Apter A, Grammer LC, Naughton B, Patterson R. Asthma in the elderly: a brief report. NER Allergy Proc 1988;9:153.

56. Burr MC, Charles D, Roy K, et al. Asthma in the elderly: an epidemiological survey. Br Med J 1979;1:1041.

57. Evans R III. Recent observations reflecting increases in mortality from asthma. J Allergy Clin Immunol 1987;80:337.

58. Blanc P. Occupational asthma in a national disability survey. Chest 1987;92:613.

59. Chan-Yeung M, Malo J-L. Occupational asthma. N Engl J Med 1995;333:107.

60. Juel K, Pedersen PA. Increasing asthma mortality in Denmark 1969–88 not a result of a changed coding practice. Ann Allergy 1992;68:180.

61. Bousquet J, Hatton F, Godard P, Michel FB. Asthma mortality in France. J Allergy Clin Immunol 1987;80:389.

62. Sly RM. Changing asthma mortality. Ann Allergy 1994;73:259.

63. Bates DV, Baker-Anderson M. Asthma mortality and morbidity in Canada. J Allergy Clin Immunol 1987;80:39S.

64. Sly MR. Changing asthma mortality and sales of inhaled bronchodilators and anti-asthmatic drugs. Ann Allergy 1994;73:439.

65. Bates DV. Airway structure and function. In: Respiratory function in disease. Philadelphia: WB Saunders, 1989:1.

66. Patterson R, McKenna JM, Suszko IM, et al. Living histamine containing cells from the bronchial lumens of humans: description and comparison of histamine content with cells of rhesus monkeys. J Clin Invest 1977;59:217.

67. Fick RB, Richerson HB, Zavala DC, Hunninghake GW. Bronchoalveolar lavage in allergic asthmatics. Am Rev Respir Dis 1987;135:1204.

68. Friedman MM, Kaliner MA. Human mast cells and asthma. Am Rev Respir Dis 1987;135:1157.

69. Barnes PJ, Cuss FM, Palmer JB. The effect of airway epithelium on smooth muscle contractability in bovine trachea. Br J Pharmacol 1985;86:685.

70. Woolcock AJ, Salmone CM, Yan K. The shape of the dose response curve to histamine in asthmatic and normal subjects. Am Rev Respir Dis 1984;130:71.

71. Richardson JB. Airways smooth muscle. J Allergy Clin Immunol 1987;80:409.

72. Reid LM. The presence or absence of bronchial mucus in fatal asthma. J Allergy Clin Immunol 1987;80:415.

73. Robin ED, Lewiston N. Unexpected, unexplained sudden death in young asthmatic subjects. Chest 1989;96:790.

74. Sur S, Grotty TB, Kephart GM, et al. Sudden-onset fatal asthma: a distinct entity with few eosinophils and relatively more neutrophils in the airway submucosa? Am Rev Respir Dis 1993;148:713.

75. Bhaskar KR, Reid L. Application of density gradient methods for the study of mucus glycoprotein and other macromolecular components of the sol and gel phases of asthmatic sputa. J Biol Chem 1981;256:7583.

76. Mavom Z, Shelhamer JH, Kaliner M. Human pulmonary macrophage-derived mucus secretagogue. J Exp Med 1984;189:844.

77. Laitinen LA, Laitinen A, Haahtela T. A comparative study of the effects of an inhaled corticosteroid, budesonide, and a β_2-agonist, terbutaline, on airway inflammation in newly diagnosed asthma: a randomized, double-blind, parallel-group controlled trial. J Allergy Clin Immunol 1992;90:32.

78. Leff AR. Endogenous regulation of bronchomotor tone. Am Rev Respir Dis 1988;137:1198.

79. Beasley R, Rocke WR, Roberts JA, Holgate ST. Cellular events in the bronchi in mild asthma and after bronchial provocation. Am Rev Respir Dis 1989;139:806.

80. Cutz E, Levison H, Cooper DM. Ultrastructure of airways in children with asthma. Histopathology 1978;2:407.

81. Flint KC, Leung KBP, Hudspith BN, Brostoff J, Pearce FL, Johnson NM. Bronchoalveolar mast cells in extrinsic asthma: a mechanism for the inhalation of antigen specific bronchoconstriction. Br Med J 1985;291:923.

82. Pearce FL, Flint KC, Leung KBT, et al. Some studies on human pulmonary mast cells obtained by bronchoalveolar lavage and by enzymatic dissociation of whole lung tissue. Int Arch Allergy Appl Immunol 1987;82:507.

83. Smith LJ, Rubin A-HE, Patterson R. Mechanism of platelet activating factor–induced bronchoconstriction in humans. Am Rev Respir Dis 1988;137:1015.

84. Wasserman SI. Platelet-activating factor as a mediator of bronchial asthma. Hosp Pract 1988;23:49.

85. Alam R, Rozniecki J, Salmaj K. A mononuclear cell-derived histamine release from basophils *in vitro*. Ann Allergy 1984;53:66.

86. Baeza ML, Reddigavi S, Haak-Frendscho M, Kaplan AP. Purification and further characterization of human mononuclear cell histamine-releasing factor. J Clin Invest 1989;83:1204.

87. Liao T-N, Hsieh K-H. Altered production of histamine-releasing factor (HRF) activity and responsiveness to HRF after immunotherapy in children with asthma. J Allergy Clin Immunol 1990;86:894.

88. Kikuchi Y, Okabe S, Tamura G, et al. Chemosensitivity and perception of dyspnea in patients with a history of near-fatal asthma. N Engl J Med 1994;330:1329.

89. McFadden ER Jr. Exertional dyspnea and cough as preludes to acute attacks of bronchial asthma. N Engl J Med 1975;292:555.

90. Rebuck AS, Pengelly LD. Development of pulsus paradoxus in the presence of airways obstruction. N Engl J Med 1973;288:66.

91. Petheram IS, Kerr IH, Collins JV. Value of chest radiographs in severe acute asthma. Clin Radiol 1981;32:281.

92. Findley LJ, Sahn SA. The value of chest roentgenograms in acute asthma in adults. Chest 1981;80:535.

93. Sherman S, Skoney JA, Ravikrishnan KP. Routine chest radiographs in exacerbations of chronic obstructive pulmonary disease: diagnostic value. Arch Intern Med 1989;149:2493.

94. Slavin RG. Sinusitis in adults and its relation to allergic rhinitis, asthma and nasal polyps. J Allergy Clin Immunol 1988;82:950.

95. Rodriquez-Roisin R, Ballester E, Roca J, Torres A, Wagner PD. Mechanisms of hypoxemia in patients with status asthmaticus. Am Rev Respir Dis 1989;139:732.

96. Allen JN, Davis WB. Eosinophilic lung diseases. Am J Respir Crit Care Med 1994;150:1423.

97. Buchanan DR, Cromwell O, Kay AB. Neutrophil chemotactic activity in acute severe asthma. Am Rev Respir Dis 1987;136:1397.

98. Backer JW, Yerger S, Segar WE. Elevated plasma antidiuretic hormone levels in status asthmaticus. Mayo Clin Proc 1976;51:31.

99. Adnot S, Chabrier PE, Andrivet P, et al. Atrial natriuretic peptide concentrations and pulmonary hemodynamics in patients with pulmonary artery hypertension. Am Rev Respir Dis 1987;136:951.

100. Benatar SR. Fatal asthma. N Engl J Med 1986;314:423.

101. Strunk RC. Death due to asthma: new insights into sudden unexpected deaths, but the focus remains on prevention. Am Rev Respir Dis 1993;148:550.

102. Birkhead G, Attaway NJ, Strunk RC, et al. Investigation of a cluster of deaths of adolescents from asthma: evidence implicating inadequate treatment and poor patient adherence with medications. J Allergy Clin Immunol 1989;84:484.

103. Robertson CF, Rubinfeld AR, Bowes G. Deaths from asthma in Victoria: a 12-month survey. Med J Aust 1990;152:511.

104. Esdaile JM, Feinstein AR, Horwitz RI. A reappraisal of the United Kingdom epidemic of fatal asthma: can general mortality data implicate a therapeutic agent? Arch Intern Med 1987;147:543.

105. Kallenbach JM, Frankel AH, Lapinsky SE, et al. Determinants of near fatality in acute severe asthma. Am J Med 1993;95:265.

106. Greenberger PA. Potentially fatal asthma. Chest 1992;101:401S.

107. Suissa S, Ernst P, Boivin J-F, et al. A cohort analysis of excess mortality in asthma and the use of inhaled β-agonists. Am J Respir Crit Care Med 1994;149:604.

108. Spitzer WO, Suissa S, Ernst P, et al. The use of β-agonists and the risk of death and near death from asthma. N Engl J Med 1992;326:501.

109. Rebuck AS, Read J. Assessment and management of severe asthma. Am J Med 1971;51:788.

110. Axelrod L. Glucocorticoids. In: Kelly WN, Harris ED, Ruddy S, Sledge CB, eds. Textbook of rheumatology. 4th ed. Philadelphia: WB Saunders, 1993:779.

111. Lowenthal M, Patterson R, Greenberger PA, et al. Malignant potentially fatal asthma: achievement of remission and the application of an asthma severity index. Allergy Proc 1993;14:333.

112. Huckauf H, Mach AN. Behavioral factors in the etiology of asthma. Chest 1987;91:141S.

113. Groves JE. Taking care of the hateful patient. N Engl J Med 1976;293:883.

114. Fitzsimons T, Patterson D, Patterson R. The allergic patient who is non-compliant and abusive: dealing with the adverse experience. Ann Allergy 1991;66:311.

115. Chandler MJ, Grammer LC, Patterson R. Noncompliance and prevarication in life-threatening adolescent asthma. NER Allergy Proc 1986;7:367.

116. McGrath KG, Greenberger PA, Patterson R, Zeiss CR. Factitious allergic disease: multiple factitious illness and familial Munchausen's stridor. Immunol Allergy Prac 1984;7:263.

117. Apter A, Grammer LC, Naughton B, Patterson R. Asthma in the elderly: a brief report. NER Allergy Proc 1988;9:153.

118. Kalliel JN, Goldstein BM, Braman SS, Settipane GA. High frequency of atopic asthma in a pulmonary clinic population. Chest 1989;96:1336.

119. Burrows B, Martinez FD, Halonen M, Barbee RA, Cline MG. Association of asthma with serum IgE levels and skin test reactivity to allergens. N Engl J Med 1989;320:271.

120. Habenicht HA, Burge HA, Muilenberg MC, et al. Allergen carriage by atmospheric aerosols. II. Ragweed-pollen determinants in submicronic atmospheric aerosols. J Allergy Clin Immunol 1984;74:64.

121. Findlay SR, Stotsky E, Lieterman K, Hermady Z, Ohman JL Jr. Allergens detected in association with airborne particles capable of penetrating into the peripheral lung. Am Rev Respir Dis 1983;128:1008.

122. Luczynska CM, Yin L, Chapman MD, Platts-Mills TAE. Airborne concentrations and particle size distribution of allergen derived from domestic cats (Felis domesticus). Am Rev Respir Dis 1990;141:361.

123. Cockcroft DW. The bronchial late response in the pathogenesis of asthma and its modulation by therapy. Ann Allergy 1985;55:857.
124. O'Hollaren MT, Yunginger JW, Offord KP, et al. Exposure to an aeroallergen as a possible precipitating factor in respiratory arrest in young patients with asthma. N Engl J Med 1991;324:359.
125. Sporik R, Holgate ST, Platts-Mills TAE, Cogswell JJ. Exposure to house-dust mite allergen (Der p I) and the development of asthma in childhood: a prospective study. N Engl J Med 1990;323:502.
126. American Thoracic Society. Environmental control and lung disease. Am Rev Respir Dis 1990;142:915.
127. Busse WW. Viral infections in humans. Am J Respir Crit Care Med 1995;151:1675.
128. Welliver RC, Wong DT, Sun M, et al. The development of respiratory syncytial virus-specific IgE and the release of histamine in nasopharyngeal secretions after infection. N Engl J Med 1981;305:841.
129. Greenberger PA, Patterson R. The diagnosis of potentially fatal asthma. NER Allergy Proc 1988;9:147.
130. Settipane GA. Adverse reactions to aspirin and related drugs. Arch Intern Med 1981;141:328.
131. Szczeklik A, Gryglewski RJ, Czerniawska-Mysik G. Relationship of inhibition of prostaglandin biosynthesis by analgesics to asthma in aspirin-sensitive patients. Br Med J 1975;1:67.
132. Stevenson DD, Pleskow WW, Simon RA, et al. Aspirin-sensitive rhinosinusitis asthma: a double-blind crossover study of treatment with aspirin. J Allergy Clin Immunol 1984;73:500.
133. Mathison DA, Stevenson DD, Simon RA. Precipitating factors in asthma: aspirin, sulfites, and other drugs and chemicals. Chest 1985;87:50S.
134. Szczeklik A, Gryglewski RJ, Czerniawska-Mysik G, Nizankowska E. Aspirin sensitive asthma and arachidonic acid transportation. NER Allergy Proc 1986;7:21.
135. Malo J-L, Cartier A, Ghezzo H, Lafrance M, McCants M, Lehrer SB. Patterns of improvement in spirometry, bronchial hyperresponsiveness and specific IgE antibody levels after cessation of exposure in occupational asthma caused by snow-crab processing. Am Rev Respir Dis 1988;138:807.
136. Brooks SM, Weiss MA, Bernstein IL. Reactive airway dysfunction syndrome (RADS): persistent asthma syndrome after high level irritant exposure. Chest 1985;88:376.
137. Promisloff PA, Lenchner GS, Cichelli AV. Reactive airway dysfunction syndrome in three police officers following a roadside chemical spill. Chest 1990;98 928.
138. Vedal S, Enarson DA, Chan H, Ochnio J, Tse KS, Chan-Yeung M. A longitudinal study of the occurrence of bronchial hyperresponsiveness in Western red cedar workers. Am Rev Respir Dis 1988;137:651.
139. Zeiss CR, Mitchell JH, Van Peenen PFD, Harris J, Levitz D. A twelve-year clinical and immunologic evaluation of workers involved in the manufacture of trimellitic anhydride (TMA). Allergy Proc 1990;11:71.
140. McFadden ER Jr. Exercise and asthma. N Engl J Med 1987;317:502.
141. Rubinstein I, Levinson H, Slutsky AS, et al. Immediate and delayed bronchoconstriction after exercise in patients with asthma. N Engl J Med 1987;317:482.
142. McFadden ER Jr, Lenner KAM, Strohl KP. Postexertional airway rewarming and thermally induced asthma: new insights into pathophysiology and possible pathogenesis. J Clin Invest 1986;78:18.
143. Smith CM, Anderson SD, Walsh S, McElrea MS. An investigation of heat and water exchange in the recovery period after exercise in children with asthma. Am Rev Respir Dis 1989;140:598.
144. Cheriyan S, Greenberger PA, Patterson R. Outcome of cough variant asthma treated with inhaled steroids. Ann Allergy 1994;73:478.
145. Patterson R, Schatz M. Factitious allergic emergencies: anaphylaxis and laryngeal "edema." J Allergy Clin Immunol 1975;56:152.
146. Shim C, Williams MH. Effects of odors in asthma. Am J Med 1986;80:18.
147. Ing AJ, Ngu MC, Breslin ABX. Pathogenesis of chronic persistent cough associated with gastroesophageal reflux. Am J Respir Crit Care Med 1994;149:160.
148. Perrin Fayolle M, Gormand F, Braillon G, et al. Long-term results of surgical treatment for gastroesophageal reflux in asthmatic patients. Chest 1989;96:40.
149. Platts-Mills TAE. Allergen-specific treatment for asthma. III. Am Rev Respir Dis 1993;148:553.
150. Brown JE, Greenberger PA. Immunotherapy and asthma. Immunol Allergy Clin North Am 1993;13:939.
151. Abramson MJ, Puy RM, Weiner JM. Is allergen immunotherapy effective in asthma? A meta-analysis of randomized controlled trials. Am J Respir Crit Care Med 1995;151:969.
152. Formgren H. The therapeutic value of oral long-term treatment with terbutaline in asthma. Scand J Respir Dis 1975;56:321.
153. Larsson S, Svedmyr N, Thiringer G. Lack of beta adrenoceptor resistance in asthmatics during long-term treatment with terbutaline. J Allergy Clin Immunol 1977;59:93.
154. Repsher LH, Anderson JA, Bush RK, et al. Assessment of tachyphylaxis following prolonged therapy of asthma with inhaled albuterol aerosol. Chest 1984;85:34.
155. Sly RM, Badiei B, Faciane J. Comparison of subcutaneous terbutaline with epinephrine in treatment of asthma in children. J Allergy Clin Immunol 1977;59:128.
156. Chapman KR, Smith DL, Rebuck AS. Hemodynamic effects of an inhaled beta-2 agonist. Clin Pharmacol Ther 1984;35:762.
157. Glass P, Dulfano MJ. Evaluation of a new β_2-adrenergic receptor stimulant, terbutaline, in bronchial asthma. I. Subcutaneous comparison with epinephrine. Curr Ther Res 1973;15:141.
158. Smith PR, Heurich AE, Leffler CT. A comparative study of subcutaneously administered terbutaline and epinephrine in treatment of acute bronchial asthma. Chest 1977;71:129.

159. Colacone A, Wolkove N, Stern E, et al. Continuous nebulization of albuterol (Salbutamol) in acute asthma. Chest 1990;97:693.

160. Shim CS, Williams MH. Effects of bronchodilator therapy administered by canister versus jet nebulizer. J Allergy Clin Immunol 1984;73:387.

161. Fanta CH, Rossing TH, McFadden ER. Glucocorticoids in acute asthma: Critical controlled trial. Am J Med 1983;74:845.

162. Svedmyr N. Action of corticosteroids on beta-adrenergic receptors. Am Rev Respir Dis 1990;141:S31.

163. Fiel SB, Swartz MA, Glanz K, et al. Efficacy of short-term corticosteroid therapy in outpatient treatment of acute bronchial asthma. Am J Med 1983;75:259.

164. Chapman KR, Verbeek PR, White JG, et al. Effect of a short course of prednisone in the prevention of early relapse after the emergency room treatment of acute asthma. N Engl J Med 1991;324:788.

165. Shapiro GG, Furukawa CT, Pierson WE, Gardinier R, Bierman CW. Double-blind evaluation of methylprednisolone versus placebo for acute asthma episodes. Pediatrics 1983;71:510.

166. Peers SH, Flower RJ. The role of lipocortin in corticosteroid actions. Am Rev Respir Dis 1990;141:S18.

167. Schleimer RP. Effects of glucocorticosteroids on inflammatory cells relevant to their therapeutic applications in asthma. Am Rev Respir Dis 1990;141:S59.

168. Falliers CJ, Ellis EF. Corticosteroids and varicella. Arch Dis Child 1965;40:593.

169. Messer J, Reitman D, Sacks HS, Smith H Jr, Chalmers TC. Association of adrenocorticosteroid therapy and peptic-ulcer disease. N Engl J Med 1983;309:21.

170. Spiro HM. Is the steroid ulcer a myth? N Engl Med 1983;309:45.

171. Schatz M, Patterson R, Kloner R, Falk J. The prevalence of tuberculosis and positive tuberculin skin tests in a steroid related asthmatic population. Ann Intern Med 1976;84:261.

172. Fauci AS, Dale DC, Balow JE. Glucocorticosteroid therapy: mechanisms of action and clinical considerations. Ann Intern Med 1976;84:304.

173. Greenberger PA, Hendrix RW, Patterson R, et al. Bone studies in patients on prolonged systemic corticosteroid therapy for asthma. Clinical Allergy 1982;12:363.

174. Lukert BP, Raisz LG. Glucocorticoid-induced osteoporosis: pathogenesis and management. Ann Intern Med 1990;112:352.

175. Reid IR, Ibberston HK. Calcium supplementation in the prevention of steroid-induced osteoporosis. Am J Clin Nutr 1986;44:287.

176. Chernow B, Alexander R, Smallridge RC, et al. Hormonal responses to graded surgical stress. Arch Intern Med 1987;147:1273.

177. Falliers CJ, Chai H, Molk L, et al. Pulmonary and adrenal effects of alternate-day corticosteroid therapy. J Allergy Clin Immunol 1972;49:156.

178. Axelrod L. Glucocorticoid therapy. Medicine 1976;55:39.

179. Greenberger PA, Chow MJ, Atkinson AJ Jr, Patterson R. Comparison of prednisolone kinetics in patients receiving daily or alternate-day prednisone for asthma. Clin Pharmacol Ther 1986;39:163.

180. Collins JV, Haris PWR, Clark TJH, et al. Intravenous corticosteroids in treatment of acute bronchial asthma. Lancet 1970;ii:1407.

181. Klein R, Waldman D, Kershnar H, et al. Treatment of chronic childhood asthma with beclomethasone dipropionate aerosols. I. A double blind crossover trial in nonsteroid-dependent patients. Pediatrics 1977;60:7.

182. Wyatt R, Waschek J, Weinberger M, et al. Effects of beclomethasone and alternate-day prednisone on children with asthma. N Engl J Med 1978;299:1387.

183. Haahtela T, Jarvinen M, Kava T, et al. Comparison of a β_2-agonist, terbutaline, with an inhaled corticosteroid, budesonide, in newly detected asthma. N Engl J Med 1991;325:388.

184. Haahtela T, Jarvinen M, Kava T, et al. Effects of reducing or discontinuing inhaled budesonide in patients with mild asthma. N Engl J Med 1994;331:700.

185. Juniper EF, Kline PA, Vanzieleghem MA, Ramsdale EH, O'Byrne PM, Hargreave FE. Effect of long-term treatment with an inhaled corticosteroid (budesonide) on airway hyperresponsiveness and clinical asthma in nonsteroid-dependent asthmatics. Am Rev Respir Dis 1990;142:832.

186. DeBaets FM, Goeteyn M, Kerrebijn KF. The effects of two months of treatment with inhaled budesonide on bronchial responsiveness to histamine and house-dust mite antigen in asthmatic children. Am Rev Respir Dis 1990;142:581.

187. Busse WW. What role for inhaled steroids in chronic asthma? Chest 1993;104:1565.

188. Newman SP, Woodman G, Clarke SW, Sackner M. Effect of Inspir-ease on the deposition of metered dose aerosols in the human respiratory tract. Chest 1986;89:551.

189. Rall TW. Drugs used in the treatment of asthma. In: Gilman AG, Rall TW, Nies AS, Taylor P, eds. The pharmacologic basis of therapeutics. 8th ed. New York: Pergamon Press, 1990:618.

190. Mitenko PA, Ogilvie RI. Rational intravenous doses of theophylline. N Engl J Med 1973;289:600.

191. Jacobs MH, Senior RM, Kessler G. Clinical experience with theophylline. JAMA 1976;235:1983.

192. Zwillich CW, Sutton FD, Neff TA, et al. Theophylline-induced seizures in adults: correlations with serum concentrations. Ann Intern Med 1975;82:784.

193. Greenberger PA, Cranberg JA, Ganz MA, Hubler GL. A prospective evaluation of elevated serum theophylline concentrations to determine if high concentrations are predictable. Am J Med 1991;91:67.

194. Newhouse MT. Is theophylline obsolete? Chest 1990;98:1.

195. Lam A, Newhouse MT. Management of asthma and chronic airflow limitation: are methylxanthines obsolete? Chest 1990;98:44.
196. Littenberg B. Aminophylline treatment in severe acute asthma: a meta-analyis. JAMA 1988;259:1678.
197. Chapman KR, Bryant D, Marlin GE, et al. A placebo-controlled dose-response study of enprofylline in the maintenance therapy of asthma. Am Rev Respir Dis 1989;139:688.
198. Alciato P, Cantone PA, Fico D, Gagliardini R, Petrella V. Bamifylline in the therapy of asthmatic syndromes: efficacy and side effects vs. delayed-action theophylline anhydride. Minerva Med 1990;81:93.
199. Howell JBL, Altounyan REC. A double-blind trial of disodium cromoglycate in the treatment of allergic bronchial asthma. Lancet 1967;ii:539.
200. Foreman JC, Garland LG. Cromoglycate and other antiallergic drugs: a possible mechanism of action. Br Med J 1976;1:820.
201. Foreman JC, Mongar JL, Gomperts BD, et al. A possible role for cyclic AMP in the regulation of histamine secretion and the action of cromoglycate. Biochem Pharmacol 1975;24:538.
202. Lavin N, Rachelefsky MD, Kaplan SA. An action of disodium cromoglycate: Inhibition of cyclic 3',5'-AMP phosphodiesterase. J Allergy Clin Immunol 1976;57:80.
203. Blumenthal MN, Selcow J, Spector S, Zeiger RS, Mellon M. A multicenter evaluation of the clinical benefits of cromolyn sodium aerosol by metered dose inhaler in the treatment of asthma. J Allergy Clin Immunol 1988;81:681.
204. DeJong JW, Teengs JP, Postma DS, et al. Nedocromil sodium versus albuterol in the management of allergic asthma. Am J Respir Crit Care Med 1994;149:91.
205. Fink JN, Forman S, Slivers WS, et al. A double-blind study of the efficacy of nedocromil sodium in the management of asthma in patients using high doses of bronchodilators. J Allergery Clin Immunol 1994;94:473.
206. O'Hickey SP, Rees PJ. High-dose nedocromil sodium as an addition to inhaled corticosteroids in the treatment of asthma. Respir Med 1994;88:499.
207. Rebuck AS, Gent M, Chapman KR. Anticholinergic and sympathomimetic combination therapy of asthma. J Allergy Clin Immunol 1983;71:317.
208. Karpel JP, Breidbart D, Fusco MJ. A comparison of atropine sulfate and metaproterenol sulfate in the emergency treatment of asthma. Am Rev Respir Dis 1986;133:727.
209. Gilman MJ, Meyer L, Carter J, Clovis C. Comparison of aerosolized glycopyrrolate and metaproterenol in acute asthma. Chest 1990;98:1095.
210. Goyal RK. Muscarinic receptor subtypes: physiology and clinical implications. N Engl J Med 1989;321:1022.
211. Israel E, Ruben P, Kemp JP, et al. The effect of inhibition of 5-lipoxygenase by zileuton in mild-to-moderate asthma. Ann Intern Med 1993;119:1059.
212. Hirsch DJ, Hirsch SR, Kalbfleisch JH. Effect of central air conditioning and meteorologic factors on indoor spore counts. J Allergy Clin Immunol 1978;62:22.
213. Habenicht HA, Burge HA, Muilenberg ML, et al. Allergen carriage by atmospheric aerosol. II. Ragweed-pollen determinants in submicronic atmospheric fractions. J Allergy Clin Immunol 1984;74:64.
214. Reisman RE, Mauriello PM, Davis DB, Georgitis JW, DeMasi JM. A double-blind study of the effectiveness of a high efficiency particulate air (HEPA) filter in the treatment of patients with perennial allergic rhinitis and asthma. J Allergy Clin Immunol 1990;85:1050.
215. Samet J. Environmental controls and lung disease. Am Rev Respir Dis 1990;142:915.
216. Benowitz NL, Hall SM, Herning RI. Smokers of low-yield cigarettes do not consume less nicotine. N Engl J Med 1983;309:139.
217. Adams SL, Mathews J, Grammer LC. Drugs that exacerbate myasthenia gravis. Ann Emerg Med 1984;13:532.
218. Dunn TL, Gerber MJ, Shen AS, Fernandez E, Iseman MD, Cherniak RM. The effect of topical ophthalmic instillation of timolol and betaxolol on lung function in asthmatic subjects. Am Rev Respir Dis 1986;133:264.
219. Prakash VBS, Rosenow EC III. Pulmonary complications from ophthalmic preparations. Mayo Clin Proc 1990;65:521.
220. Lipworth BJ, McMurray JJ, Clark RA, Struthers AD. Development of persistent late onset asthma following treatment with captopril. Eur Respir J 1989;2:586.
221. Levey BA. Angiotensin-converting enzyme inhibitors and cough. Chest 1990;98:1052.
222. May CD. Objective clinical laboratory studies of immediate hypersensitivity reactions to foods in asthmatic children. J Allergy Clin Immunol 1976;58:500.
223. Johnstone DE, Dutton A. The value of hyposensitization therapy for bronchial asthma in children: a 14 year study. Pediatrics 1968;42:793.
224. Stevenson DD. Oral challenges to detect aspirin and sulfite sensitivity in asthma. NER Allergy Proc 1988;9:135.
225. Patterson R, DeSwarte RD, Greenberger PA, et al. Drug allergy and protocols for management of drug allergies. Allergy Proc 1994;15:243.
226. Stevenson DD, Pleskow WW, Simon RA, et al. Aspirin-sensitive rhinosinusitis asthma: a double-blind crossover study of treatment with aspirin. J Allergy Clin Immunol 1984;73:500.
227. Ruffin RE, Latimer KM, Schembri DA. Longitudinal study of near fatal asthma. Chest 1991;99:77.
228. Klein JJ, Lefkowitz MS, Spector SL, et al. Relationship between serum theophylline levels and pulmonary function before and after inhaled beta agonist in "stable" asthmatics. Am Rev Respir Dis 1983;127:413.
229. Gautrin P, D'Aquino LC, Gagnon G, et al. Comparison between peak expiratory flow rates (PEFR) and FEV$_1$ in the monitoring of asthmatic subjects at an outpatient clinic. Chest 1994;106:1419.

230. Ogirala RG, Aldrich TK, Prezant DJ, Sinnett MJ, Enden JB, Williams MH. High-dose intramuscular triamin-cinolone in severe, chronic, life-threatening asthma. N Engl J Med 1991;324:585.
231. Mullarkey MF, Blumenstein BA, Andrade WP, Bailey GA, Olason I, Wetzel CE. Methotrexate in the treatment of corticosteroid-dependent asthma: a double blind crossover study. N Engl J Med 1988;318:603.
232. Ezrurum SC, Leff JA, Cochran JE, et al. Lack of benefit of methotrexate in severe, steroid-dependent asthma. Ann Intern Med 1991;114:353.
233. Dykewicz MS, Greenberger PA, Patterson R, Halwig JM. Natural history of asthma in patients requiring long-term systemic corticosteroids. Arch Intern Med 1986;146:2369.
234. Klaustermeyer WB, Noritake DT, Kwong FK. Chrysotherapy in the treatment of corticosteroid-dependent asthma. J Allergy Clin Immunol 1987;79:720.
235. Corrigan CJ, Brown PH, Barnes NC, et al. Glucocorticoid resistance in chronic asthma: glucocorticoid pharmacokinetics, glucocorticoid receptor characteristics, and inhibition of peripheral blood T cell proliferation by glucocorticoids *in vitro*. Am Rev Respir Dis 1991;144:1016.
236. Corrigan CJ, Brown PH, Barnes NC, et al. Glucocorticoid resistance in chronic asthma: peripheral blood T lymphocyte activation and comparison of the T lymphocyte inhibitory effects of glucocorticoids and cyclosporin A. Am Rev Respir Dis 1991;144:1026.
237. Corbridge TC, Hall JB. The assessment and management of adults with status asthmaticus. Am J Respir Crit Care Med 1995;151:1296.
238. Mountain RD, Sahn SA. Clinical features and outcome in patients with acute asthma presenting with hypercapnia. Am Rev Respir Dis 1988;138:535.
239. Kurland G, Williams J, Lewiston NJ. Fatal myocardial toxicity during continous infusion intravenous isoproterenol therapy of asthma. J Allergy Clin Immunol 1979;63:407.
240. Cotton EK, Parry W. Treatment of status asthmaticus and respiratory failure. Pediatr Clin North Am 1975;22:163.
241. Steichen Kabalin C, Yarnold PR, Grammer LC. Low complication rate of corticosteroid-treated asthmatics undergoing surgical procedures. Arch Intern Med 1995;155:1379.
242. Greenberger PA, Miller TP, Lifschultz B. Circumstances surrounding deaths from asthma in Cook County (Chicago) Illinois. Allergy Proc 1993;14:321.
243. Manning PJ, Watson RM, Margolskee DJ, Williams VC, Schwartz JI, O'Byrne PM. Inhibition of exercise-induced bronchoconstriction by MK-571, a potent leukotriene D_4-receptor antagonist. N Engl J Med 1990;323:1736.

Allergic Diseases, 5th Edition,
edited by Roy Patterson, Leslie Carroll Grammer, and
Paul A. Greenberger. Lippincott–Raven Publishers, Philadelphia, © 1997.

23

Hypersensitivity Pneumonitis

Jordan N. Fink

*J.N. Fink: Department of Allergy-Immunology,
Medical College of Wisconsin, Milwaukee, WI 53226.*

Pearls for Practitioners
Roy Patterson

- Hypersensitivity pneumonitis should be considered in chronic or acute noninfectious pneumonitis. It is uncommon but important since lung destruction can occur.
- The list of potential causes is long. Just run through the list. Most of them can be excluded by using common sense.
- Keeping the causative source of antigen in the home is dangerous as lung destruction progresses. Deaths have resulted from prolonged exposure to birds in the house.
- The diagnosis of hypersensitivity pneumonitis in a worker where litigation is involved can be a real problem.
- Some people would rather risk lung destruction than give up their birds.
- Treating a patient with corticosteroids when the antigen remains in the environment is dangerous.
- Unfortunately, serodiagnosis by some laboratories results in false-negative results. Know the laboratory you use.
- Positive prescriptions against antigens may only indicate exposure, not hypersensitivity pneumonitis. Clinical skill is required.

Most of the hypersensitivity diseases of the respiratory tract in humans are asthma or rhinitis, and are caused by the release of pharmacologic mediators from mast cells and the recruitment of inflammatory cells as a result of IgE antigen-initiated reactions. The inhaled antigens usually are common pollen grains, mold spores, or animal proteins, and the resulting reaction induces bronchospasm, mucosal edema, increased secretions, and inflammation. However, allergic respiratory reactions may take other forms, and additional immunologic processes involving precipitating antibodies, circulating antigen–antibody complexes, and cellular mechanisms may play a role in the pathogenesis of the disorders. Although asthma and rhinitis occur most often in individuals with atopic constitutions, the diseases discussed in this chapter can be seen in both atopic and nonatopic patients. The disorders may be grouped under the general term of *hypersensitivity pneumonitis* but are also referred to as *extrinsic allergic alveolitis*. These diseases occur as the result of immunologic inflammation after the inhalation of any of several organic dusts.[1–25] They present in several clinical forms, depending on the patient's immunologic responsiveness and intensity of exposure to the offending dust, as well as the antigenicity of the inhaled biologic dust.

ETIOLOGY

Almost any inhaled organic dust can sensitize and result in the development of hypersensitivity pneumonitis; a list of antigenic materials associated with the disorders is shown in Table 23-1. The diameters of the inhaled particles that reach the terminal airways where lesions are initiated are no larger than 3 to 5 μm. The dusts may be derived from animal proteins; for example, in pigeon breeder's disease, the inhaled antigens are contained in dried avian droppings.[3,13,23] In pituitary snuff-taker's disease, the offending material is the pituitary powder containing bovine or porcine proteins. The inhalation of vegetable dusts contaminated with various microorganisms also causes hypersensitivity reactions such as farmer's lung, bagassosis, and mushroom picker's disease. In these disorders, the inhaled dusts from the moldy vegetation are contaminated with thermophilic actinomycetes such as *Micropolyspora faeni*, *Thermoactinomyces vulgaris*, *Thermoactinomyces viridis*, or *Thermoactinomyces candidus*, whose spores are smaller than 1 mm and can reach terminal airways, causing sensitization and subsequent immunologic inflammatory lung disease. These thermophilic bacteria are ubiquitous and grow best at temperatures of 45° to 50°C, which commonly occur in decomposing hay, sugar cane, or mushroom compost. Thermophilic actinomycetes also have been

TABLE 23-1. *Sensitivity materials in hypersensitivity pneumonitis*

Etiology	Disease entity	Antigenic material inhaled	antigen
Induced by serum proteins	Bird breeder's lung	Avian dust	Avian proteins
	Pituitary snuff taker's lung	Pituitary powder	Bovine or porcine proteins
	Pearl oyster shell pneumonitis	Pearl oyster shell dust	Oyster shell glycoprotein
Induced by microorganisms	Farmer's lung	Moldy hay	*Micropolyspora faeni* or *Thermoactinomyces vulgaris, T sacchari, T viridis, T candidus, Micropolyspora* sp
	Bagassosis	Moldy sugar cane	
	Mushroom picker's lung	Mushroom compost	
	Pneumonitis from contaminated air conditioner, humidifier, or heating system (forced air system disease)	Dust from air conditioners, humidifier, or furnace	
	Maple bark disease	Moldy maple bark	
	Sequoiosis	Redwood dust	
	Suberosis	Moldy cork dust	
	Cheese washer's lung	Cheese particles	
	Paprika splitter's lung	Paprika dust	*Cryptostroma corticale*
	Malt worker's lung	Malt dust	*Graphium* sp
	Summer pneumonitis	House dust	*Penicillium frequentans* *Penicillium caseii* *Mucor stolonifer* *Aspergillus clavatus* *Trichosporon cutaneum*
Similar diseases	Smallpox handler's lung	Smallpox scab dust	Unknown
	Enzyme worker's lung	Enzyme dust	*Bacillus subtilis*
	Bathtub refinisher's lung	Chemical catalyst	Toluene diisocyanate
	Epoxy resin lung	Heated epoxy resin	Phthalic anhydride
	Plastic worker's lung	Plasticizer	Trimellitic anhydride
	Drug induced	Pharmacologic agents	Gold, thiazides, penicillin, tetracyclines, hydroxyurea

shown to contaminate forced air heating, humidification, or air-conditioning systems of commercial or residence buildings where hypersensitivity pneumonitis can occur as a result of sensitization to these and other contaminants.[2,12]

The inhalation of other antigens also may result in hypersensitivity pneumonitis. Workers removing the bark from maple logs and inhaling the spores of *Cryptostroma corticale*,[11] woodworkers exposed to redwood dust that contains the mold *Graphium* sp,[8] individuals working in cheese factories in which *Penicillium caeseii* spores may be inhaled, and brewers working in malt factories where spores of *Aspergillus clavatus*[21] may be present also develop disease. A similar pneumonitis also may occur in workers exposed to the enzyme of *Bacillus subtilis* used in detergent manufacturing,[14] and after exposure to organic chemicals such as phthalic anhydrides[24] or toluene diisocyanate.[25] Recently, pneumonitis occurring only in the summer in Japan has been traced to homes contaminated with *Trichosporon cutaneum*.[15] The list of inhaled organic dusts that result in a hypersensitivity pneumonitis grows as exposure to new antigens increases.

In addition to the presence of an organic dust in the environment, other factors play a role in the development of a hypersensitivity pneumonitis in the exposed individual. The frequency and extent of exposure as well as the immunologic reactivity of the host are likely to influence the response to the dust, as are factors such as ciliary transport mechanisms, alveolar macrophage phagocytosis, and other coexisting pulmonary inflammatory processes.

CLINICAL FEATURES

The clinical manifestations of these respiratory disorders may present in several forms, depending on the immunologic response to the inhaled antigen, the antigenicity of the dust, and the frequency and intensity of exposure (Table 23-2). In general, the manifestations are similar, regardless of organic dust inhaled, and hypersensitivity pneumonitis may be considered as a syndrome with a spectrum of clinical features, although each specific disease may be caused by a different organic dust. The atopic individual may demonstrate typical bronchospasm or rhinorrhea immediately after inhalation of the dust; this reaction may be followed hours later by clinical features of a hypersensitivity pneumonitis. The nonatopic patient, however, usually responds with the late-type reaction characteristic of these disorders.

TABLE 23-2. *Clinical features of hypersensitivity pneumonitis*

Feature	Acute form	Subacute form	Chronic form
Relation of symptoms to exposure	+	+	−
Chills, fever	+	±	−
Cough, dyspnea	+	+	+
Malaise, myalgia, arthralgia	+	+	±
Anorexia, weight loss	±	+	+
Interstitial rales heard	+	+	±
Clubbing	−	−	±
Chest x-ray	Nodular infiltrates	Nodular infiltrates	Fibrosis honeycombing
Pulmonary function	Restriction	Restriction	Restriction or obstruction
Serum precipitins	+	+	+
Reversible with avoidance	Rapid	Slow	None
Reversible with corticosteroids	Rapid	Rapid	None

Acute Form

The most common and most easily recognized form of hypersensitivity pneumonitis follows intermittent exposure to a specific organic dust. Within 4 to 6 hours of exposure, the sensitized patient develops symptoms of cough, dyspnea, fever, chills, myalgia, and malaise, resembling a systemic viral or bacterial infection. The symptoms persist for 8 to 12 hours, but the patient recovers spontaneously, only to experience a recurrence of symptoms with reexposure. Numerous attacks may be associated with weight loss and anorexia. Between the acute attacks and in the absence of further antigen exposure, the patient often feels normal. Clinical examination during an attack reveals an acutely ill, dyspneic patient with prominent bibasilar moist rales. Although the patient appears to recover within a few hours, the rales may persist for a few days.

During the attack, laboratory studies usually demonstrate a leukocytosis with the white blood cell count as high as 25,000. Eosinophilia is unusual but may be as high as 10%. Often, levels of total serum IgG are elevated, but in some patients all of the major immunoglobulin classes are increased. Levels of IgE are elevated only in patients with atopic diseases; IgE levels usually are normal in hypersensitivity pneumonitis.

Results from pulmonary function studies done during the asymptomatic period of the acute form of a hypersensitivity pneumonitis usually are normal. Measurable changes occur 4 to 6 hours after exposure to the offending antigen (Fig. 23-1). There is a reduction in vital capacity, a decrease in gas transfer across the alveolar wall (as measured by diffusing capacity), and a

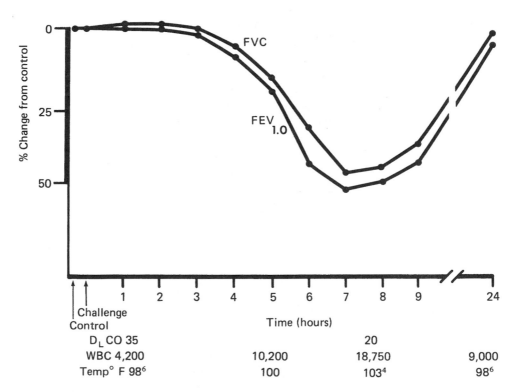

FIG. 23-1. Pulmonary function changes in an acute episode of hypersensitivity pneumonitis. Notice the time delay from challenge. FVC, forced vital capacity; $FEV_{1.0}$, forced expiratory volume in 1 second; DL_{CO}, diffusion capacity.

decrease in pulmonary compliance. Some patients also demonstrate decreases in expiratory flow rates and 1-second forced vital capacity, indicating airway obstruction. Chest x-rays may show fine nodular densities and peripheral infiltrates suggestive of interstitial and alveolar involvement (Figure 23-2), but a normal chest roentgenogram finding does not exclude the disease. With avoidance of exposure to the offending materials or therapy with corticosteroids, all symptoms disappear and abnormal laboratory test results return to normal. Continued intermittent exposure to the offending organic dust, however, may lead to permanent pulmonary function and radiographic abnormalities associated with progressive respiratory insufficiency. Fatalities because of progressive hypersensitivity pneumonitis have been reported.[26,27]

Subacute Form

Some patients have a more insidious type of disease with rare acute attacks. These individuals usually are exposed to small amounts of antigen over long periods (e.g., lovebird or parakeet fanciers). The symptoms resemble those of a progressive bronchitis: dyspnea, chronic productive cough with scanty sputum, anorexia, fatigue, and weight loss. Pulmonary function

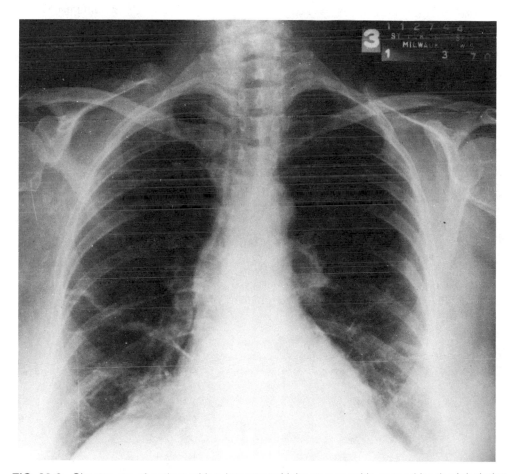

FIG. 23-2. Chest x-ray of patient with a hypersensitivity pneumonitis caused by the inhalation of thermophilic actinomycetes contaminating her furnace humidifier.

abnormalities of progressive restriction, diffusion defect, and increased stiffness of the lung are seen. These patients often are diagnosed as having chronic bronchitis, recurrent episodes of influenza, idiopathic pulmonary fibrosis, or Hamman-Rich syndrome. Although the clinical laboratory abnormalities respond to corticosteroids or prolonged avoidance of exposure to the offending dust, the response is much less prompt than in the acute form. If sufficient fibrosis is present, the pulmonary function abnormalities become irreversible.

Chronic Form

In some cases, chronic irreversible lung damage may occur. This may take the form of irreversible fibrosis and pulmonary insufficiency, and is seen in long-standing cases of farmer's lung and in persons who keep parakeets, budgerigars, or lovebirds. These persons have symptoms of progressive dyspnea and may develop irreversible pulmonary function abnormalities or restriction, diffusion defects, and "stiff" lungs that do not respond to corticosteroids. Lung biopsy specimens from these patients demonstrate interstitial fibrosis with granulomas and thickening of alveolar walls.

In a few patients with farmer's lung, pigeon breeder's disease, or bagassosis, pulmonary function tests show persistently marked elevation of the residual volume, diminished flow rates, and loss of pulmonary elasticity, suggestive of emphysema. Histologic examination of these lungs shows obstructive bronchitis with distal destruction of alveoli. Such patients usually do not respond to corticosteroids or avoidance of exposure, even if these measures are pursued for prolonged periods.

Although avoidance of exposure usually is followed by resolution of signs and symptoms, this does not always occur. Patients with the chronic form of hypersensitivity pneumonitis manifest progressive pulmonary impairment. Patients with multiple acute episodes of farmer's lung may continue to have respiratory impairment, even long after avoidance.[19]

IMMUNOLOGIC FEATURES

The characteristic immunologic feature of these disorders is the presence of precipitins against the offending antigen in the sera of affected individuals (Fig. 23-3). These antibodies may be demonstrated by gel diffusion techniques using the patient's serum and the suspected antigen. Immunoelectrophoresis has shown these precipitating antibodies to be of the IgG class, although other studies have demonstrated antibody activity in other classes of immunoglobulins.[28,29] A few patients have low titers of precipitins, and it may be necessary

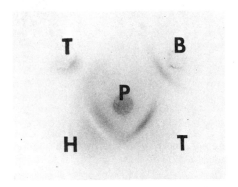

FIG. 23-3. Immunodiffusion studies of serum of patient (P) in Figure 23-2 against thermophilic antigens (T), bagasse (B), and moldy hay (H).

to concentrate their serum to detect the antibodies, but relatively high titers of these antibodies have been seen in the sera of most symptomatic patients studied. As many as 50% of asymptomatic individuals exposed to the same antigen also may have precipitins, but usually of lesser titer. Thus, the finding of precipitins must be considered in light of the clinical history when the diagnosis of hypersensitivity pneumonitis is considered.

Skin tests with suspected thermophile antigens have been shown to be unreliable because of nonspecific irritation-type reactions. In the disorders caused by inhalation of serum proteins, however, such as pigeon breeder's disease, skin tests may be of value. Both immediate wheal-and-flare and late (4- to 6-hour) skin reactions may be observed. The immediate reactions are the same type as seen with the common inhalant allergens, but the late reactions resemble the Arthus phenomenon, indicative of a vasculitis because of a precipitin–antigen reaction. The late reaction begins with a variable of edema and erythema of the injected area; it can progress to central necrosis, but it usually subsides in 24 hours unless necrosis has occurred. Histologic examination of biopsy specimens of such skin reactions has demonstrated lesions consistent with Arthus-type reactions, with a mild vasculitis consisting of polymorphonuclear and plasma cell infiltration of the vessels in the area.[1,17]

RADIOGRAPHIC FEATURES

Hypersensitivity pneumonitis cannot be distinguished radiographically from other nonimmunologic interstitial disorders. Roentgenogram findings may be normal or they may show recurrent interstitial nodular infiltrations or fibrotic changes, depending on the stage of the disease.[5,17]

PATHOLOGIC FEATURES

The histologic features of the lung in the hypersensitivity disorders depend on the stage of the disease at the time of biopsy (Fig. 23-4). In early stages of farmer's lung, bagassosis, mushroom picker's disease, and some hypersensitivity pneumonitis caused by antigens other than thermophilic organisms, the alveolar walls are infiltrated with lymphocytes. Plasma cells and histocytes containing foamy cytoplasm also may be seen within the alveolar spaces. Later, the interstitium becomes infiltrated with mononuclear cells and scattered giant cell granulomata. In still later stages, fibrosis of these areas occurs, and an organizing bronchiolitis obliterans may be seen.

In biopsy specimens from cases of pigeon breeder's disease, similar interstitial and alveolar granulomatous and infiltrative changes may be seen.[10,30,31] In addition, foamy macrophages, possibly derived from alveolar macrophages, may be found in the interstitial areas and within the alveoli. The interstitial position of these foamy cells may be unique for pigeon breeder's disease because this feature is not common in the other hypersensitivity pneumonitides.

Bronchiolitis obliterans can be observed with peripheral destruction of alveoli in some chronic cases of farmer's lung, bagassosis, or pigeon breeder's disease. The interstitial and intraalveolar infiltrate in these cases is less distinctive, and there are fewer foam-laden macrophages than in the other forms of the disorder.[30,31]

DIFFERENTIAL DIAGNOSIS

The diagnosis of a typical case of a hypersensitivity pneumonitis usually can be made by evaluating the environmental history, by examining results of appropriate laboratory and

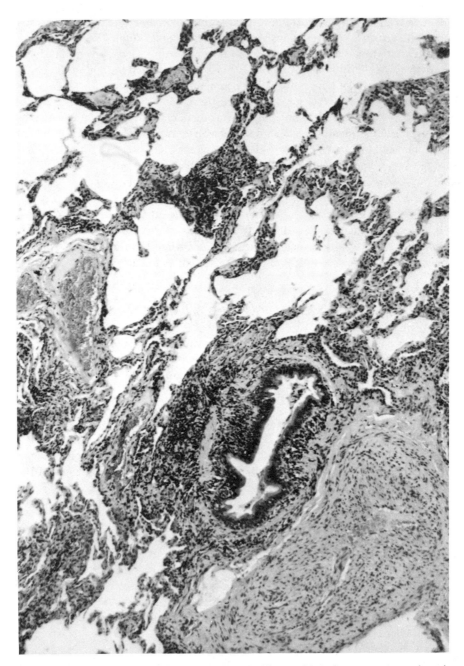

FIG. 23-4. Lung biopsy specimen of the patient in Figure 23-2 demonstrates a lymphocytic interstitial pneumonitis with early granuloma formation (×250).

serologic studies, and by using a trial of avoidance and reexposure where possible (Table 23-3). The more insidious and progressive forms of hypersensitivity pneumonitis may be difficult to diagnose. Chest x-ray and pulmonary function abnormalities of other interstitial pulmonary disorders such as chronic eosinophilic pneumonia, the collagen vascular diseases, lymphogenous spread of carcinoma, desquamative interstitial pneumonia, and sarcoid may be similar. The finding of extrapulmonary involvement (such as generalized lymphadenopathy or abdominal organomegaly) rules out a hypersensitivity pneumonitis. At times, however, a lung biopsy may be necessary to make a definitive diagnosis. Biopsy also may be necessary to differentiate these disorders from diffuse idiopathic pulmonary fibrosis, which clinically resembles the fibrotic stage of hypersensitivity pneumonitis.

CONTROLLED EXPOSURE TO ANTIGENS

On occasion, the patient may be exposed cautiously to the suspected antigen, and the reaction carefully observed. This may be done during an asymptomatic period by allowing the farmer to enter the barn or the pigeon breeder to enter the coop. The patient then should be brought to the hospital and observed frequently over the next 8 hours for symptoms or signs of hypersensitivity pneumonitis.

Some reactions may be diagnosed by careful inhalation exposure to nonirritating sterile extracts of the suspected antigen, although this is less desirable than observation after natural exposure. This purposeful exposure of an individual, however, either in the appropriate environment or by direct airway challenge, must be considered an experimental technique to be done with great caution by experienced physicians. With dilute extracts—previously shown not to induce any changes in normal individuals—minimal abnormalities in pulmonary function tests or a rise in temperature of a few degrees 4 to 6 hours after exposure may clarify the diagnosis. Corticosteroids may be needed in these cases to abort severe attacks that were induced inadvertently.

TABLE 23-3. *Diagnostic methods of hypersensitivity pneumonitis*

History
Suspicious of environmentally induced symptoms

Chest X-Ray
Abnormalities depend on stage of disease and proximity to exposure
Normal finding on chest x-ray is possible

Pulmonary Function
Abnormalities depend on stage of disease and proximity to exposure
Usually ↓FVC, ↓DLCO, ↓Pao_2
Normal function is possible

Precipitins
Usually present to offending environmental agents

Trial of Avoidance
Results in relief of symptoms and return to normal function

Bronchoalveolar Lavage
Lymphocytosis with predominance of suppression T cells

Lung Biopsy
Features characteristic of hypersensitivity pneumonitis

FVC, forced vital capacity; DLCO, diffusion capacity of the lungs for carbon monoxide; Pao_2, arterial partial pressure of oxygen.

PATHOGENESIS

Evaluation of pulmonary cell populations from patients with hypersensitivity pneumonitis has revealed activation of macrophages and release of proinflammatory cytokines and CD8 or suppressor cell attractants from those cells.[32,33] Further, the alveolitis of hypersensitivity pneumonitis is lymphocytic and is largely composed of CD8 suppressor cells, which appear to have decreased functional capacity.[34–38] The results of these processes likely are the major pathogenetic mechanisms of the inflammatory response seen in this disease.

THERAPY

As in all other allergic disorders, the primary therapy should be avoidance of the offending antigen once it is known. Because many of these disorders are occupational, certain measures may be necessary, such as the use of masks with filters capable of removing the antigen, appropriate ventilation of working areas, or even a change of occupation.

Drug therapy may be needed in the acute or subacute forms of these disorders when avoidance cannot be carried out immediately. Although antihistamines or bronchodilators have no effect on the symptom pattern, patients usually respond to the administration of corticosteroids. Moderate doses of these drugs may be necessary for prolonged periods, along with avoidance, to determine if reversibility of the clinical abnormalities is possible. Hyposensitization should be avoided because toxic immune complexes may be formed when the injected antigen combines with the precipitating IgG, and systemic vasculitis or serum sickness may result.

REFERENCES

1. Avila R, Villar TG. Suberosis: respiratory disease in cork workers. Lancet 1968;i:620.
2. Banaszak EF, Thiede WH, Fink JN. Hypersensitivity pneumonitis due to contamination of an air conditioner. N Engl J Med 1970;283:271.
3. Barboriak JJ, Sosman AJ, Reed CE. Serologic studies in pigeon breeders' disease. J Lab Clin Med 1965;65:600.
4. Barrowcliff DR, Arblaster PG. Farmer's lung: a study of an early acute fatal case. Thorax 1968;23:49.
5. Bringhurst LS, Byrne RN, Gershon-Cohen J. Respiratory disease of mushroom workers. JAMA 1959;171:15.
6. Buechner HA, Prevatt AL, Thompson J, et al. Bagassosis: a review with further historical data studies of pulmonary function and results of adrenal steroid therapy. Am J Med 1958;25:234.
7. Campbell JN. Acute symptoms following work with hay. Br Med J 1932;2:1143.
8. Cohen Hi, Merigan TC, Kosek JC, et al. A granulomatous pneumonitis associated with redwood sawdust inhalation. Am J Med 1967;43:758.
9. Cross T, MacIver AM, Lacey J. The thermophilic actinomycetes in moldy hay. J Gen Microbiol 1968;50:351.
10. Emanuel DA, Wenzel FJ, Bowerman CI, Lawton BR. Farmer's lung: clinical, pathologic and immunologic study of twenty-four patients. Am J Med 1964;37:392.
11. Emanuel DA, Wenzel FJ, Lawton BR. Pneumonitis due to *Cryptostroma corticale* (maple-bark disease). N Engl J Med 1966;274:1413.
12. Fink JN, Banaszak EF, Thiede WH, et al. Interstitial pneumonitis due to hypersensitivity to an organism contaminating a heating system. Ann Intern Med 1971;74:80.
13. Fink JN, Sosman AJ, Barboriak JJ, et al. Pigeon breeders' disease: a clinical study of a hypersensitivity pneumonitis. Ann Intern Med 1968;68:1205.
14. Flindt MLH. Pulmonary disease due to inhalation of *Bacillus subtilis* containing proteolytic enzyme. Lancet 1969;i:1177.
15. Kawai T, Tamura M, Murao M. Summer-type hypersensitivity pneumonitis: a unique disease in Japan. Chest 1984;85:311.
16. Norris-Evans WH, Foreman WH. Smallpox handler's lung. Proc R Soc Med 1963;56:274.
17. Pepys J. Hypersensitivity disease of the lungs due to fungi and other organic dusts. Monogr Allergy 1969;4:44.
18. Pepys J, Jenkins PA, Lachmann PJ, et al. An iatrogenic autoantibody: immunological response to pituitary snuff in patients with diabetes insipidus. Clin Exp Immunol 1966;1:377.

19. Rankin J, Kobayashi M, Barbee RA, et al. Pulmonary granulomatoses due to inhaled organic antigens. Med Clin North Am 1967;51:459.
20. Reed CE, Sosman A, Barbee RA. Pigeon breeders' lung. JAMA 1965;193:261.
21. Riddle HFV, Grant JWB. Allergic alveolitis in a malt worker. Thorax 1968;23:271.
22. Salvaggio JE, Buechner HA, Seabury JH, et al. Bagassosis. I. Precipitins against extracts of crude bagassee in the serum of patients with bagassosis. Ann Intern Med 1966;64:748.
23. Hargreave FE, Pepys J, Longbottom JL, et al. Bird breeder's (fancier's) lung. Lancet 1966;i:44.
24. Schlueter DP, Banaszak EF, Fink JN, et al. Occupational asthma due to tetrachlorophthalic andydride. J Soc Occup Med 1978;20:183.
25. Fink JN, Schlueter DP. Bathtub refinisher's lung: an unusual response to toluene diisocyanate. Am Rev Respir Dis 1978;118:955.
26. Ghose T, Landrigan P, Killeen R, et al. Immunopathologic studies in patients with farmer's lung. Clin Allergy 1974;4:119.
27. Greenberger PA, Pien LC, Patterson R, Robinson P, Roberts M. End stage lung and ultimately fatal disease in a bird fancier. Am J Med 1989;86:119.
28. Patterson R, Roberts M, Roberts RR, et al. Antibodies of different immunoglobulin classes against antigens causing farmer's lung 1976;114:315.
29. Patterson R, Schatz M, Fink JN, et al. Pigeon breeder's disease: serum immunoglobulins concentrations: IgG, IgM, IgA, and IgE antibodies against pigeon serum. Am J Med 1976;60:144.
30. Hensley GT, Garancis JC, Cherayil GD, Fink JN. Lung biopsies of pigeon breeder's disease. Arch Pathol 1969;87:572.
31. Kawanami O, Basset F, Barrios R, Lacronique JG, Ferrans VJ, Crystal RG. Hypersensitivity pneumonitis in man: light and electron microscopic studies of 18 lung biopsies. Am J Pathol 1983;110:275.
32. Denis M. Proinflammatory cytokines in hypersensitivity pneumonitis. Am J Resp Crit Care Med 1995;151.164.
33. Reynolds HY, Fulmer JD, Kazmierowski JA, Roberts W, Frank MM, Crystal RG. Analysis of cellular and protein content of bronchoalveolar lavage fluid from patients with idiopathic pulmonary fibrosis and chronic hypersensitivity pneumonitis. J Clin Invest 1977;59:165.
34. Fink JN, Moore VL, Barboriak JJ. Cell-mediated hypersensitivity in pigeon breeders. Int Arch Allergy Appl Immunol 1975;49:83.
35. Mornex JF, Cordier G, Pages J, et al. Activated lung lymphocytes in hypersensitivity pneumonitis. J Allergy Clin Immunol 1984;74:719.
36. Keller RH, Swartz S, Schlueter DP, Bar-Sela S, Fink JN. Immunoregulation in hypersensitivity pneumonitis phenotypic and functional studies of bronchoalveolar lavage lymphocytes. Am Rev Respir Dis 1984;130:766.
37. Barquin N, Sansores R, Chapela R, Perez-Tamayo R, Selman M. Immunoregulatory abnormalities in patients with pigeon breeder's disease. Lung 1990;168:103.
38. Moore VL, Pedersen GM, Hauser WC, Fink JN. A study of lung lavage materials in patients with hypersensitivity pneumonitis. J Allergy Clin Immunol 1980;65:365.

Allergic Diseases, 5th Edition,
edited by Roy Patterson, Leslie Carroll Grammer, and
Paul A. Greenberger. Lippincott–Raven Publishers, Philadelphia, © 1997.

24

Allergic Bronchopulmonary Aspergillosis

Paul A. Greenberger

*P.A. Greenberger: Division of Allergy-Immunology,
Northwestern University Medical School, Chicago, IL 60611-3008.*

Pearls for Practitioners
Roy Patterson

- Negative results from prick and intradermal skin tests for *Aspergillus fumigatus* exclude allergic bronchopulmonary aspergillosis (ABPA).
- ABPA may yield only positive serologic findings without any other features of ABPA. This is ABPA-serologics.
- Four serologic tests are necessary to exclude or diagnose ABPA, but positive results from three of four tests can make a diagnosis.
- Stage IV (corticosteroid-dependent asthma) ABPA generally requires only inhaled corticosteroids. Moderate- to low-dose alternate-day prednisone is needed in some patients.
- ABPA should be excluded in all asthmatics.
- Inhaled antifungal agents are not needed for ABPA. Prednisone controls the acute phase or exacerbations.
- Rarely, a patient who has all of the clinical findings of ABPA will have elevated total IgE but negative serologic findings for *Aspergillus* infections. This is allergic bronchopulmonary mycosis (ABPM). ABPM should be treated like ABPA. Finding the fungus responsible is a research project.
- In a newly diagnosed case of ABPA, the total serum IgE will decline 35% to 75% with prednisone therapy. The goal should be treatment with prednisone until the IgE level reaches a plateau, not to reach the "normal" level of IgE, because this requires excessive use of prednisone.
- ABPA serologic findings may remain positive for decades in stage IV (corticosteroid-dependent) ABPA. This does not indicate a poor prognosis.
- ABPA serologic findings may become negative with high-dose prednisone therapy.
- Most patients with fibrotic (stage V) ABPA die. Stage V is rarely found since ABPA is being diagnosed before progression to stage V.

Allergic bronchopulmonary aspergillosis (ABPA) is characterized by immunologic reactions to antigens of *Aspergillus fumigatus* (Af) that are present in the bronchial tree and result in pulmonary infiltrates and proximal bronchiectasis. ABPA was first described in England in 1952 in patients with asthma who had recurrent episodes of fever, roentgenographic infiltrates, peripheral blood and sputum eosinophilia, and sputum production containing Af hyphae.[1] The first case of an adult with ABPA in the United States was described in 1968,[2] and the first childhood case was reported in 1970.[3] Since then, the increasing recognition of ABPA in children,[4–8] adults,[9,10] corticosteroid-dependent asthmatics,[11] and patients with cystic fibrosis[11–16] is probably the result of the increasing awareness by physicians of this complication of asthma and the available serologic aids such as total serum IgE,[17] serum IgE and IgG antibodies to Af,[18,19] and precipitating antibodies.[20]

ABPA was identified in 6.0% of 531 patients in Chicago with asthma and immediate cutaneous reactivity to an *Aspergillus* mix,[21] whereas 28% of such patients in Cleveland had ABPA.[22] These surprisingly high prevalence figures were generated from the ambulatory setting of allergist–immunologists and suggest that the overall prevalence of ABPA in patients with chronic asthma is 1% to 2%.[21] ABPA has been identified on an international basis, and because of its destructive potential, should be confirmed or excluded in all patients with chronic asthma.

Aspergillus species are ubiquitous, thermotolerant, and can be recovered on a perennial basis.[23] Spores are 2 to 3.5 μm and can be cultured on Sabouraud's agar slants incubated at 37° to 40°C. *Aspergillus* hyphae may be identified in tissue by hematoxylin and eosin staining, but identification and morphologic features are better appreciated with silver methenamine or periodic acid-Schiff stains. Hyphae are 7 to 10 μm in diameter, septate, and classically branch at 45-degree angles. *Aspergillus* species, particularly *Aspergillus flavus* and Af, produce some toxic metabolites, of which aflatoxin is the most widely known. Af produces proteolytic enzymes that may contribute to lung damage when Af hyphae are present in bronchial mucus. *A flavus* and Af have been incriminated in avian aspergillosis, a major economic concern in the poultry industry. For example, aspergillosis is common in turkey poults and causes 5% to 10% mortality rates in production flocks.[24] *Aspergillus* infections as a cause of abortions in sheep are well recognized, as are infections in horses, cattle, and camels.

Aspergillus terreus is used in the pharmaceutical industry for synthesis of the cholesterol-lowering drug levostatin. For use in the baking industry, *Aspergillus* species produce amylase, cellulase, and hemicellulase. Because these enzymes are powdered, some bakery workers may develop IgE-mediated rhinitis and asthma.[25]

Organisms of the genus *Aspergillus* may produce different types of disease, depending on the immunologic status of the patient. In nonatopic patients, *Aspergillus* hyphae may grow in damaged lung and cause a fungus ball (aspergilloma). Morphologically, an aspergilloma contains thousands of tangled *Aspergillus* hyphae in pulmonary cavities and can complicate sarcoidosis, tuberculosis, carcinoma, cystic fibrosis, or even ABPA.[26] Hypersensitivity pneumonitis may result from inhalation of large numbers of Af or *Aspergillus clavatus* spores by malt workers. These spores also may produce farmer's lung disease. *Aspergillus* species may invade tissue in the immunologically compromised (neutropenic) host, causing sepsis and death.[27,28] *Aspergillus* species have been associated with emphysema, colonization of cysts, pulmonary suppurative reactions, and necrotizing pneumonia in other patients.[29] In the atopic patient, fungal spore asthma may be seen secondarily to IgE-mediated bronchospasm in response to inhalation of *Aspergillus* spores. Why some of these patients with asthma develop ABPA remains a subject for speculation. In patients without asthma, *Aspergillus* hyphae have been identified in mucoid impactions of sinuses, a condition that morphologically resembles mucoid impaction of bronchi in ABPA.[30,31] Such allergic *Aspergillus* sinusitis may occur in patients with ABPA.[32]

DIAGNOSTIC CRITERIA AND CLINICAL FEATURES

The criteria used for diagnosis of classic ABPA consist of five essential criteria; other criteria may be present, depending on the classification and stage of disease. The minimal essential criteria are (1) asthma, even cough variant asthma or exercise-induced asthma; (2) central bronchiectasis; (3) elevated total serum IgE ($\geq$1000 ng/mL); (4) immediate cutaneous reactivity to *Aspergillus*; and (5) elevated serum IgE or IgG antibodies, or both, to Af. Central bronchiectasis in the absence of distal bronchiectasis, as occurs in cystic fibrosis, is pathognomonic for ABPA. Such patients are labeled ABPA-CB (for central bronchiectasis). Other features of ABPA are often present. For example, the expected diagnostic criteria of ABPA-CB include (1) asthma; (2) immediate cutaneous reactivity to Af; (3) precipitating antibodies to Af; (4) elevated total serum IgE; (5) peripheral blood eosinophilia ($\geq$1000/mm^3); (6) a history of either transient or fixed roentgenographic infiltrates; (7) proximal bronchiectasis; and (8) elevated serum IgE-Af and IgG-Af.[33] These diagnostic criteria may not apply to ABPA-S (seropositive) where bronchiectasis cannot be detected by hilar tomography or chest tomography. Patients who have all of the criteria for ABPA, but in whom central bronchiectasis is not present, have ABPA-S.[10,34] The minimal essential criteria for ABPA-S include (1) asthma, (2) immediate cutaneous reactivity to *Aspergillus*, (3) elevated total serum IgE, and (4) elevated serum IgE and IgG antibodies to Af compared with sera from patients with asthma without ABPA.[10] Other features of ABPA include positive sputum cultures for Af, a history of expectoration of golden brown plugs containing Af hyphae, and late (Arthus-type) skin reactivity to intracutaneous testing with Af. Patients with asthma without ABPA may have positive cutaneous test reactions to Af, peripheral blood eosinophilia, and a history of roentgenographic infiltrates (from atelectasis from inadequately controlled asthma). *Aspergillus* precipitins are not diagnostic of ABPA, and sputum cultures may be negative for Af or even unobtainable if the patient has little bronchiectasis. In ABPA-S, bronchiectasis cannot be detected by high-resolution computed tomography. Serologic measurements have proven useful in making the diagnosis of ABPA. A marked elevation in total serum IgE as well as IgE and IgG antibodies to Af are of value in making the diagnosis.[19] Furthermore, the decline in total serum IgE by at least 35% after institution of prednisone has been shown to occur in ABPA.[35]

ABPA should be suspected in all patients with asthma who have immediate cutaneous reactivity to Af.[21] The absence of a documented roentgenographic infiltrate does not exclude ABPA-CB. Familial ABPA has been described, which emphasizes the need for screening family members for evidence of ABPA if they have asthma. Clearly, ABPA should be suspected in patients with a history of roentgenographic infiltrates, pneumonia, or abnormal findings on chest films. Increasing severity of asthma without other cause may indicate evolving ABPA, but some patients present solely with asymptomatic pulmonary infiltrates. Consolidation on the chest roentgenogram caused by ABPA often is not associated with the rigors, chills, as high a fever, and overall malaise, as would be a bacterial pneumonia that causes the same degree of roentgenographic consolidation. The time of onset of ABPA may precede recognition by many years,[36] or there may be early diagnosis of ABPA before significant lung destruction and roentgenographic infiltrates have occurred.[10] ABPA must be considered in the patient older than 40 years with chronic bronchitis, bronchiectasis, or interstitial fibrosis. Further lung damage may be prevented by treatment. The dose of corticosteroids necessary for controlling chronic asthma may be inadequate to prevent the emergence of ABPA, although the total serum IgE may be only moderately elevated because of suppression by systemic corticosteroids.

Patients with ABPA manifest multiple allergic conditions. For example, just 1 of 50 patients diagnosed and managed at Northwestern University Medical School (Chicago) has isolated cutaneous reactivity to Af.[35] Other atopic disorders usually are present in patients with ABPA.[35] The severity of asthma ranges from mild, which requires occasional bronchodilators, to corticosteroid dependent. Four patients denied developing wheezing or dyspnea on exposure to raked leaves, moldy hay, or damp basements, but they noticed nonimmunologic triggering factors such as cold air, infection, or weather changes. These findings emphasize that ABPA may be present in patients who appear to have no obvious IgE-mediated bronchospasm.

The number of diagnostic criteria vary depending on the classification (ABPA-CB or ABPA-S) and stage of ABPA. Furthermore, prednisone therapy causes clearing of the chest roentgenographic infiltrates, decline of total serum IgE, disappearance of precipitating antibodies, peripheral blood or sputum eosinophilia, and absence of sputum production.

PHYSICAL EXAMINATION

The physical examination in ABPA may be completely unremarkable in the asymptomatic patient, or it may show crackles, bronchial breathing, or wheezing, depending on the degree and quality of lung disease. An acute flare-up in ABPA may be associated with temperature elevation to 39°C (103°F; although this is uncommon) with malaise, wheezing, and sputum production. Viral or bacterial infections in patients with asthma may simulate exacerbations of ABPA. In some cases of ABPA, extensive pulmonary consolidation on roentgenography may be accompanied by few or no clinical symptoms, in contrast to the usual manifestations of a patient with a bacterial pneumonia and the same degree of consolidation. When extensive fibrosis has occurred from ABPA, posttussive crackles are present. ABPA has been associated with collapse of a lung from a mucoid impaction, and in one patient, it was associated with a spontaneous pneumothorax.[37] The physical examination gives evidence for these diagnoses. When ABPA infiltrates affect the periphery of the lung, pleuritis may occur, and it may be associated with restriction of chest wall movement on inspiration and a pleural friction rub. Some patients with end-stage ABPA (fibrotic—stage IV) have digital clubbing and cyanosis.[36,38]

RADIOLOGY

Roentgenographic changes may be transient or permanent[39–42] (Figs. 24-1 through 24-6). Transient roentgenographic changes, which may clear with or without corticosteroid therapy, seem to be the result of parenchymal infiltrates or mucoid impactions or secretions in damaged bronchi. These nonpermanent findings include (1) perihilar infiltrates simulating adenopathy; (2) air–fluid levels from dilated central bronchi filled with fluid and debris; (3) massive consolidation, which may be unilateral or bilateral; (4) roentgenographic infiltrates; (5) "toothpaste" shadows, which result from mucoid impactions in damaged bronchi; (6) "gloved-finger" shadows from distally occluded bronchi filled with secretions; and (7) "tramline" shadows, which are two parallel hairline shadows extending out from the hilum. The width of the transradiant zone between the lines is that of a normal bronchus at that level.[39] Tramline shadows, which represent edema of the bronchial wall, may be seen in asthma without ABPA, in cystic fibrosis, and in left ventricular failure with elevated pulmonary venous pressure. Permanent roentgenographic findings related to proximal bronchiectasis have been shown to occur in sites of previous infiltrates, which are often, but not exclusively, in the upper lobes. This is in contrast to postinfectious bronchiectasis, which is associated with distal abnormalities and normal proximal bronchi. When permanent lung damage occurs to large bronchi, parallel-line shadows and ring-shadows are seen. These do not change with corticosteroid treatment. Parallel-line shadows are dilated tramline shadows that result from bronchiectasis; the transradient zone between the lines is wider than that of normal bronchus. These shadows are believed to be permanent, representing bronchial widening. The ring-shadows, 1 to 2 cm in diameter, are dilated bronchi en face. Pulmonary fibrosis may occur and be irreversible. Late

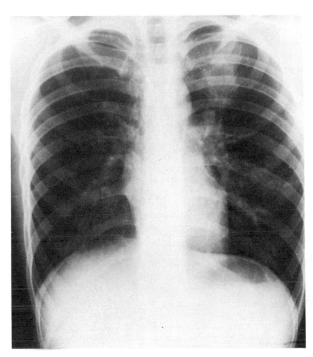

FIG. 24-1. Presentation chest radiograph of an 11-year-old boy with far-advanced allergic bronchopulmonary aspergillosis. Massive homogeneous consolidation in left upper lobe is shown. (Mintzer RA, Rogers LF, Kruglick GD, Rosenberg M, Neiman H, Patterson R. The spectrum of radiologic findings in allergic bronchopulmonary aspergillosis. Radiology 1978;127:301.)

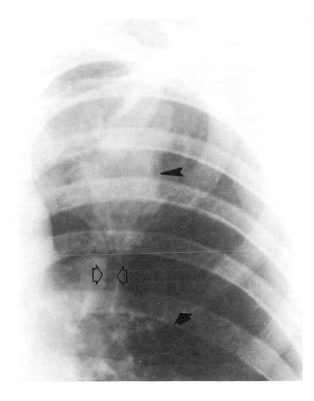

FIG. 24-2. Magnified view of the left upper lobe shows massive homogenous consolidation (narrow arrowhead), parallel lines (open broad arrowheads), and ring shadows (closed broad arrowheads). (Mintzer RA, Rogers LF, Kruglick GD, Rosenberg M, Neiman H, Patterson R. The spectrum of radiologic findings in allergic bronchopulmonary aspergillosis. Radiology 1978;127:301.)

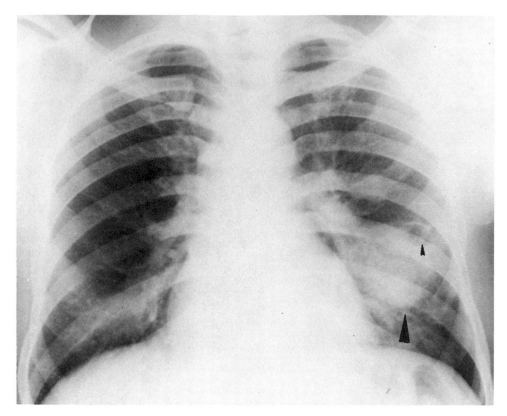

FIG. 24-3. Presentation chest radiograph of a 31-year-old man with far-advanced allergic bronchopulmonary aspergillosis. Notice the massive homogeneous consolidation (*large arrowhead*) and air–fluid level (*small arrowhead*). (Mintzer RA, Rogers LF, Kruglick GD, Rosenberg M, Neiman H, Patterson R. The spectrum of radiologic findings in allergic bronchopulmonary aspergillosis. Radiology 1978;127:301.)

findings in ABPA include cavitation, contracted upper lobes, and localized emphysema. When bullous changes are present, a spontaneous pneumothorax may occur.[36]

With high clinical suspicion of ABPA (bronchial asthma, high total serum IgE, immediate cutaneous reactivity to Af, precipitating antibody against Af) and a negative finding on chest roentgenogram, central bronchiectasis may be demonstrated by thin-section hilar linear tomography or computed tomography.[40–43]

Computed tomography should be done as an initial radiologic test beyond the chest roentgenogram (Figs. 24-7 through 24-9). If findings are normal, studies should be repeated in 1 year for highly suspicious cases.

High-resolution computed tomography using 1.5-mm section cuts has proved valuable in the detection of bronchiectasis in ABPA.[42] The thin-section cuts were obtained every 1 to 2 cm. Bronchial dilatation was present in 41% of lung lobes in eight ABPA patients compared with 15% of lobes in patients with asthma without ABPA. Bronchiectasis may be cylindrical, saccular, or varicose. From the axial perspective, central bronchiectasis was present when it occurred in the inner two thirds of the lung. Thin-layer anteroposterior hilar tomography has been effective in identifying central bronchiectasis.[40] In contrast to the axial perspective of computed tomography, hilar tomography identifies dilated bronchi in the coronal plane.

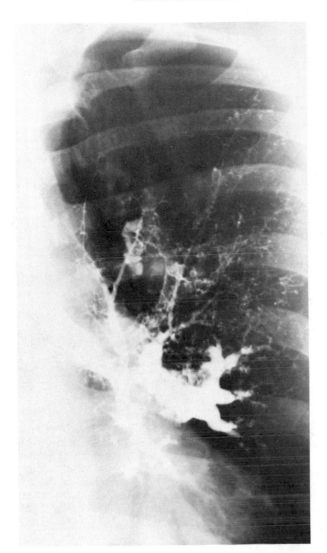

FIG. 24-4. Bronchogram showing classic proximal bronchiectasis with normal peripheral airways in a 25-year-old woman with allergic bronchopulmonary aspergillosis. (Mintzer RA, Rogers LF, Kruglick GD, Rosenberg M, Nelman H, Patterson R. The spectrum of radiologic findings in allergic bronchopulmonary aspergillosis. Radiology 1978;127: 301.)

STAGING

Five stages of ABPA have been identified[9]: acute, remission, exacerbation, corticosteroid-dependent asthma, and fibrotic. The acute stage (stage I) is present when all of the major criteria of ABPA can be documented. These criteria are asthma, immediate cutaneous reactivity to Af, precipitating antibody to Af, elevated serum IgE, peripheral blood eosinophilia, history of or presence of roentgenographic infiltrates, and proximal bronchiectasis, unless the patient has ABPA-S. If measured, sera from stage I patients have elevated serum IgE and IgG antibodies to Af compared with sera from patients with asthma and immediate cutaneous reactivity to *Aspergillus* but insufficient criteria for ABPA. After therapy with prednisone, the chest roentgenogram clears and the total serum IgE declines substantially. Remission (stage II) is defined as clearing of the roentgenographic lesions and decline in total serum IgE for at least 6 months. Exacerbation (stage III) of ABPA is present when, after the remission that follows prednisone therapy, the patient develops a new roentgenographic infiltrate, total IgE

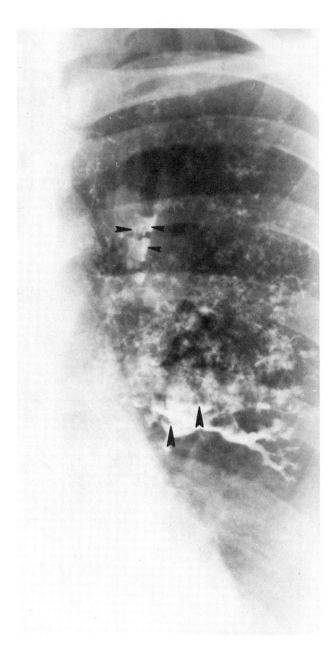

FIG. 24-5. Posttussive films after bronchography. Air–fluid levels (*large arrowheads*) are present in several partially filled ectatic bronchi. A bronchus in the left upper lobe is filled after the tussive effort, confirming that a portion of the density seen in this area is a filled ectatic proximal bronchus (*small arrowheads*). (Mintzer RA, Rogers LF, Kruglick GD, Rosenberg M, Neiman H, Patterson R. The spectrum of radiologic findings in allergic bronchopulmonary aspergillosis. Radiology 1978;127:301.)

rises over baseline, and the other criteria of stage I appear. Corticosteroid-dependent asthma (stage IV) includes patients whose prednisone cannot be terminated without occurrence of severe asthma or new roentgenographic infiltrates. Despite prednisone administration, most patients have elevated total serum IgE, precipitating antibody, and elevated serum IgE and IgG antibodies to Af. Roentgenographic infiltrates may occur. Stage V ABPA is present when extensive cystic or fibrotic changes are demonstrated on the chest roentgenogram. Patients in the fibrotic stage have some degree of irreversible obstructive flow rates on pulmonary function testing. A reversible obstructive component requires prednisone therapy, but high-dose prednisone does not reverse the roentgenographic lesions or irreversible obstructive disease.

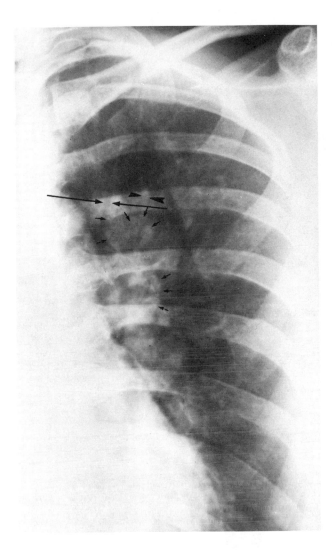

FIG. 24-6. Magnified view of the left upper lung of the patient shown in Figures 24-4 and 24-5 demonstrates parallel lines (*long arrows*) and toothpaste shadows (*arrowheads*). Perihilar infiltrates (pseudohilar adenopathy) and a gloved-finger shadow are seen (*small arrows*). (Mintzer RA, Rogers LF, Kruglick GD, Rosenberg M, Neiman H, Patterson R. The spectrum of radiologic findings in allergic bronchopulmonary aspergillosis. Radiology 1978;127:301.)

At the time of the initial diagnosis, the stage of ABPA may not be defined, but it becomes clear after several months of observation and treatment.

Patients with ABPA-S can be in stages I through IV but not V.

LABORATORY FINDINGS

All patients exhibit immediate cutaneous (wheal-and-flare) reactivity to Af antigen. Because of the lack of standardized Af antigens for clinical testing, differences in skin reactivity have been reported by different authors[33,44 47] (Table 24-1). Approximately 25% of patients with asthma without ABPA demonstrate immediate skin reactivity to Af, and about 10% show precipitating antibodies against Af.[47]

Some ABPA patients display a diphasic skin response to the intradermal injection of *Aspergillus* antigen. This consists of a typical immediate wheal and flare seen within 20 minutes, which subsides, to be followed in 4 to 8 hours by erythema and induration that resolves

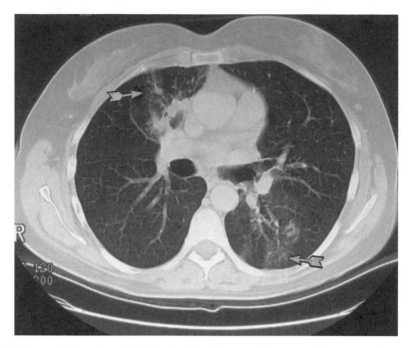

FIG. 24-7. Computed tomographic image of a 42-year-old woman demonstrating right upper lobe and left lower lobe infiltrates—the latter not seen on the posteroanterior and lateral radiographs. Dilated bronchioles are present in areas of infiltrates (*arrows*).

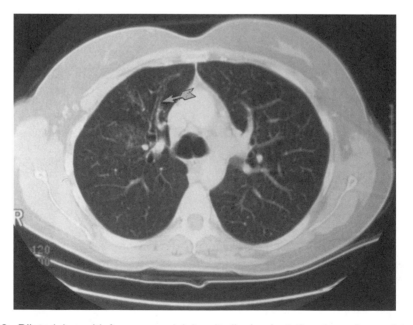

FIG. 24-8. Dilated bronchi from an axial longitudinal orientation (*arrow*) consistent with bronchiectasis. (Same patient as in Fig. 24-7).

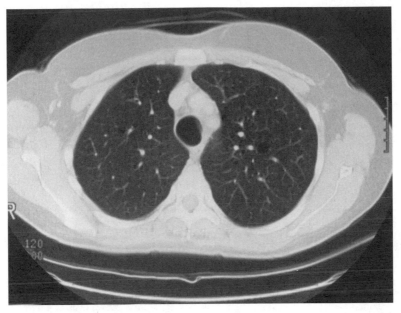

FIG. 24-9. Cystic (dilated) bronchi and bronchioles. (Same patient as in Fig. 24-7).

in 24 hours. Biopsy of this late reaction has shown IgG, IgM, IgA, and C3, suggesting an Arthus (type III) immune response.[48] IgE antibodies are also likely to participate in the late reactions. Few ABPA patients treated at Northwestern University Medical School have biphasic skin reactivity despite the presence of anti-Af IgE antibodies and precipitating antibodies. Conversely, these patients are not tested by intradermal injection, because prick test results are positive in virtually all patients. As shown in Table 24-1, precipitating antibody to Af is common in patients without ABPA and likely represents previous exposure to the Af antigens. In ABPA, however, these antibodies seem to be important in the pathogenesis of the disease, although exactly how they contribute is unclear.

After rocket immunoelectrophoresis of Af mycelia and addition of Af antisera raised in rabbits, 35 different bands have been detected, documenting the large number of components in Af. A potential antigen (an acidic glycoprotein) has been purified from mycelial cell sap of Af that has four polypeptides of 45,000 daltons (d) linked by disulfide bonds.[49] This glycoprotein reacted with 75% of sera from aspergilloma and ABPA patients, but not with normal human sera or with sera from patients with other fungal diseases.

Using crossed immunoelectrophoresis of an *Aspergillus* culture filtrate with sera from patients with ABPA demonstrated 35 arcs, from which 8 to 10 had reactivity with IgE antibodies.[50] Concanavalin A nonbinding components of Af culture filtrates or mycelium have been found to react with sera from ABPA patients, and other components have molecular weights to 200,000 d.[50,51]

An Af polypeptide called *Asp f I* that is 18,000 d and generated from a culture filtrate was found to react with IgE and IgG antibodies and was toxic to lymphocytes.[52,53] *Asp f I* is a member of the mitogillin family, which has ribonuclease (ribotoxic) activity. Sera from ABPA patients react with several ribotoxins, and far greater quantities of IgE and IgG antibodies to ribotoxins from *Aspergillus* are present in patients with ABPA compared with nonatopic patients or with patients with asthma.[53]

TABLE 24-1. *Incidence of immunologic reactions to* Aspergillus fumigatus

Patients studied	Immediate skin reactivity (%)	Precipitins (%)
Normal population	1–4	0–3
Hospitalized patients		2.5–6
Asthma without aspergillosis	12–38	9–25
Asthma without aspergillosis*		
London	23	10.5
Cleveland	28	7.5
ABPA	100	100[†]
Aspergilloma	25	100
Cystic fibrosis	39	31

ABPA, allergic bronchopulmonary aspergillosis.
*Similar antigenic material was used for both groups.
[†]May be negative at times.
Data from Hoehne JH, Reed CE, Dickie HA. Allergic bronchopulmonary aspergillosis is not rare. Chest 1973;63:177; Longbottom JL, Pepys J. Pulmonary aspergillosis: diagnostic and immunologic significance of antigens and C-substance in *Aspergillus fumigatus.* J Pathol Bacteriol 1964;88:141; Reed C. Variability of antigenicity of *Aspergillus fumigatus.* J Allergy Clin Immunol 1978;61:227; Rosenberg M, Patterson R, Mintzer R, et al. Clinical and immunologic criteria for the diagnosis of allergic bronchopulmonary aspergillosis. Ann Intern Med 1977;86:405; and Schwartz HJ, Citron KM, Chester EH, et al. A comparison of the prevalence of sensitization to *Aspergillus* antigens among asthmatics in Cleveland and London. J Allergy Clin Immunol 1978;62:9.

In the double-gel diffusion technique, most patients show at least one to three bands to Af. Some sera must be concentrated five times to demonstrate precipitating antibody. A precipitin band with no immunologic significance may be seen, caused by the presence of C-reactive protein in human sera that cross-reacts with a polysaccharide antigen in *Aspergillus*. This false-positive band can be avoided by adding citric acid to the agar gel.

Because of the high incidence of cutaneous reactivity and precipitating antibodies to Af in patients with cystic fibrosis and transient roentgenographic infiltrates attributed to *Aspergillus*, there is concern that *Aspergillus* could contribute to the ongoing lung damage of cystic fibrosis. The question also has been raised whether ABPA might be a variant form of the latter. In the patient population at Northwestern University Medical School, all patients tested had normal sweat chloride concentrations in the absence of cystic fibrosis. There is increasing evidence that ABPA can complicate cystic fibrosis, and it must be considered in that population because up to 10% of patients with cystic fibrosis have ABPA.[11–16]

Serum IgE concentrations in patients with ABPA are elevated, but the degree of elevation varies markedly. Af growing in the respiratory tract without tissue invasion, as in ABPA, can provide a potent stimulus for production of total "nonspecific" serum IgE.[54] The serum IgE antibody to Af can be determined by radioimmunoassay or enzyme-linked immunoassay. When serum IgE or serum IgG antibodies, or both, against Af are elevated compared with sera from prick test–positive asthmatic patients without evidence for ABPA, ABPA is highly probable or definitely present.[7,22] With prednisone therapy and clinical improvement, the total IgE and IgE-Af decrease although at different rates. Presumably, this drop is associated with a decrease in the number of Af organisms in the bronchi. It is possible, but unlikely, that the reduction in IgE results directly from prednisone without an effect on Af in the lung, because in other conditions such as atopic dermatitis and asthma, corticosteroids did not lower total serum IgE concentrations significantly.[55,56]

Because of wide variation of total serum IgE concentrations in atopic patients with asthma, some difficulty exists in differentiating the patient with ABPA from the patient with asthma and cutaneous reactivity to Af, with or without precipitating antibody to Af and a history of an abnormal finding on chest roentgenogram. Detection of elevated serum IgE and IgG antibodies to Af has proved useful to identify patients with ABPA.[6,7,16,22] Sera from patients with ABPA have at least twice the level of antibody activity to Af than do sera from asthmatics with prick-positive skin reactions to Af. During other stages of ABPA, the indices have diagnostic value if results are elevated but are not consistently positive in all patients.[57] In patients with suspected ABPA, serodiagnosis should be attempted before corticosteroid therapy is started. Hyperimmunoglobulinemia E should raise the possibility of ABPA in any patient with asthma, although other causes include parasitism, atopic dermatitis, hyper-IgE syndrome, immune deficiency, Churg-Strauss vasculitis, and remotely IgE myeloma.

Lymphocyte transformation is present in some cases but is not a diagnostic feature of ABPA.[33] Delayed hypersensitivity (type IV) reactions occurring 48 hours after administration of intradermal *Aspergillus* antigens typically are not seen.[58]

T- and B-cell analysis of selected patients with ABPA has not shown abnormal numbers of B cells, CD4 (helper) cells, or CD8 (suppressor) cells. However, some patients have evidence for B-cell activation (CD19+, CD23+) or T-cell activation (CD25+).

Circulating immune complexes have been described during an acute flare-up of ABPA with activation of the classic pathway.[59] Although C1q precipitins were present in patient sera, it was not proven that *Aspergillus* antigen was present in these complexes. ABPA is not considered to be characterized by circulating immune complexes as in serum sickness. It has been demonstrated that Af can convert C3 proactivator to C3 activator, a component of the alternate pathway.[60] It is known that secretory IgA can activate the alternate pathway, and that *Aspergillus* in the bronchial tract can stimulate IgA production.[61]

In vitro basophil histamine release resulted from exposure to an *Aspergillus* mix, anti-IgE, and other fungi in patients with ABPA and fungi-sensitive asthma (with immediate cutaneous reactivity to Af).[62] There was much greater histamine release to *Aspergillus* and anti-IgE from basophils of patients with ABPA than there was from fungi-sensitive asthmatics. Further, patients with stage IV and stage V ABPA demonstrated greater histamine release to *Aspergillus* than did patients in stages I, II, or III. There was greater histamine release to other fungi from cells from ABPA patients than there was from patients with asthma. These data document a cellular difference in ABPA patients when compared with fungi-sensitive asthmatics. There was no difference between ABPA patients and patients with asthma in terms of cutaneous end-point titration using a commercially available *Aspergillus* mix.

A positive sputum culture for Af is a helpful, but not pathognomonic, feature of ABPA. Repeated positive cultures may be significant. Whereas some patients produce golden brown plugs of mucus containing *Aspergillus* mycelia, others produce no sputum at all, even in the presence of roentgenographic infiltrates. Sputum eosinophilia usually is found in patients with significant sputum production, but is not essential for the diagnosis and clearly is not specific.

Peripheral blood eosinophilia is seen in untreated patients, but need not be extremely high, and often is about 10% to 25% of the differential in patients who have not received oral corticosteroids.

Bronchial inhalational challenges with *Aspergillus* are not required to confirm the diagnosis and are not without risk. Nevertheless, a dual reaction usually occurs after bronchoprovocation. An immediate reduction in flow that resolves, to be followed in some cases by a recurrence of obstruction after 4 to 10 hours, has been described.[48] Pretreatment with beta agonists prevents the immediate reaction, pretreatment with corticosteroids prevents the late reaction, and cromolyn sodium has been reported to prevent both. Inhalational challenge with Af in a patient with asthma sensitive to *Aspergillus* produces the immediate response only. Aspergilloma patients may respond only with a late pattern.

LUNG BIOPSY

Because of the increasing recognition of ABPA and the availability of serologic tests, the need for lung biopsy in confirming the diagnosis seems unnecessary unless other diseases must be excluded. Bronchiectasis in the affected lobes in segmental and subsegmental bronchi, with sparing of distal branches, characterizes the pattern of proximal or central bronchiectasis.[63-65] Bronchi are tortuous and dilated. Histologically, bronchi contain tenacious mucus, fibrin, Curschmann's spirals, Charcot-Leyden crystals, and inflammatory cells (mononuclears and eosinophils). Fungal hyphae can be identified in the bronchial lumen, and *Aspergillus* can be isolated in culture. No evidence exists for invasion of the bronchial wall, despite numerous hyphae in the lumen. Bronchial wall damage is associated with the presence of mononuclear cells and eosinophils, and in some cases with granulomata. Organisms of *Aspergillus* may be surrounded by necrosis, or acute or chronic inflammation. In other areas, fibrous tissue replaces the submucosa. It is not known why bronchial wall destruction is focal with uninvolved adjacent areas.

A variety of morphologic lesions have been described in patients meeting criteria of ABPA.[63-65] These include *Aspergillus* in granulomatous bronchiolitis, exudative bronchiolitis, *Aspergillus* in microabscess, eosinophilic pneumonia, lipid pneumonia, lymphocytic interstitial pneumonia, desquamative interstitial pneumonia, pulmonary vasculitis, and pulmonary fibrosis. Some patients with ABPA may show pathologic features consistent with bronchocentric granulomatosis. Mucoid impaction related to ABPA may cause proximal bronchial obstruction with distal areas of bronchiolitis obliterans. Examples of microscopic sections from ABPA patients are shown in Figures 24-10 through 24-12.

PATHOGENESIS

In some patients who had a normal bronchogram finding before they developed ABPA, bronchiectasis has been found to occur at the sites of roentgenographic infiltrates. Currently, it is thought that inhaled *Aspergillus* spores grow in the patient's tenacious mucus and release antigenic materials that react with bronchial mast cells, lymphocytes, macrophages, and antibodies, followed by tissue damage that is associated with subsequent bronchiectasis or roentgenographic infiltrates. *Aspergillus* spores are thermophilic; therefore, growth is feasible in bronchi. It is unclear whether *Aspergillus* spores are trapped in the viscid mucus, or whether they have a special ability to colonize the bronchial tree. Proteolytic enzymes or possibly ribotoxins produced by Af growing in the bronchial tree may contribute to lung damage on a nonimmunologic or immunologic basis. Immunologic injury could occur because the release of antigenic material is associated with production of IgE, IgA, IgG, and cytokines from mononuclear cells. Although peripheral blood lymphocytes from stable ABPA patients have not been found to form excess IgE in vitro compared with nonatopic patients, at the time of an ABPA flare-up, these cells produced significantly increased amounts of IgE.[66] This suggests that during an ABPA flare-up, IgE-forming cells are released into the systemic circulation, presumably from the lung. The diphasic skin reaction requires IgE and possibly IgG, and it has been suggested that a similar reaction occurs in the lung. Nevertheless, the lack of immunofluorescence in vascular deposits is against an immune complex vasculitis as cause of bronchial wall damage.

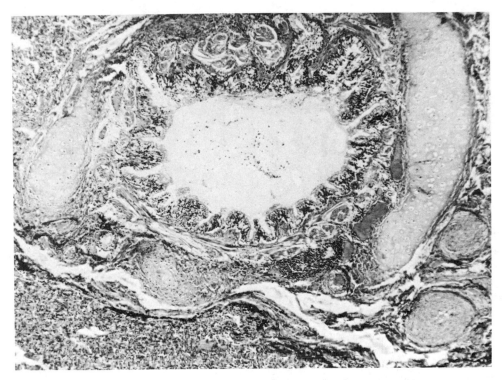

FIG. 24-10. Cross-section of bronchus (right middle lobe section) shows mural thickening, cellular infiltration, and mucous material filling the lumen. Eosinophils are abundant in the airway wall and in the peribronchial infiltrate (Hematoxylin & eosin stain, ×10). (Imbeau SA, Nichols D, Flaherty D, et al. Allergic bronchopulmonary aspergillosis. J Allergy Clin Immunol 1978·62:243, from the specimen collection of Enrique Valdivia.)

The passive transfer of serum containing IgG and IgE antibodies from a patient with ABPA to a monkey, followed by bronchial challenge with *Aspergillus*, has been associated with pulmonary lesions in the monkey.[2]

Slavin and associates[67] immunized monkeys with Af and detected IgG antibodies. Normal human serum was infused into both immunized and nonimmunized monkeys, and allergic human serum from a patient with ABPA (currently without any precipitating antibody) was infused into other monkeys, immunized and nonimmunized. All animals were challenged with aerosolized Af, and lung biopsies were performed on the fifth day. Only the monkey with precipitating antibody (IgG) to *Aspergillus* who received human allergic serum (IgE) showed biopsy changes consistent with ABPA. Mononuclear and eosinophilic infiltrates were present, with thickening of alveolar septa, but without evidence of vasculitis. These findings confirm that IgE and IgG directed against *Aspergillus* are necessary for the development of pulmonary lesions.

Similarly, a murine model of ABPA was developed that resulted in blood and pulmonary eosinophilia[68] Af particulates simulating spores were inoculated by the intranasal route. If Af in alum was injected into the peritoneal cavity, anti–Af-IgG$_1$ and total IgE concentrations increased. However, pulmonary and peripheral blood eosinophilia did not occur. In contrast, intranasal inoculation of Af resulted in perivascular eosinophilia, pulmonary lymphocytes, plasma cells, histocytes, and eosinophils, consistent with ABPA. A true model of ABPA where animals develop spontaneously occurring pulmonary infiltrates has yet to be described.

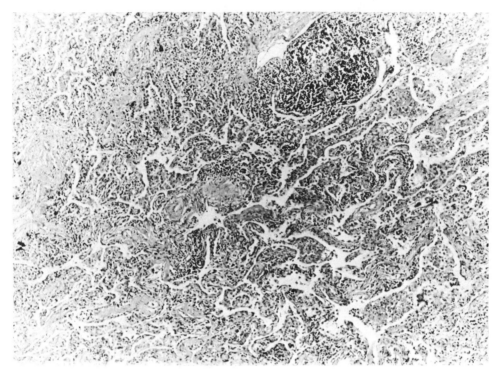

FIG. 24-11. Typical microscopic appearance representing eosinophilic pneumonia. The collapsed alveoli contain a predominance of large mononuclear cells, few lymphocytes, plasma cells, and clumps of eosinophils. Similar cells infiltrate the alveolar walls. Superior segment of the upper lobe was resected for cavitary and infiltrative lesion (Hematoxylin & eosin stain, ×120). (Imbeau SA, Nichols D, Flaherty D, et al. Allergic bronchopulmonary aspergillosis. J Allergy Clin Immunol 1978:62:243, from the speciment collection of Enrique Valdivia.)

Lymphocytes likely produce interleukin (IL)-4 (or IL-13) and IL-5 to support IgE synthesis and eosinophilia, respectively. An elevated level of soluble IL-2 receptors suggests lymphocyte activation.[69] Evidence for types I, III, and IV hypersensitivity exists, and it is likely that differing degrees of each contribute to lung destruction in the individual patient. The demonstration of hyperreleasibility of mediators from basophils of patients with stage IV and V ABPA[62] is consistent with the hypothesis that a subgroup of patients may be the most susceptible to immunologic injury if peripheral blood basophils are representative bronchial mast cells. The fact that patients with any stage of ABPA have increased in vitro histamine release, if it can be applied to bronchial mast cells, suggests that mast cell mediator release to various antigens (fungi) may contribute to lung damage in ABPA.

Analysis of bronchoalveolar lavage fluid from stages II and IV ABPA patients who had no current chest roentgenographic infiltrates revealed evidence for local antibody production of IgA-Af and IgE-Af compared with peripheral blood.[70] Bronchial lavage IgA-Af levels were 96 times that of peripheral blood, and IgE-Af in lavage fluid was 48 times that found in peripheral blood. Although total serum IgE was elevated, there was no increase in bronchial lavage total IgE corrected for albumin. These results suggest that the bronchoalveolar space is not the source of the markedly elevated total IgE in ABPA. Perhaps pulmonary interstitium or nonpulmonary sources are sites of total IgE production in ABPA.

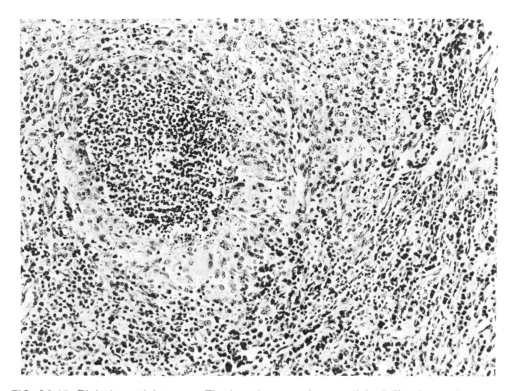

FIG. 24-12. Right lower lobectomy. The lung has prominent cellular infiltration and an area of early bronchocentric granulomatosis, with leukocytes and a crown of epithelioid cells. Infection with *Aspergillus* is demonstrated in the center of the lesions with special stains (Hematoxylin & eosin stain, x240). (Imbeau SA, Nichols D, Flaherty D, et al. Allergic bronchopulmonary aspergillosis. J Allergy Clin Immunol 1978:62:243, from the specimen collection of Enrique Valdivia.)

Serial analysis of serum IgA-Af in ten patients showed sharp elevations over baseline before (five patients) or during (five patients) roentgenographic exacerbations of ABPA for IgA_1-Af.[61] Serum IgA_2-Af was found elevated before the exacerbation in two patients and during the exacerbation in five patients. Immunoblot analysis of sera showed heterogeneous polyclonal antibody responses to seven different molecular weight bands of Af.[71] Band intensity increased during ABPA exacerbations, and patients' sera often had broader reactivity with Af bands from 24- to 90-kd molecular weights during disease flare-ups.

The many immunologic and other abnormalities identified in ABPA likely participate directly or indirectly in lung destruction both in bronchi and distally. The basis of the effectiveness of prednisone in treatment of ABPA requires greater clarification as well.

DIFFERENTIAL DIAGNOSIS

The differential diagnosis of ABPA includes disease states associated primarily with transient or permanent roentgenographic lesions, asthma, and peripheral blood or sputum eosinophilia. The asthma patient with a roentgenographic infiltrate may have atelectasis from inadequately controlled asthma. Bacterial, viral, or fungal pneumonia must be excluded in addition to tuberculosis and the many other causes of roentgenographic infiltrates. Eosinophilia may occur with parasitism, tuberculosis, Churg-Strauss vasculitis, pulmonary infiltrates from drug allergies, neoplasm, eosinophilic pneumonia, and rarely, avian-hypersensitivity pneumonitis. Mucoid impaction of bronchi may occur without ABPA. All patients with a history of mucoid impaction syndrome or with collapse of a lobe or lung, however, should have ABPA excluded. Similarly, although the morphologic diagnosis of bronchocentric granulomatosis is considered by some to represent an entity distinct from ABPA, ABPA must be excluded in such a patient. Although the sweat test for cystic fibrosis is within normal limits in ABPA patients, unless concomitant cystic fibrosis is present, the patient with cystic fibrosis and asthma or changing roentgenographic infiltrates should have ABPA excluded. The genetics of ABPA are just beginning to be studied to determine similarities with cystic fibrosis. Many patients with a history of pulmonary infiltrates with eosinophilia are likely to have ABPA.

In the patient without a history of roentgenographic infiltrates, ABPA should be suspected on the basis of (1) a positive, immediate cutaneous reaction to *Aspergillus*, with or without a late (4- to 8-hour) reaction; (2) elevated total serum IgE; (3) increasing severity of asthma; (4) abnormalities on chest roentgenogram; (5) repeatedly positive sputum cultures for *Aspergillus* sp, or (6) bronchiectasis.

A rare patient with asthma, roentgenographic infiltrates, and bronchiectasis or a history of surgical resection for such may present with peripheral eosinophilia, elevated total serum IgE, but other negative serologic results for ABPA. Some other allergic bronchopulmonary fungosis may be present. For example, illnesses consistent with allergic bronchopulmonary candidiasis, curvulariosis, dreschleriosis, stemphyliosis, and pseudallescheriosis have been described.[72,73] Positive sputum cultures, precipitating antibodies, or in vitro assays for an organism other than *Aspergillus* or for different *Aspergillus* species suggest a causative source of the allergic bronchopulmonary fungosis.

The presence of bronchiectasis from ABPA has been associated with colonization of bronchi by atypical mycobacteria.[74] The identification of atypical mycobacteria in the sputum should at least raise the possibility of ABPA in patients with asthma who do not have acquired immunodeficiency syndrome.

NATURAL HISTORY

Although most patients are diagnosed before 40 years of age and an increasing number are diagnosed before 20 years of age, the diagnosis of ABPA must not be overlooked in older patients previously characterized as having chronic asthma or chronic bronchiectasis. Late sequelae of ABPA include irreversible pulmonary function abnormalities, symptoms of chronic bronchitis, and pulmonary fibrosis.[36] Death results from respiratory failure and cor pulmonale. ABPA has been associated with respiratory failure in the second or third decade of life. Most patients who have ABPA do not progress to the end-stage disease, especially if there is early diagnosis and appropriate treatment. Patients who present in the acute stage (I) of ABPA may enter remission (stage II), recurrent exacerbation (stage III), or may develop corticosteroid-dependent asthma (stage IV). One patient who had a single roentgenographic infiltrate when her ABPA was diagnosed entered a remission stage that lasted for 8 years until an exacerbation occurred.[75] Thus, a remission does not imply permanent cessation of disease activity. This case may be the exception, but it emphasizes the need for longer term observation of patients with ABPA. Patients who have corticosteroid-dependent asthma (stage IV) at the time of diagnosis may evolve into pulmonary fibrosis (stage V). Because prednisone does not reverse bronchiectasis or the pulmonary fibrotic changes in the lung, every effort should be made by physicians managing patients with asthma to suspect and confirm cases of ABPA before significant structural damage to the lung has developed.

In managing patients with ABPA, a lack of correlation exists between clinical symptoms and chest roentgenographic lesions. Irreversible lung damage may occur without the patient seeking medical attention. In Great Britain, ABPA exacerbations were reported to occur between October and February during elevations of fungal spore counts.[20] In Chicago, 38 of 49 (77.5%) ABPA exacerbations (new roentgenographic infiltrate with elevation of total serum IgE) occurred from June through November in association with increased outdoor fungal spore counts.[76]

Acute and chronic pulmonary function changes have been studied in a series of ABPA cases, during which time all patients received corticosteroids and bronchodilators.[77] There appeared to be no significant correlation between duration of ABPA (mean follow-up period, 44 months), duration of asthma, and diffusing capacity of the lungs for carbon monoxide (DLCO), total lung capacity (TLC), vital capacity (VC), and forced expiratory volume in 1 second (FEV_1), and $FEV_{1\%}$. In six patients with acute exacerbations of ABPA, a significant reduction in TLC, VC, FEV_1, and DLCO occurred, which returned to baseline during steroid treatment. Thus, early recognition and prompt effective treatment of flare-ups seem to reduce the likelihood of irreversible lung damage. The prognosis for stage V patients is less favorable than for patients classified into stages I through IV.[38] Although prednisone has proven useful in patients with end-stage lung disease, 6 of 17 stage V patients (observed for a mean 4.9 years) died. When the FEV_1 was 0.8 L or less after aggressive initial corticosteroid administration, the outcome was poor.[38] In contrast, when stage IV patients are managed effectively, deterioration of respiratory function parameters or status asthmaticus does not occur.

Safirstein and colleagues,[78] in a 5-year follow-up of ABPA cases, reported that a daily prednisone dose of 7.5 mg was required to maintain clinical improvement and roentgenographic clearing in 80% of patients, compared with 40% of those treated with either cromolyn or bronchodilators alone.[78] In a study of patients from Northwestern University who had periodic blood sampling, both immunologic and clinical improvement occurred with prednisone therapy. Individuals with ABPA have high initial total serum IgE concentrations, and those patients previously never requiring oral steroids for control of asthma have the highest concentrations. Treatment with prednisone causes roentgenographic and clinical improvement, as well as decreases in total serum IgE. Total IgE and IgE-Af may increase before and during a flare-up.

Prognostic factors remain to be established that may identify patients at risk of developing stage IV or V ABPA. The roentgenographic lesion at the time of diagnosis does not appear to provide prognostic data about long-term outcome unless the patient is stage V.

TREATMENT

Prednisone is the drug of choice but need not be administered indefinitely. Multiple agents have been tried, including intrabronchial instillation of amphotericin B, nystatin, cromolyn, beclomethasone dipropionate, and triamcinolone by inhalation. Itraconazole may have an adjunctive role,[79] but prednisone therapy often eliminates or diminishes sputum plug production. Although the exact pathogenesis of ABPA is unknown, oral corticosteroids have been demonstrated to reduce the clinical symptoms, incidence of positive sputum cultures, and roentgenographic infiltrates. Corticosteroids may be effective by decreasing sputum volume by making the bronchi a less suitable culture media for *Aspergillus* sp and by inhibiting *Aspergillus*–pulmonary immune system interactions. The total serum IgE declines by at least 35% within 2 months of initiating prednisone therapy.[17] Failure to observe this reduction suggests noncompliance of patients or an exacerbation of ABPA.

The current treatment regimen at Northwestern University Medical School is to clear the roentgenographic infiltrates with daily prednisone, usually at 0.5 mg/kg. Most infiltrates clear within 2 weeks, at which time the same dose, given on a single alternate-day regimen, is begun and maintained for 2 months until the total serum IgE, which should be followed every 4 to 8 weeks for the first year, has reached a baseline concentration. The baseline total serum IgE concentration can remain elevated despite clinical and radiographic improvement. Slow reductions in prednisone, at no faster than 10 mg/month, can be carried out once a stable baseline of total IgE has been achieved. Acute exacerbations of ABPA often are preceded by a 100% rise in total serum IgE and must be treated promptly with increases in prednisone and reinstitution of daily steroids. Certainly, the physician must exclude other causes for roentgenographic infiltrates. Pulmonary functions should be measured yearly or as necessary for stages IV and V and as required for asthma.

If prednisone can be discontinued, the patient is in remission (Stage II) and perhaps just an inhaled corticosteroid is needed for management of asthma. Alternatively, if the patient has asthma that cannot be managed without prednisone despite avoidance measures and maximal antiinflammatory medications, alternate-day prednisone is necessary. The dose of prednisone required to control asthma may be less than 0.5 mg/kg on alternate days, which usually is adequate to prevent ABPA radiologic exacerbations. For corticosteroid-dependent patients (stages IV or V) with ABPA, an explanation of prednisone risks and benefits is indicated, as is the discussion that untreated ABPA infiltrates result in bronchiectasis[39,43] and irreversible fibrosis. Specific additional recommendations regarding possible estrogen supplementation for women, adequate calcium ingestion, bronchial hygiene, and physical fitness should be considered.

Immunotherapy with *Aspergillus* sp probably should not be administered in patients with ABPA, but instances of adverse effects aside from injection reactions have not occurred. It is not expected that immunotherapy with *Aspergillus* extract would result in immune complex formation.

Inhaled corticosteroids should be used to control asthma but cannot be depended on to prevent exacerbations of ABPA.

The exact role of environmental exposure of *Aspergillus* spores in the pathogenesis of ABPA remains unknown. *Aspergillus* spores are found regularly in crawl spaces, "unfinished" compost piles, manure, and fertile soil. Acute inhalation of heavy spore burdens may be deleterious and should be avoided. Attempts should be made to repair leaky basement walls to minimize moldy basements.

REFERENCES

1. Hinson KFW, Moon AJ, Plummer NS. Bronchopulmonary aspergillosis: a review and report of eight new cases. Thorax 1952;73:317.
2. Patterson R, Golbert T. Hypersensitivity disease of the lung. Univ Mich Med Cent J 1968;34:8.
3. Slavin RG, Laird TS, Cherry JD. Allergic bronchopulmonary aspergillosis in a child. J Pediatr 1970;76:416.
4. Chetty A, Bhargava S, Jain RK. Allergic bronchopulmonary aspergillosis in Indian children with bronchial asthma. Ann Allergy 1985;54:46.
5. Turner ES, Greenberger PA, Sider L. Complexities of establishing an early diagnosis of allergic bronchopulmonary aspergillosis in children. Allergy Proc 1989;10:63.
6. Kiefer TA, Kesarwala HH, Greenberger PA, Sweeney JR, Fischer TJ. Allergic bronchopulmonary aspergillosis in a young child: diagnostic confirmation by serum IgE and IgG indices. Ann Allergy 1986;56:233.
7. Greenberger PA, Liotta JL, Roberts M. The effects of age on isotypic antibody responses to *Aspergillus fumigatus*: implications regarding *in vitro* measurements. J Lab Clin Med 1989;114:278.
8. Imbeau SA, Cohen M, Reed CE. Allergic bronchopulmonary aspergillosis in infants. Am J Dis Child 1977;131:1127.
9. Patterson R, Greenberger PA, Radin RC, Roberts M. Allergic bronchopulmonary aspergillosis: staging as an aid to management. Ann Intern Med 1982;96:286.

10. Greenberger PA, Miller TP, Roberts M, Smith LL. Allergic bronchopulmonary aspergillosis in patients with an without evidence of bronchiectasis. Ann Allergy 1993;70:333.

11. Basich JE, Graves TS, Baz MN, et al. Allergic bronchopulmonary aspergillosis in steroid dependent asthmatics. J Allergy Clin Immunol 1981;68:98.

12. Laufer P, Fink JN, Bruns W, et al. Allergic bronchopulmonary aspergillosis in cystic fibrosis. J Allergy Clin Immunol 1984;73:44.

13. Maguire S, Moriarty P, Tempany E, Fitzgerald M. Unusual clustering of allergic bronchopulmonary aspergillosis in children with cystic fibrosis. Pediatrics 1988;82:835.

14. Nelson L, Callerame ML, Schwartz R. Aspergillosis and atopy in cystic fibrosis. Am Rev Respir Dis 1979;120:863.

15. Zeaske R, Bruns WT, Fink JN, et al. Immune responses to *Aspergillus* in cystic fibrosis. J Allergy Clin Immunol 1988;82:73.

16. Knutsen AP, Hutchinson PS, Mueller KR, Slavin RG. Serum immunoglobulins E and G anti-*Aspergillus fumigatus* antibody in patients with cystic fibrosis who have allergic bronchopulmonary aspergillosis. J Lab Clin Med 1990;116:724.

17. Rosenberg M, Patterson R, Roberts M, et al. The assessment of immunologic and clinical changes occurring during corticosteroid therapy for allergic bronchopulmonary aspergillosis. Am J Med 1978;64:599.

18. Wang JLF, Patterson R, Rosenberg M, Roberts M, Cooper BJ. Serum IgE and IgG antibody activity against *Aspergillus fumigatus* as a diagnostic aid in allergic bronchopulmonary aspergillosis. Am Rev Respir Dis 1978;117:917.

19. Greenberger PA, Patterson R. Application of enzyme linked immunosorbent assay (ELISA) in diagnosis of allergic bronchopulmonary aspergillosis. J Lab Clin Med 1982;15:93.

20. Pepys J. Hypersensitivity disease of the lungs due to fungi and organic dusts. Monogr Allergy 1969;4.

21. Greenberger PA, Patterson R. Allergic bronchopulmonary aspergillosis and the evaluation of the patient with asthma. J Allergy Clin Immunol 1988;81:646.

22. Schwartz HJ, Greenberger PA. The prevalence of allergic bronchopulmonary aspergillosis in patients with asthma, determined by serologic and radiologic criteria in patients at risk. J Lab Clin Med 1991;117:138.

23. Solomon WR, Burge HP, Boise JR. Airborne *Aspergillus fumigatus* levels outside and within a large clinical center. J Allergy Clin Immunol 1978;62:56.

24. Chute HL. Fungal infections. In: Hafstad MS, ed. Aspergillosis in diseases of poultry. 7th ed. Ames, IA: Iowa State University Press, 1978;367.

25. Quirce S, Cuevas M, Diez-Gomez ML, et al. Respiratory allergy to *Aspergillus*-derived enzymes in bakers' asthma. J Allergy Clin Immunol 1992;90:970.

26. Rosenberg IL, Greenberger PA. Allergic bronchopulmonary aspergillosis and aspergilloma: long-term follow-up without enlargement of a large multiloculated cavity. Chest 1984;85:123.

27. Weiner MH, Talbot GH, Gerson SL, Felice G, Cassileth PA. Antigen detection in the diagnosis of invasive aspergillosis. Ann Intern Med 1983;99:777.

28. Johnson TM, Kurup VP, Resnick A, Ash RC, Fink JN, Kalbfleisch J. Detection of circulating *Aspergillus fumigatus* antigen in bone marrow transplant patients. J Lab Clin Med 1989;114:700.

29. Binder RE, Faling J J, Pugatch RE, Mahasaen C, Snider GL. Chronic necrotizing pulmonary aspergillosis: a discreet clinical entity. Medicine 1982;151:109.

30. Katzenstein AL, Salc SR, Greenberger PA. Allergic *Aspergillus* sinusitis: a newly recognized form of sinusitis. J Allergy Clin Immunol 1983;72:89.

31. Goldstein MF, Atkins PC, Cogan FC, Kornstein MJ, Levine RS, Zweiman B. Allergic *Aspergillus* sinusitis. J Allergy Clin Immunol 1985;76:515.

32. Sher TH, Schwartz HJ. Allergic *Aspergillus* sinusitis with concurrent allergic bronchopulmonary *Aspergillus*: report of a case. J Allergy Clin Immunol 1988;81:844.

33. Rosenberg M, Patterson R, Mintzer R, Cooper BJ, Roberts M, Harris KE. Clinical and immunologic criteria for the diagnosis of allergic bronchopulmonary aspergillosis. Ann Intern Med 1977;86:405.

34. Patterson R, Greenberger PA, Halwig JM, Liotta JL, Roberts M. Allergic bronchopulmonary aspergillosis: natural history and classification of early disease by serologic and roentgenographic studies. Arch Intern Med 1986;146:916.

35. Ricketti AJ, Greenberger PA, Patterson R. Immediate type reactions in patients with allergic bronchopulmonary aspergillosis. J Allergy Clin Immunol 1983;71:541.

36. Greenberger PA, Patterson R, Ghory AC, et al. Late sequelae of allergic bronchopulmonary aspergillosis. J Allergy Clin immunol 1980;66:327.

37. Ricketti AJ, Greenberger PA, Glassroth J. Spontaneous pneumothorax in allergic bronchopulmonary aspergillosis. Arch Intern Med 1984;144:151.

38. Lee TM, Greenberger PA, Patterson R, Roberts M, Liotta JL. Stage V (fibrotic) allergic bronchopulmonary aspergillosis: a review of 17 cases followed from diagnosis. Arch Intern Med 1987;147:319.

39. Mintzer RA, Rogers LF, Kruglick GD, Rosenberg M, Neiman H, Patterson R. The spectrum of radiologic findings in allergic bronchopulmonary aspergillosis. Radiology 1978;127:301.

40. Fisher MR, Mendelson EB, Mintzer RA, Ricketti AJ, Greenberger PA. Use of linear tomography to confirm the diagnosis of allergic bronchopulmonary aspergillosis. AJR 1984;87:499.

41. Mendelson EB, Fisher MR, Mintzer RA, Halwig JM, Greenberger PA. Roentgenographic and clinical staging of allergic bronchopulmonary aspergillosis. Chest 1985;87:334.

42. Neeld DA, Goodman LR, Gurney JW, Greenberger PA, Fink JN. Computerized tomography in the evaluation of allergic bronchopulmonary aspergillosis. Ann Rev Respir Dis 1990;142:1200.

43. Goyal R, White CS, Templeton PA, et al. High attenuation mucous plugs in allergic bronchopulmonary aspergillosis: CT appearance. J Comput Assist Tomog 1992;16:649.

44. Hoehne JH, Reed CE, Dickie HA. Allergic bronchopulmonary aspergillosis is not rare. Chest 1973;63:177.

45. Longbottom JL, Pepys J. Pulmonary aspergillosis: diagnostic and immunologic significance of antigens and C-substance in *Aspergillus fumigatus*. J Pathol Bacteriol 1964;88:141.

46. Reed C. Variability of antigenicity of *Aspergillus fumigatus*. J Allergy Clin Immunol 1978;61:227.

47. Schwartz HJ, Citron KM, Chester EH, et al. A comparison of the prevalence of sensitization to *Aspergillus* antigens among asthmatics in Cleveland and London. J Allergy Clin Immunol 1978;62:9.

48. McCarthy DS, Pepys J. Allergic bronchopulmonary aspergillosis: clinical immunology. II. Skin, nasal, and bronchial tests. Clin Allergy 1971;1:26.

49. Calvanico JN, DuPont BL, Huang CJ, Patterson R, Fink JN, Kurup VP. Antigens of *Aspergillus fumigatus*. I. Purification of a cytoplasmic antigen reactive with sera of patients with *Aspergillus*-related disease. Clin Exp Immunol 1981;45:662.

50. Kurup VP, Ramasamy M, Greenberger PA, Fink JN. Isolation and characterization of a relevant *Aspergillus fumigatus* antigen with IgG and IgE binding activity. Int Arch Allergy Appl Immunol 1988;86:176.

51. Longbottom JL, Austwick PKC. Antigens and allergens of *Aspergillus fumigatus*. I. Characterization by quantitative immunoelectrophoretic techniques. J Allergy Clin Immunol 1986;78:9.

52. Arruda LK, Mann BJ, Chapman MD. Selective expression of a major allergen and cytotoxin, *Asp fI*, in *Aspergillus fumigatus*: implications for the immunopathogenesis of *Aspergillus*-related diseases. J Immunol 1992;149:3354.

53. Kurup VP, Kumar A, Kenealy WR, Greenberger PA. *Aspergillus* ribotoxins react with IgE and IgG antibodies of patients with allergic bronchopulmonary aspergillosis. J Lab Clin Med 1994;123:749.

54. Patterson R, Rosenberg M, Roberts M. Evidence that *Aspergillus fumigatus* growing in the airway of man can be a potent stimulus of specific and nonspecific IgE formation. Am J Med 1977;63:257.

55. Johnansson SGO, Juhlin L. lmmunoglobulin E in "healed" atopic dermatitis and after treatment with corticosteroids and azathioprine. Br J Dermatot 1970;82:10.

56. Settipane GA, Pudupakkam RK, McGowan JH. Corticosteroid effect on immunoglobulins. J Allergy Clin Immunol 1978;62:163.

57. Patterson R, Greenberger PA, Ricketti AJ, Roberts M. A radioimmunoassay index for allergic bronchopulmonary aspergillosis. Ann Intern Med 1983;99:18.

58. Slavin RG, Hutcheson PS, Knutsen AP. Participation of cell-mediated immunity in allergic bronchopulmonary aspergillosis. Int Arch Allergy Appl Immunol 1987;83:337.

59. Geha PS. Circulating immune complexes and activation of the complement sequence in acute allergic bronchopulmonary aspergillosis. J Allergy Clin Immunol 1977;60:357.

60. Marx JJ, Flaherty DK. Activation of the complement sequence by extracts of bacteria and fungi associated with hypersensitivity pneumonitis. J Allergy Clin Immunol 1976;57:328.

61. Apter AJ, Greenberger PA, Liotta JL, Roberts M. Fluctuations of serum IgA and its subclasses in allergic bronchopulmonary aspergillosis. J Allergy Clin Immunol 1989;84:367.

62. Ricketti AJ, Greenberger PA, Pruzansky JJ, Patterson R. Hyperreactivity of mediator releasing cells from patients with allergic bronchopulmonary aspergillosis as evidenced by basophil histamine release. J Allergy Clin Immunol 1983;72:386.

63. Chan-Yeung M, Chase WH, Trapp W, Grzybowski S. Allergic bronchopulmonary aspergillosis. Chest 1971;59:33.

64. Imbeau SA, Nichols D, Flaherty D, et al. Allergic bronchopulmonary aspergillosis. J Allergy Clin Immunol 1978;62:243.

65. Bosken CH, Myers JL, Greenberger PA, Katzenstein A-LA. Pathologic features of allergic bronchopulmonary aspergillosis. Am J Surg Pathol 1988;12:216.

66. Ghory AC, Patterson R, Roberts M, Suszko IM. In vitro IgE formation by peripheral blood lymphocytes from normal individuals and patients with allergic bronchopulmonary aspergillosis. Clin Exp Immunol 1980;40:581.

67. Slavin RG, Fischer VW, Levin EA, Tsai CC, Winzenburger P. A primate model of allergic bronchopulmonary aspergillosis. Int Arch Allergy Appl Immunol 1978;56:325.

68. Kurup VP, Mauze S, Choi H, et al. A murine model of allergic bronchopulmonary aspergillosis with elevated eosinophils and IgE. J Immunol 1992;148:3783.

69. Brown JE, Greenberger PA, Yarnold PR. Soluble serum interleuken 2 receptors in patients with asthma and allergic bronchopulmonary aspergillosis. Ann Allergy Asthma Immunol 1995;74:484.

70. Greenberger PA, Smith LJ, Hsu CCS, Roberts M, Liotta JL. Analysis of bronchoalveolar lavage in allergic bronchopulmonary aspergillosis: divergent responses in antigen-specific antibodies and total IgE. J Allergy Clin Immunol 1988;82:164.

71. Bernstein JA, Zeiss CR, Greenberger PA, Patterson R, Marhoul JL, Smith LL. Immunoblot analysis of sera from patients with allergic bronchopulmonary aspergillosis: correlation with disease activity. J Allergy Clin Immunol 1990;86:532.

72. Greenberger PA. Allergic bronchopulmonarv aspergillosis and fungoses. Clin Chest Med 1988;9:599.

73. Miller MA, Greenberger PA, Palmer J, et al. Allergic bronchopulmonary pseudallescheriosis in a child with cystic fibrosis. Am J Asthma Allergy Pediatr 1993;6:177.

74. Greenberger PA, Katzenstein A-LA. Lipoid pneumonia with atypical mycobacterial colonization in allergic bronchopulmonary aspergillosis: a complication of bronchography and a therapeutic dilemma. Arch Intern Med 1983;143:2003.

75. Halwig JM, Greenberger PA, Levin M, Patterson R. Recurrence of allergic bronchopulmonary aspergillosis after 7 years of remission. J Allergy Clin Immunol 1984;74:738.

76. Radin R, Greenberger PA, Patterson R, Ghory AC. Mold counts and exacerbations of allergic bronchopulmonary aspergillosis. Clin Allergy 1983;13:271.

77. Nichols D, Dopico GA, Braun S, Imbeau S, Peters ME, Rankin J. Acute and chronic pulmonary function changes in allergic bronchopulmonary aspergillosis. Am J Med 1979;67:631.

78. Safirstein BH, D'Souza MF, Simon G, Tai EH-C, Pepys J. Five-year follow-up of allergic bronchopulmonary aspergillosis. Am Rev Respir Dis 1973;108:450.

79. Denning DW, Van Wye JE, Lewiston NJ, et al. Adjunctive therapy of allergic bronchopulmonary aspergillosis with itraconazole. Chest 1991;100:813.

Allergic Diseases, 5th Edition,
edited by Roy Patterson, Leslie Carroll Grammer, and
Paul A. Greenberger. Lippincott–Raven Publishers, Philadelphia, © 1997.

25

Occupational Immunologic Lung Disease

Leslie C. Grammer

*L.C. Grammer: Division of Allergy-Immunology,
Northwestern University Medical School, Chicago, IL 60611-3008.*

Pearls for Practitioners
Roy Patterson

- Diagnosing immunologic lung disease often is complicated by occupationally related factors such as emotional concerns of workers and potential litigation. This makes the clinical evaluation far more complex than for other immunologic lung disease.
- The reactive airway disease syndrome, (RADS), suggested as resulting from inhalational exposure to irritant chemicals, may or may not exist. I have never seen a case that I accepted as RADS.
- I do not believe that true allergy to formaldehyde exists. Irritation above 3 ppm occurs in most humans.
- The experienced allergist can work out occupational allergy to proteins. The problem of allergy to low molecular weight chemicals generally is a major research endeavor.

It has been known for many years that a wide variety of occupational respiratory disorders are caused by immunologic mechanisms.[1] Moreover, increasing industrialization has led to the production of numerous materials capable of inducing immunologically mediated lung disease in the working population. This is of concern to physicians who diagnose and treat these diseases, and to labor, management, and various governmental agencies.

Two major subdivisions of diseases constitute occupational immunologic lung disease (OILD): (1) immunologically mediated asthma, and (2) hypersensitivity pneumonitis.[2] This chapter organizes the various exposures into the most relevant disease category. However, various overlaps and uncertainties exist in OILD. First, some exposures cause more than one disease. For instance, some antigens, such as trimellitic anhydride (TMA) and various fungal antigens, cause more than one immunologic pulmonary disease, including asthma or hypersensitivity pneumonitis.[3] Second, many reactive chemicals, such as TMA, cause disease either by irritant or immunologic mechanisms. Finally, some pulmonary responses have not been definitely established as immunologically or nonimmunologically mediated. An example is certain isocyanate responses.

EPIDEMIOLOGY

Incidence and prevalence figures for OILD are difficult to obtain for several reasons. First, there is often a high turnover rate in jobs associated with OILD, thus selecting workers who have not become sensitized. For instance, there is a high turnover rate among platinum workers.[4] In a study of an electronics industry, a substantial proportion of workers who left reported respiratory disease as the reason.[5] Second, occupationally related diseases generally are underreported.[6] For instance, although the incidence of work-related illness is thought to be upward of 20 per 100, only 2% of these illnesses were recorded in employers' logs, as is required by the Occupational Safety and Health Administration (OSHA).[7] Finally, the incidence of disease varies with the antigen exposure. For example, the incidence rate of occupational lung disease among animal handlers is estimated at 6%,[8] whereas that of workers exposed to proteolytic enzymes can be as high as 45%.[9]

About 2% of all cases of asthma in industrialized nations is occupationally related.[10] In a U.S. Social Security Disability Survey, approximately 15% of asthma was classified as occupational in origin.[11]

MEDICOLEGAL ASPECTS

Most sensitizing agents that have been reported to cause occupational asthma are proteins of plants, animal, or microbial derivation and are therefore not specifically regulated by OSHA. Some of the low molecular weight sensitizers such as isocyanates, anhydrides, and platinum are regulated by OSHA; published standards for airborne exposure can be found in the Code of Federal Regulations (CRF 29.1910.1000).[12] OSHA, a division of the U.S. Department of Labor, is responsible for determining and enforcing these legal standards. The National Institute of Occupational Health and Safety (NIOSH), a division of the U.S. Department of Health and Human Services, is responsible for reviewing available research data on exposure to hazardous agents and providing recommendations to OSHA relative to airborne exposure limits. However, NIOSH has no regulatory or enforcement authority in this regard. More than 200 different substances have been reported to act as respiratory sensitizers and causes of occupational asthma.[13] In only a few European countries are such occupational respiratory illnesses recognized by law with rights of compensation. In France, such etiologic agents as isocyanates, biologic enzymes, and tropical wood dusts are recognized.[13] In the United Kingdom, such agents as platinum salts, isocyanates, colophony, and epoxy resins are recognized. In countries where legislation involving compensation exists, implementation may be extremely difficult because of the lack of explicit criteria for the diagnosis of a given occupational disease.[14]

In the last decade in the United States, hazard communication and worker's right-to-know legislation has been passed at the federal, state, and local level.[15] Substances that are capable of inducing respiratory sensitization generally are considered hazardous, and thus workers exposed to such substances are covered in most legislation. The common elements that exist in most hazard communication legislation are as follows: (1) that the employer apprise a governmental agency relative to its use of hazardous substances; (2) that the employer inform the employee of the availability of information on hazardous substances to which the employee is exposed; (3) that there be availability to the employee of alphabetized lists of material safety data sheets for hazardous substances in the workplace; (4) that there be labeling of containers of hazardous substances; and, (5) that training be provided to employees relative to health hazards, methods of detection, and protective measures to be used in handling hazardous substances. This sort of hazard communication legislation may make workers more aware of the potential that exists to develop respiratory sensitization and OILD syndromes from certain exposures. Whether this awareness will have any impact on the incidence of OILD remains to be seen.

ASTHMA

Pathophysiology

The pathophysiology of asthma is reviewed in Chapter 22. The major pathophysiologic abnormalities of asthma, occupational or otherwise, are bronchoconstriction, excess mucus production, and inflammatory infiltration, including activated T cells, mast cells, and eosinophils of the bronchial walls.[16] These abnormalities are at least partly explained by neurogenic mechanisms and release of inflammatory mediators and cytokines such as interleukins and interferons. Type 1 hypersensitivity involving crosslinking IgE on the surface of mast cells and basophils, thus resulting in release of mediators such as histamine, leukotrienes, cytokines such as IL-3, IL-4, and IL-5, is believed to be the triggering mechanism in most types of immediate-onset asthma. There is increasing evidence that cellular mechanisms are important in asthma.[17,18]

Reaction Patterns

Several patterns of asthma may occur after a single inhalation challenge[19] (Table 25-1). The *immediate* reaction is mediated by IgE, occurs within minutes of challenge, presents as large airway obstruction, and is preventable with cromolyn and reversible by bronchodilators. The *late* response occurs several hours after inhalation challenge, presents as small airway obstruction in which wheezing may be mild and cough and dyspnea may predominate, lasts for several hours, is usually preventable with steroids[20] or cromolyn, and is only partly reversed by bronchodilators.

The *dual* response is a combination of the immediate and late asthmatic responses. It is partially prevented by steroids or bronchodilators. After a single challenge study with certain antigens like western red cedar, the patient may have repetitive asthmatic responses occurring over several days. This repetitive asthmatic response can be reversed with bronchodilators.

TABLE 25-1. *Types of respiratory responses to inhalation challenge*

	Immediate	Late	Repetitive
Asthma			
Onset	10–20 min	4–6 h	Periodic after initial attack
Duration	1–2 h	2–6 h	Days
Abnormality	FEV_1	FEV_1	FEV_1
Immune mechanism	IgE	IgE (IgG)	?
Symptoms	Wheezing	Wheezing, dyspnea	Recurrent wheezing
Therapy	Bronchodilators	Bronchodilators, corticosteroids	Bronchodilators

FEV_1, forced expiratory volume in 1 second.

Other atypical patterns—square wave, progressive, and progressive and prolonged immediate—have been described after diisocyanate challenges; the mechanisms resulting in these patterns have not been elucidated.[21] There is increasing evidence implicating immunologic mechanisms, in particular, cellular mechanisms, in the pathophysiology of asthmatic responses to isocyanates.[22–24]

Etiologic Agents

Most of the 200 agents that have been described to cause occupational asthma are high molecular weight ($\geq$3 kd) heterologous proteins of plant, animal, or microorganism origin.[25] Low molecular weight chemicals can act as irritants and aggravate preexisting asthma. They also act as allergens if they are capable of haptenizing autologous proteins in the respiratory tract.[26] Numerous reviews of occupational asthma have information on etiologic agents.[6,27,28] A representative list of agents and industries associated with OILD is found in Table 25-2.

Etiologic Agents of Animal Origin

Proteolytic enzymes are known to cause asthmatic symptoms on the basis of type I immediate hypersensitivity. Examples are pancreatic enzymes, hog trypsin[29] used in the manufacture of plastic polymer resins, and *Bacillus subtilis* enzymes[30] incorporated into laundry detergents. Positive skin test results, in vitro IgE antibody, and inhalation challenges have been demonstrated with *B subtilis* enzymes, which are no longer used in the United States.[31] Papain, which is a proteolytic enzyme of vegetable origin used in brewing beer and manufacturing meat tenderizer, has been noted to cause similar symptoms by IgE-mediated mechanisms.[32]

Animal dander causes asthma in a variety of workers, including veterinarians, laboratory workers, grooms, shepherds, breeders, pet shop owners, farmers, and jockeys.[33] This is even a problem for people whose work takes them to homes of clients who have pets, such as real estate salespeople, interior designers, and domestic workers.

Immediate asthmatic reactions and late interstitial response have been reported after inhalation challenge with avian proteins in persons who raise birds for profit.[34] Positive skin test results and in vitro IgE have been demonstrated.

A variety of insect scales have been associated with asthma. Occupational exposure to insect scales occurs in numerous circumstances.[3] Bait handlers can become sensitized to mealworms used as fishing bait.[35] Positive skin test results, in vitro IgE antibody, and inhalation challenges have been demonstrated to mealworms. Positive skin test results have been shown in various workers who have asthma on insect exposure: to screw worm flies in insect control personnel,[36] to moths in fish bait workers,[37] and to weevils in grain dust workers.[38]

Asthma has been noted in workers who crush oyster shells to remove the meat.[39] On the basis of skin test results to various allergens, the researchers determined that the allergen was the primitive organisms that attached to the oyster shell surface. Similarly, asthma may occur from sea squirt body fluids in workers who gather pearls and oysters[40] and in snow crab workers.[41]

Etiologic Agents of Vegetable Origin

In terms of plant protein antigens, exposure to latex antigens, particularly that dispersed by powder in gloves, has become an important cause of occupational asthma in the health care

TABLE 25-2. *Occupational allergens*

Agent	Industries and occupations
Animal proteins	
Proteolytic enzymes	Plastic polymer resin manufacturing, detergent industry, pharmaceutical industry, meat tenderizer manufacturing, beer clearing
Animal dander, saliva, urine	Lab researchers, veterinarians, grooms, breeders, pet shop owners, farmers
Avian protein	Poultry breeders, bird fanciers
Insect scales	Beekeepers, insect control workers, bait handlers, mushroom workers, entomologists
Vegetable proteins	
Latex	Health care workers
Flour or contaminants (insects, molds)	Bakers
Green coffee beans, tea, garlic, soybeans	Workers in processing plants
Grain dust	Farmers, workers in processing plants
Castor beans	Fertilizer workers
Vegetable gums	Printing industry workers
Wood dusts: boxwood, mahogany, oak, redwood, Western red cedar	Carpenters, sawyers, wood pulp workers, foresters, cabinet makers
Penicillium caseii	Cheese workers
Orris root, rice flour	Hairdressers
Thermophilic molds	Mushroom workers
Chemicals	
Antibiotics	Hospital and pharmaceutical personnel
Other drugs: piperazine hydrochloride, alpha-methyldopa, amprolium hydrochloride	Hospital and pharmaceutical personnel
Platinum	Workers in processing plants
Nickel	Nickel-plating workers
Anhydrides (TMA, PA, TCPA)	Workers in manufacture of curing agents, plasticizers, anticorrosive coatings
Azo dyes	Dye manufacturers
Ethylenediamine	Shellac/lacquer industry workers
Isocyanates	Production of paints, surface coatings, insulation polyurethane foam
Soldering fluxes, colophony	Welders
Chloramine T	Sterilization

Lab, laboratory; TMA, trimellitic anhydride; PA, phthalic anhydride; TCPA, tetra chloro phthalic anhydride.

setting.[42] In the baking industry, flour proteins are well recognized as causing occupational asthma.[43] Numerous other plant foodstuff proteins have been described as causing occupational asthma with inhalational exposure, including tea,[44] garlic,[45] coffee beans,[46] and soybeans.[47] Other plant protein sources reported to cause occupational asthma include castor beans,[48] vegetable gums,[49] wood dusts,[50] and dried flowers.[51] Wood dust from western red cedar is a well-recognized cause of occupational asthma, but the antigen appears to be the low molecular weight chemical, plicatic acid, not a high molecular weight plant protein.[52]

A variety of microbes have been reported to be sensitizing agents in occupational asthma. Among these are molds[53] and bacteria such as thermophilic actinomycetes.[54]

Chemicals

Asthma has been described in pharmaceutical workers and hospital personnel exposed to pharmacologic products. Numerous antibiotics are known to cause asthma, positive skin test results, or specific IgE, including ampicillin, penicillin, spiramycin, and sulfa drugs.[55] Other pharmaceuticals, including amprolium hydrochloride, alpha-methyldopa, and piperazine hydrochloride, cause asthma on an immunologic basis.[6]

Workers in platinum-processing plants may have rhinitis, conjunctivitis, and asthma.[56] Positive results to bronchial challenges and specific IgE have been demonstrated in affected workers. Another metal, nickel sulfate, also has been reported to cause IgE-mediated asthma.[57]

The manufacture of epoxy resins requires a curing agent, usually an acid anhydride or a polyamine compound. Workers thus may be exposed to acid anhydrides in the manufacture of curing agents, plasticizers, and anticorrosive coating material. Studies have shown that three different patterns of immunologic respiratory response may occur[3] (Table 25-3).

Initially, it was presumed that the antibody in affected workers would be directed only against the trimellityl (TM) haptenic determinant. However, studies of antibody specificity demonstrate that there is antibody directed against both hapten and TM–protein determinants that are considered new antigen determinants.[58]

Other acid anhydrides described as causing similar problems include phthalic anhydride, hexahydrophthalic anhydride, and pyromellitic anhydride.

Isocyanates are required catalysts in the production of polyurethane foam, vehicle spray paint, and protective surface coatings. Approximately 5% to 10% of isocyanate workers develop asthma from exposure to subtoxic levels after a variable period of latency.[59] The isocyanates described as causing occupational asthma include toluene diisocyanate, hexamethylene diisocyanate, diphenylmethyl diisocyanate, and isopherone diisocyanate.[59] The histologic features of bronchial biopsy specimens from workers with isocyanate asthma appears similar to that from patients with immunologic asthma, and thus is suggestive of an immunologic mechanism.[60,61] Compared with isocyanate workers with a negative response to bronchial challenges, workers with a positive response to challenges have a higher incidence and level of antibodies against isocyanate–protein conjugates.[62] However, most isocyanate

TABLE 25-3. *TMA-induced respiratory diseases and immunologic correlates*

Disease	Mechanism	Immunologic tests
Asthma or rhinitis	IgE	Immediate skin test IgG against TM–protein conjugate
Late respiratory systemic syndrome (LRSS)	IgG and IgA	IgG, IgA, or total antibody against TM–protein conjugate
Pulmonary disease, anemia syndrome	Complement-fixing antibodies	Complement-fixing antibodies against TM cells

TMA, trimellitic anhydride; TM, trimellityl.

workers with positive challenge responses do not have detectable specific IgE in their serum. Hypersensitivity pneumonitis[63] and hemorrhagic pneumonitis[64] from isocyanates have been reported to be caused by immunologic mechanisms. HLA class II alleles have been studied in isocyanate asthma[65]; a positive association was reported. Formaldehyde, a respiratory irritant at ambient concentrations of 1 ppm or more, often is cited as a cause of occupational asthma; however, documented instances of formaldehyde-induced IgE-mediated asthma are almost nonexistent.[66] A bifunctional aldehyde, glutaraldehyde has been reported to cause occupational asthma.[67] Ethylenediamine, a chemical used in shellac and photographic developing industries, has been reported to cause occupational asthma.[68] Chloramine T,[69] reactive azo dyes,[70] piperazine, and dimethyl ethanolamine are other chemicals also reported to be causes of occupational asthma.[71]

HYPERSENSITIVITY PNEUMONITIS

The signs, symptoms, immunologic features, pulmonary function abnormalities, pathologic features, and laboratory findings of hypersensitivity pneumonitis are reviewed in Chapter 23. No matter what the etiologic agent, the presentation follows one of two patterns. In the acute form, patients have fever, chills, chest tightness, dyspnea without wheezing, and nonproductive cough 4 to 8 hours after exposure. The acute form resolves within 24 hours. In the chronic form, which results from prolonged low-level exposure, patients have mild coughing, dyspnea, fatigue, and weight loss. Either form can lead to pulmonary fibrosis with irreversible change; thus, this disease must be recognized early so that irreversible lung damage does not occur.

A variety of organic dusts from fungal, bacterial, or serum protein sources in occupational settings have been identified as etiologic agents of hypersensitivity pneumonitis[72] (Table 25-4). Several chemicals, including anhydrides and isocyanates (discussed previously), have been reported to cause hypersensitivity pneumonitis.

DIAGNOSIS

The diagnosis of OILD is not complex in the individual worker if symptoms appear at the workplace shortly after exposure to a well-recognized antigen. However, diagnosis can be difficult in patients whose symptoms occur many hours after exposure, for instance, late asthma from TMA. Because of the increasing importance of OILD, it is essential to evaluate patients with respiratory syndromes for a possible association between their current disease states, their pulmonary function test results, and their immunologic exposure in the work environment.[73]

In the case of the well-established OILD syndrome, a careful history and physical examination may suffice. The history and physical examination findings in asthma and hypersensitivity pneumonitis are discussed in Chapters 22 and 23, respectively. In less obvious situations, however, it is often necessary to demonstrate the presence of antibodies and clinical sensitivity.[74]

Immunologic evaluations may provide important information about the cause of the respiratory disease. Skin tests, with antigens determined to be present in the environment, may detect IgE antibodies and suggest a causal relation.[75] Haptens may be coupled to carrier proteins, such as human serum albumin, and used in skin tests[76,77] or radioimmunoassays.[78] In cases of interstitial lung disease, double gel immunodiffusion techniques may be used to determine the presence of precipitating antibody, which would indicate antibody production against antigens known to cause disease.[79]

TABLE 25-4. *Occupational hypersensitivity pneumonitides*

Disease	Exposure	Specific inhalant
Farmer's lung	Moldy hay	*Micropolyspora faeni*
		Thermoactinomyces vulgaris
Malt worker's disease	Fungal spores	*Aspergillus clavatus*
		Aspergillus fumigatus
Maple-bark stripper's disease	Moldy logs	*Cryptostroma corticale*
Wood-pulp worker's disease	Moldy logs	*Alternaria* sp
Sequoiosis	Moldy redwood sawdust	*Graphium* sp
		Aureobasidium pullulans
Humidifier/air conditioner disease	Fungal spores	Thermophilic actinomycetes
		Naegleria gruberi
Bird breeder's disease	Avian dust	Avian serum
Bagassosis	Moldy sugarcane	*T vulgaris*
Mushroom worker's disease	Mushroom compost	*M faeni*
		T vulgaris
Suberosis	Moldy cork dust	*Penicillium frequetans*
Isocyanate disease	Isocyanates	Toluene diisocyanate
		Diphenylmethane diisocyanate

It may be necessary to attempt to reproduce the clinical features of asthma or interstitial lung disease by bronchial challenge, followed by careful observation of the worker. Challenge may be conducted by natural exposure of the patient to the work environment, comparing results of both preexposure and postexposure pulmonary function studies with those of similar studies on nonwork days. Another technique used for diagnosis of OILD is controlled bronchoprovocation in the laboratory with preexposure and postexposure pulmonary function measurements.[80] The intensity of exposure must not exceed that ordinarily encountered on the job, and the appropriate personnel and equipment must be available to treat respiratory abnormalities that may occur.

If the analysis of OILD is not for an individual patient but for a group of workers afflicted with a respiratory illness, the approach is different. The initial approach to an epidemiologic evaluation of OILD is usually a cross-sectional survey using a well-designed questionnaire.[81] The questionnaire should include a chronologic description of all past job exposures, symptoms, chemical exposures and levels, length of employment, and protective respiratory equipment used. Analysis of the survey can establish possible sources of exposure. All known information about the sources of exposure should be sought in the form of previously reported toxic or immunologic reactions. Ultimately, immunologic tests and challenges may be done selectively.

PROGNOSIS

Unfortunately, many workers with occupational asthma do not completely recover even though they have been removed from exposure to a sensitizing agent. Prognostic factors that have been examined include specific IgE, duration of symptomatology, pulmonary function testing, and nonspecific bronchial hyperreactivity (BHR). An unfavorable prognosis has been associated with a persistent high level of specific IgE,[82] long duration of symptoms (more than 1 to 2 years), abnormal pulmonary function test results, and a high degree of BHR.[83] The obvious conclusion from these studies is that early diagnosis and removal from exposure are requisites for the goal of complete recovery. In workers who remain exposed after a diagnosis of occupational asthma is made, further deterioration of lung function and increase in BHR have been reported.[84] Life-threatening attacks and even deaths have been reported when exposure continues after diagnosis.[85]

TREATMENT

The management of OILD consists of controlling the worker's exposure to the offending agent. This can be accomplished in various ways. Sometimes the worker can be moved to another station; or efficient dust and vapor extraction can be instituted; or the ventilation can be improved, so that a total job change is not required. Consultation with an industrial hygienist familiar with exposure levels may be helpful in this regard. Remember that levels of exposure below the legal limits that are based on toxicity still may cause immunologic reactions. Filtering-type face masks are not especially efficient or well tolerated. Ideally, the working environment should be designed to limit concentration of potential sensitizers to safe levels. Unfortunately, this is impractical in many manufacturing processes, and even in a carefully monitored facility recommended thresholds may be exceeded.[86] Thus, avoidance may entail retraining and reassigning a worker to another job.

Pharmacologic management of OILD rarely is helpful in the presence of continued exposure on a chronic basis. Certainly, in acute hypersensitivity pneumonitis, a short course of corticosteroids (see Chap. 23) is useful in conjunction with avoidance. However, chronic administration of steroids for occupational hypersensitivity pneumonitis is not recommended. Asthma resulting from contact with occupational exposures responds to therapeutic agents such as theophylline, beta agonists, and steroids (see Chap. 22). As exposure continues, sensitivity may increase, making medication requirements prohibitive.

Immunotherapy has been used with various occupational allergens that cause asthma, including treatment of laboratory animal workers,[87] bakers,[88] and oyster gatherers, with reported success. Immunotherapy may be feasible in a limited number of patients, with certain occupational allergens of the same nature as the common inhalant allergens; however, it is difficult and hazardous with many agents that cause occupational immunologic asthma.

PREVENTION

The key principle in OILD is that prevention, rather than treatment, must be the goal. Such preventative measures as improved ventilation and adhering to threshold limits (as discussed in *Treatment*) would be helpful in this regard. Efforts should be made to educate individual workers and managers in high-risk industries so that affected workers can be recognized early. Right-to-know legislation will hopefully be useful in this regard.

No preemployment screening criteria have been shown to be useful in predicting the eventual appearance of OILD. It is known that atopy is a predisposing factor to a worker developing IgE-mediated disease.[54] Whether cigarette smoking is a risk factor for OILD is unclear.

Prospective studies, such as that of Zeiss and colleagues[89] of TMA workers, may demonstrate that serial immunologic studies are useful in predicting which workers are likely to develop immunologically mediated diseases. Those workers then could be removed from the offending exposure and retrained before any illness develops. Thus far, this approach has been studied only in TMA workers. Two other prospective studies of TMA workers show that decreasing the airborne levels reduces disease prevalence.[90,91] This may prove to be the best approach to preventing OILD from other agents.

REFERENCES

1. Goldstein RA. Foreword to symposium proceedings on occupational immunologic lung disease. J Allergy Clin Immunol 1982;70:4.
2. Salvaggio JE. Overview of occupational immunologic lung disease. J Allergy Clin Immunol 1982;70:5.
3. Patterson R, Zeiss CR, Pruzansky JJ. Immunology and immunopathology of trimellitic anhydride pulmonary reactions. J Allergy Clin Immunol 1982;70:19.
4. Roberts AE. Platinosis: a five year study of the effects of soluble platinum salts on employees in a platinum laboratory and refinery. Arch Ind Hyg 1951;4:549.
5. Perks WH, Burge PS, Rehahn M, et al. Work-related respiratory disease in employees leaving an electronic factory. Thorax 1979;34:19.
6. Bernstein IL. Occupational asthma. Clin Chest Med 1981;2:255.
7. Discher DP, Feinberg HC. Pilot study for development of an occupational disease surveillance method. HEW publication (NIOSH) no. 75-162, 1975.
8. Carroll KB, Pepys J, Longbottom JL, Hughes, DT, Benson HG. Extrinsic allergic alveolitis due to rat serum proteins. Clin Allergy 1975;5:443.
9. Brooks SM. The evaluation of occupational airways disease in the laboratory and workplace. J Allergy Clin Immunol 1982;70:56.
10. Salvaggio J, ed. NIAID Task Force report: asthma and other allergic diseases. US Department of Health, Education and Welfare, NIH publication no. 79-387, 1979:330.
11. Blanc P. Occupational asthma in a national disability survey. Chest 1987;92:613.
12. Office of the Federal Register National Archives and Records Administration. Code of Federal Regulations 1900–1910. Washington, DC: Federal Register, 1993.
13. Chan-Yeung M, Malo J-L. Aetiological agents in occupational asthma. Eur Respir J 1994;7:346.
14. Miller AC, Green M. Occupational asthma. J R Soc Med 1982;75:225.
15. Olishifski JB. Industrial hygiene. In: Zenz C, ed. Occupational medicine. Chicago: Mosby-Year Book Medical Publishers, 1988:13.
16. Glassroth J, Smith LJ: Asthma-pathophysiology. In: Patterson R, Zeiss CR, Grammer LC, Greenberger PA, eds. Allergic diseases: diagnosis and management. 4th ed. Philadelphia: JB Lippincott, 1993:611.
17. Gratziou C, Carroll M, Walls A, Howarth PH, Holgate ST. Early changes in T lymphocytes recovered by bronchoalveolar lavage after local allergen challenge of asthmatic airways. Am Rev Respir Dis 1992;145:1259.
18. Azzawi M, Johnston PW, Majundar S, Kay AB, Jeffery PK. T lymphocytes and activated eosinophils in airway mucosa in fatal asthma and cystic fibrosis. Am Rev Respir Dis 1992;145:1477.
19. Fink JN. Evaluation of the patient for occupational immunologic lung disease. J Allergy Clin Immunol 1982;70:11.
20. Boschetto P, Fabbri LM, Zocca E, et al. Prednisone inhibits late asthmatic reactions and airway inflammation induced by toluene diisocyanate in sensitized subjects. J Allergy Clin Immunol 1987;80:261.
21. Cartier A, Malo J-L. Occupational challenge tests. In: Bernstein IL, Chan-Yeung M, Malo J-L, Bernstein DI, eds. Asthma in the workplace. 1st ed. New York: Marcel Dekker, 1993;215.
22. Vandenplas O, Malo J-L, Saetta M, Mapp CE, Fabrri LM: Occupational asthma and extrinsic alveolitis due to isocyanates: current status and perspectives. Br J Ind Med 1993;50:213.
23. Di Stefano A, Saetta M, Maestrelli P, et al. Mast cells in the airway mucosa and rapid development of occupational asthma induced by toluene diisocyanate. Am Rev Respir Dis 1993;147:1005.
24. Maestrelli P, Calcagni PG, Saetta M, et al. Sputum eosinophilia after asthmatic responses induced by isocyantes in sensitized subjects. Clin Exp Allergy 1994;24:29.
25. Bush RK, Kagen SL. Guidelines for the preparation and characterization of high molecular weight allergens used for the diagnosis of occupational lung disease. J Allergy Clin Immunol 1989;84:814.
26. Aguis RM, Elton RA, Sawyer L, Taylor P. Occupational asthma and the chemical properties of low molecular weight organic substances. Occup Med 1994;44:34.
27. Bernstein DI, Bernstein IL. Occupational asthma. In: Middleton E Jr, Reed CE, Ellis EF, Adkinson NF Jr, Yunginger JW, Busse WW, eds. Allergy: principles and practice. 4th ed. St Louis: Mosby-Year Book Medical Publishers, 1993:1369.

28. Cockcroft D. Occupational asthma. Ann Allergy 1990;65:169.
29. Colten HR, Polakoff PL, Weinstein SF, Strieder DJ. Immediate hypersensitivity to hog trypsin resulting from industrial exposure. N Engl J Med 1975;292:1050.
30. Slavin RG. Asthma in adults. III. Occupational asthma. Hosp Pract 1978;13:133.
31. Slavin RG, Lewis GR. Sensitivity to enzyme additives in laundry detergent workers. J Allergy Clin Immunol 1971;48:262.
32. Novey HS, Keenan WJ, Fairshter RD, et al. Pulmonary disease in workers exposed to papain: clinicophysiological and immunological studies. Clin Allergy 1980;10:721.
33. Gross NJ. Allergy to laboratory animals: epidemiologic, clinical and physiologic aspects and a trial of cromolyn in its management. J Allergy Clin Immunol 1980;66:158.
34. Hargreave FE, Pepys J. Allergic respiratory reactions in bird fanciers provoked by allergen inhalation provocation tests. J Allergy Clin Immunol 1972;50:157.
35. Bernstein DI, Gallagher JS, Bernstein IL. Meal worm asthma: clinical and immunologic studies. J Allergy Clin Immunol 1983;72:475.
36. Gibbons HL, Dillie JR, Cauley RG. Inhalant allergy to the screw worm fly. Arch Environ Health 1965;10:424.
37. Stevenson DD, Mathews KP. Occupational asthma following inhalation of moth particles. J Allergy 1967;39:274.
38. Lunn JA. Millworkers' asthma: allergic responses to the grain weevil (*Sitophilus granarius*). Br J Ind Med 1966;23:149.
39. Wada S, Nishimoto Y, Nakashima T, Shigenobu T, Onori K. Clinical observation of bronchial asthma in workers who culture oysters. Hiroshima J Med Sci 1967;16:255.
40. Jyo T, Katsutani T, Inoko T, et al. Studies on oyster shucker's asthma and asthma-like disease affecting oyster shuckers in Hiroshima prefecture. Jpn J Allergol 1964;13:88.
41. Malo J-L, Cartier A, Ghezzo H, Lafrance M, McCants M, Lehrer SB. Patterns of improvement in spirometry, bronchial hyperresponsiveness, and specific IgE antibody levels after cessation of exposure in occupational asthma caused by snow crab processing. Am Rev Respir Dis 1988;138:807.
42. Slater JE. Continuing medical education: latex allergy. J Allergy Clin Immunol 1994;94:139.
43. Blanco Carmona JG, Juste Picon S, Garces Sotillos M. Occupational asthma in bakeries caused by sensitivity to alpha-amylase. Allergy 1991;46:274.
44. Cartier A, Malo J-L. Occupational asthma due to tea dust. Thorax 1990;45:203.
45. Falleroni AF, Zeiss CR, Levitz D. Occupational asthma secondary to inhalation of garlic dust. J Allergy Clin Immunol 1981;68:156.
46. Lehrer SB. Bean hypersensitivity in coffee workers' asthma: a clinical and immunological appraisal. Allergy Proc 1990;11:65.
47. Ferrer A, Torres A, Roca J, Sunyer J, Anto JM, Rodriguez Roisin R. Characteristics of patients with soybean dust-induced acute severe asthma requiring mechanical ventilation. Eur Respir J 1990;3:429.
48. Coombs RR, Hunter A, Jonas WE, Bennich H, Johannson SG, Panzani R. Detection of IgE (IgND) specific antibody (probably reagin) to castor bean allergen by the red cell linked antigen antiglobulin reaction. Lancet 1968;i:1115.
49. Lagier F, Cartier A, Somer J, Dolovich J, Malo J-L. Occupational asthma caused by guar gum. J Allergy Clin Immunol 1990;85:785.
50. Godnic-Cvar J, Gomzi M. Case report of occupational asthma due to palisander wood dust and bronchoprovocation challenge by inhalation of pure wood dust from a capsule. Am J Ind Med 1990;18:541.
51. Schroeckenstein DC, Meier-Davis S, Yunginger JW, Bush RK. Allergens involved in occupational asthma caused by baby's breath (*Gypsophila paniculata*). J Allergy Clin Immunol 1990;86:189.
52. Chan-Yeung M. Immunologic and non-immunologic mechanisms in asthma due to western red cedar (*Thuja plicata*). J Allergy Clin Immunol 1982;70:32.
53. Gottlieb SJ, Garibaldi E, Hutcheson PS, Slavin RG. Occupational asthma to the slime mold *Dictyostelium discoideum*. J Occup Med 1993;35:1231.
54. Brooks SM. Occupational and environmental asthma. In: Rom WN, ed. Environmental and occupational medicine, 2d ed. Boston: Little, Brown, 1992:393.
55. Charpin J. Occupational asthma. In: Yamamura Y, Frick OL, Hariuchi Y, et al, eds. Allergology. Amsterdam: Excerpta Medica, 1974:120.
56. Cromwell O, Pepys J, Parish WE, Hughes EG. Specific IgE antibodies to platinum salts in sensitized workers. Clin Allergy 1979;9:109.
57. Malo J-L, Cartier A, Doepner M, Nieboer E, Evans S, Dolovich J. Occupational asthma caused by nickel sulfate. J Allergy Clin Immunol 1982;69:55.
58. Patterson R, Suszko IM, Zeiss CR, Pruzansky JJ. Characterization of hapten-human serum albumins and their complexes with specific human antisera. J Clin Immunol 1981;1:181.
59. Balaan MR, Banks DE. The respiratory effects of isocyanates. In: Rom WN, ed. Environmental and occupational medicine. 2d ed. Boston: Little, Brown, 1992:967.
60. Saetta M, di Stefano A, Maestrelli P, et al. Airway mucosal inflammation in occupational asthma induced by toluene diisocyanate. Am Rev Respir Dis 1992;145:160.
61. Saetta M, Maestrelli P, di Stefano A, et al. Effect of cessation of exposure to toluene diisocyanate (TDI) on bronchial mucosa of subjects with TDI-induced asthma. Am Rev Respir Dis 1992;145:169.

62. Grammer LC, Harris KE, Malo J-L, Cartier A, Patterson R. The use of an immunoassay index for antibodies against isocyanate human protein conjugates and application to human isocyanate disease. J Allergy Clin Immunol 1990;86:94.

63. Walker CL, Grammer LC, Shaughnessy MA, Duffy M, Stotlzfus VD, Patterson R. Diphenylmethan diisocyanate hypersensitivity pneumonitis: a serologic evaluation. J Occup Med 1994;31:315.

64. Patterson R, Nugent KM, Harris KE, Eberle ME. Case reports: immunologic hemorrhagic pneumonia caused by isocyanates. Am Rev Respir Dis 1990;141:225.

65. Bignon JS, Aron Y, Ju LY, et al. HLA class II alleles in isocyanate-induced asthma. Am J Respir Crit Care Med 1994;149:71.

66. Dykewicz MS, Patterson R, Cugell DW, Harris KE, Wu AF. Serum IgE and IgG to formaldehyde-human serum albumin: lack of relation to gaseous formaldehyde exposure and symptoms. J Allergy Clin Immunol 1991;87:48.

67. Chan-Yeung M, McMurren T, Catonio-Begley F, Lam S. Clinical aspects of allergic disease: occupational asthma in a technologist exposed to glutaraldehyde. J Allergy Clin Immunol 1993;91:974.

68. Lam S, Chan-Yeung M. Ethylenediamine-induced asthma. Am Rev Respir Dis 1980;121:151.

69. Blasco A, Joral A, Fuente R, Rodriguez M, Garcia A, Domingues A. Bronchial asthma due to sensitization to chloramine T. J Invest Allergol Clin Immunol 1992;2:167.

70. Nilsson R, Nordlinder R, Wass U, Meding B, Belin L. Asthma, rhinitis, and dermatitis in workers exposed to reactive dyes. Br J Ind Med 1993;50:65.

71. Vallieres M, Cockcroft DW, Taylor DM, Dolovich J, Hargreave FE. Dimethyl ethanolamine-induced asthma. Am Rev Respir Dis 1977;115:867.

72. Fink JN. Hypersensitivity pneumonitis. In: Middleton E, Reed CE, Ellis ER, Adkinson NF, Yunginger JW, Busse WW, eds. Allergy: principles and practice. St Louis: CV Mosby, 1993:1415.

73. Bernstein DI. Clinical assessment and management of occupational asthma. In: Berstein IL, Chan-Yeung M, Malo J-L, Bernstein DI, eds. Asthma in the workplace. New York: Marcel Dekker, 1993:103.

74. Grammer LC, Patterson R. Immunologic evaluation of occupational asthma. In: Bernstein IL, Chan-Yeung M, Malo J-L, Bernstein DI, eds. Asthma in the workplace. New York: Marcel Dekker, 1993:125.

75. Grammer LC, Patterson R, Zeiss CR. Guidelines for the immunologic evaluation of occupational lung disease. J Allergy Clin Immunol 1989;84:805.

76. Butcher BT, Salvaggio JE, Weill H, Ziskind MM. Toluene diisocyanate (TDI) pulmonary disease: immunologic and inhalation challenge studies. J Allergy Clin Immunol 1976:58:89.

77. Zeiss CR, Patterson R, Pruzansky JJ, Miller MM, Rosenberg M, Levitz D. Trimellitic anhydride (TMA)-induced airway syndromes: clinical and immunologic studies. J Allergy Immunol 1977;60:96.

78. Zeiss CR, Pruzansky JJ, Patterson R. A solid phase radioimmunoassay for the quantitation of human reaginic antibody against ragweed antigen E. J Immunol 1973;110:414.

79. Richerson HB, Bernstein IL, Fink JN, et al. Guidelines for the clinical evaluation of hypersensitivity pneumonitis. J Allergy Clin Immunol 1989;84:839.

80. Cartier A, Bernstein IL, Burge PS, et al. Guidelines for bronchoprovocation on the investigation of occupational asthma. J Allergy Clin Immunol 1989;84:823.

81. Smith AB, Castellan RM, Lewis D, Matt T. Guidelines for the epidemiologic assessment of occupational asthma. J Allergy Clin Immunol 1989;84:794.

82. Grammer LC, Shaughnessy MA, Henderson J, et al. A clinical and immunologic study of workers with trimellitic-anhydride–induced immunologic lung disease after transfer to low exposure. Am Rev Resp Dis 1993;148:54.

83. Hudson P, Cartier A, Pineau L, et al. Follow-up of occupational asthma caused by crab and various agents. J Allergy Clin Immunol 1985;76:682.

84. Marabini A, Dimich-Ward H, Kwan SY, Kennedy SM, Waxler-Morrison N, Chan-Yeung M. Clinical and socioeconomic features of subjects with red cedar asthma: a follow-up study. Chest 1993;104:821.

85. Chan-Yeung M, Lam S. State of the art-occupational asthma. Am Rev Respir Dis 1986;137:686.

86. Diem JE. Five year longitudinal study of workers employed in a new toluene diisocyanate manufacturing plant. Am Rev Respir Dis 1982;126:420.

87. Wahn U, Siraganian RP. Efficacy and specificity of immunotherapy with laboratory animal allergen extracts. J Allergy Clin Immunol 1980;65:413.

88. Thiel H, Ulmer WT. Baker's asthma: development and possibility for treatment. Chest 1978;78:400.

89. Zeiss CR, Wolkonsky P, Chacon R, et al. Syndromes in workers exposed to trimellitic anhydride: a longitudinal clinical and immunologic study. Ann Intern Med 1983;98:9.

90. Boxer MB, Grammer LC, Harris KE, Roach DE, Patterson R. Six-year clinical and immunologic follow-up of workers exposed to trimellitic anhydride. J Allergy Clin Immunol 1987;80:147.

91. Grammer LC, Harris KE, Sonenthal KR, Ley C, Roach DE. A cross-sectional survey of 46 employees exposed to trimellitic anhydride. Allergy Proc 1992;13:139.

Allergic Diseases, 5th Edition,
edited by Roy Patterson, Leslie Carroll Grammer, and
Paul A. Greenberger. Lippincott–Raven Publishers, Philadelphia, © 1997.

26

Controversial and Unproven Methods in Allergy Diagnosis and Treatment

Abba I. Terr

A.I. Terr: Division of Immunology, Stanford University Medical Center, Stanford, CA 94305.

Pearls for Practitioners
Roy Patterson

- In any chronic medical condition where chronic management is necessary, there are always non-scientific approaches that may have psychological impact but no other benefit. They may be costly, possibly dangerous, and may delay or even prevent the application of useful therapies. When one such useless approach fades away, others arise to replace it. Will "health care reform" help?
- At times, it is difficult for a physician not to become angry about the use of grossly inappropriate treatment regimens with no benefit that drain funds from patients. Keep your cool and do your best to give appropriate guidance.
- Ingesting pollen is a nonscientific treatment can cause anaphylaxis in an allergic patient, and the therapeutic value is nonexistent
- Some board-certified allergists drift into the use of unproven techniques, perhaps because of the frustration of dealing with chronic, noncurable disease.

The state of the art in allergy diagnosis and treatment provides the practicing physician with the means for successfully managing most patients with allergic diseases. The immunologic and pathophysiologic mechanisms of these diseases, as revealed from many years of experimental and clinical research, form the foundation of scientifically based management. Although future research in allergy will refine and extend current diagnostic and therapeutic procedures and probably will offer dramatically new methods of treatment, there is little justification for an empirical approach to the allergic patient.

Nevertheless, unconventional and unproven procedures and theories are used by some practitioners as "alternatives" to a rational allergy practice based on scientific principles. Those who use these controversial methods often are unwilling to accept evidence contrary to their beliefs, and they often make exaggerated claims of efficacy, citing enthusiastic testimonies from their patients or clients.

Allergists encounter many patients who believe or have been told that they have allergies when they do not. A false diagnosis of "allergy" or "hypersensitivity" may be especially appealing to persons with functional or psychophysiologic illness.[1] Legitimate concern over the current state of environmental pollution has created a climate for unsupported claims of allergy to trace amounts of environmental chemicals in the atmosphere and foods. The changing pattern of financing medical care in the United States that encourages competition to reduce medical costs also encourages unscientific practices to "compete" with scientifically based medical care. Ironically, this increases cost while lowering overall quality.

This chapter describes some of the methods and theories of unproven value in allergy practice. The clinician who treats patients with allergy must be knowledgeable about both accepted and unproven techniques and theories to practice rationally and effectively.

DEFINITIONS

Certain terms have been used for different forms of medical practice:

• Standard practice
• Accepted practice
• Conventional (or unconventional methods
• Proven (or unproven) methods
• Controversial methods
• Experimental (investigational) procedures
• Alternative medicine
• Complementary medicine
• Fraud
• Quackery
• Standard of care

Standard practice is generally defined as the methods of diagnosis and treatment that are used by reputable physicians in a particular specialty (or primary care practice). Standard practice is not rigid. It involves a range of options, and procedures must be tailored to the individual patient. Physicians who are knowledgeable, trained, and experienced in allergy may prefer certain diagnostic and therapeutic methods while at the same time recognizing that other methods are acceptable.

Acceptable methods are those that are based on, or consistent with, the current knowledge of the immunologic and physiologic pathogenesis of allergic diseases. In addition, they have "stood the test of time," because a sufficient period of usage and evaluations by properly conducted, scientifically based clinical trials have revealed their efficacy and safety.

Experimental procedures refer to potentially new methods of practice arising from the results of scientific studies or from chance empirical observation. The term experimental should be reserved for those methods of diagnosis and treatment that are undergoing clinical trials on subjects who are informed of the experimental nature of the procedure, their potential risks, and their potential benefits. Subjects must give informed consent to participate in experimental trials.

Controversial methods refer to procedures that lack scientific credibility and have not been shown to have clinical efficacy. They are promoted and used by few physicians, not by the majority of practicing allergists. Most of the controversial methods discussed in this chapter have been evaluated in clinical trials and shown to be ineffective. In some cases, there are insufficient data to establish effectiveness. Some controversial procedures are being used for which no supporting data exist other than anecdotal testimonies.

The terms *alternative* or *complementary* often are used by those who practice controversial methods to distinguish their methods from those used by "traditional" or "classic" practitioners. These terms are not used here, because they obscure the real issue of whether a particular procedure has been validated for clinical use by proper scientific scrutiny.

The terms *fraud* and *quackery* generally equate to medical practices performed by individuals who knowingly, deliberately, and deceitfully use controversial methods for profit. Many physicians who use controversial procedures in allergy practice, however, do so because they sincerely believe that these practices are worthwhile and are unwilling to accept evidence to the contrary.

Standard of care is a term usually used in the course of litigation. The definition varies according to jurisdiction. In California, for example, it is defined for purpose of jury instruction as follows:

> In performing professional services for a patient, a physician has the duty to have that degree of learning and skill ordinarily possessed by reputable physicians practicing in the same or similar locality and under similar circumstances. The further duty of the physician is to use the care and skill ordinarily exercised in like cases by reputable members of the profession practicing in the same or similar locality under similar circumstances, and to use reasonable diligence and his or her best judgment in the exercise of skill and the application of learning, in an effort to accomplish the purpose for which the physician is employed. A failure to fulfill any such duty is negligence.

UNCONVENTIONAL DIAGNOSTIC METHODS

Experienced allergists recognize that a thorough history and physical examination are the critical elements in allergy diagnosis. Laboratory testing is used selectively to supplement the history and physical findings, especially where objective measurement of a functional abnormality such as airway obstruction is desired, or where other diseases must be ruled out of further consideration. "Allergy tests" such as skin prick or intradermal tests, patch tests, or in vitro antibody tests are tests for the presence of an immune response of a particular type (e.g., IgE antibody or cell-mediated immunity) to a specific allergen. These tests alone do not diagnose or predict an allergic disease, but they do assist the clinician in diagnosis when the results are correlated with the patient's history.

Inappropriate diagnostic tests fall into three categories:

1. Ineffective
2. Effective but misused
3. Effective but misinterpreted

Ineffective diagnostic tests are procedures that are of no possible diagnostic value under any circumstance. While giving the appearance of a "test," these procedures are not in accord with current knowledge of allergy pathophysiology, and there is no scientific evidence to support their use for any condition, allergy or otherwise. They produce responses indistinguishable from placebo responses in double-blind evaluation.

Effective but misused diagnostic tests are procedures that are intrinsically capable of a valid measurement, but are not appropriate for use in allergy diagnosis. They may have diagnostic and therapeutic value for certain other clinical conditions, but they have no value for the particular allergic disease for which they are being used.

Effective but misinterpreted diagnostic tests are procedures that are intrinsically capable of being used in allergy diagnosis but are not appropriate for general clinical use because of expense, low sensitivity or specificity, or lack of general availability. For example, the in vitro histamine release test has been widely used in allergy research where it has been invaluable in furthering knowledge of disease, but it cannot be recommended for clinical use. It may be modified to assume a place in allergy practice in the future.

"Diagnostic" Procedures of No Value Under Any Circumstance

The procedures included in this category are not based on sound scientific principles, and they have not been shown by proper controlled clinical trials to be capable of assisting in diagnosis for any condition.

The Cytotoxic Test

The cytotoxic test is also known as the leukocytotoxic test or Bryan's test.[2,3] It is performed by placing a drop of whole blood or buffy coat as an unstained mount on a microscope slide coated with a food extract. A drop of water sometimes is added to the blood cells. The technician observes the unstained cells to observe any change in shape or appearance of leukocytes. The subjective impression of swelling, vacuolation, crenation, or other changes in the morphologic features of leukocytes constitutes a "positive" test result, and this is considered evidence of allergy to the food. The procedure has not been standardized for time of incubation, pH, osmolarity, temperature, or other conditions. Therefore, it is unlikely that leukocyte morphologic features can be accurately assessed. The procedure is advertised as a test for allergy to foods or drugs.

There are no known allergic diseases caused by food-induced leukocyte cytotoxicity. Although some drugs do cause immunologically mediated cytotoxicity of leukocytes, no studies show that this phenomenon can be demonstrated in vitro using Bryan's test. Several controlled clinical trials have shown that the cytotoxic test is not reproducible, and it does not correlate with any clinical evidence of food allergy.[4,5]

Provocation–Neutralization

Provocation–neutralization is a procedure that is claimed by its proponents to diagnose allergy to foods, inhalant allergens, and environmental chemicals. It is also used to "diagnose" allergy to hormones and microorganisms, particularly *Candida albicans*.

The test is performed by administering to the patient a test dose of an extract of one of these substances by either intracutaneous injection, subcutaneous injection, or sublingual drop. The patient then records any subjective sensations appearing during the subsequent 10 minutes. Any such report by the patient constitutes a positive test result, which is considered as evidence for allergy to the substance. If the test result is negative, it is repeated with higher concentrations of the test substance until the patient reports any sensation or symptom. The patient is then given a lower concentration of the extract, and if fewer or no symptoms are reported, the reaction is said to be "neutralized."[6–13] The neutralization dose is then used by the patient as a form of therapy (see later). When the test is performed by intradermal injection, increasing wheal diameter with increasing dose is considered corroborative evidence of a positive test result. In provocation–neutralization, the test result is graded as positive even if the reported sensations are different from those in the history of the patient's illness.[14,15] Some proponents measure the pulse rate during the test, but there is disagreement about its significance. The substances most commonly tested in this way are food extracts; chemicals such as phenol, formaldehyde, and ethanol; inhalant allergen extracts; hormones; inflammatory mediators such as histamine and serotonin; and even saline or water.

Published reports of provocation–neutralization testing yield conflicting results.[16] These reports included patients with varying clinical manifestations, used different testing methods, and had variable criteria for a positive test result. Many lack placebo controls. These studies therefore reflect the lack of standardization and the subjective nature of provocation–neutralization.

Modern concepts of immunologic disease do not provide a rationale for the presumed provocation of subjective symptoms and their immediate neutralization under the conditions used in this procedure.[17] One well-designed, placebo-controlled double-blind evaluation of provocation–neutralization for the diagnosis of food allergy in 18 patients showed that symptoms were provoked with equal frequency by food extracts and by placebo,[18] showing that results are based on suggestion.[19] Furthermore, there is a potential danger of causing oral mucosal edema or even a systemic reaction[20] in any patient with a significant IgE sensitivity to the allergen being tested. The procedure can be extremely time-consuming, because only one concentration of a single allergen can be tested at one time.

An Environmental Control Unit in which patients are tested to airborne exposure to chemicals in testing booths has been described.[21] However, unlike bronchial provocation testing in asthma, a positive test result is based on self-reported symptoms only. There are no published reports of controlled studies of this method of testing.

Electrodermal Diagnosis

Electrodermal diagnosis purports to measure changes in skin resistance after the patient is exposed to an allergen.[22] The allergen extract, usually a food, is placed in a container that is then put on a metal plate inserted into an electrical circuit that includes the patient's skin and a galvanometer. A change in skin electrical resistance is said to be a positive test indicating allergy to the food.

This procedure has no rational physiologic basis, and no studies have supported its use. Proponents use acupuncture points on the skin when performing this bizarre procedure.

Applied Kinesiology

In applied kinesiology, the muscle strength of a limb is measured before and after the patient is exposed to a test allergen.[23] Exposure to the allergen, usually a food, is done by placing a vial of the allergen extract on the patient's skin, and the measurement of the muscle strength is estimated subjectively by a technician. A loss or weakening of muscle strength is considered a positive test result, supposedly indicating allergy to the test food.

No scientific rationale justifies the concept that allergy to a food or to any other allergen weakens skeletal muscle, and the belief that exposure to the allergen could occur through a vial in contact with the skin is clearly untenable.

Diagnostic Procedures Misused for Allergy "Diagnosis"

The procedures included in this category are ineffective for allergy diagnosis, although they may be useful for diagnosis of other conditions. They are considered under two categories: (1) nonimmunologic tests, and (2) immunologic tests.

Nonimmunologic Tests That Are Inappropriate for Allergy Diagnosis

Certain procedures are valid diagnostic tests, but not for allergy. Those discussed here are the pulse test and quantification of chemicals in body fluids and tissues. These tests have been promoted for allergy diagnosis based on erroneous concepts of the pathogenesis of allergy.

Pulse Test

Measuring change in pulse rate, either an increase or decrease, has been proposed as a method for diagnosing allergy when a test substance is ingested or injected.[24] A change in pulse rate occurs from a variety of normal physiologic conditions, and it occurs in the course of many diseases well known to physicians. There is no reason to believe that an increase or decrease in the heart rate by itself can be used to diagnose allergy.

Testing for Environmental Chemicals in the Body

A few physicians subscribe to the unsubstantiated belief that a wide range of synthetic chemicals at low dosage are toxic to the human immune system, resulting in "sensitivities" to numerous chemicals, foods, drugs, and other agents.[25,26] Samples of whole blood, erythrocytes, serum, urine, fat, and hair are analyzed for the presence of a variety of environmental chemicals. The list of chemicals commonly includes organic solvents, various hydrocarbons, and pesticides. Analytical methods and instrumentation are available for quantitating almost any chemical at levels as low as parts per billion, and in some cases parts per trillion. Indeed, many environmental chemicals can be detected at this low level in almost everyone because of the ubiquitous presence of these substances in the world. Under some circumstances, it may be appropriate to detect toxic quantities of a suspected chemical where poisoning is suspected, but the presence of such chemicals in the body, regardless of quantity, bears no relation to allergic disease. The concept of an immunotoxic cause of allergic sensitivity is unproven.

Immunologic Tests That Are Inappropriate in Allergy Diagnosis

The immunologic pathogenesis of allergy is firmly established. The mechanisms of allergy caused by IgE antibodies, immune complexes, and cell-mediated hypersensitivity are described elsewhere in this book, as are the clinical manifestations of immunologically mediated hypersensitivity and the appropriate immunologic tests for diagnosis. Unfortunately, some clinical laboratories promote the use of certain tests for allergy diagnosis, although they are not appropriate *for this purpose*. Notice that the tests discussed here may be technically correct, but they are irrelevant in the clinical evaluation of allergic disease. In some cases, the test results may be important in the diagnosis of other diseases; in other cases, the results reflect normal physiologic conditions.

Serum IgG Antibodies

IgG antibodies to atopic allergens such as foods or inhalants are not involved in the pathogenesis of atopy. Although some allergists have speculated that delayed adverse reactions to foods may be caused by circulating immune complexes containing IgG or IgE antibodies to foods,[27–29] this concept is still unproven. IgG antibodies and postprandial circulating immune complexes to foods are probably normal phenomena and not indicative of disease.[30] They are found in low concentrations in normal serum compared with the quantity of circulating antibodies and immune complexes required to evoke inflammation in serum sickness. Circulating IgG antibodies to the common inhalant allergens can be detected in the serum of patients receiving allergen immunotherapy (hyposensitization). Although these therapeutically induced specific antibodies are referred to as "blocking antibodies," their protective role in injection therapy of atopic respiratory disease is uncertain. Some information indicates that the level of IgG blocking antibody to Hymenoptera venom generated by desensitization of patients who had experienced anaphylaxis from the venom may correlate with clinical protection by the treatment. However, measurement of IgG antibodies or immune complexes has no proven diagnostic or prognostic value in the management of atopic patients. Detection of a specific IgG antibody to the clinically relevant antigen may be diagnostically useful in serum sickness and in allergic bronchopulmonary aspergillosis.

Total Serum Immunoglobulin Levels

Quantifying the total serum levels of IgG, IgA, IgM, and IgE can be accomplished easily and accurately in the clinical laboratory. Significant reductions of the serum levels of one or more immunoglobulin classes characterize the immunoglobulin deficiency diseases.[31] Polyclonal increases in these immunoglobulins are common in certain chronic infections and autoimmune diseases. Monoclonal hyperproduction occurs in multiple myeloma and Waldenström's macroglobulinemia. Alterations in the total serum level of IgG, IgA, or IgM is not a feature of allergic diseases, even in diseases involving IgG antibodies such as serum sickness. Conversely, serum IgE levels generally are higher in atopic patients than in nonatopic controls. Patients with allergic asthma have higher levels than do those with allergic rhinitis, and some patients with atopic dermatitis have high levels. The total serum IgE is not a useful "screen" for atopy, however, because numerous atopic patients have levels that fall within the range of nonatopic persons. Furthermore, the total level of any immunoglobulin gives no information about antibody specificity. Immunologic specificity is the cornerstone of allergy diagnosis. In allergic bronchopulmonary aspergillosis, the total serum IgE level has prognostic significance because it correlates with disease activity.[32]

Lymphocyte Subset Counts

Monoclonal antibody technology and flow cytometric study have made it possible to obtain accurate counts of each of the many lymphocyte subsets that are identified by specific cell surface markers, termed *clusters of differentiation* (CD). For example, the CD4 marker identifies lymphocytes with helper–inducer activity, and the CD8 marker identifies T cells that function in cytotoxicity or immune suppression. Quantifying lymphocytes with certain cell markers is useful in diagnosis of lymphocyte cellular immunodeficiencies and lymphocytic leukemias, but not in allergy. There is a wide normal range for many subsets of lymphocytes, and the circulating levels may fluctuate significantly in the healthy state.

Food Immune Complex Assay

Some commercial clinical laboratories offer tests that detect circulating immune complexes that are specific for food antigens and antibodies. They claim or imply that the test can be used for the diagnosis of allergy to foods. A certain amount of ingested food protein is normally absorbed intact through the gastrointestinal tract, permitting the formation of an immune response and low levels of circulating antibody to these food proteins.[30] Some allergists have proposed that a variety of allergic reactions are caused by the formation of immune complexes containing food antigens and IgE or IgG antibodies,[27–29] but more investigation is necessary to accept this concept. Food immune complexes are more likely to be a normal mechanism for clearing the food antigens from the circulation.[33]

The method for detection involves a two-site recognition system in which an antibody to the food is bound to a solid-phase absorbent.[33,34] This antibody, when incubated with the test serum, fixes the antigen–antibody complex, and the bound complex is detected and quantified by a labeled antiimmunoglobulin. The simplicity of the assay has allowed its modification for commercial application.

There is no proof that circulating food immune complexes cause any form of human disease. Patients with IgA deficiency may have high circulating concentrations of immune complexes to bovine albumin, but the pathophysiologic role of these complexes is unknown.[35,36] No support exists for the use of assays for food immune complexes in the diagnosis of allergic disease.

UNCONVENTIONAL TREATMENT METHODS

Effective management of the patient with allergic disease must be based on an accurate diagnosis. Once this is accomplished, the three principal forms of treatment are (1) allergen avoidance, (2) medications to reverse the symptoms and pathophysiologic abnormalities, and (3) allergen immunotherapy. The total management of the patient with allergy (or any other disease) must take into account the physical, emotional, and social conditions of the patient. Therefore, each program must be individualized. All forms of treatment—including allergen avoidance—are subject to undesired adverse effects, so monitoring the course of treatment should be part of the overall program.

This section covers specific forms of inappropriate allergy treatment that fall into two categories: (1) treatments that have not been shown to be effective for any disease, and (2) treatments that are not appropriate for allergy but may be effective in other conditions.

Treatment Methods of No Value

The modalities discussed here include some that are directed specifically toward allergy and others that are promoted for allergy and for other chronic conditions. All of these are without any proven therapeutic effect, although they may be widely used and in some cases may result in temporary symptomatic improvement or sense of well-being. The placebo effect may accompany any therapeutic maneuver, regardless of whether that maneuver has a disease-modifying result.

Neutralization

Neutralizing (also called symptom-relieving) therapy is an extension of the provocation–neutralization testing procedure.[6,37–39] The patient is supplied with a set of treatment extracts consisting of allergens, foods, or chemicals at a concentration deemed from the prior testing to neutralize symptoms. The patient injects or applies sublingually a certain small amount of these neutralizing extracts to either relieve symptoms or to prevent symptoms in anticipation of an environmental exposure. They are also recommended as a continuous maintenance program. There is no rational mechanism based on current immunologic theory that could account for immediate symptom neutralization of allergens. The published studies of this form of therapy are either anecdotal, or they indicate that a beneficial effect cannot be attributed to anything other than suggestion.[16] The treatment usually is prescribed for "chemical and food hypersensitivity," but it is also offered for true allergic diseases.

Acupuncture

The ancient Chinese method of acupuncture has been used over the centuries to treat virtually every disease, although modern medical science offers little theoretical support for its continued use. Nevertheless, acupuncture has become a significant alternative to medical therapy in the western world. It is used exclusively by some practitioners, and by others as an adjunct to medications, homeopathy, naturopathy, and psychotherapy. Numerous allergic patients in the United States are likely to have turned to acupuncture at some time for relief of asthma, allergic rhinitis, and allergic dermatoses. It is also used by patients who have other medical problems or symptoms that they consider to be allergic. Although some patients report temporary benefit, no reported studies have documented either symptomatic improvement or long-term benefit in allergic disease.

Homeopathic Remedies

Homeopathy is an alternative form of "healing" based on treating "like with like," that is, the causative agent of a disease presumably cures the disease when administered in exceedingly small amounts. Since this concept has a superficial resemblance to allergen immunotherapy or desensitization, it is not surprising that homeopathic practitioners offer their remedies in the treatment of allergy. Homeopathic remedies consist of extracts of several natural substances, including plants, animal products, and insects. These extracts are serially diluted through a process known as succussion, which is simply the vigorous shaking of a container of diluted extract. Homeopathists also prescribe "natural" hormones in the form of extracts of endocrine glands, including adrenal cortex, thyroid, thymus, pancreas, and spleen. These are taken orally. There is no evidence that homeopathic remedies have any therapeutic effect for any disease, including allergy.

Detoxification

A program purported to achieve detoxification is used as a method of allergy treatment by those who subscribe to the unfounded theory that an allergic state can be induced by toxic damage to the immune system from exposure to lipid-soluble environmental chemicals stored in body fat.[25,26]

The method consists of exercise and sauna. Exercise is done by running outdoors to increase circulation, followed by a sauna at a temperature of 60° to 82°C (140° to 180°F). Body fluids are replenished by drinking water, and oral sodium and potassium repletion is offered at the patient's discretion. The patient also takes supplements of vitamins, calcium, and magnesium. High-dose niacin therapy is used to induce erythema. A mixture of four "essential" oils (i.e., soy, walnut, peanut, and safflower) also is given, presumably to help deplete the adipose tissue of fat-soluble chemical contaminants. This procedure takes about 5 hours and is repeated daily for 20 to 30 days, although some patients continue this regimen much longer.

The theory of immunotoxicity as a cause of allergic disease is contrary to an extensive body of clinical experience. The concept that increased circulation, vasodilation, and oral ingestion of vegetable oils can mobilize "toxins" from fat into sweat is unproven. The potential dangers of this detoxification program have not been adequately studied.

Injection of Food Extracts

Elsewhere in this book are detailed descriptions of the technique and effectiveness of specific allergen immunotherapy using injections of inhalant allergens causing respiratory disease or Hymenoptera venom causing anaphylaxis. This form of therapy has been shown to be effective in these IgE-mediated diseases. Anaphylaxis and urticaria also can occur as a result of IgE antibodies to foods. Although the prevalence of IgE-mediated food allergy is considerably lower than that of inhalant allergy, some patients experience life-threatening anaphylactic reactions from ingestion of exceedingly minute amounts of the food allergen. Fatalities from food anaphylaxis have been reported most commonly in cases of peanut allergy. Peanut protein is found in a variety of food products, so that strict avoidance is difficult for even the most conscientious patient. Elimination or reduction of this dangerous form of sensitivity by allergen immunotherapy would be a desirable goal, but there have been no reports that injections of food extracts are effective and safe in IgE-mediated food allergy. Such treatment at this time should be considered investigational.

Nevertheless, some practitioners do prescribe food extract injections, often consisting of a combination of foods based on skin test results or the patient's report of intolerance to foods. This form of treatment must be considered unproven as to efficacy and potential danger until appropriate clinical trials have been carried out.

Urine Injection

The drinking of urine was an ancient healing practice. The modern medical literature contains a single paper published in 1947 on "urine therapy" in which intramuscular injections of the patient's own urine was recommended for a long list of symptoms and illnesses, including allergy.[40] Recently, some medical and alternative practitioners have revived this bizarre procedure, claiming that urine contains unspecified chemicals produced by the patient during an allergic reaction and that these chemicals inhibit or neutralize future allergic reactions when injected back into the same patient. No scientific evidence supports autogenous urine injections, nor are there clinical studies indicating that the treatment is effective.

The risk of injecting urine is potentially great. Soluble renal tubular and glomerular antigens are normally excreted in the urine. Repeated injections of these antigens could theoretically induce autoimmune nephritis.

Enzyme-Potentiated Desensitization

A recent unproven "modification" of allergen immunotherapy for patients with atopic allergy, called enzyme-potentiated desensitization, has appeared. It consists of a single preseasonal subcutaneous injection of pollen extract mixed with a minute quantity of the enzyme beta glucuronidase. It is offered as an alternative to the usual extended course of immunotherapy, which requires a program of graduated increasing doses of allergen and several years of monthly maintenance injections. Although a single low-dose injection of an allergen is certainly less likely than conventional immunotherapy to cause a systemic reaction, there is no evidence that enzyme-potentiated desensitization is efficacious in atopic disease.[41]

Inappropriate Treatment Methods

The forms of therapy discussed in this section have been recommended for treatment of allergic diseases. Each has a specific role in the management of certain diseases, but not for the treatment of allergy.

Vitamin, Mineral, and Nutrient Supplementation

A variety of "supplements" have been recommended for patients with allergies. In some cases, these supplements are promoted to relieve allergy symptoms, and in other cases they are promoted as a cure. A variety of unsubstantiated theories have arisen to rationalize their use.

Vitamins, minerals, and amino acids are among the more common items prescribed by practitioners of alternative medicine to treat patients with allergy or allergy-like symptoms. Deficiency of these substances as a cause of allergy is the usual explanation, although there is no scientific basis for such a statement. Neither have there been controlled clinical trials demonstrating a therapeutic effect. Fortunately, most patients taking such supplements suffer no harm, although excessive intake of fat-soluble vitamins could result in dangerous toxicity. Therapy with antioxidants—such as vitamin C and E and glutathione—is justified by assuming that allergic inflammation generates free radicals causing oxidative damage to tissues.[42] Although it is true that toxic oxygen metabolites are activated during the course of certain inflammatory reactions, the kinetics and localization of these events and the availability of endogenous antioxidants make it unlikely that ingesting these dietary supplements would be effective. Furthermore, no reported clinical trials document effectiveness in any allergic disease.

Diets

Avoidance is the only certain method for treating food allergy. Although any food has the potential for being allergenic, food allergy in adults is uncommon. The individual patient with food allergy usually has a sensitivity to one or at most a few foods. Food allergy is more common among allergic infants and small children. In all age groups, however, avoidance therapy only rarely requires the use of an extensive elimination diet, and adequate food substitutes usually are available.

Unfortunately, the unsubstantiated concept of multiple food allergies as a cause of vague subjective symptoms, behavioral problems, and emotional illness has resulted in the unnecessary restriction of many foods. The risk of nutritional deficiency is obvious, although in practice many patients abandon highly restrictive diets because of the lack of long-term benefit.

Proponents of the concept of multiple food allergies sometimes recommend a "rotary diversified diet," in which the patient rotates foods so that the same food is eaten only once every 4 to 5 days.[43] To do this, it is necessary to keep extensive and accurate records, causing further unnecessary and time-consuming preoccupation with diet and symptoms.[44]

Environmental Chemical Avoidance

The concept of "multiple food and chemical sensitivities" discussed later carries with it a recommendation for extensive avoidance of environmental "chemicals." Allergists recommend a reasonable program of allergen avoidance for patients with respiratory allergy. Simple measures to reduce exposure to house dust and dust mites through the elimination of bedroom carpeting and special casings for pillows and mattress are clinically effective and pose no undue hardship on the patient and family. Similar measures to reduce indoor air levels of mold spores and other allergens also can be done efficiently and cheaply. Reduction of occupational exposure to proven workplace allergens and irritants, such as animals, isocyanate fumes, acid anhydrides, wood dusts, and grain dusts, are mandatory for patients with documented occupational asthma or hypersensitivity pneumonitis caused by these agents.

In contrast, the recommendation to avoid any exposure, even minute amounts, of multiple chemicals[45,46] such as pesticides, organic solvents, vehicle exhaust fumes, gasoline fumes, household cleaners, glues and adhesives, and new carpets is a recommended "treatment" for a group of patients with multiple chronic vague symptoms who are diagnosed as having chemical sensitivity based on unproven diagnostic methods, primarily provocation–neutralization. This extensive form of chemical avoidance usually requires drastic lifestyle changes. Patients who accept this form of treatment often wear masks in public, live in stripped-down homes or trailers, and avoid synthetic clothing. Some of them move away to isolated communities.[14,15] Not only is there no proof that these drastic measures help these people, there is evidence for significant psychological harm.[47,48]

Antifungal Medications

The unsubstantiated theory of "*Candida* hypersensitivity syndrome" discussed later proposes the existence of allergic sensitivities brought on by a presumed immunotoxic effect of normal colonization of the gastrointestinal and genitourinary tracts by the yeast *C albicans*. Physicians who believe in this theory use a treatment program consisting of a special diet and antifungal medications. Nystatin usually is prescribed first in a powder form given orally in minute dosage followed by ketoconazole or diflucan if the desired effect is not achieved. Although these drugs are indicated in the treatment of cutaneous and systemic candidiasis, their use in the nebulous *Candida* hypersensitivity syndrome cannot be justified. One controlled clinical trial showed that nystatin did not differ from placebo in its effect on such patients.[49]

Immunologic Manipulation

Allergic diseases represent an inappropriate response by the immune system to environmental allergens. These diseases affect a minority of the population exposed to allergens. Most forms of allergy arise from complex interactions of genetic and environmental factors. Allergen avoidance prevents disease but does not eliminate the underlying immunologically induced hypersensitive state. In theory, it would be desirable to be able to manipulate the immune system therapeutically in such a way as to ablate the specific allergic sensitivity without inhibiting the other necessary functions of the immune system. Much of the current basic research on the immunology of allergy is directed toward such a goal. Allergen immunotherapy, discussed elsewhere in this book, approaches but does not achieve this ideal therapeutic aim, although it is clinically beneficial in most cases.

Immunologic manipulation through the use of immunosuppressive drugs, immunostimulating drugs, therapeutic monoclonal antibodies with specificity for certain components of the immune system, and immunoregulatory cytokines is under investigation in clinical trials in many other diseases, particularly in autoimmunity and cancer.

Therapeutic gamma globulin injections are standard treatment for documented IgG antibody deficiency, and they have been proven effective for this purpose. Gamma globulin injections also have been used empirically for other diseases, and there is evidence that they are effective in idiopathic thrombocytopenic purpura and in Kawasaki's disease. The mechanism of efficacy in these two diseases is unknown. Gamma globulin injections are being recommended by some practitioners for allergy, but until effectiveness is shown by proper double-blind studies, such treatment should be considered experimental.

CONTROVERSIAL THEORIES ABOUT ALLERGY

The clinical practice of allergy rests on a firm foundation of established immunologic and physiologic principles. These are discussed elsewhere in this book. Some unconventional methods of diagnosis and treatment are based on unconventional theories, others arose empirically and spawned a variety of unsubstantiated theories, and still others lack any theoretical basis. Some of the unconventional theories are discussed in this section.

Allergic Toxemia

Allergic diseases are characterized by focal inflammation in certain target organs, such as the bronchi in asthma, the nasal mucosa and conjunctivae in allergic rhinitis, the gastrointestinal mucosa in allergic gastroenteropathy, and the skin in atopic dermatitis, urticaria, and allergic contact dermatitis. Multiple target organs are involved in systemic anaphylaxis and in serum sickness. During the course of illness, the patient may experience systemic symptoms such as fatigue or other localized symptoms (i.e., headache) in parts of the body not directly involved in the allergic inflammation. These collateral symptoms sometimes are explainable pathophysiologically, for example, as secondary effects of hypoxemia and hyperventilation in asthma or from cranial and neck muscle tension because of excessive sneezing in rhinitis.

Furthermore, it is possible that locally released inflammatory mediators and cytokines may produce systemic effects, although direct proof is lacking.

For many years, certain allergists have proposed that a variety of systemic, often vague, complaints such as fatigue, drowsiness, weakness, body aching, nervousness, irritability, mental confusion or sluggishness, and poor memory *in the absence* of any clinical sign of allergic inflammation could be caused by exposure to environmental allergens. The allergens implicated in this concept most often are foods, but recently chemical additives in foods and drugs also have been implicated. This "syndrome" has been referred to as allergic toxemia,[49] allergic tension fatigue syndrome,[50] or cerebral allergy.[51] The literature on this subject is extensive but largely anecdotal. No definitive controlled studies have shown the existence of such a syndrome.[16] Although there are claims of dramatic improvement from the elimination of certain foods or chemicals, these claims are not supported by scientific evidence.

An extension of the allergic toxemia concept is the idea that allergy is the cause of certain psychiatric conditions. According to one theory, childhood attention-deficit/hyperactivity disorder (previously called hyperactivity and learning disability) is caused by food colors and preservatives.[52] This concept was quickly accepted by certain physicians and parents who recommended and used food additive-free diets for hyperactive children. Controlled studies, however, do not support this concept.[53] Several published studies claim that ingestion of certain foods, particularly wheat, causes or aggravates adult schizophrenia.[54,55] These studies are not definitive, however, and there has been no confirmatory research.

Multiple Chemical Sensitivities

In the last 40 years, a small number of physicians have evolved a system of practice based on the theory that a wide range of environmental chemicals cause a variety of physical and psychological illnesses and a host of nonspecific complaints in patients who often have no objective physical signs. Multiple food sensitivities also are implicated in many of these patients. The practice based on these ideas is known as clinical ecology.[46,56,57]

The first clinical ecology theory of disease postulated that these patients suffer from failure of the human species to adapt to synthetic chemicals.[58] Another theory proposes that symptoms represent an exhaustion of normal homeostasis caused by ingestion of foods and inhalation of chemicals. Still another concept implicates environmental substances as toxic to the human immune system, perhaps by interfering with the function of T lymphocytes in regulation of the immune response.[59] Clinical ecology practitioners invoke other unique concepts, such as a maximum total-body load of antigen, masked food hypersensitivity, and a spreading phenomenon. A recently proposed theory explains multiple vague symptoms on the basis of toxicity to the central nervous system by low-level exposure to environmental chemicals.[60]

This form of practice centers on a diagnosis of "environmental illness," which has also been called multiple chemical sensitivities, ecologic illness, chemical hypersensitivity syndrome, total allergy syndrome, and 20th century disease. The diagnosis is applied to patients having a wide range of clinical symptoms. In some cases, the diagnosis is used to describe patients with a single problem, such as asthma, migraine headaches, premenstrual syndrome, arthralgias, or recurrent abdominal pain,[14,15] although most often it is applied to patients with multiple long-standing symptoms rather than to those with a circumscribed physical illness. It is also used as a diagnosis for patients with bizarre conversion reactions, anxiety and depression, or psychosomatic illness. Some patients are asymptomatic.[14] No specific physical abnormality or laboratory abnormality is required for diagnosis.

Because of the lack of a characteristic history or pathognomonic physical sign or laboratory test, the diagnosis often is made on the strength of the provocation–neutralization procedure described earlier. Some clinical ecologists also employ measurement of serum immunoglobulins, complement components, blood level of lymphocyte subsets, and blood or tissue level of pesticides as a supplement to provocation–neutralization for diagnosis. It is not clear, however, how these test results indicate the presence of environmental illness. The few published reports show a variable and often conflicting set of abnormalities of dubious clinical significance, because these reports lack proper controls or evidence of reproducibility.[16]

The principal methods of treatment advocated by clinical ecologists are avoidance and neutralization therapy. Avoidance of foods believed to cause or aggravate illness is accomplished by a rotary diversified diet, which is based on the belief that multiple food sensitivities occur in this illness. Avoidance of all food additives, environmental synthetic chemicals, and even some natural chemicals usually is recommended, but the level of avoidance varies with the enthusiasm of the patient and physician. Most commonly, patients eliminate scented household products, synthetic fabrics and plastics, and pesticides. They generally try to limit exposure to air pollutants, gasoline fumes, and vehicle exhaust fumes. In the United States, several isolated communities have been established for patients deemed unsuitable for the urban environment.

Neutralization therapy is achieved by self-administered sublingual applications or subcutaneous injections of food and chemical extracts, as described earlier. None of these forms of treatment—either singly or in combination—has been evaluated in properly controlled studies to determine efficacy or potential adverse effects, although clinical ecologists and their patients claim that these methods are successful. Treatment also may include megadose vitamin therapy, mineral or amino acid supplements, and antioxidants on the premise that these treatments strengthen the immune system and enhance immune responses. Supportive experimental or clinical evidence has not been presented. Drug therapy generally is condemned as a form of chemical exposure, although oxygen, mineral salts, and antifungal drugs frequently are prescribed.

Candida Hypersensitivity Syndrome

Recently, environmental illness has been linked causally with the yeast *C albicans*, which is normally resident in the microflora of the gastrointestinal and female genitourinary mucous membranes. Many persons with no clinical evidence of *Candida* infection and no evidence of defective local or systemic immunity, pregnancy, diabetes mellitus, endocrine diseases, or medications known to cause opportunistic candidiasis are said to have an illness known as *Candida* hypersensitivity syndrome.[61,62] The syndrome is otherwise indistinguishable from environmental illness. Proponents of this concept believe that *C albicans* causes behavioral and emotional diseases and a variety of physical illnesses and symptomatic states. Individuals who have ever received antibiotics, corticosteroids, birth control pills, or have ever been pregnant, even in the remote past, are said to be susceptible to this syndrome. Diagnosis is made by history and not by diagnostic testing. The recommended treatment is avoidance of sugar, yeast, and mold in the diet, and the use of a rotary diversified diet. Nystatin, ketoconazole, caprylic acid, and vitamin and mineral supplements are recommended. This syndrome is reminiscent of the concept of "autointoxication" that was popular 100 years ago. In the opinion of some practitioners in that era, the bacterial component of the normal intestinal flora was considered to cause numerous physical and psychological disabilities.[63]

REMOTE PRACTICE OF ALLERGY

In allergy practice, the proper diagnosis and treatment for each patient is based on a thorough history and physical examination by a physician knowledgeable about allergic diseases. In many cases, testing for specific sensitivities by skin or in vitro tests and other laboratory tests and x-rays may be indicated to supplement the findings from the history and physical examination. The results of allergy skin tests and in vitro tests for IgE antibodies do not distinguish whether the patient currently has symptomatic disease or will in the future, and therefore test results alone provide potential sensitivities that cannot be used as the basis for recommending drug therapy or allergy immunotherapy without knowledge of the clinical findings.

Unfortunately, because skin and in vitro testing for IgE antibody sensitivities are relatively easy to perform, some practitioners do provide a diagnosis and recommend treatment based solely on these test results. This is known as the remote practice of allergy.[64] It is clearly unacceptable because allergic *disease* occurs through a complex interplay of constitutional, environmental, and allergic factors, all of which must be known to the treating physician to avoid unnecessary, inappropriate, and potentially dangerous treatment.

POSITION STATEMENTS

Many national and local medical societies have published position statements or papers dealing with certain facets of medical practice. Most of these position statements cover one of two areas of medical practice: (1) methods that are unproven, controversial, and unscientific, such as those described in this chapter; and (2) promising new methods that have undergone sufficient clinical trial to suggest that they may be ready for general use by the practicing community. Position statements usually are the response of the organization to inquiries by its members or by third parties responsible for payment of medical fees.

There are several such position statements on controversial allergy practices.[16,64-68] They provide a scholarly review of the controversy, documentation through citations of the medical literature, and a position that reflects the best scientific clinical interpretation of all of the existing information about the particular procedure in question. Although some members of the organization may disagree with the position, it generally does reflect the prevailing opinion of most members. Position statements obviously do not by themselves establish a standard of care in diagnosis or treatment of disease. They have informational value for the individual practitioner, however, in selecting the best care for their patients.

The Health Care Financing Administration has published an extensive review of cytotoxic testing and provocation–neutralization testing and treatment, concluding that these procedures are not effective. They are therefore excluded from reimbursement under the Medicare program.[69,70]

REFERENCES

1. Stewart DE, Raskin J. Psychiatric assessment of patients with "20th century disease" ("total allergy syndrome"). Can Med Assoc J 1985;133:1001.
2. Bryan WTK, Bryan M. The application of in vitro cytotoxic reactions to clinical diagnosis of food allergy. Laryngoscope 1960;70:810.
3. Bryan MP, Bryan WTK. Cytologic diagnosis of allergic disorders. Otolaryngol Clin North Am 1974;7:637.
4. Lieberman P, Crawford L, Kjelland J, et al. Controlled study of the cytotoxic food test. JAMA 1974;231:728.
5. Lehman CW. The leukocytic food allergy test: a study of its reliability and reproducibility. Effect of diet and sublingual food drops on this test. Ann Allergy 1980;45:150.

6. Lee CH, Williams RI, Binkley EL. Provocative inhalant testing and treatment. Arch Otolaryngol 1969;90:81.
7. Lehman CW. A double-blind study of sublingual provocative food testing: a study of its efficacy. Ann Allergy 1980;45:144.
8. Draper LW. Food testing in allergy: intradermal provocative vs. deliberate feeding. Arch Otolaryngol 1972;95:169.
9. Crawford LV, Lieberman P, Harfi HA, et al. A double-blind study of subcutaneous food testing sponsored by the Food Committee of the American Academy of Allergy. J Allergy Clin Immunol 1976;57:236. Abstract.
10. King DS. Can allergic exposure provoke psychological symptoms? A double-blind test. Biol Psychiatry 1981;16:3.
11. Willoughby JW. Provocative food test technique. Ann Allergy 1965;23:543.
12. Rinkel RH, Lee CH, Brown DW, et al. The diagnosis of food allergy. Arch Otolaryngol 1964;79:71.
13. Lee CH, William RI, Binkley EL. Provocative inhalation testing and treatment. Arch Otolaryngol 1969;90:173.
14. Terr AI. Environmental illness: clinical review of 50 cases. Arch Intern Med 1986;146:145.
15. Terr AI. Clinical ecology in the workplace. J Occup Med 1989;31:257.
16. American College of Physicians. Clinical ecology. Ann Intern Med 1989;111:168. Position paper.
17. Terr AI. "Multiple chemical hypersensitivities": immunologic critique of clinical ecology theories and practice. Occup Med 1987;2:683.
18. Jewett DL, Fein G, Greenberg MH. A double-blind study of symptom provocation to determine food sensitivity. N Engl J Med 1990;323:429.
19. Ferguson A. Food sensitivity or self-deception? N Engl J Med 1990;323:476.
20. Green M. Sublingual provocative testing for food and FD and C dyes. Ann Allergy 1974;33:274.
21. Rea WJ, Peters DW, Smiley RE, et al. Recurrent environmentally triggered thrombophlebitis: a five-year follow-up. Ann Allergy 1977;38:245.
22. Tsuei JJ, Lehman CW, Lam FMK, et al. A food allergy study utilizing the EAV acupuncture technique. Am J Acupuncture 1984;12:105.
23. Garrow JS. Kinesiology and food allergy. Lancet 1988;296:1573.
24. Coca A. The pulse test. New York: Carol Publishing, 1982.
25. Laseter JL, DeLeon IR, Rea WJ, et al. Chlorinated hydrocarbon pesticides in environmentally sensitive patients. Clin Ecol 1983;2:3
26. Rousseaux CG. Immunologic responses that may follow exposure to chemicals. Clin Ecol 1987;5:33.
27. Paganelli R, Levinsky RJ, Brostoff J, et al. Immune complexes containing food proteins in normal and atopic subjects after oral challenge and effect of sodium cromoglycate on antigen absorption. Lancet 1979;i:1270.
28. Delire M, Cambiaso CL, Masson PL. Circulating immune complexes in infants fed on cow's milk. Nature 1979;272:632.
29. Paganelli R, Atherton DJ, Levinsky R. The differences between normal and milk allergic subjects in their immune response after milk ingestion. Arch Dis Child 1983;58:201.
30. Husby S, Oxelius V-A, Teisner B, et al. Humoral immunity to dietary antigens in healthy adults: occurrence, isotype and IgG subclass distribution of serum antibodies to protein antigens. Int Arch Allergy Appl Immunol 1985;77:416.
31. Ammann A. Antibody (B cell) immunodeficiency disorders. In: Stites DP, Terr AI, Parslow TG, eds. Basic and clinical immunology. 8th ed. Norwalk, CT: Appleton & Lange, 1994:766.
32. Greenberger PA, Patterson R. Allergic bronchopulmonary aspergillosis and the evaluation of the patient with asthma. J Allergy Clin Immunol 1988;81:646.
33. Haddad ZH, Vetter M, Friedman J, et al. Detection and kinetics of antigen-specific IgE and IgG immune complexes in food allergy. Ann Allergy 1983;51:255.
34. Leary HL, Halsey JF. An assay to measure antigen-specific immune complexes in food allergy patients. J Allergy Clin Immunol 1984;74:190.
35. Cunningham-Rundels C, Brandeis WE, Good RA, et al. Milk precipitins, circulating immune complexes and IgA deficiency. Proc Natl Acad Sci USA 1978;75:3387.
36. Cunningham-Rundels C, Brandeis WE, Good RA, et al. Bovine proteins and the formation of circulating immune complexes in selective IgA deficiency. J Clin Invest 1979;64:272.
37. Morris DL. Use of sublingual antigen in diagnosis and treatment of food allergy. Ann Allergy 1969;27:289.
38. Rea WJ, Podell RN, Williams ML, et al. Intracutaneous neutralization of food sensitivity: a double-blind evaluation. Arch Otolaryngol 1984;110:248.
39. Kailin EW, Collier R. "Relieving" therapy for antigen exposure. JAMA 1971;217:78. Letter.
40. Plesch J. Urine therapy. Med Press 1947;218:128.
41. Fell P, Brostoff J. A single dose desensitization for summer hay fever: results of a double-blind study—1988. Eur J Clin Pharmacol 1990;38:77.
42. Levine SA, Reinhardt JH. Biochemical-pathology initiated by free radicals, oxidant chemicals, and therapeutic drugs in the etiology of chemical hypersensitivity disease. J Orthomol Psychiatry 1983;12:166.
43. Rinkel HJ. Food allergy: function and clinical application of the rotary diversified diet. J Pediatr 1948;32:266.
44. Terr AI. Clinical ecology. J Allergy Clin Immunol 1987;79:423. Editorial.
45. Rea WJ, Bell IR, Suits CW, et al. Food and chemical susceptibility after environmental chemical overexposure: case histories. Ann Allergy 1978;41:101.
46. Dickey LD. Clinical ecology. Springfield, IL: Charles C Thomas, 1976.

47. Randolph TG. Human ecology and susceptibility to the chemical environment. Springfield, IL: Charles C Thomas, 1962.
48. Brodsky CM. "Allergic to everything": a medical subculture. Psychosomatics 1983;24:731.
49. Dismukes WE, Wade JS, Lee JY, et al. A randomized double-blind trial of nystatin therapy for the candidiasis hypersensitivity syndrome. N Engl J Med 1990;323:1717.
50. Speer F. The allergic tension–fatigue syndrome. Pediatr Clin North Am 1954;1:1029.
51. Miller JB. Food allergy: provocative testing and injection therapy. Springfield, IL: Charles C Thomas, 1972.
52. Feingold B. Why your child is hyperactive. New York: Random House, 1975.
53. Defined diets and childhood hyperactivity. JAMA 1982;248:290. Consensus conference.
54. Dohan FC, Grasberger JC. Relapsed schizophrenics: earlier discharge from the hospital after cereal-free, milk-free diet. Am J Psychiatry 1973;130:685.
55. Singh MM, Kay SR. Wheat gluten as a pathogenic factor in schizophrenia. Science 1976;191:401.
56. Bell IR. Clinical ecology: a new medical approach to environmental illness. Bolinas, CA: Common Knowledge Press, 1982.
57. Randolph TG, Moss RW. An alternative approach to allergies. New York: Lippincott & Cromwell, 1980.
58. Randolph TG. Sensitivity to petroleum including its derivatives and antecedents. J Lab Clin Med 1952;40:931. Abstract.
59. Levin AS, Byer VS. Environmental illness: a disorder of immune regulation. Occup Med 1987;2:669.
60. Ashford NA, Miller CS. Chemical exposures. New York: Van Nostrand Reinhold, 1991.
61. Truss CO. Tissue injury induced by *Candida albicans*: mental and neurologic manifestations. J Orthomol Psychiatry 1978;7:17.
62. Truss CO. The role of *Candida albicans* in human illness. J Orthomol Psychiatry 1981;10:228.
63. Bassler A. Intestinal toxemia (autointoxication) biologically considered. Philadelphia: FA Davis, 1930.
64. American Academy of Allergy and Immunology. The remote practice of allergy. J Allergy Clin Immunol 1986;77:651. Position statement.
65. American Academy of Allergy and Immunology. Clinical ecology. J Allergy Clin Immunol 1986;78:269. Position statements.
66. American Academy of Allergy and Immunology. Candidiasis hypersensitivity syndrome. J Allergy Clin Immunol 1986;78:271. Position statements.
67. California Medical Association Scientific Board Task Force on Clinical Ecology. Clinical ecology: a critical appraisal. West J Med 1986;144:239.
68. Allergy: conventional and alternative concepts. London: Royal College of Physicians of London, 1992.
69. Health Care Financing Administration. Medicare programs: exclusion from Medicare coverage of certain food allergy tests and treatments. Fed Reg 1983;48:37,716.
70. Health Care Financing Administration. Medicare programs: exclusion of certain food allergy tests and treatments from Medicare coverage. Fed Reg 1990;55:35,466.

Allergic Diseases, 5th Edition,
edited by Roy Patterson, Leslie Carroll Grammer, and
Paul A. Greenberger. Lippincott–Raven Publishers, Philadelphia, © 1997.

27

Allergic Disorders and Pregnancy

Paul A. Greenberger

*P.A. Greenberger: Division of Allergy-Immunology,
Northwestern University Medical School, Chicago, IL 60611-3008.*

Pearls for Practitioners
Roy Patterson

- Every allergic patient can be managed comfortably during pregnancy with medications proven safe for use during pregnancy. The physician managing the pregnancy may have to be educated regarding this.
- Corticosteroids, inhaled or used by inhalation with oral prednisone on alternate days, can successfully and safely control asthma in every pregnant patient.
- Rhinitis of pregnancy is uncommon and can be severe, but is manageable so that the patient is comfortable during pregnancy.
- Allergen immunotherapy can safely be continued during pregnancy.
- Inadequate prenatal care may have an unfortunate outcome for child, mother, or both. This is even more unfortunate for the pregnant patient with asthma.

Many of the major conditions the allergist-immunologist treats can occur in the context of gestation or in anticipation of pregnancy. Specific conditions include asthma, urticaria, angioedema, anaphylaxis, rhinitis, sinusitis, and nasal polyposis. Goals of managing gravidas should include effective control of underlying allergic-immunologic conditions, proper avoidance measures, limitation on medications to those considered appropriate for use during gestation, planning for possible allergic emergencies such as status asthmaticus or anaphylaxis, and communication between the physician managing the allergic-immunologic conditions and the physician managing the pregnancy.

ASTHMA

Asthma occurs in 1% to 4% of pregnancies.[1,2] In some cases, asthma has its onset during gestation and may be severe in that status asthmaticus occurs or wheezing dyspnea results in interrupted sleep, persistent coughing, and hypoxemia. The effects of ineffectively managed asthma on the gravida can be devastating: maternal deaths may occur with repeated episodes of severe asthma.[3] Other untoward effects from asthma include fetal loss (stillbirths or abortions), increased rate of preterm deliveries (less than 37 weeks' gestation), intrauterine growth retardation (less than 2400 g), and gestational hypertension.[4–11] Fortunately, not all studies report all of these complications. Repeated episodes of status asthmaticus during gestation have resulted in hypoxemic effects on the fetus. Termination of a pregnancy has been deemed necessary because of life-threatening status asthmaticus.[12] Conversely, with cooperation between the gravida and physician managing asthma and effective asthma management, there can be successful pregnancy outcomes.[6–10,13] Prevention of status asthmaticus has been associated with pregnancy outcomes approaching that of the general population.[6–10,13–16] Use of inhaled beclomethasone dipropionate[6,7,9] has been effective in addition to prednisone[6–9] to manage even the most severe cases of asthma.

PHYSIOLOGIC CHANGES DURING GESTATION

Pulmonary

Tidal volume increases during gestation, whereas the frequency of respiration is unchanged.[2,17] This combination produces a 19% to 50% increase in minute ventilation.[18,19] Oxygen consumption increases 20% to 32%. The increase in minute ventilation produces a respiratory alkalosis attributable to increases in progesterone. These changes occur before significant uterine enlargement takes place. Arterial blood gas concentrations reflect a compensated respiratory alkalosis, with pH ranging from 7.40 to 7.47 and partial pressure of carbon dioxide (PCO_2) ranging from 25 to 32 mm Hg.[20] The maternal partial pressure of oxygen (PO_2) has been reported to be from 91 to 106 mm Hg.[20] The near-term alveolar–arterial oxygen gradient is 14 mm Hg in the sitting position compared with 20 mm Hg in the supine position. An explanation for the larger alveolar–arterial oxygen gradient in the supine position is decreased cardiac output because compression of the inferior vena cava by the uterus reduces venous return.

Total lung capacity is unchanged or reduced by 4% to 6%, and vital capacity is preserved in the absence of exacerbations of asthma. The gravida breathes at reduced lung volumes because residual volume and functional residual capacity are reduced. The diaphragm moves cephalad.[17] As with the development of maternal hyperventilation, the residual volume and functional residual capacity decline before significant uterine enlargement occurs. The diaphragm flattens during gestation, and there is less negative intrathoracic pressure reported in some studies. It seems that early airway closure would occur if there were less negative intrathoracic pressure, but such a finding has not been demonstrated, at least in nonasthmatic gravidas. In that during acute asthma episodes, the patient with asthma generates large negative intrathoracic pressures to apply radial bronchodilating traction, any decline in ability to develop more negative inspiratory pressures would predispose gravidas with asthma to more sudden deteriorations.

Bronchial responsiveness to methacholine does not change to a large degree, although a statistically significant change has been reported with PC_{20} increasing from 0.35 to 0.72 mg/mL from preconception to postpartum.[21] In this study of gravidas with mild asthma, the forced expiratory volume in 1 second (FEV_1) improved by 150 mL, and FEV_1 increased from 82% to 87%.[21] The increase in serum progesterone concentration during gestation did not correlate with improvement in bronchial responsiveness.[22] This observation suggests that factors other than progesterone contribute to changes in bronchial responsiveness, although progesterone relaxes smooth muscles of the uterus and gastrointestinal tract.

Other Physiologic Changes

Cardiac output increases by 30% to 60%, because of an increase in heart rate, yet stroke volume increases little.[23] The fall in systemic vascular resistance is accompanied by a rise of the heart rate from 10 to 20 beats per minute. Uterine blood flow increases tenfold from 50 to 500 mL/minute at term.[20] The blood volume increases an average of 1600 mL, and gravidas appear vasodilated as total-body water expands by 1 to 5 L.[20,23,24] Gravidas are sensitive to overzealous fluid administration. Although correcting any dehydration is indicated, injudicious fluid replacement has resulted in acute pulmonary edema with normal cardiac function. During the latter half of gestation, these changes become manifest because the gravida has increased preload (mild volume overload), increased chronotropy, and reduced afterload.[23]

The maternal hemoglobulin concentration decreases, although during gestation there is a 20% to 40% increase in erythrocyte mass.[23] Such an increase is offset by the even larger increase of plasma volume, resulting in relative anemia.

FETAL OXYGENATION

The vascular resistance of uterine vessels (progesterone effect) declines so that there can be the large increase in uterine blood flow.[20] The fetus survives in a low-oxygen environment with little reserve oxygen stores, should the supply of oxygen-rich uterine blood be compromised. Animal and human studies demonstrate reduced fetal oxygenation if there is reduced uterine blood flow such as occurs with severe maternal hypotension, hypocarbia, or shock.[20] Maternal hyperventilation can reduce venous return and also shift the maternal oxyhemoglobin dissociation curve to the left. Modest declines in maternal oxygenation seem to be tolerated by the fetus, but substantial degrees of maternal hypoxemia can threaten fetal survival. Uterine vessels during gestation are dilated maximally based on experimental data primarily from pregnant sheep and some human studies. Uterine vessels do not undergo vasodilation after β-adrenergic agonist stimulation, but do undergo vasoconstriction from α-adrenergic agonists. Some obstetric anesthesiologists administer intravenous ephedrine, 25 to 50 mg, for hypotension during epidural anesthesia. The β-adrenergic effects of ephedrine result in increased cardiac output, which raises systolic pressure and maintains uterine perfusion. Subcutaneous epinephrine provides primarily β-adrenergic stimulation, whereas intravenous epinephrine results in both α- and β-adrenergic effects.

The fetal hemoglobin is 16.5 g/L and the P_{50}, or oxygen pressure at which hemoglobin is 50% saturated, is 22 mm Hg in the fetus, in contrast to 26 to 28 mm Hg in the gravida.[20] Fetal umbilical venous PO_2 measurements at term average about 32 mm Hg, with a PCO_2 of 49 mm Hg. When the gravida inspires 100% oxygen in the absence of acute asthma, fetal umbilical venous PO_2 increases to 40 mm Hg and PCO_2 to 48 mm Hg.[25] For the fetus in distress, such changes can be important, but clearly the uteroplacental circulation is a large shunt. The leftward shift of the fetal hemoglobin oxygen dissociation curve results in larger increases in fetal PO_2 than in maternal blood for incremental rises in arterial PO_2.

EFFECTS OF PREGNANCY ON ASTHMA

For the individual gravida, it is not possible to predict the effects of pregnancy on asthma. Studies in the literature report varying degrees of improvement, deterioration, or no change in clinical course. In one review of nine studies involving 1059 pregnancies, 49% of gravidas were unchanged in terms of severity of asthma, 29% improved, and 22% worsened.[26] A prospective study of 198 pregnancies recorded similar results in that 40% of gravidas had no change in antiasthma medications, 42% required more medications, and 18% of gravidas requires less medications.[10] Similarly, using medication and symptom diary cards, during 366 gestations in 330 gravidas with mild or moderate asthma, asthma was unchanged in 33%, improved in 28%, and worsened in 35%.[15]

Adolescence with pregnancy in gravidas with asthma has been associated with many emergency room visits and hospitalizations for asthma.[27] Accurate serial data were not available to compare preconception and gestational asthma events. Adolescents with severe asthma may not benefit from antiinflammatory medications such as inhaled beclomethasone dipropionate because of their poor compliance with physician advice and medications.

PREGNANCY OUTCOMES IN THE GENERAL POPULATION

The mean birth weight from 1983 data from the National Center for Health Statistics was 3370 g.[7] The incidence rate of miscarriage was 11.8% to 13.8% in a study of women medical residents and wives of male residents.[28] Preterm deliveries (less than 37 weeks' gestation) occurred in 6.0% to 6.5% of study gravidas compared with 9.6% in the general population.[7] Intrauterine growth retardation (birth weight less than 2500 g) occurred in 6.8% of gestations[7] in the general population and in 5.3% to 5.8% of women residents or wives of male residents.[28] The incidence rate of gravidas requiring cesarean deliveries was about 20%.

CHOICE OF THERAPY

Avoidance Measures

As in management of the nonpregnant patient with asthma, general avoidance measures and those specific to the individual are indicated. General avoidance measures include smoking cessation; minimal or no alcoholic beverages; cessation of illicit drug use; and avoidance of tetracyclines (discoloration of infant's teeth), sulfonamides (G6PD deficiency could cause hemolytic anemia), troleandomycin, and newer antibiotics like clarithromycin and azithromycin until safety data become available. Methotrexate is contraindicated. Individual avoidance measures relate to animals, birds, dust mites, and fungi, which may cause IgE-mediated asthma. Aspirin and nonsteroidal antiinflammatory drugs should be withheld in the aspirin-intolerant gravida. Concomitant rhinitis, sinusitis, or nasal polyps should be treated.

Medications

It is preferable to recommend antiasthma medications for which established data from human pregnancies are available. Further, inhaled drugs are favored since the potential drug dosage that would cross the placenta is reduced. Organogenesis in human pregnancies is relatively short (days 12 to 56) compared with animals. The time for fetal growth and development is much longer in humans whereas it is shorter in animals. Drugs are infrequent causes of major congenital malformations.[29] Congenital malformations occur in about 2% to 6.5% of pregnancies. Although a few congenital malformations—up to 5%—are attributable to environmental factors like drug effects, maternal infections, and radiation, 65% to 70% of malformations result from unknown factors. About 25% of major malformations are genetically related, and 3% are caused by recognized chromosomal abnormalities.

Examples of teratogenic agents include ethanol, isotretinoin, phenytoin, carbamazepine, valproic acid, diethylstilbestrol (vaginal carcinoma), thalidomide, inorganic iodides, lithium carbonate, tetracycline, streptomycin, and some antineoplastic drugs that have not caused abortions earlier. Most antiasthma medications are considered appropriate for use in pregnancy. The FDA classification system for drug administration during gestation must be considered in the context of drug advertising by manufacturers and is not an absolute prohibition on prescription of a drug during gestation with the exception of a class X agent.

Human data from use of most antiasthma medications are available and have not identified increased teratogenic risks for oral corticosteroids such as prednisone or methylprednisolone, or the intravenous preparations hydrocortisone or methylprednisolone.[2,6–9,27] Experience with inhaled beclomethasone dipropionate has not identified fetal abnormalities in 71 pregnancies where therapeutic dosages were used at conception or during the first trimester.[6,7,9,27] These corticosteroids are considered appropriate during gestation. Published experience from Northwestern University (Chicago) with prednisone, beclomethasone dipropionate, or both totals over 250 pregnancies without an increased risk of teratogenesis.

Another antiinflammatory drug, cromolyn, has not been associated with an increased risk of congenital malformations in a series of 296 cases[30] as well as during use in the United States since 1973.[2] Nedocromil, which blocks early and late allergic-induced bronchial reactions and has antieosinophil activity, has meager first trimester reported experience. However, animal studies are negative for teratogenicity.

Theophylline is considered appropriate for use during gestation, should it be required.[13,20] The hepatic elimination clearance of theophylline has been shown to decrease in the third trimester by approximately 4% to 6%.[31] Protein binding decreases in the second and third trimesters, so more free theophylline is available for elimination. Further, increased glomerular filtration rate increases renal clearance of theophylline during gestation. These changes offset reduced hepatic clearance.[31] The last trimester may be associated with 10% increases in the theophylline serum concentrations. Aiming for maximal theophylline serum concentrations of 8 to 15 μg/mL should reduce the likelihood of accumulations of theophylline during pregnancy. However, theophylline is not essential with the use of 8 to 20 daily inhalations of beclomethasone dipropionate.

Controversy remains regarding which β-adrenergic agonist to administer during gestation. Drugs considered appropriate for human use include epinephrine, terbutaline, and ephedrine.[32] The latter is rarely indicated. Other drugs such as albuterol may be appropriate, but published human data are limited. Albuterol, pirbuterol, and metaproterenol were listed as appropriate by the National Institutes of Health Working Group on asthma and pregnancy.[2] Overuse must be avoided. The inhaled route should minimize drug delivered to the placenta.

Specific drugs to avoid include troleandomycin, methotrexate, triamcinolone, inorganic iodides, and ciprofloxacin. Influenza immunization is advisable for gravidas with long-term asthma. It is administered during the second or third trimester.

Allergen Immunotherapy

Allergen immunotherapy can be continued or initiated during pregnancy. The only recognized risk from this modality is the well-recognized risk of anaphylaxis.[31] No data suggest that gravidas are more likely to experience anaphylaxis from allergen immunotherapy. Data from the 121 pregnancies in 90 gravidas receiving allergen immunotherapy showed a low incidence of anaphylaxis.[33] Immunotherapy should be administered with the usual precautions to avoid anaphylaxis, or it should be withheld until postpartum. Anaphylaxis during gestation can cause abortions (as in beekeepers' wives[34] who are stung), shock,[35] or perinatal death.[35] Allergen immunotherapy does not protect the fetus from subsequent development of atopic disorders.[33,36]

ACUTE ASTHMA

As in managing the nonpregnant patient with asthma, acute asthma should be reversed as quickly and effectively as possible. Status asthmaticus has been associated with intrauterine growth retardation,[6,7] stillbirths, maternal deaths, and additional untoward effects on the fetus such as cerebral palsy. The goal in treating acute asthma is to minimize maternal hypoxemia, hypocarbia, or respiratory acidosis and to maintain adequate oxygenation for the fetus.

Beta-adrenergic agonists remain the drugs of choice for acute asthma. I prefer subcutaneous epinephrine for moderate or severe bronchospasm.[20] The dose may be given every 20 minutes if needed in the first hour. Alternatively, subcutaneous terbutaline can be administered and repeated in 30 minutes.[32] There are no reports of teratogenic effects from terbutaline. Terbutaline may be administered by metered dose inhaler also. The justification for using epinephrine is as follows: (1) it is synthesized endogenously, (2) it is not teratogenic when given in recommended doses subcutaneously, (3) it is metabolized rapidly, (4) it is readily available, and (5) variables associated with drug delivery by inhalation do not have to be considered. When epinephrine is administered by the subcutaneous route, its effects are primarily β-adrenergic stimulation. There is a fear that epinephrine causes fetal loss by decreasing uterine blood flow. The use of subcutaneous epinephrine increases cardiac output, which can maintain uterine perfusion. The adverse effects of acute asthma can be a real threat to the gravida and fetus; therefore, effective control of acute asthma is necessary.

Inhaled β-adrenergic therapy, primarily with metaproterenol or albuterol, has not been associated with adverse effects and is considered acceptable therapy by some investigators.[2,37]

When the gravida presents with moderate or severe acute wheezing dyspnea, oral corticosteroids should be administered with initial β-adrenergic agonists. For example, prednisone, 40 to 60 mg orally, is an appropriate dose. Corticosteroids have several beneficial effects in acute asthma, although an effect in the first 6 hours may not be detectable.[38]

When the gravida has not improved substantially after epinephrine or terbutaline administration (two doses) or nebulized albuterol, theophylline can be administered with admonitions (see Chap. 22). The use of theophylline in the nonpregnant patient with asthma is controversial because some studies have not documented benefit when theophylline is added to β-adrenergic agonists in treating acute asthma.[39–41] For the severely dyspneic gravida, theophylline may be administered as adjunctive therapy to β-adrenergic agonists and corticosteroids, but this is controversial.

When assessing a gravida in the emergency room, if hospitalization is required for status asthmaticus, an arterial blood gas measurement is indicated, as is supplemental oxygen administration. The physician managing the pregnancy should assess the gravida from the obstetric perspective. Some gravidas require fetal heart monitoring, for example, before discharge.

Excessive fluid replacement is not indicated, but volume depletion should be corrected. The gravida can develop acute pulmonary edema (noncardiac) from excessive crystalloid administration because of the volume expansion that occurs during gestation.

If the gravida can be discharged from the emergency room, a short course of oral corticosteroids should be given to prevent continued asthma symptoms and signs.[42] Planning an outpatient follow-up visit in 1 week is advised.

In the rare setting of acute respiratory failure during status asthmaticus, an emergency cesarean delivery may be necessary.[12] If mechanical ventilation[43] is indicated, the physician managing the asthma and the obstetrician must plan for when a cesarean delivery might be indicated.

CHRONIC ASTHMA

The following lists some types of chronic asthma that occur during gestation:

- Allergic
- Nonallergic
- Mixed
- Potentially fatal asthma
- Malignant potentially fatal asthma
- Adolescent asthma
- Asthma and allergic bronchopulmonary aspergillosis
- Aspirin intolerant asthma

Should gravidas require daily medication, an allergy-immunology consultation is indicated to identify IgE-mediated triggers of asthma, to determine if allergic bronchopulmonary aspergillosis is present, and to provide expertise in diagnosis and treatment of nasal polyps, rhinitis, or sinusitis. Avoidance measures are indicated to reduce bronchial hyperresponsiveness and the need for antiasthma medications.

The goals of chronic management include maintaining a functional respiratory status and minimizing wheezing dyspnea, nocturnal asthma, exercise intolerance, emergency room visits, and status asthmaticus.

Dyspnea can be sensed during gestation in the absence of asthma during the first two trimesters.[44] A respiratory rate greater than 18/minute has been considered a warning sign for pulmonary disease complicating "dyspnea during pregnancy."[44]

Many gravidas can be managed effectively with inhaled beclomethasone dipropionate[7,9] and inhaled epinephrine or terbutaline for symptomatic relief.[6,9,32] For severe asthma, beclomethasone dipropionate can be inhaled up to 20 times daily (840 μg). Proper inhalation technique is necessary and should be assessed periodically. Should asthma be managed ineffectively with avoidance measures and this combination of medications, using cromolyn or theophylline can be considered. If the gravida has wheezing on examination or nocturnal asthma, however, a short course of prednisone may be indicated to relieve symptoms.[20] If the gravida has improved after 1 week of prednisone, either the prednisone can be discontinued or it can be converted to an alternate-day regimen and tapered.[6,7,9,32] The most effective antiasthma medications for chronic administration during gestation in order of efficacy (highest to lowest) are prednisone, inhaled beclomethasone dipropionate, inhaled β-adrenergic agonists (epinephrine or terbutaline), theophylline, or cromolyn.

For noncorticosteroid-requiring asthma, inhaled beclomethasone dipropionate, cromolyn, or possibly theophylline are appropriate during gestation. If these drugs are ineffective because of worsening asthma such as from an upper respiratory infection, a short course of prednisone such as 40 mg daily for 5 to 7 days may be administered. Antibiotics can be prescribed for purulent rhinitis, bronchitis, or sinusitis. Erythromycin, ampicillin, amoxicillin, or cefaclor are appropriate initial antibiotics. No data support the claim of teratogenicity of penicillins or cephalosporins.[45]

A summary of appropriate medications during gestation is given in Table 27-1. These medications have been used throughout gestation without an increased risk of reported teratogenicity.

Most patients can be managed successfully during gestation. Some patients with potentially fatal asthma are unmanageable because of noncompliance with physician advice, medications, or in keeping ambulatory clinical appointments. Such gravidas are considered to have malignant potentially fatal asthma. Long-acting methylprednisolone is of value to prevent repeated episodes of status asthmaticus or respiratory failure.[46] This approach should be instituted to prevent fetal loss or maternal death in the nearly impossible to manage gravida. Adequate documentation in the medical record is needed. Evaluations should be obtained from the psychologist, psychiatrist, and social worker. Gravidas with malignant potentially fatal asthma, however, may refuse evaluation or necessary therapy. The serum glucose should be determined regularly because of hyperglycemia produced by long-acting methylprednisolone. Other antiasthma medications should be minimized to simplify the medication regimen.

TABLE 27-1. *Appropriate therapy during gestation in the ambulatory patient*

Mild Asthma

Inhaled beclomethasone dipropionate

Inhaled epinephrine or terbutaline

Inhaled cromolyn

Theophylline (optional)

Moderate or Severe Asthma

Inhaled beclomethasone dipropionate (up to 840 µg daily)

Prednisone: short daily course, then alternate day

Inhaled epinephrine or terbutaline

Theophylline (optional)

Long-acting methylprednisolone (selected cases)

Rhinitis

Chlorpheniramine

Tripelennamine

Diphenhydramine

Intranasal beclomethasone dipropionate

Allergen immunotherapy for severe allergic rhinitis

Purulent Rhinitis, Bronchitis, Sinusitis

Erythromycin

Ampicillin, amoxicillin

Cefaclor

Intranasal beclomethasone dipropionate

LABOR AND DELIVERY

When asthma is controlled effectively, the gravida is able to participate in prepared childbirth methods such as Lamaze without limitation. Minute ventilation increases to as much as 20 L/minute during labor and delivery.[25] Should cesarean delivery be necessary, complications from anesthesia should not create difficulty if asthma is well controlled. When the gravida has used inhaled beclomethasone dipropionate or oral corticosteroids during gestation, predelivery corticosteroid coverage should include 100 mg hydrocortisone every 8 hours until postpartum, and other medications can be used. Parenteral corticosteroids suppress any asthma that might complicate anesthesia required for cesarean delivery. The prior use of inhaled beclomethasone dipropionate or alternate-day prednisone should not suppress the surge of adrenal corticosteroids associated with labor or during anesthesia.

When the gravida has a planned cesarean delivery, preoperative prednisone can be administered for 3 to 5 days before anesthesia. The gravida should be examined 1 to 2 weeks before delivery to confirm stable respiratory status and satisfactory pulmonary function. In gravidas with mild asthma whose antiasthma medications consisted of theophylline, cromolyn, or inhaled β-adrenergic agonists, additional preanesthetic therapy can consist of 5 days of inhaled corticosteroid.

When the gravida presents in labor in respiratory distress, emergency measures such as subcutaneous epinephrine or terbutaline or inhaled albuterol should be administered promptly. Intravenous corticosteroids and possibly aminophylline should be administered to try to prevent the worsening of asthma. Adequate oxygenation and fetal monitoring are essential.

RHINITIS DURING PREGNANCY

Intranasal obstruction and nasal secretions can be troublesome during gestation and can interfere with sleep. An estimated 30% to 72% of gravidas experience symptoms of rhinitis during gestation.[47] Nasal congestion during gestation can be influenced by (1) increased blood volume, (2) progesterone's effects of smooth muscle relaxation of nasal vessels, and (3) estrogen's effects causing mucosal edema.[48] Nasal biopsy results from symptom-free gravidas showed glandular hyperactivity manifested by swollen mitochondria and an increased number of secretory granules.[49] Special stains demonstrated increased metabolic activity, increased phagocytosis, and increased acid mucopolysaccharides, thought to be attributed to high concentrations of estrogens. Similar findings were present in gravidas with nasal symptoms. Additional findings included increased (1) goblet cell numbers in the nasal epithelium, (2) cholinergic nerve fibers around glands and vessels, and (3) vascularity and transfer of metabolites through cell membranes.[49] Women using oral contraceptives but in whom no nasal symptoms had occurred have similar histopathologic and histochemical changes, as do symptom-free gravidas.[50] Oral contraceptive use in women who developed nasal symptoms was associated with interepithelial cell edema, mucus gland hyperplasia, and proliferation of ground substance analogous to symptomatic gravidas.[50] Serum concentrations of estradiol, progesterone, and vasoactive intestinal polypeptide did not differentiate symptomatic from asymptomatic gravidas.[51]

Nasal congestion that causes symptoms is likely to occur in the second and third trimesters.[47] The differential diagnosis for rhinitis of pregnancy includes allergic rhinitis, nonallergic rhinitis including vasomotor rhinitis or nonallergic rhinitis with eosinophilia, nasal polyposis, and sinusitis or purulent rhinitis. Rhinitis medicamentosa may be present when topical decongestants have been used excessively.

Treatment of nasal symptoms during gestation requires an accurate diagnosis, effective pharmacotherapy, and avoidance measures in some cases. For example, smoking and illicit drugs should be discontinued, as should topical decongestants. Intranasal beclomethasone dipropionate is valuable to relieve nasal obstruction. If large nasal polyps are present and topical corticosteroids are ineffective, a short course of prednisone should be prescribed. The blood glucose should be monitored because the gravida is prone to hyperglycemia. Antihistamines help gravidas with milder degrees of allergic rhinitis and some nonallergic types of rhinitis occasionally. Long-term experience and the Collaborative Perinatal Project have demonstrated safety for chlorpheniramine (1070 exposures), diphenhydramine (595 exposures), and tripelennamine (121 exposures).[52] Too few data support the use of brompheniramine, and surprisingly, in the Collaborative Perinatal Project, its use in 65 pregnancies was associated with an increased risk of congenital malformations.[52] I avoid treating with pseudoephedrine to avoid potential α-adrenergic stimulation of uterine vessels, although it has been recommended by others.[2,48] Phenylpropanolamine in 726 exposures was associated with significantly greater risk of malformations (ear and eye), whereas this risk was not detected with pseudoephedrine (39 exposures) or phenylephrine (1249 exposures).[52]

Intranasal cromolyn can be used for mild allergic rhinitis, based on experience with 296 gravidas with asthma.[3]

Antibiotics for infectious sinusitis or purulent rhinitis are listed in Table 27-1. Ampicillin, amoxicillin, erythromycin, and cefaclor are antibiotics to be given initially, depending on the prior therapy of the gravida. Sulfonamides are contraindicated because of the possibility of G6PD deficiency in the fetus. Tetracyclines are contraindicated because of maternal fatty liver during gestation (third trimester) and staining of teeth in the infant. Human data with clavulanic acid, a beta-lactamase inhibitor combined with amoxicillin, are not available.

Allergen immunotherapy reduces the need for medications in cases of allergic rhinitis. This therapy can be continued in pregnancy and, if symptoms are severe and the gravida agrees, immunotherapy may be initiated during gestation. During immunotherapy in 121 pregnancies in 90 gravidas, six gravidas experienced anaphylaxis.[33] No abortions or other adverse effects occurred.[33] Often, the decision to begin immunotherapy after delivery is made for the convenience and ability of the woman to present for injections in a timely fashion. Severe allergic rhinitis symptoms during gestation can be reduced with intranasal corticosteroids and antihistamines.

URTICARIA, ANGIOEDEMA, AND ANAPHYLAXIS

Urticaria or angioedema should be evaluated and treated during gestation with little change from the nongravid state. Causes for urticaria and angioedema include foods, medications, infections (viral), and underlying conditions such as collagen vascular disorders. Some episodes of urticaria are attributable to dermatographism or other physical urticarias, chronic urticaria, or idiopathic acute urticaria. The differential diagnosis during gestation includes hereditary angioedema (HAE),[53,54] pruritic urticaria papules and plaques of pregnancy (PUPPP),[55] and herpes gestationis.[56]

In the series of Frank and colleagues,[54] only during 2 of 25 gestations was there an increased frequency of attacks of HAE. No acute episodes of HAE occurred during delivery. Chappatte and deSwiet[53] reported unpredictability of HAE during gestation and a maternal fatality. The concentration of C_1 inhibitor declines in normal pregnancy because of increased plasma volume. Some gravidas have worsening clinical symptoms and create major management problems. Contraception is advisable as a rule. Stanozolol or danazol result in a fourfold to fivefold increase in the concentration of C_1 inhibitor and C_4. Although stanozolol has been administered during gestation without masculinizing fetal effects or fetal loss,[53] its use is discouraged in gravidas with HAE. Contraception should be used if a woman is receiving attenuated androgens for HAE.

For acute severe central episodes of HAE, rapid administration of subcutaneous epinephrine has been used, but additional specific therapy must include stanozolol, 4 mg four times a day, and airway care measures (intubation or tracheostomy). Although unavailable in the United States, a concentrate of C_1 inhibitor for parenteral administration has proven effective, with onset of action in 30 to 60 minutes.[57] Antifibrinolytic agents are considered unwise to use in pregnancy because of their potential thrombotic effects. Nevertheless, three pregnancies in one gravida occurred uneventfully despite the use of epsilon-amino-caproic acid.[57]

During gestation, no specific maintenance therapy is necessary in gravidas with peripheral HAE. Based on the series of Frank and associates[54] of gravidas with peripheral or central HAE, exacerbations during the time of tissue trauma (i.e., delivery) did not occur. If an episode of upper airway obstruction occurs during a cesarean delivery, epinephrine, stanozolol, and intubation are indicated. Use of C_1 inhibitor concentrates, if available and of low risk, otherwise would be of value acutely.

The PUPPP syndrome occurs in the last trimester and begins on the abdomen with numerous extremely pruritic erythematous urticarial plaques and papules surrounded by pale halos.[55,56] Topical corticosteroids are of value, and maternal or fetal complications are unlikely. Herpes gestationis consists of intense pruritus followed by lesions that may be bullous, papulovesicular, or pustular.[56] Some gravidas develop tense grouped vesicles on the abdomen or extremity.

Pharmacologic treatment of chronic urticaria or angioedema often is required. Despite its long-term use, there are few data regarding appropriateness of hydroxyzine in the first trimester. The established appropriateness of diphenhydramine, chlorpheniramine, or tripelennamine favors their use. Ephedrine or oral terbutaline may be added for more difficult cases, but often prednisone, 20 to 30 mg daily, may be necessary to control moderate to severe urticaria or angioedema.

Anaphylaxis during gestation has been described after penicillin, cefotetan,[58] Hymenoptera stings,[34] oxytocin,[59] phytomenadione,[60] fentanyl,[61] iron dextran,[62] anti-snakebite venom,[63] and even bupivacaine.[64] The latter is unexpected, based on current knowledge of local anesthetic reactions, and may have been an untoward effect of using a dose of 23 mL. Fetal distress or even death have been described, and gravidas have experienced profound shock with reduced uterine blood flow during anaphylaxis in pregnancy. As in other cases of anaphylaxis, prevention as well as emergency medications and therapy are needed. Epinephrine subcutaneously should be administered promptly. If the gravida is hypotensive, then usual resuscitative measures should be instituted to maintain blood pressure and the airway. Obstetric assistance should be obtained immediately should cesarean delivery be indicated.

VENOM IMMUNOTHERAPY

Venom immunotherapy is a highly efficacious form of therapy to prevent future episodes of Hymenoptera anaphylaxis. Graft[65] reported a successful pregnancy in a gravida treated with maintenance dosages of wasp and mixed vespid venoms. Subsequently, the Committee on Insects of the American Academy of Allergy and Immunology reported 63 pregnancies in 26 gravidas with no definite systemic reactions.[66] Five of 43 gestations resulted in spontaneous abortions, thought to be unrelated to stings or immunotherapy. One term infant (2.7%) had multiple congenital cardiovascular malformations; this incidence is within the range of expected congenital malformations. The use of venom immunotherapy appears to be appropriate.[66] Other issues should be discussed with the gravida, such as avoidance measures and personal use of epinephrine.

REFERENCES

1. deSwiet M. Diseases of the respiratory system. Clin Obstet Gynecol 1977;4:287.
2. National Institutes of Health, National Heart, Lung and Blood Institute Working Group on Asthma and Pregnancy, National Asthma Education Program, Management of Asthma during pregnancy. Public Health Service, U.S. Department of Health and Human Services, NIH publication no. 93-3279, 1993.
3. Gordon M, Niswander KR, Berendes H, Kantor AG. Fetal morbidity following potentially anoxigenic obstetric conditions. VII. Bronchial asthma. Am J Obstet Gynecol 1970;106:421.
4. Schaefer G, Silverman F. Pregnancy complicated by asthma. Am J Obstet Gynecol 1961;82:182.
5. Bahna SL, Bjerkedal J. The course and outcome of pregnancy in women with bronchial asthma. Acta Allergology 1972;27:397.
6. Greenberger PA, Patterson R. The outcome of pregnancy complicated by severe asthma. Allergy Proc 1988;9:539.
7. Fitzsimmons R, Greenberger PA, Patterson R. Outcome of pregnancy in women requiring corticosteroids for severe asthma. J Allergy Clin Immunol 1986;78:349.
8. Schatz M, Patterson R, Zeitz S, O'Rourke J, Melam H. Corticosteroid therapy for the pregnant asthmatic patient. JAMA 1975;23:804.
9. Greenberger PA, Patterson R. Beclomethasone dipropionate for severe asthma during pregnancy. Ann Intern Med 1983;98:478.
10. Stenius-Aarniala R, Piirila P, Teramo K. Asthma and pregnancy: a prospective study of 198 pregnancies. Thorax 1988;43:12.
11. Perlow JH, Montgomery D, Morgan MA, et al. Severity of asthma and perinatal outcome. Am J Obstet Gynecol 1992;167:963.
12. Gelber M, Sidi Y, Gassner S, et al. Uncontrollable life-threatening status asthmaticus: an indication for termination of pregnant by cesarean section. Respiration 1984;46:320.
13. Stenius-Aarniala B, Riikonen S, Teramo K. Slow-release theophylline in pregnant asthmatics. Chest 1995;107:642.
14. Gluck JC, Gluck PA. The effects of pregnancy upon asthma: a prospective study. Ann Allergy 1976;37:164.
15. Schatz M, Harden K, Forsythe A, et al. The course of asthma during pregnancy, postpartum, and with successive pregnancies: a prospective analysis. J Allergy Clin Immunol 1988;81:509.
16. Schatz M, Zeiger RS, Harden KM, et al. The safety of inhaled β-agonist bronchodilators during pregnancy. J Allergy Clin Immunol 1988;82:686.
17. Gilroy RJ, Mangura BT, Lavietes MH. Rib cage and abdominal volume displacements during breathing in pregnancy. Am Rev Respir Dis 1988;137:668.
18. Alaily AB, Carrol KB. Pulmonary ventilation in pregnancy. Br J Obstet Gynaecol 1978;85:518.
19. Cugell DW, Frank NR, Gaensler EA, Badger TL. Pulmonary function in pregnancy. I. Serial observations in normal women. Am Rev Tuberc 1953;67:568.
20. Greenberger PA, Patterson R. Management of asthma during pregnancy. N Engl J Med 1985;312:897.
21. Juniper EF, Daniel EE, Roberts RS, Kline PA, Hargreave FE, Newhouse MT. Improvement in airway responsiveness and asthma severity during pregnancy. Am Rev Respir Dis 1989;140:924.
22. Juniper EF, Daniel EE, Roberts RS, Kline PA, Hargreave FE, Newhouse MT. Effect of pregnancy on airway responsiveness and asthma severity: relationship to serum progesterone. Am Rev Respir Dis 1991;143:S78.
23. Sullivan JM, Ramanathan KB. Management of medical problems in pregnancy: Severe cardiac disease. N Engl J Med 1985;313:304.
24. Clark SL, Cotton DB, Lee W, et al. Central hemodynamic assessment of normal term pregnancy. Am J Obstet Gynecol 1989;161:1439.
25. Wulf KH, Kunzel W, Lehmann V. Clinical aspects of placental gas exchange. In: Longo LD, Bartels H, eds. Respiratory gas exchange and blood flow in the placenta. Bethesda, MD: Public Health Service, 1972:505. DHEW publication no. (NIH) 73-361.
26. Turner ES, Greenberger PA, Patterson R. Management of the pregnant asthmatic patient. Ann Intern Med 1980;93:905.
27. Apter AJ, Greenberger PA, Patterson R. Outcomes of pregnancy in adolescents with severe asthma. Arch Intern Med 1989;149:2571.
28. Klebanoff MA, Shiono PH, Rhoads GG. Outcomes of pregnancy in a national sample of resident physicians. N Engl J Med 1990;323:1040.
29. Warkany J. Congenital malformations: notes and comments. Chicago: Year Book Publishers, 1971:38.
30. Wilson J. Utilisation du cromolyglycate de sodium au cours de la grosse. Acta Ther (Suppl) 1982;8:45.

31. Frederiksen MC, Ruo TI, Chow MJ, Atkinson AJ Jr. Theophylline pharmacokinetics in pregnancy. Clin Pharmacol Ther 1986;40:321.
32. Patterson R, Greenberger PA, Frederiksen MC. Asthma and pregnancy: responsibility of physicians and patients. Ann Allergy 1990;65:469.
33. Metzger WJ, Turner E, Patterson R. The safety of immunotherapy during pregnancy. J Allergy Clin Immunol 1978;61:268.
34. Bousquet J, Miuller UR, Dreborg S, et al. Immunotherapy with hymenoptera venoms: position paper of the Working Group on Immunotherapy of the European Academy of Allergy and Clinical Immunology. Allergy 1987;42:401.
35. Entman SS, Moise KJ. Anaphylaxis in pregnancy. South Med J 1984;77:402.
36. Settipane RA, Chafee FH, Settipane GA. Pollen immunotherapy during pregnancy: long-term follow-up of offsprings. Allergy Proc 1988;9:555.
37. Schatz M, Zeiger RS. Treatment of asthma and allergic rhinitis during pregnancy. Ann Allergy 1990;65:427.
38. Svedmyr N. Action of corticosteroids on beta-adrenergic receptors: clinical aspects. Am Rev Respir Dis 1990;141:S31.
39. Self TH, Abou-Shala N, Burns R, et al. Inhaled albuterol and oral prednisone therapy in hospitalized adult asthmatics. Does aminophylline add any benefit? Chest 1990;98:1317.
40. Fanta CH, Rossing TH, McFadden ER. Treatment of acute asthma: is combination therapy with sympathomimetics and methylxanthines indicated? Am J Med 1986;80:5
41. Siegel D, Sheppard D, Gelb A, Weinberg PF. Aminophylline increases the toxicity but not the efficacy of an inhaled beta adrenergic agonist in the treatment of acute exacerbations of asthma. Am Rev Respir Dis 1985;132:283.
42. Chapman KR, Verbeek PR, White JG, Rebuck AS. Effect of a short course of prednisone in the prevention of early relapse after the emergency room treatment of acute asthma. N Engl J Med 1991;324:788.
43. Schreier L, Cutler RM, Saigal V. Respiratory failure in asthma during the third trimester: report of two cases. Am J Obstet Gynecol 1989;160:80.
44. Tenholder MF, South-Paul JE. Dyspnea in pregnancy. Chest 1989;96:381.
45. American Medical Association. Drug Evaluation Annual 1994, Department of Drugs, Division of Drugs and Toxicology. 6th ed. Chicago: American Medical Association, 1993:1359.
46. Chandler MJ, Grammer LC, Patterson R. Noncompliance and prevarication in life-threatening adolescent asthma. NER Allergy Proc 1986;7:367.
47. Bende M, Hallgarde V, Sjogren C. Occurrence of nasal congestion during pregnancy. Am J Rhinol 1989;3:217.
48. Schatz M, Zeiger RS. Diagnosis and management of rhinitis during pregnancy. Allergy Proc 1988;9:545.
49. Toppozada H, Michaels L, Toppozada M, El-Ghazzawi I, Talaat M, Elwany S. The human respiratory nasal mucosa in pregnancy: an electron microscopic and histochemical study. J Laryngol Otol 1982;96:613.
50. Toppozada H, Toppozada M, El-Ghazzawi I, Elwany S. The human respiratory nasal mucosa in females using contraceptive pills: an ultramicroscopic and histochemical study. J Laryngol Otol 1984;98:43.
51. Bende M, Hallgarde M, Sjogren V, Uvnas-Moberg K. Nasal congestion during pregnancy. Clin Otolaryngol 1989;14:385.
52. Heinonen OP, Sloan D, Shapiro S. Birth defects and drugs in pregnancy. Littleton, MA: PSG Publishing, 1977:1.
53. Chappatte O, deSwiet M. Hereditary angioneurotic oedema and pregnancy: case reports and review of the literature. Br J Obstet Gynaecol 1988;95:938.
54. Frank MM, Gelfand JA, Atkinson JP. Hereditary angioedema: the clinical syndrome and its management. Ann Intern Med 1976;4:580.
55. Lawley T, Hertz K, Wade TR, Ackerman AB, Katz SI. Pruritic urticarial papules and plaques of pregnancy. JAMA 1979;241:1696.
56. Smith A, Burkhart CG. Pruritus of pregnancy. Cutis 1984;34:486.
57. Logan RA, Greaves MW. Hereditary angio-edema: treatment with C₁ esterase inhibitor concentrate. J R Soc Med 1987:77:1046.
58. Bloomberg RJ. Cefotetan-induced anaphylaxis. Am Obstet Gynecol 1988;159:125.
59. Kawarabayaski T, Narisawa Y, Nakamura K, Sugimori H, Oda M, Taniquchi Y. Anaphylactoid reaction to oxytocin during cesarean section. Gynecol Obstet Invest 1988;25:277.
60. Anderson TH, Hindsholm KB, Fallingborg J. Severe complication to phytomenadione after intramuscular injection in woman in labor. Acta Obstet Gynecol Scand 1989;68:381.
61. Zucker-Pinchoff B, Ramanathan S. Anaphylactic reaction to epidural fentanyl. Anesthesiology 1989;71:599.
62. Sharpe O, Hall EG. Renal impairment, hypertension and encephalomacia in an infant surviving severe intrauterine anoxia. Proc R Soc Med 1953;46:1063.
63. Schatz M. Asthma and pregnancy. J Asthma 1990;27:335.
64. Emmott RS. Recurrent anaphylactoid reaction during cesarean section. Anesthesiology 1990;45:62. Letter.
65. Graft DF. Venom immunotherapy during pregnancy. Allergy Proc 1988;9:563.
66. Schwartz HJ, Golden DBK, Lockey RF. Venom immunotherapy in the Hymenoptera-allergic pregnant patient. J Allergy Clin Immunol 1990;85:709.

Index

Page numbers followed by *f* indicate figures; those followed by *t* indicate tables.